Anesthesia for infants and children

Third edition

Anesthesia for infants and children

Robert M. Smith, M.D.

Anesthesiologist, The Children's Medical Center,
Boston, Mass.; Associate Clinical Professor of Anesthesia,
Harvard Medical School, Boston, Mass.; Consultant in
Anesthesia, Peter Bent Brigham Hospital, Boston, Mass.,
Boston Lying-in Hospital, and U. S. Naval Hospital,
Chelsea, Mass.

Foreword by
Robert E. Gross, M.D.

With 240 illustrations

The C. V. Mosby Company

Saint Louis   1968

Dedicated to my wife
Margaret Louise Smith
and to 100,000 brave young patients
about whom this book is written

Foreword

During the past decade surgery has made important strides in providing safer and improved methods for handling various problems in infancy and childhood, indeed now making it possible to correct some conditions which were previously thought to be entirely hopeless. Many factors have contributed to these dramatic advances in pediatric surgery. Outstanding among them is the work of anesthesiologists who have focused on the field and have provided well-standardized procedures for carrying small and critically ill patients through operations on literally all portions and every system of the body. The surgeon realizes that his chances for success or failure are determined in great measure by the capabilities of the person at the head of the table who is administering the anesthetic.

In some medical circles there seems to be an attitude that the surgical operator is managing the show; in others, the anesthetist has an overly possessive feeling toward the patient. Neither approach is proper. It is best for each to be cognizant of his own problems and also to know of the other's difficulties; both must work together for total care of the patient. Certainly this is the most pleasant way to work, and surely it is the most effective way to conduct a child through a surgical ordeal.

It has been my good fortune to have Dr. Smith as the head of our anesthesiology service. He has managed in an expert and harmonious way a large department, carrying a heavy clinical load. In addition, he has been inquisitive and desirous of developing new ideas and bringing forth new technical advances. He has been an excellent teacher of doctors, nurses, and students. He has written this book to summarize and put on record the anesthetic methods which have been found to be most practical and useful. The volume will doubtless prove to be of great value to all readers who are interested in strengthening their knowledge of anesthesia for infants and children.

Robert E. Gross, M.D.

WILLIAM E. LADD PROFESSOR OF CHILDREN'S SURGERY
HARVARD MEDICAL SCHOOL

Preface

The succession of three editions of this book within ten years may call for some explanation.

The first edition (1959) was intended to be a basic text stating fundamentals that would be useful to anyone who might be called upon to give anesthesia to an infant or child. Ether was considered the safest agent, and techniques employing maximum simplicity were stressed as being most reliable and almost always preferable. The precordial stethoscope, spontaneous respiration, and a rational approach to intravenous therapy seemed the bulwarks of pediatric anesthesia.

By 1963 several changes had taken place. Ether was still the most widely used anesthetic, but the field was shared with cyclopropane, relaxants, and especially halothane, which was rapidly growing in popularity. Endotracheal techniques and assisted or controlled respiration often took precedence over spontaneous respiration. The stethoscope remained the sine qua non of pediatric anesthesia.

Between 1963 and 1968 several more changes took place. Because of the increasing fear of explosion of ether and cyclopropane and the versatility of halothane, the latter agent gained overwhelming lead over all other agents for pediatric use, and with it brought widespread adoption of nonrebreathing techniques for smaller patients.

The wide acceptance of halothane came only after considerable doubt, and now after a short period of unlimited use, fear has again been aroused concerning toxicity caused by halogenated agents. Although rare, acute hepatic necrosis appears to be associated with repeated use of halogenated agents, due probably to a sensitizing process. This leads one to believe that the goal is yet to be won, and that we should press on in our search for a better and safer agent or combination of agents.

Monitoring by stethoscope remains fundamental. Blood pressure, especially in infants, has gained in significance, and temperature has recently become a matter of serious concern to neonatologists as well as pediatric anesthetists.

Although anesthesia for infants, and for children undergoing open-heart surgery, has undergone important development, problems outside of the operating room have demanded great attention. Management of ventilatory problems, whether in postoperative patients or in medical patients such as those with status asthmaticus, has become a major responsibility and represents an area in which great progress has been made, but much more is needed.

In the preparation of this edition once again I owe much to Professor Charles D. Cook and to his associate, Dr. Etsuro K. Motoyama, for Chapter 3, which has always been the most valuable feature of the book. I have been most fortunate in gaining help from many sides in obtaining illustrations. Dr. Paul Holinger has most graciously loaned me two of his unique endoscopic color photographs and Drs. Colodny, Schuster, and Matson, among others, have contributed many of their illustrations. Mr. Janis Cirulis furnished me with excellent sketches in record time. Mr. Ferdinand Harding produced photographs of equipment and clinical material with his usual skill.

To authors and publishers whose illustrations I have borrowed, I am deeply grateful. The children and parents who have cooperated in the production of illustrations certainly deserve credit for their important part.

For secretarial assistance, Miss Earlene Cone deserves the entire credit.

Robert M. Smith, M.D.

Contents

Anesthesia for infants and children

Chapter 1

Basic requirements in pediatric anesthesia

Perspective
Information
Safety
Simplicity—when possible
Technical skill
Flexibility
Interest in children

There are several basic requirements or principles that are of importance throughout all phases of pediatric anesthesia. A consideration of these principles will explain the point of view taken and will make possible a logical approach to the subject as a whole.

PERSPECTIVE

An anesthetist will be of maximum value if he can see the relative importance of events about him. An over-all concept of the present position of pediatric anesthesia should be of assistance in this, as should be an appreciation of the place of the anesthetist as an individual.

The development of pediatric anesthesia has naturally been closely associated with that of pediatric surgery. As a specialty pediatric surgery is relatively new. Prior to 1930 children underwent tonsillectomy, appendectomy, and various orthopedic procedures, but the operations were performed with the methods used upon adults and were performed by surgeons more accustomed to adult patients. With rare exception the anesthetic used for children was ether, administered either by the open-drop or by the insufflation technique.

The first major development in pediatric surgery consisted of the introduction of new operative techniques devised for children and especially for infants. More extensive abdominal procedures were undertaken, and the scope of general surgery in young children was considerably extended. Ladd and Gross supplied much of the impetus for this development and for the evolution of a school of men specifically trained in children's surgery.

1

Interest in the field grew rapidly and was greatly accelerated by the introduction of surgery for congenital heart disease by Gross, Blalock, and Potts (1938-1944). At present pediatric surgery commands wide attention, both because of the remarkable progress it has been making and because of its potentiality in reshaping young lives.

The growth of pediatric surgery to its present state was facilitated by three other developments—the introduction of antibiotics, knowledge of fluid and electrolyte therapy, and improved anesthesia. Other factors contributed in varying degrees, but the picture as a whole is one of combined achievement in which anesthesia played one of the important supporting roles.

The main improvements in anesthesia have consisted of a better understanding of the responses of children to anesthesia, the introduction of specially devised apparatus and methods, and the application of a much wider variety of agents to suit specific needs. Among the first to contribute significantly to the development of modern pediatric anesthesia were Leigh, Belton, Stephen, McQuiston, Deming, and Slater in North America, and Anderson, Rees, and others in England.

The position of the anesthetist as an individual has been strengthened by supplemental services rendered in the fields of oxygen and inhalation therapy, fluid therapy, resuscitation, and pain control. Certainly the anesthetist should play a major role in the postoperative recovery room and in the intensive therapy unit. Whether he actually is in charge of such a unit or acts as a team member will depend on the local situation. In spite of such other activities, I believe that the chief responsibility of the anesthetist should continue to remain in the operating room, to help the surgeon.

The use of perspective is especially important in surgeon-anesthetist relationships. The success of many operations depends upon the efficiency of a smoothly working team; consequently maximum cooperation is essential. In procedures on small children and babies, when the anesthetist and the surgeon often must share an extremely small field of operation, there is additional need for consideration of the other's problems.

INFORMATION

Although progress has been marked in technical improvements, the knowledge we have of our patients is still in a relatively primitive state. The prolonged and critical operations now undertaken make it imperative that we know more about the children we anesthetize. Three types of information are needed: (1) that concerning the individual child being anesthetized, (2) that about specific diseases of patients coming to operation, and (3) information relating to infants and children in general. We can all learn about the individual by studying his history and by examining him prior to anesthesia as well as by studying him during and after anesthesia. Most anesthetists need to learn more about conditions peculiar to the pediatric group, such as omphalocele, pyloric stenosis, pancreatic fibrosis, and hydrocephalus. Much of this information is available in the literature. Anyone engaged in pediatric anesthesia should be familiar with such texts as Nelson's[1] *Textbook of pediatrics,* Gross'[2] *The surgery of infancy and childhood,*

Pediatric surgery edited by Benson and associates,[3] as well as current pediatric journals.

Our greatest over-all need for information lies in our general understanding of physiology in both normal and abnormal children. Until we learn more about the control of respiration and circulation, about temperature regulation, and about the development of the nervous and endocrine systems, we can only continue to grope along on an empirical basis. Investigation is difficult, and as yet few have devised methods of study that are adaptable to small patients. Dr. Clement Smith's[4] classic text, *The physiology of the newborn infant,* summarizes most of the known data of studies of this aspect of the field but of necessity leaves many of our problems unanswered.

The main purpose of this book will be to assemble as much of the practical information as is available concerning the basic response of children to anesthesia. Techniques and agents will be described, but it is hoped that these will soon be made obsolete by the introduction of better methods. The patient and his reactions will remain the same, however, and it is upon these that attention should be centered.

SAFETY

To say that safety is the first principle in actual patient management seems obvious and trite, but to omit it would be inexcusable. The subject deserves special consideration in pediatric anesthesia because (1) mortality at present is unreasonably high and (2) there is often considerable difficulty in deciding which approach is safest. Safety in anesthesia is a relative thing, dependent upon many factors. If any generalization is made, it immediately must be modified to suit individual cases. Reference to maximum safety here will mean that which in the hands of the average anesthetist will entail least danger in a large number of cases. Opinions are based on experience of many years in which large numbers of infants and children have been anesthetized by a rapidly changing group of residents.

There are several anesthetists who have developed special skills and techniques with children. Spinal and local anesthetics, relaxants, and intravenous agents that might be inadvisable in the hands of the inexperienced may be used with special advantages by those who have had adequate experience. Consequently there are few if any techniques that can be completely condemned.

At the present stage of development, however, the criterion for most should not be "What can I get away with?" or "What will look most impressive?" but "What will get me into least real trouble in 100 cases?"

SIMPLICITY—WHEN POSSIBLE

In general, simplicity affords greater safety in anesthesia, and this applies especially to pediatric anesthesia. Our aim should be to strip away unnecessary details and try to make difficult procedures look easy, rather than to introduce complicated methods and make easy procedures appear difficult. No procedure should be added unless it is clearly indicated. This applies to minor details such as hot-water bottles, as well as involved techniques such as hypothermia. Any added maneuver or device carries its own risk and also divides the anesthetist's attention. There are times, obviously, when simple techniques will not be adequate, as in more extensive operations, or procedures on extremely poor-risk patients. Such conditions will demand use of more sophisticated methods for accurate control of anesthesia and supportive therapy.

TECHNICAL SKILL

The term technician has been used among anesthetists with a derogatory implication; however, technical ability is of first-line priority in the anesthetic management of infants and children. Regardless of the extent of his scientific background, an anesthetist who fumbles about in the operating room impresses no one.[5] Dexterity, meticulous attention to detail, and constant close scrutiny of the patient should be characteristics of all anesthetists—characteristics that are invaluable in dealing with children.

FLEXIBILITY

Small patients change from moment to moment, and no two are quite alike. The most carefully planned approach many turn out to be unsatisfactory for that particular child, and it is far better to change the approach than to try to force the child into a pattern he does not fit. Much of the success of an operation can depend upon the induction of anesthesia, and here especially the anesthetist must have a variety of techniques at hand. One child may accept a mask readily, while another will be horrified by it and will not even lie down on the operating table. Imagination, enthusiasm, tact, and insight also may be helpful in some instances.

INTEREST IN CHILDREN

Finally, it goes without saying that one should be able to enjoy working with children.[6] Since children are naturally attractive and responsive, most anesthetists are happy to work with them. In addition, some individuals seem to be born with a special gift that combines sincerity, enthusiasm, and gentleness. These people can quickly grasp the attention and the confidence of a child and thereby change many hospital procedures from frightening experiences to relatively pleasant ones. An anesthetist who has such a gift enjoys a great advantage.

REFERENCES

1. Nelson, W. E., editor: Textbook of pediatrics, ed. 7, Philadelphia, 1959, W. B. Saunders Co.
2. Gross, R. E.: The surgery of infancy and childhood, Philadelphia, 1953, W. B. Saunders Co.
3. Benson, C. D., Mustard, W. T., Ravitch, M. M., Snyder, W. H., and Welch, K. W., editors: Pediatric surgery, Chicago, 1962, Year Book Medical Publishers, Inc.
4. Smith, C. A.: The physiology of the newborn infant, ed. 3, Springfield, Ill., 1959, Charles C Thomas, Publisher.
5. Mushin, W. W.: The teaching of anesthesia, Anesthesiology 19:131-140, 1958.
6. Potts, W. J.: Pediatric surgery is growing up, J.A.M.A. 166:462-466, 1958.

Chapter 2

Biology and behavior, or factors determining the child's response to anesthesia

Unless it can be shown that anesthesia for infants and children has definite problems or situations that place it apart as different from anesthesia for adults, there is little purpose in setting forth on a prolonged dissertation.

For years people have assumed or suspected certain underlying differences but have failed to define them. In reply to repeated questions such as "Is the child a poor risk?" or "How do children differ from adults?" the answers have consisted of such generalizations as "The child has a narrow margin of safety" or that much overworked phrase "The child is not a little man." Occasionally these catchwords carry some truth, but usually the meaning is not clear, and often the implications are false. Surely it is time that evidence was produced that could confirm such statements and thereby justify pediatric anesthesia as an entity.

How, then, is the child different?

First, it should be pointed out that whereas a child 6 or 8 years old is obviously different from an adult, there is even greater difference between an infant and that child. This will be emphasized repeatedly but never sufficiently. The term "child" and "pediatric" are often used with the idea that they represent a "standard" child. Nothing could be further from the truth. These terms, as ordinarily used, include all ages from birth to 12 years, and no more heterogeneous assortment could be imagined.

Now, then, when we step back and try to point out the precise factors that make infants and children different from grown patients, we find that there are many and that for the most part they fall into five categories: (1) anatomic differences, which may relate to differences in gross over-all size, to differences in proportion, or to differences in the structure of individual organ systems; (2) psychologic differences, including the uncontrolled emotions and behavior of the young child; (3) physiologic factors, relating both to general metabolism and to function of various organ systems; (4) pathologic factors, in which are included the special lesions seen only in infants and children, as well as the characteristic way in which children react to illness, infection, and other types of general disease; and (5) differences in response to pharmacologic agents, as seen in altered tolerance to relaxants and analgesic drugs.

ANATOMIC FACTORS

Difference in size. The most obvious difference between child and adult is in size, but the degree of difference and the variation even within the pediatric age group is hard to appreciate. The contrast between a 3-pound infant and an overgrown 150-pound youth perhaps is more impressive when it is stated that by weight the 150-pound boy is 50 times, or 5,000%, the size of the baby.

Difference in proportion or relative size. Less obvious than the difference in over-all size is the difference in proportion or relative size of body structures in the pediatric group. The infant's head is large and bulky, and his neck is so short that there often appears to be no neck at all, the chin meeting the chest at the level of the second costal interspace (Fig. 2-1). The chest is relatively small, the abdomen is weak, and the legs are short and poorly developed. Such disproportions are of special consequence when they involve respiratory exchange, as many of them do.

In comparing size it makes considerable difference whether one uses weight, height, or surface area as the basis of comparison. As pointed out by Harris,[1] the normal 7-pound newborn baby is 1/3.3 the size of the adult in length but 1/9 adult size by body surface and 1/21 adult size by weight (Fig. 2-2).

Of the body measurements that of *surface area* is probably most significant

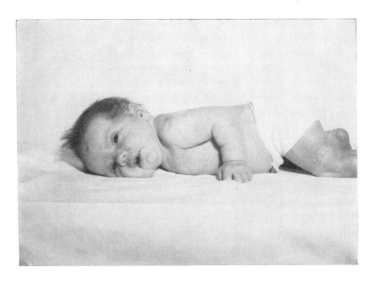

Fig. 2-1. A normal infant has a large head, short neck, narrow shoulders and chest, and a large abdomen.

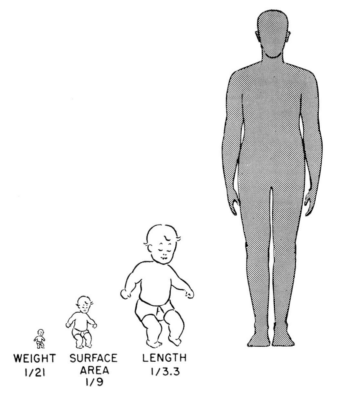

WEIGHT   SURFACE   LENGTH
1/21   AREA   1/3.3
             1/9

Fig. 2-2. Proportions of newborn infant to adult with respect to weight, surface area, and length. (From Harris, J. S.: Ann. N. Y. Acad. Sci. 66:966, 1957.)

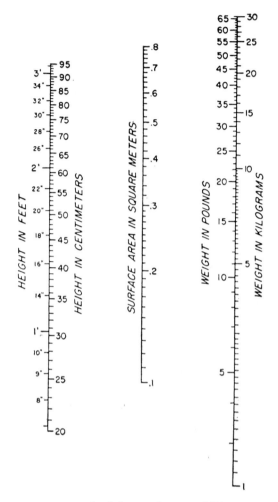

Fig. 2-3. Body surface area nomogram for infants and young children. (Reprinted by permission of the publishers and The Commonwealth Fund, from Talbot, N. B., Sobel, E. H., McArthur, J. W., and Crawford, J. D.: Functional endocrinology from birth through adolescence, Cambridge, Mass., Harvard University Press; copyright, 1952, by The Commonwealth Fund.)

since the curve of surface area as related to body weight is very similar to the curve of basal metabolic activity measured in calories per hour per square meter. For this reason surface area is believed a better criterion than age or weight in judging basal fluid and nutritional requirements. For clinical use this practice appears somewhat difficult, but reference to the nomogram of Talbot and associates[2] (Fig. 2-3) facilitates the procedure considerably. In general, the smaller the patient the greater is the relative surface area of the body. At birth the body surface averages 0.2 sq.M., whereas in the adult it averages 1.75 sq.M. A table of average weight, height, and surface area is presented for reference (Table 2-1).

Differences in organic structure. In addition to differences in gross anatomic features the structure of several individual organ systems deserves mention. Con-

Table 2-1. *Relationship of body surface area to age, weight, and height*

Age	Height (in.)	Weight (lb.)	Surface area of body (sq.M.)
Newborn	20	6.6	0.20
3 mo.	21	11.0	0.25
1 yr.	31	22.0	0.45
3 yr.	38	32.0	0.62
6 yr.	48	46.0	0.80
9 yr.	53	66.0	1.05
15 yr.	63	110.0	1.50
Adult	68	154.0	1.75

cerning the *central nervous system,* it is chiefly of academic interest that the cortical sulci are relatively undeveloped at birth.[3,4]

Myelination of the nerve tracts is known to be incomplete at birth, and it is generally agreed that function does not reach full development until myelination occurs.[5,6] Sensory tracts of the spine are myelinated at birth, but motor tracts are not completely myelinated until the child is about 2 years old.[7]

In the brain itself, the cortex of the newborn infant shows very meager distribution of cellular elements.[8] When this area is compared to the same area in an infant only 6 months of age, the contrast is striking (Fig. 2-4).

Myelination occurs more slowly along the fiber tracts of the brain, gradually extending through the connecting areas of the midbrain and the reticular system. It is believed that the process continues until middle life.

Of some interest to those using spinal anesthesia in infants is consideration of the level to which the spinal cord extends in the dural sheath. At birth it extends to the third lumbar vertebra, and by the time the child is 1 year old the cord has assumed its permanent position, ending at the first lumbar vertebra.[3]

Poor development of bodily support by *bone and muscle* may combine with disproportion to create problems for the child. Some of these problems become especially evident when children are positioned for operation. In the prone position the shoulders are too small to give adequate support in spite of attempts to build them up with padding. If the child is made to sit up for a pneumoencephalogram, the neck makes a very weak stem for the heavy head.

The *thoracic cage* of the infant consists of a classic combination of structural handicaps. The thorax is small, and the sternum is soft, affording an unstable base for the ribs. In the premature infant the sternum may be deeply retracted with each inspiration. The ribs of the infant are horizontally positioned, reducing the bucket-handle motion upon which thoracic respiration depends (Fig. 2-5). The diaphragm rides high, and its motion is embarrassed by the large abdomen characteristic of healthy babies. Intercostal muscles of normal respiration are poorly developed, and accessory muscles appear to give relatively little assistance in times of need. Although exchange has been shown to be efficient under normal conditions,[9] these factors make it extremely difficult to meet increased demands imposed by illness or surgery.

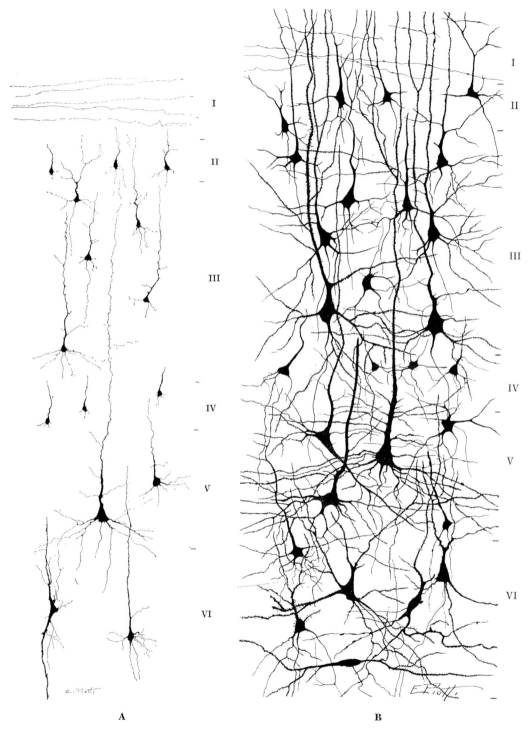

Fig. 2-4. Cellular structure of the occipitotemporal zone (area PH). **A,** At birth. **B,** Same area at 6 months of age. (Reprinted by permission of the publishers, from Conel, J. L.: The postnatal development of the human cerebral cortex, vols. 1 and 4, Cambridge, Mass., Harvard University Press; copyright, 1939, 1951, by The President and Fellows of Harvard College.)

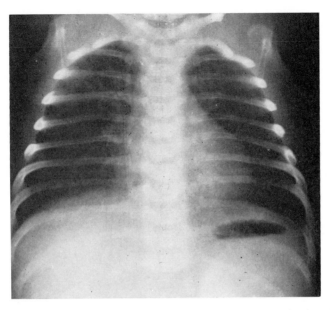

Fig. 2-5. The structure of the infant thorax is relatively weak, and expansion is reduced by horizontally positioned ribs. (From Harris, G. B., and Wittenborg, M. H.: Int. Anesth. Clin. 1:53, 1962.)

The *upper respiratory tract* in children is predisposed to obstruction because of the narrowness of nasal passages, glottis, and trachea. Abundant secretions and a large tongue may be expected, whereas hypertrophied tonsils and adenoids and other pathologic lesions are often superimposed.

There are important differences in the structural relationships in the airways of infants when compared to the adult (Fig. 2-6). As noted by Eckenhoff[10] the larynx of the newborn infant is more cephalad, the rima glottidis lying opposite the interspace of the third and fourth cervical vertebrae, whereas in the adult it lies opposite the interspace of the fourth and fifth vertebrae. In addition the vocal cords slant upward and backward, due to approximation of the hyoid to the thyroid cartilage. The structure of the epiglottis is characteristic in being narrow and U shaped, while the loose areolar tissue of the glottis makes it especially susceptible to the formation of edema following trauma or simply as a result of overhydration.

The actual dimensions of the respiratory tract are of importance. The findings of Engel[11] were summarized and tabulated by Hall [12] (Table 2-2).

Eckenhoff[10] has emphasized Engel's findings that the narrowest area of the upper respiratory tract may be at the cricoid ring rather than at the rima glottidis. This has been found to be true in several cases,[13] but whether it is the rule remains questionable. When noted, it has usually been associated with several congenital anomalies, especially those involving abnormal skull development, as craniosynostosis and Apert's syndrome (Chapter 21).

Studies of the structure of the trachea and bronchi have been somewhat con-

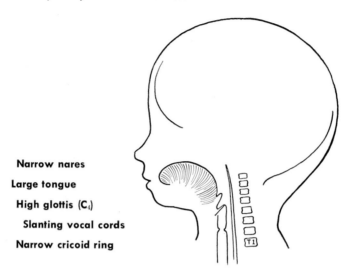

Narrow nares

Large tongue

High glottis (C₄)

Slanting vocal cords

Narrow cricoid ring

Fig. 2-6. Characteristic differences of the infant airway.

Table 2-2. *Dimensions of respiratory tract components in children**

Age	Lung volume (ml.)	Alveolar surface area (sq.cm.)	Tracheal length (cords to carina) (cm.)	Tracheal diameter (mm.)
Birth	100	16,000	4.0	6.0
3 mo.	150	16,250	4.0	6.8
6 mo.	230	57,000	4.2	7.2
1 yr.	400		4.3	7.8
18 mo.	470	111,000	4.5	8.8
2 yr.	500	184,000	5.0	9.5
3 yr.	550	236,000	5.3	
4 yr.	600		5.4	11.0
5 yr.	700		5.6	
6 yr.	800		5.7	

*From Hall, J. E.: Proc. Roy. Soc. Med. **48:**761, 1955.

tradictory. Adriani and Griggs[14] observed that both the left and right bronchi of small infants branch at a 55° angle from the trachea, whereas careful investigation by Smith[15] demonstrated the configuration to be similar to that in adults—the right bronchus branching at 25°, the left at approximately 70°.

Estimation of dead space and the relative proportion of alveolar surface in the infant has brought some disagreement. Although it has been thought that the infant's ventilation was handicapped by a relative increase in dead space, it is now believed that the relationship of dead space to weight remains the same through life. As it happens, this relationship is 1 ml. of dead space per pound of body weight in persons of normal body build.

There is still uncertainty concerning the actual amount of alveolar surface area in the infant as related to that in the adult. The varied respiratory patterns of the infant have been interpreted by some to be due to increased alveolar surface and by others to be due to decreased alveolar surface. More evidence will be necessary before either statement is substantiated.

Although the gross development of the *kidney* is complete at birth, the development of glomeruli and tubules is not mature until the child is several months old.[16] There is a parallel delay in functional development.

The *thymus gland* is relatively large during infancy; however, the concept of thymic death, or status lymphaticus, has fallen into disrepute, as has the more recently held view that an enlarged thymus can contribute to respiratory obstruction.

The *adrenal glands* are greatly enlarged at birth, measuring some twenty times their relative size in the adult. However, the enlargement is almost entirely due to tissue of little functional value that undergoes involution early in infancy.[17,18]

PSYCHOLOGIC DIFFERENCES
BETWEEN CHILD AND ADULT

Next to size and gross anatomic differences, the emotional pattern of the child is most striking in contrast to the adult patient. In everyday experience the excited child is one of the most trying problems that the anesthetist faces, and one he handles with least success. Much greater understanding of the child's psyche is necessary before we can become proficient in this field.[19,20]

The exact age at which infants can become frightened is difficult to determine, but they appear to be startled by noises shortly after birth, and it does not seem unreasonable to imagine that the sensation of inhaling raw ether vapor might arouse strong if primitive emotions. While these reactions may be instinctive at first, the element of fear and apprehension undoubtedly develops at an earlier age than we realize. Psychologists generally agree that fear and emotional disturbances are greatest in children just before they are able to talk. Following that time, upsetting experiences are not uncommon, but they are eased by the child's ability to express himself.

The reaction of the young infant to anything that startles or displeases him is uncontrolled release of vocal and physical resistance. The vehemence of these outbursts may increase up to the age of 2 or 3 years, after which time it should gradually diminish, although many exceptions are seen.

The effect of these mental and physical paroxysms is known to be important during both the operative and postoperative periods. It is sufficient here to mention this aspect of the child's makeup, which is so different from that of the adult. The many approaches to better patient preparation now being attempted certainly are greatly needed.[21-23]

PHYSIOLOGIC CHARACTERISTICS
OF INFANT AND CHILD

Physiologic factors have greatest significance in determining the child's reaction to anesthesia. Factors of concern are energy metabolism, central and au-

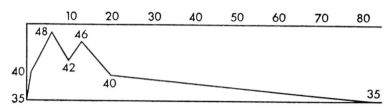

Fig. 2-7. Guedel's curve of the normal metabolic rate throughout life. (From Guedel, A. E.: Inhalation anesthesia, New York, 1937, The Macmillan Co.)

tonomic nervous system activity, temperature control, fluid and electrolyte balance, and the responses of cardiovascular, respiratory, gastrointestinal, hepatorenal, and endocrine systems—in other words, most of the bodily functions.

Energy metabolism. The rate of metabolic activity or oxygen consumption sets the patterns for many of the child's reactions to everyday life, as well as to anesthesia, surgery, illness, and medical therapy. This pattern in the child is one of raised basal activity plus the capacity for further elevation in response to various stimuli.

Certain estimates have been made of basal metabolic activity in infants and children. In 1943 Guedel,[24] in his classic textbook *Inhalation anesthesia,* published a metabolic curve derived from the tables of DuBois[25] and others (Fig. 2-7). This curve has been widely copied throughout literature on anesthesia and has been of great value in establishing the importance of basal metabolism in relation to anesthetic requirements. Guedel's curve (Fig. 2-7) shows the child's metabolism to be maximum at 6 years of age, with a second peak at 12 years of age. The highest point in Guedel's curve is 48 calories per hour per square meter.

More recent studies by Lewis, Duval, and Iliff,[26] and Lee and Iliff[27] at the University of Colorado have resulted in somewhat different curves in which the maximal point is reached between 6 and 18 months of age (Fig. 2-8). The highest point in their mean curves for both boys and girls is approximately 58 calories per hour per square meter. Following the first peak there is a gradual fall in metabolic rate until puberty is approached. Immediately prior to puberty there may be a definite rise in metabolic activity, with a postpuberal fall, but this deflection is not marked and may occur at any time between 11 and 15 years of age. A composite of several individual curves will consequently show a plateau effect in place of a prepuberal peak. These findings have been confirmed by other recent studies[28,29] and suggest that Guedel's curve be modified in two respects: (1) the first maximal peak should occur early in infancy rather than at 6 years of age and (2) the prepuberal peak occurs at a variable age and does not approach the level of the primary peak.

Basal oxygen requirements at birth are estimated to be approximately 6 ml. per kilogram per minute and that of the adult 4 ml. per kilogram per minute.[30] Considerable attention has been called to the correlation of basal oxygen consumption with that of surface area. Although it is true that surface area is a better guide to basal metabolic energy than is age, height, or weight, it must be remembered that the child is seldom at basal conditions. It is well known that fever

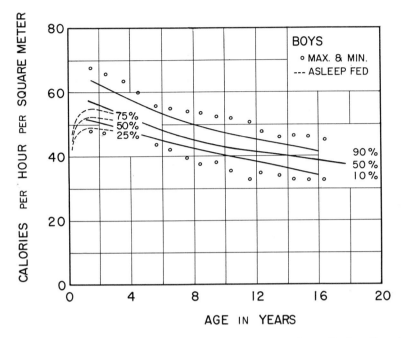

Fig. 2-8. Basal metabolic activity in boys from birth to 21 years of age. Broken lines indicate studies on infants fed and asleep; solid lines show studies done on children in a fasting, awake condition. (Unpublished graph, courtesy Dr. Alberta Iliff, Child Research Council, University of Colorado School of Medicine, Denver, Colo.)

raises the oxygen requirement 7% per degree of temperature elevation, that illness and emotion add further need, and that muscular activity may raise it an additional 300% to 400%. The situation fluctuates widely from day to day and from moment to moment, depending upon the state of health or the state of mind of the child.

This characteristic variability makes it practically impossible to gauge bodily needs by any fixed measurement of age, weight, or even body surface, since none of these changes with temperature, shock, or excitement. In general, it may be assumed that during childhood relatively larger doses of sedatives will be required in view of elevated basal metabolism, but fluid and nutritional needs must be estimated very largely on a short-term basis, with greatest reliance upon changing clinical signs.

Physiology of the central and the autonomic nervous systems. In explaining the child's reaction to anesthesia, nervous system activity would appear to be next in importance to energy metabolism. An outstanding characteristic of infant physiology is *variability* and *lack of control,* as seen in respiration, muscular activity, or temperature regulation. Much of this instability may be traced to inadequate neurologic function, either the result of incomplete anatomic development of nerve pathways or lack of functional experience in neuromuscular cordination.[16]

An explanation of several characteristic reactions in the young child lies in the current belief that the infant has *decreased nervous system irritability*. Although Guedel considered the child's nervous irritability to be elevated and to follow the same curve as basal metabolic activity, this would not necessarily be true, since basal metabolism depends upon muscular tone, body surface, growth, and other factors over and above that of nervous system activity. It has also been implied that increased nervous system activity might be an underlying factor in the child's predisposition to convulsions.[31] McQuarrie[32] points out, however, that the infant actually has decreased irritability, as shown by elevation of the threshold for electrical stimulation. This applies to the cerebral cortex as well as to peripheral nerves.

When one considers the infant's decreased sensitivity to pain, the increased tolerance of hypoxia,[17] and the lower levels of conscious behavior, all seem to fit nicely into this concept that the infant has decreased nervous irritability.

Sensory and motor development do not appear to progress in parallel relationship in the child. Although the disparity has been attributed to difference in myelination, some disagreement still exists on this point.

Anatomic end organs and nerve tracts for smell, taste, touch, hearing, sight, and pain sensations are present at birth. McGraw[5] goes so far as to say that these sensations actually exist at birth "though discrimination is poorly developed."

At what age an infant is first able to feel pain is a matter of considerable practical interest to an anesthetist. Clinically, it appears that newborn infants have decreased feeling of pain, since they tolerate considerable operative trauma with surprising lack of concern. It may be that in such situations pain is felt, but due to decreased irritability and poor correlation of response, the reaction is damped or lost completely.

In order to limit the use of meaningless words the term pain should be defined. If we start by stating that "pain is the consciousness of an uncomfortable sensation," we know what we are talking about. "Consciousness" or "perception" of a sensation such as pain depends upon cortical activity. In the newborn infant cortical activity is not developed and subcortical centers remain dominant.[7] Consequently, although pain can be felt without demonstration of motor reaction under certain circumstances (curarized adult), failure of reaction in small infants is probably due to actual inability of the cortex to perceive or register pain.

McGraw[5] investigated the reaction of infants to pinprick. She found that some newborn infants do not react to such a stimulus at all until 1 week old and make only mass responses until 1 month old, being unable to localize or identify the source. Undoubtedly, considerable variation exists, but in general it seems safe to say that an infant's perception of pain is determined by the degree of his cortical development. The response and cortical activity of the baby may be compared to that of a patient receiving thiopental anesthesia. A baby with an undeveloped cortex and a deeply anesthetized patient both lack cortical activity, and both are unable to feel pain. A baby with partial cortical development and a patient under light thiopental anesthesia will show mass, undirected responses, still without "consciousness" of pain. When a baby cries on stimulation, and the patient first complains, the pain may be felt but not remembered (amnesia), whereas complete cortical development of the baby and full awakening are neces-

ALL TO C₂

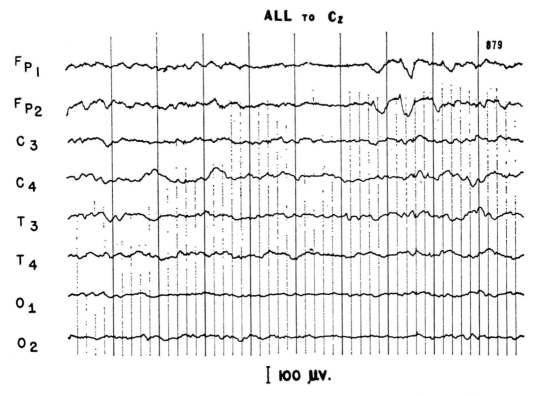

[**100 μv.**

Fig. 2-9. Electroencephalogram of 4-day-old infant. Interval between heavy lines equals 1 second. (From Brechner, V. L., Walter, R. D., and Dillon, J. B.: Practical electroencephalography for the anesthesiologist, Springfield, Ill., 1962, Charles C Thomas, Publisher.)

sary for normal consciousness and remembrance of pain. How long it takes an infant ot reach this stage is not definitely known; however, there is evidence that cortical development adequate for pain perception may be present in infants 1 week old.

As will be pointed out, there is evidence that *rapid fatigability of nervous response* is a characteristic of the child's general reaction. This may explain the child's short bursts of activity, his increased need for sleep, and his decreased tolerance of respiratory obstruction.

Control and coordination of motor function. Control and coordination of motor function develop slowly, but the progress is more easily followed than that of sensation. In young infants lack of fine control is typical in both central and autonomic nervous systems. Neuromuscular control depends upon balanced, correctly timed responses that enable the individual to sense minute stimuli and make equally minute counteractions. Lacking such ability, the infant does not react until the stimulus is heavy, and then a full-scale response is evoked. The widely overshooting responses and the lack of finer elements of control typical of the infant resemble those of a microscope that has a coarse adjustment but no fine adjustment.

The changing cortical activity as traced through infancy and childhood shows pronounced basic differences. At birth the infant's electroencephalogram is undifferentiated, irregular, and variable (Fig. 2-9). This state of marked reduction of cortical activity persists for 2 to 3 months and then gradually shows increasing developmental change (Fig. 2-10). The infant also shows an ever-changing pattern of reflex responses that can be used to evaluate his rate of neurologic maturation.[33,34]

The child's susceptibility to convulsive disorders is well known but has not been clearly explained. McQuarrie[32] believes that it probably is due to the infant's characteristic structure of brain tissue noted previously—"lack of myeline, greater water content, and more rapid metabolism." The immature development of central inhibitory mechanisms may be responsible in part for the tendency for convulsions to arise at the lower brain levels in younger patients.

The autonomic nervous system, being more primitive than the central nervous system, is relatively well developed at birth. Visceral functions are characteristically variable, however, since the finer mechanisms of control are absent here also. In infants the general reaction to stress has been found to be comparable to that of the adult, but the reaction is believed to become exhausted more quickly.[35] The development of autonomic control differs in the various organ

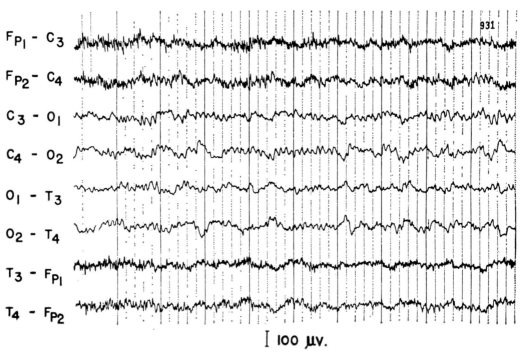

Fig. 2-10. Electroencephalogram of 1-year-old child showing considerably faster activity and reduced amplitude. (From Brechner, V. L., Walter, R. D., and Dillon, J. B.: Practical electroencephalography for the anesthesiologist, Springfield, Ill., 1962, Charles C Thomas, Publisher.)

systems, the cardiovascular system being under better regulation than is the respiratory system.[36]

The vagus nerve appears to play an important but inconsistent role in the young infant. At birth strong vagal tone seems evident in the rapid onset of bradycardia with hypoxia or cyclopropane anesthesia; yet there is little or no gagging or bradycardia when the larynx is stimulated by intubation of the trachea without anesthesia. Furthermore, whether due to inactivity of vagus or vomiting centers, infants rarely vomit during or after anesthesia.

When an infant holds his breath until deeply cyanotic and then continues to do so until the heart slows, one wonders about the state of carotid body activity. Cross[35] studied carotid body activity in the newborn infant and believes that although fatigue of the reflex may play a part, it is more probable that the medullary centers are acutely sensitive to oxygen want, and, as soon as oxygenation falls perceptibly, the medulla fails to react to signals from the carotid body.

Cardiovascular system. Fortunately the child's cardiovascular system is resilient and dependable. Although subject to some variability of control, this is less marked than other functions such as respiration or temperature regulation. The myocardium is strong and not subject to the degenerative process of older persons. Sudden or overwhelming insults may cause alarming responses of cyanosis, bradycardia, or shock, but with removal of the cause the return of activity often is spectacular.

It is of chief concern to know the normal range of activity for the hearts of young children. The infant's blood volume is relatively high in proportion to body mass. The figure accepted as most reliable at this time is 84 ml. per kilogram of body weight in the newborn infant as compared to 65 ml. per kilogram for the adult.[37] The normal 7-pound infant would thus have a blood volume of about 290 ml. Both the red blood cell count and the hemoglobin vary considerably during infancy, being elevated at birth, then falling sharply until the child is about 3 months old, then gradually rising again until adult levels are reached at 8 to 10 years of age (Fig. 2-11).

Heart rhythm. An infant's heart rhythm is relatively stable. The electrocardiographic tracing shows right ventricular predominance until the child is about 6 months old but otherwise is not remarkable.[38] Children frequently show sinus arrhythmia, and although variations in rate are common, serious disturbances in rhythm are relatively rare.

Blood pressure. A child's blood pressure is slightly less than that of an adult. At birth, the systolic pressure varies between 75 and 85 mm. Hg and usually rises 5 to 10 mm. Hg within 2 weeks. Table 2-3 shows average blood pressures for children. Although blood pressure is difficult to determine in infants, the anesthetist must bear in mind that infants develop shock very readily. Observation of the blood pressure actually is more important in infants and children than in adults.

Heart rate. The heart rate is rapid in young infants and may vary widely without serious consequences. Table 2-4 shows the normal heart rate of conscious infants and children. At birth the heart rate of a resting infant may be 90 to 110, and then upon crying or struggling there will be a sudden rise to 170 or 180 per

Table 2-3. *Average blood pressure of children**

Age	Systolic (mm. Hg)	Diastolic (mm. Hg)
Newborn	75-85	40-50
2 wk.-4 yr.	85	60
5 yr.	87	60
6 yr.	90	60
7 yr.	92	62
8 yr.	95	62
9 yr.	98	64
10 yr.	100	65
11 yr.	105	65
12 yr.	108	67
13 yr.	110	67
14 yr.	112	70
15 yr.	115	72
16 yr.	118	75

*From Kaplan, Samuel: In Nelson, W. B., editor: Textbook of pediatrics, ed. 7, Philadelphia, 1959, W. B. Saunders Co., p. 822.

Table 2-4. *Average pulse rate at different ages**

Age	Lower limits of normal	Average	Upper limits of normal
Newborn	70	120	170
1-11 mo.	80	120	160
2 yr.	80	110	130
4 yr.	80	100	120
6 yr.	75	100	115
8 yr.	70	90	110
10 yr.	70	90	110

*From Kaplan, Samuel: In Nelson, W. B., editor: Textbook of pediatrics, ed. 7, Philadelphia, 1959, W. B. Saunders Co., p. 821.

minute. After the administration of atropine, infants often show pulse rates of 170 to 190 prior to induction of anesthesia. This represents almost complete vagal release, and more atropine or the effect of subsequent anesthesia rarely results in appreciable increase of pulse beyond that level. Rates of 200 to 230 occasionally may be seen in infants without evident complications.

Fig. 2-12 shows the variation in pulse rate of 100 patients of different ages under atropine premedication and ether anesthesia. It is evident that younger patients show more rapid rates and greater variation than do older patients.

Under cyclopropane anesthesia the child's heart responds rather quickly with definite bradycardia unless a vagolytic agent such as atropine has been administered. Once the vagal action is effectively blocked, the child's heart tolerates cyclopropane extremely well.

Congenital heart disease. The anesthetist's most frequent cause of concern

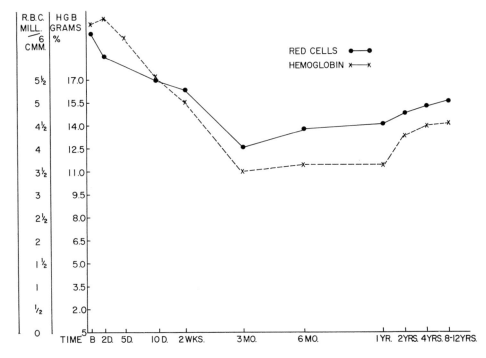

Fig. 2-11. Normal variation in hemoglobin and red blood cell count during infancy and child-hood. (From Kaplan, Samuel: In Nelson, W. E., editor: Textbook of pediatrics, ed. 7, Philadel-phia, 1959, W. B. Saunders Co.)

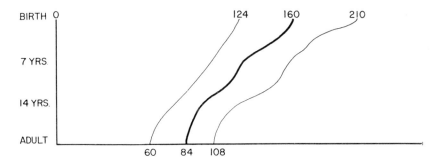

Fig. 2-12. Variations in the response of pulse rate to ether anesthesia (100 patients). Curves rep-resent minimum, average, and maximum rates during anesthesia.

in relation to the cardiovascular system in children is associated with congenital heart lesions. The response of the abnormal heart will be discussed in Chapter 18.

Respiratory physiology. It is of maximum importance to clarify the under-standing of respiratory function in pediatric patients. Respiration in the child and especially in the infant is notoriously subject to irregularities of all types that combine to form the greatest source of difficulty for the pediatric anesthetist.

At present, investigation of respiratory physiology in children is being carried on with vigor, and enough information has already been accumulated to be of considerable value to anesthetists. This material will be presented in Chapter 3 by Drs. Cook and Motoyama.

Liver and kidney function. The functional development of the liver may be incomplete at birth. Yudkin and Gellis[39] have shown that excretion of bromsulphalein is delayed in newborn infants. Other liver function tests, however, were found to be normal, and the deficiency of the liver is not believed to be great. Pseudocholinesterase is known to be decreased in the newborn[17]; however, the metabolism of succinylcholine is considerably more rapid in the infant than in the adult (Chapter 14).

As previously stated, histologic development of the kidney is not complete until the child is several months old. Barnett,[40] McCance,[41] and others have demonstrated that by standard renal function tests, such as urea clearance, urinary concentration, and glomerular filtration rate, the child's kidney is delinquent for several months after birth. Certainly it is true that infants run greater risk of developing water intoxication, sodium retention, or sudden dehydration than do adults. However, a more tolerant view of the infant kidney is now being suggested.[42] Considering the great demand made upon it by the rapid water turnover, the infant kidney appears to do a rather commendable job.

Endocrine function. In assessing the child's reaction to anesthesia and surgery the function of the *adrenal glands* should be an important consideration. This aspect has been the object of much attention recently. The large size of the adrenal cortex at birth has been noted. However, studies of Lanman[43] and of Klein[44] suggest that the adrenal cortex of the infant produces very little steroid until 2 or 3 weeks after birth. The infant's reaction to stress during the newborn period depends almost entirely upon the steroids endowed to him by his mother. It may follow that infants born after a stressful labor receive more steroids and are better prepared to face life than those born under less trying conditions. After any normal infant is 1 month old, his reaction to stress is believed to be at least as effective as that of an adult.

It may be of some importance to know that at birth the adrenal medulla produces little or no epinephrine, the entire catechol output consisting of norepinephrine.[45]

The *thyroid gland* is perhaps of more significance than is commonly believed. Although this gland is not large during early childhood, the rate of thyroxin metabolism is greatly increased.[46]

Fluid and electrolyte metabolism. In pointing out important differences between the adult and child, that of fluid and electrolyte balance is of primary importance. This subject is discussed in Chapter 26. It may be said here that fluid requirements follow a pattern similar to that of oxygen requirements, being minimal at birth, rapidly accelerating to a maximum between 9 and 18 months of age, then gradually receding throughout childhood and adult life.

The increased fluid metabolism that exists throughout most of childhood plays a large part in causing the increased dangers of both dehydration and fluid excess. The inadequate buffering mechanisms[47] and elevated chloride level combine to set the stage for edema and acidosis.

Metabolic response to anesthesia. The investigation of Bunker and associates[48] suggested that although adult human beings did not develop acidosis during ether anesthesia, infants, like dogs, did show some acidosis. Reynolds,[49] and Graff, Holzman, and Benson,[50] in more recent work, did not find any acidosis during infant anesthesia using nonrebreathing techniques. The differences in results were relatively small, and probably were due to use of dissimilar anesthetic methods.

Metabolic response to surgery. Studies of the metabolic response of newborn infants to surgery have been made by Rickham.[51] His findings were based on study of only 9 patients, but his methods were extremely painstaking. The outstanding difference he found to be in potassium metabolism. Contrary to expectation the infants studied lost no more potassium following extensive surgery than might have been caused by simple starvation. Other differences noted were the decreased incidence of ileus and the short duration and slight degree of postoperative weight loss. Rickham emphasized the great resistance of the newborn infant in the first day of life, and he too placed much of the credit on the presence of adrenocorticoid hormones derived from the mother. McLean and Paulsen[52] observed that the primary difference in the postoperative response of the infant was in the absence of water or sodium retention.

Temperature regulation. The regulation of body heat is still another function that has exaggerated responses during childhood. Temperature regulation is of special interest at present for several reasons: (1) small infants often suffer marked loss of body heat during anesthesia, exposing them to numerous hazards and complications[53,54]; (2) older children, especially those with fever or in an overheated environment, run the risk of hyperthermic reactions[55] (Chapter 27); and (3) the continuing problems of the value and techniques of induced hypothermia[56] (Chapter 16).

During fetal existence, body temperature is maintained at approximately 0.5° C. above that of the mother.[57] At birth, it is normal for the infant's rectal temperature to fall when exposed to ideal conditions, which are believed to be room temperature 32° to 34° C., relative humidity 50%, and air velocity not greater than 5 cm./sec.

The infant at birth is homeothermic and possesses a number of heat-controlling mechanisms. His normal heat production or basal metabolic activity at birth, measured and expressed in oxygen consumption, is 4 to 5 ml. of O_2/kg./min.[58] Heat loss, like that of older humans, occurs chiefly through radiation and convection, each of which accounts for approximately 50%. Under usual circumstances the human heat loss through conduction is almost negligible.

The importance of radiant heat loss is rather striking. An infant lying uncovered in a room heated to 85° F. will lose heat by radiation to a black wall 15 feet distant.[59]

When exposed in a cool environment infants lose heat rapidly because of relatively greater surface area and lack of protective subcutaneous tissue. The protective mechanism of vasoconstriction is present from birth, but shivering, although it has been observed, is seldom an effective heat-producing mechanism. Two possible mechanisms for nonshivering thermogenesis have been discovered in the neonate. In 1960 Moore and Underwood[60] suggested that norepinephrine could

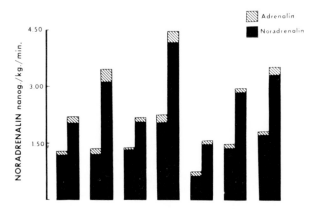

Fig. 2-13. Mechanism of infant response to cold. Chart shows urinary catecholamine levels of infants at normal temperature, paired with response upon cooling. Note that norepinephrine (Noradrenalin) is major factor at normal temperature and plays predominant role in response to cooling. (From Stern, L., Lees, M. H., and Leduc, J.: Pediatrics 36:367, 1965.)

be a factor in neonatal thermogenesis. It has been known that norepinephrine plays a more important role than epinephrine in neonatal life. Upon exposure of neonates to cold Stern, Lees, and Leduc[61] showed that catechol response consists chiefly of norepinephrine (Fig. 2-13), but the mechanism by which it increases heat production has not been completely defined. It may involve acceleration of carbohydrate and lipid metabolism, increased cardiovascular work, or decreased neuromuscular activity. The catecholamines appear to be intimately involved in temperature regulation at all ages. In older humans it has been observed that shivering is inhibited by anesthetic agents that stimulate catechol excretion, but that it is prominent with agents such as thiopental and halothane, which do not evoke adrenocortical response. Injection of epinephrine or norepinephrine into the cerebral ventricles reduces body temperature, while administration of 5-hydroxytryptamine raises the temperature, probably by action on hypothalamic thermoregulation centers.[62]

The second heat-producing mechanism in neonates is thought to exist in the brown adipose tissue known to play an important role in hibernating animals. It has been demonstrated by Johansson,[63] Dawkins and Scopes,[64] Joel,[65] and Aherne and Hull[66] that infants possess a specialized layer of adipose tissue that is distributed along the spine, nape of the neck, axillae, and perirenal area and that contains an increased vascular, nervous, and mitochondrial content, which in turn holds a high concentration of norepinephrine (Fig. 2-14). This tissue has a high oxygen requirement, and it is believed that it plays the part of an active heat-producing center in the newborn.

In studying the thermal factors that influence the neonate, Adamsons[57] found that the rectal temperature and oxygen consumption bear no correlation. An infant with a rectal temperature of 95° F. might have the same oxygen consumption if the temperature rose to 98° F. On the other hand, a very close correlation was found between oxygen consumption and the difference between rectal tem-

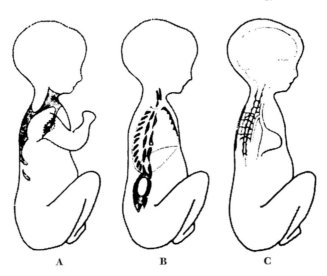

A   B   C

Fig. 2-14. Brown adipose tissue in superficial, **A,** and deep, **B,** sites in the newborn infant. **C,** Diagrammatic representation of the venous drainage from the interscapular pad. (From Aherne, W., and Hull, D.: Proc. Roy. Soc. Med. **57:**1172, 1964.)

perature and skin temperature, suggesting that peripheral receptors have much to do with bodily temperature control, actually more than the hypothalamic centers (Figs. 2-15 and 2-16).

During operation severe cooling will increase the danger of myocardial depression especially during rapid blood transfusion. Since gases become more soluble in cooler blood, a patient breathing a given anesthetic mixture will be in danger of passing to a deeper and more depressing plane if he becomes colder. Following operation temperatures below 95° F. may seriously depress respiration, as well as prolong recovery and delay resumption of normal fluid intake.

In older children abnormal elevation of temperature is more to be feared. Because of increased metabolic activity or environmental factors, a child's temperature may rise to 104° or 105° F., when there will be danger of convulsions and death.

Anesthetic agents have not been shown to have a specific temperature-elevating effect. Most agents, including ether, depress the central control and, by dilating peripheral vasculature and at the same time blocking shivering and sweating mechanisms, give up the control of temperature to the environment. The environmental factors of room temperature and humidity (plus additional controlling devices) will be the greatest determining factors in causing rise or fall of temperature during anesthesia.[67,68] To prevent temperature elevation during surgery in larger children the operating room temperature should be not more than 70° F.

PATHOLOGIC FACTORS

The fourth group of factors that differentiate pediatric from adult anesthesia consists of pathologic differences, including (1) conditions seen only in child-

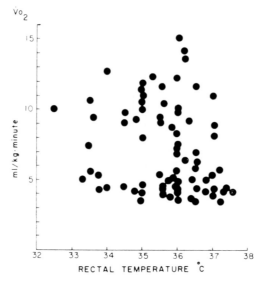

Fig. 2-15. Relationship of oxygen requirement to rectal temperature. Complete lack of correlation is obvious. (From Adamsons, K., Jr., Gandy, G. M., and James, L. S.: J. Pediat. **66:**495, 1965.)

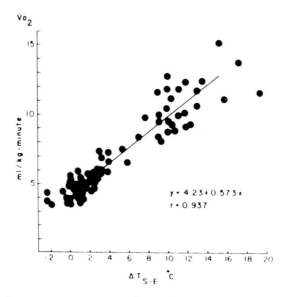

Fig. 2-16. Relation between oxygen consumption and the temperature gradient between skin and environment of mature human newborn infants with varying deep body skin temperatures. The term environmental temperature denotes that ambient air and radiating surface temperatures did not differ by more than 2° C. (From Adamsons, K., Jr., Gandy, G. M., and James, L. S.: J. Pediat. **66:**495, 1965.)

Table 2-5. *Pathologic conditions peculiar to childhood*

Prematurity	
Congenital anomalies	*Disturbances of growth or metabolism*
Hydrocephalus	Adrenogenital syndrome
Meningocele	Amyotonia
Fanconi's syndrome	Arachnodactyly
Harelip, cleft palate	Chondrodystrophy
Cystic hygroma	Gargoylism
Congenital heart disease	Mongolism
Atresias of the bowel	Pancreatic fibrosis
Omphalocele	Phenylketonuria
Teratoma	Niemann-Pick disease

hood and (2) the characteristic manner in which infants and children react to general illness as compared to the response of adults to similar diseases.

Conditions limited to the pediatric age group. A variety of diseases or lesions may be listed, each of which brings somewhat peculiar problems. The patients may come to operation for correction of the lesion, or the lesion may be merely a complicating factor. The variety is tremendous, but only a few need be mentioned as illustrations (Table 2-5).

A standard textbook of pathology should be available for information concerning unusual syndromes. That of Potter[69] is excellent for pathology of the newborn, whereas Anderson's[70] text includes all age groups.

Characteristic response of children to illness. Smith[71] pointed out that the newborn infant has an extremely vague and indefinite response to insult or illness. In the presence of pneumonia or peritonitis he may show little reaction in the way of temperature elevation or leukocytosis.

The power of survival of a normal infant, however, has long been thought to be greater during the first 24 hours of life than in the subsequent 2 weeks. This feeling is based on the concept that adrenal response, immune factors, and energy stores are fortified by heritage from the mother and will diminish gradually until the infant builds up his own resources. Many believe, therefore, that the best time to operate upon a young infant is during the first day of life.

There appear to be some faults in this point of view. Infants are known to lack maturity of several organ systems at birth and are burdened by an excess of body fluid. The lungs are believed to be expanded within 2 or 3 hours after birth if normal, but, unless observed for a reasonable period of time, such conditions as atelectasis, hyaline membrane disease, or pneumonia may not be recognized, and severe congenital heart lesions frequently are not evident until a baby is 3 or 4 days old. It might prove wiser to wait, when possible, to allow the infant to adjust himself to his new environment and to show the extent of his abnormalities before operation is attempted.

As the infant grows in strength and activity, the pattern of his reaction to disease reverses itself. An exaggerated response to infection and disease is shown in rapid temperature elevation, leukocyte rise, high pulse, and respiratory rates, with increased incidence of vomiting, convulsions, and similar manifestations. These rapid and extreme fluctuations are characteristic of most infants over 1 month of age.

RESPONSE TO PHARMACOLOGIC AGENTS

An area that has recently received well-deserved attention is that of pediatric pharmacology. The reaction of the child, and especially the infant, often is vastly different than that of the adult, involving *alteration in intensity of action,* or the appearance of *side effects* or *toxicity.* Determination of appropriate dosage of pharmacologic agents is also complicated and poorly understood, and often requires individual consideration of patient and agent.

Factors affecting response to drugs. The action of any drug may be altered at several stages in its passage through the body. Its *uptake* by lungs, digestive tract, and circulation may be affected by age, activity, and pathologic conditions present. An outstanding example of delayed uptake is the slow induction by inhalation agents in patients with tetralogy of Fallot or other types of decreased pulmonary circulation. The *distribution* of drugs depends primarily upon the cardiovascular system. In children the altered proportions of intracellular and extracellular fluid compartments also may play a part in the response to agents such as the muscle relaxants. The *metabolism* of chemical agents, whether by conjugation or degradation, is often dependent upon enzyme activity. Several enzymes are known to be deficient in neonates, and this defect is directly responsible for increased action or toxic effects of chloramphenicol and several antibiotics.[74,75] Finally, *excretion* of agents may be altered by inadequate renal function, and delayed elimination of active products naturally will prolong or intensify their action.

Additional considerations enter the picture. In use of sedatives, it is well known that *emotional and metabolic activity* is greatest in the child 1 to 3 years old. This must be considered in shaping the size of the dose.

Complications and side effects. The infant's often reported sensitivity to nondepolarizing muscle relaxants has not been explained satisfactorily, nor has the tolerance to depolarizing drugs (Chapter 14). Although Way, Costley, and Way[77] reported increased sensitivity of infants to respiratory depression with narcotics, the dosage often employed by cardiologists is surprisingly large (0.5 mg. at 1 month).

Toxic effects of several drugs have caused reasonable concern. Few of these have been anesthetic agents, but any physician should be aware of their occurrence. Chloramphenicol caused many deaths before it was realized that neonates were unable to detoxify it. Sulfonamides are known to disrupt bilirubin metabolism and cause kernicterus,[78] while novobiocin and vitamin K also may cause hyperbilirubinemia in small neonates.[79]

Numerous types of toxic and undesired effects are seen in neonates due to medications given the mother. These may cause either developmental faults or functional depression.[79,80]

Determination of dosage. None of the traditional guides for dose determination can be applied for all drugs. Age will fail when children are underdeveloped or overdeveloped, and weight is not reliable when children are obese. Body surface area has been regarded as the most reasonable basis for determining dosage of fluid requirements and some drugs,[81] but it has definite limitations. Obviously, no measurement of size signifies the child's emotional status. The agents used in anesthesia act on several different body mechanisms—muscular, cardiovascular, respiratory, and central and autonomic nervous systems being our primary concern.

We have developed patterns of dosage for many agents based on clinical experience rather than formula. As concluded by Shirkey,[74] the correct dose for all ages of man is enough, but not too much. This inexact state of affairs is what we continue to accept and defend by calling ours the "art" of medicine.

REFERENCES

1. Harris, J. S.: Special pediatric problems in fluid and electrolyte therapy in surgery, Ann. N. Y. Acad. Sci. **66:**966-975, 1957.
2. Talbot, N. B., Sobel, E. H., McArthur, J. W., and Crawford, J. D.: Functional endocrinology from birth through adolescence, Cambridge, Mass., 1952, Harvard University Press.
3. Gray, Henry: Anatomy of the human body, ed. 22 (revised and reedited by Lewis, W. H.), Philadelphia, 1930, Lea & Febiger.
4. Arey, L. B.: Developmental anatomy, Philadelphia, 1944, W. B. Saunders Co.
5. McGraw, M. B.: The neuromuscular maturation of the human infant, New York, 1943, Columbia University Press.
6. Langworthy, O. R.: Development of behavior patterns and myelinization of the nervous system in the human fetus and infant, Contrib. Embryol. **24:**3-60, 1933.
7. Thomas, A.: Etudes neurologiques sur le nouveau-ne et le jeune nourrison, Paris, 1952, Masson & Cie.
8. Conel, J. L.: The postnatal development of the human cerebral cortex, Cambridge, Mass., 1939, Harvard University Press.
9. Cook, C. D., Sutherland, J. M., Segal, S., Cherry, R. B., McIlroy, M. B., and Smith, C. A.: Studies of respiratory physiology in the newborn infant. III. Measurements of mechanics of respiration, J. Clin. Invest. **36:**440-448, 1957.
10. Eckenhoff, J.: Some anatomic considerations of the infant larynx influencing endotracheal anesthesia, Anesthesiology **12:**401-410, 1951.
11. Engel, S.: The child's lung, ed. 2, London, 1962, Edward Arnold & Co.
12. Hall, J. E.: The physiology of respiration in infants and young children, Proc. Roy. Soc. Med. **48:**761-764, 1955.
13. Colgan, F. J., and Keats, A. S.: Subglottic stenosis; a cause of difficult intubation, Anesthesiology **18:**265-269, 1957.
14. Adriani, H., and Griggs, T. S.: An improved endotracheal tube for pediatric use, Anesthesiology **15:**466-470, 1954.
15. Smith, C.: The bifurcation of the trachea in infancy; a statistical study; paper delivered at International Anesthesia Research Society, Bal Harbor, Fla., March 18-22, 1962.
16. Nelson, W. E., editor: Textbook of pediatrics, ed. 7, Philadelphia, 1959, W. B. Saunders Co.
17. Smith, C. A.: The physiology of the newborn infant, ed. 3, Springfield, Ill., 1959, Charles C Thomas, Publisher.
18. Lanman, J. T., editor: Physiology of prematurity, New York, 1957. Josiah Macy, Jr. Foundation.
19. Jackson, K.: Psychological preparation as a method of reducing emotional trauma of anesthesia in children, Anesthesiology **12:**293-300, 1951.
20. Eckenhoff, J. E.: Relationship of anesthesia to postoperative personality changes in children, Amer. J. Dis. Child. **86:**587-591, 1953.
21. Artusio, J. F., Jr., and Trousdell, M.: Comparative study of rectal Pentothal and morphine for basal anesthesia upon children for tonsillectomy, Anesthesiology **11:**443-451, 1950.
22. Betcher, A. M.: Hypno-induction techniques in pediatric anesthesia, Anesthesiology **19:**279-281, 1958.

23. Francis, W., and Cutler, R. P.: Psychological preparation and premedication for pediatric anesthesia, Anesthesiology 18:106-109, 1957.
24. Guedel, A. E.: Inhalation anesthesia, New York, 1943, The Macmillan Co.
25. DuBois, E. F.: Basal metabolism in health and disease, Philadelphia, 1927, Lea & Febiger.
26. Lewis, R. C., Duval, A. M., and Iliff, A.: Standards for the basal metabolism of children from 2 to 15 years of age inclusive, J. Pediat. 23:1-18, 1943.
27. Lee, V. A., and Iliff, A.: The energy of infants and young children during postprandial sleep, Pediatrics 18:739-749, 1956.
28. Shock, N. W.: Physiological changes in adolescence. Part I, Forty-third Year Book for the National Society for the Study of Education, 1944, pp. 56-79.
29. Duncan, G. G.: Diseases of metabolism, ed. 3, Philadelphia, 1953, W. B. Saunders Co.
30. Cross, K. W., Tizard, J. P. M., and Trythall, D. A. H.: The gaseous metabolism of the newborn infant, Acta Paediat. 46:265-285, 1957.
31. Stephen, C. R.: Elements of pediatric anesthesia, Springfield, Ill., 1954, Charles C Thomas, Publisher.
32. McQuarrie, I.: Convulsive disorders. In Nelson, W. E., editor: Textbook of pediatrics, ed. 7, Philadelphia, 1959, W. B. Saunders Co.
33. Glaser, G. H.: The neurological status of the newborn: neuromuscular and electroencephalographic activity, Yale J. Biol. & Med. 32:173-191, 1959.
34. Paine, R. S.: Detection of neurologic abnormalities in young infants, Int. Anesth. Clin. 1:1-33, 1962.
35. Cross, K. W.: Respiratory control in the neonatal period, Cold Spring Harbor Symposia on Quantitative Biology, vol. 19. The mammalian fetus; physiological aspects of development, New York, 1954, The Biological Laboratory.
36. Lipton, E. L., Steinschneider, A., and Richmond, J. B.: Autonomic nervous system in early life, New Eng. J. Med. 273:147-154; 201-208, 1965.
37. Friis-Hansen, B. J., Holaday, M., Stapleton, T., and Wallace, W. M.: Total body water in children, Pediatrics 7:321-327, 1951; Friis-Hansen, B. J.: Changes in body water compartments during growth, Acta Paediat., supp. 110, pp. 1-68, 1957.
38. Nadas, A. S.: Pediatric cardiology, ed. 2, Philadelphia, 1963, W. B. Saunders Co.
39. Yudkin, S., and Gellis, S.: Liver function in newborn infants, Arch. Dis. Child. 24:12-14, 1949.
40. Barnett, H. L.: Kidney function in young infants, Pediatrics 5:171-179, 1950.
41. McCance, R. C.: Renal physiology in infancy, Amer. J. Med. 9:229-241, 1950.
42. Barnett, H. L., Vestordal, J., McNamara, H., and Lauson, H. D.: Renal water excretion in premature infants, J. Clin. Invest. 31:1069-1073, 1952.
43. Lanman, J. T.: I. Function of adrenal cortex in premature infants without recognized disease, Pediatrics 11:120-128, 1953. II. ACTH-treated infants and infants born of toxemic mothers, Pediatrics 12:62-71, 1953.
44. Klein, R.: Neonatal adrenal physiology, Pediat. Clin. N. Amer. 1:321-334, 1954.
45. West, G. B., Shepard, D. M., and Hunter, R. B.: Adrenalin and noradrenalin concentrations in adrenal glands at different ages and in some diseases, Lancet 2:966-969, 1951.
46. Brewster, W. R.: Personal communication.
47. James, L. S., Weisbrot, I. M., Prince, C. F. Holaday, D. A., and Apgar, V.: The acid-base status of human infants in relation to birth asphyxia and the onset of respiration, J. Pediat. 33:379-394, 1958.
48. Bunker, J. P., Brewster, W. R., Smith, R. M., and Beecher, H. K.: Metabolic effects of anesthesia in man. III. Acid-base balance in infants and children during anesthesia, J. Appl. Physiol. 5:233-241, 1952.
49. Reynolds, R. N.: Acid-base equilibrium during cyclopropane anesthesia and operation in infants, Anesthesiology 27:127, 1966.
50. Graff, T. D., Holzman, R. S., and Benson, D. W.: Acid-base balance in infants during halothane anesthesia with the use of an adult circle absorption system, Anesth. Analg. 43:583-589, 1964.
51. Rickham, P. P.: The metabolic response to neonatal surgery, Cambridge, Mass., 1957, Harvard University Press.

52. McLean, E. C., and Paulsen, E. P.: The response of the newborn to major surgery: urinary electrolyte, nitrogen, and water losses, Amer. J. Dis. Child. 96:473-474, 1958.
53. Stephen, C. R., Dent, S. J., Hull, K. D., Knox, P. R., and North, N. C.: Body temperature regulation during anaesthesia in infants and children, J.A.M.A. 174:1579-1585, 1960.
54. Lewis, G. B., Jr., Leigh, M. D., and Belton, M. K.: Hypothermia in 363 pediatric surgical procedures, Anesth. Analg. 37:20-28, 1958.
55. Hogg, S., and Renwick, W.: Hyperpyrexia during anaesthesia, Canad. Anaesth. Soc. J. 13:429-436, 1966.
56. Terry, R.: Indications for cooling in pediatric anesthesia, New York J. Med. 57:105-107, 1957.
57. Adamsons, K., and Towell, M.: Thermal homeostasis in the fetus and newborn, Anesthesiology 26:531-548, 1965.
58. Scopes, J. W.: Metabolic rate and temperature control in the human baby, Brit. Med. Bull. 22:88-91, 1966.
59. Silverman, W. A., and Sinclair, J. C.: Temperature regulation in the newborn infant, New Eng. J. Med. 274:92-94, 146-148, 1966.
60. Moore, R. E., and Underwood, M. C.: Possible role of noradrenaline in control of heat production in the newborn mammal, Amer. J. Physiol. 190:240, 1957.
61. Stern, L., Lees, M. H., and Leduc, J.: Temperature, oxygen and catecholamine excretion in newborn infants, Pediatrics 36:367-374, 1965.
62. Feldberg, W., and Myers, R. D.: Effects on temperature of amines injected into the cerebral ventricles. A new concept of temperature regulation, J. Physiol. 173:226, 1964.
63. Johansson, B.: Brown fat; a review, Metabolism 8:221-240, 1959.
64. Dawkins, M. J. R., and Scopes, J. W.: Non-shivering thermogenesis in the human newborn infant, Nature 206:201-202, 1965.
65. Joel, C. D.: The physiological role of brown adipose tissue. In Renold, A. E., and Cahill, G. F., section editors: Handbook of physiology, Washington, D. C., 1965, American Physiological Society, vol. 5, chap. 9, pp. 59-85.
66. Aherne, W., and Hull, D.: Section of pediatrics. Site of heat production in the newborn infant, Proc. Roy. Soc. Med. 57:1172-1175, 1964.
67. Clark, R. E., Orkin, I. R., and Rovenstine, E. A.: Body temperature studies in anesthetized man: effect of environmental temperature, humidity, and anesthesia system, J.A.M.A. 154:311-319, 1954.
68. Searles, P. W., and Seymour, D. G.: Body temperature variation and effects during surgery, anesthesia and hypothermia, Anesth. Analg. 36:50-53, 1957.
69. Potter, E. L.: Pathology of the fetus and the newborn, Chicago, 1952, Year Book Medical Publishers, Inc.
70. Anderson, W. A. D.: Pathology, ed. 4, St. Louis, 1961, The C. V. Mosby Co.
71. Smith, C. A.: The newborn patient, Pediatrics 16:254-263, 1955.
72. Done, A. K.: Developmental pharmacology, Clin. Pharmacol. Ther. 5:432-479, 1965.
73. Done, A. K.: Drugs for children. In Modell, W., editor: Drugs of choice 1966-1967, St. Louis, 1966, The C. V. Mosby Co., pp. 48-55.
74. Shirkey, H. C.: Drug dosage for infants and children, J.A.M.A. 193:443-446, 1965.
75. Nyhan, W. L., and Lampert, F.: Response of the fetus and newborn to drugs, Anesthesiology 26:487-501, 1966.
76. Driscoll, S. G., and Hsia, D. YiYung.: The development of enzyme systems during early infancy, Pediatrics 22:785-845, supp., October, 1958.
77. Way, W. L., Costley, E. C., and Way, E. L.: Respiratory sensitivity of the newborn infant to meperidine and morphine, Clin. Pharmacol. Ther. 6:454-461, 1965.
78. Silverman, W. A.: Sulfonamides in the neonate. In May, C. D., editor: Perinatal pharmacology. Report of 41st Ross Laboratories Conference on Pediatric Research, Columbus, Ohio. 1962.
79. Schnider, S.: A review. Fetal and neonatal effects of drugs in obstetrics, Anesth. Analg. 45:372-378, 1966.
80. Moya, F., and Thorndike, S.: The effects of drugs used in labor on the fetus and newborn, Clin. Pharmacol. Ther. 5:628-653, 1965.
81. Shirkey, H. C.: Tables of dosages. In Pediatric therapy, St. Louis, 1965, The C. V. Mosby Co.

Chapter 3

Respiratory physiology in infants and children

Charles D. Cook, M.D.* and Etsuro K. Motoyama, M.D.†

Symbols commonly used in respiratory physiology
Anatomic and physiologic subdivisions of the respiratory system
Control of respiration
Lung volumes
Mechanics of respiration
Ventilation
Gas diffusion
Pulmonary circulation
Ventilation-perfusion relationships
Surface activity and lung function
Ciliary activity
Neonatal respiratory adaptation
Measurement of pulmonary function in children
Lung biopsy
Examples of respiratory abnormalities in infants and children

Anesthesiology is intimately concerned with the physiology of respiration. This is most apparent when general anesthesia is used but is also true with regional anesthesia and preanesthetic medication. In the patient subjected to general anesthesia there is usually partial and at times complete interference with the control of respiration. In addition, such factors as the loss of the cough reflex and sigh mechanism, encroachment on airway patency due to the positioning of the patient, equipment, laryngospasm, bronchospasm, and increased secretions impair respiratory function. Frequently the ventilatory requirements of patients vary during anesthesia and surgery, and the resistance

*Professor of Pediatrics and Chairman of the Department of Pediatrics, Yale University School of Medicine, New Haven, Conn.
†Assistant Professor of Anesthesiology and Pediatrics, Yale University School of Medicine, New Haven, Conn.

and dead space of anesthetic apparatus, including endotracheal tubes, accentuate the changing needs, especially in small infants. Open chest surgery, the use of muscle relaxants, and hypothermia necessitate the regulation of ventilation by the anesthesiologist for maintenance of oxygenation and normal acid-base balance (P_{co_2} and pH). Postoperative management of respiration is also an important task for the anesthesiologist. Finally, the intensive care units, recently developed in many hospitals, require active participation of the anesthesiologist and offer additional responsibilities involving resuscitation and cardiorespiratory management of critically ill patients.

This chapter will present some of the practical aspects of respiratory physiology and their application to the administration of anesthetics in children and to certain pulmonary diseases seen in the pediatric age group. Also included is a brief review of perinatal respiratory adaptation, since knowledge of events at birth is important for proper management of respiration in newborn infants in respiratory failure or for those undergoing surgery and anesthesia. As the sections that follow will indicate, there are many similarities between the respiration of infants and children on the one hand and adults on the other, but it will become apparent that both qualitative and quantitative differences exist.

SYMBOLS COMMONLY USED IN RESPIRATORY PHYSIOLOGY

Standardized symbols indicating various parameters in respiratory physiology are used to eliminate confusion. The most frequently used symbols are as follows:

Principal variables:
V : gas volume
$\dot{V}$: gas volume per minute or gas flow
P : gas pressure
F : fractional concentration in dry gas
Q : volume of blood
$\dot{Q}$: volume flow of blood per minute
S : percent saturation of hemoglobin with gas

Small subscript initials specify the preceding variables:

A : alveolar gas   as $\dot{V}_A$, alveolar ventilation usually expressed in milliliters (ml.) per minute or liters (L.) per minute

  I : inspired gas   as $F_{I_{O_2}}$, fraction of O_2 in the inspired gas

  E : expired gas   as $\dot{V}_E$, minute volume of ventilation (ml./min. or L./min.)

T : tidal gas   as V_T, tidal volume (ml. or L.)
D : deadspace gas   as V_D, volume of deadspace gas
a : arterial   as $P_{a_{O_2}}$, arterial O_2 tension (mm. Hg)
$\overline{v}$: mixed venous
c : capillary
D : diffusing capacity (ml./mm. Hg/min.)
C_1 : lung compliance (ml./cm. H_2O)
R : flow resistance (cm. H_2O/L./sec.)

ANATOMIC AND PHYSIOLOGIC SUBDIVISIONS
OF THE RESPIRATORY SYSTEM

The respiratory system is made up of the respiratory centers in the brain stem, the central and peripheral chemoreceptors, the phrenic and intercostal (efferent)

and vagal (afferent) nerves, the thoracic cage, including the musculature of the chest and abdomen and abdominal contents, the upper and lower air passages, the lungs, and the pulmonary vascular system. The following headings suggest the functional subdivisions of the respiratory system:

1. Control of respiration
2. Lung volumes
3. Mechanics of respiration
4. Ventilation
5. Gas diffusion
6. Pulmonary circulation
7. Ventilation-perfusion relationships
8. Surface activity and lung function
9. Ciliary activity

The principal desired result of these functions in all age groups is to maintain the body in oxygen and carbon dioxide equilibrium. The lungs also contribute importantly to the regulation of acid-base balance. The maintenance of a stable body temperature (by loss of water through the lungs), although occasionally important, is, on the whole, a secondary function.

CONTROL OF RESPIRATION

The activity of the respiratory center is affected by multiple impulses arising from other parts of the central nervous system as well as from the periphery. However, the primary factors controlling respiration in normal persons of all ages are chemical.

Regulation of alveolar ventilation and maintenance of normal arterial P_{o_2}, P_{co_2}, and pH are the principal functions of the medullary and peripheral chemoreceptors.[1,2] The medullary chemoreceptors, located near the surface of ventrolateral medulla, are anatomically separated from the medullary respiratory center. They respond to changes in hydrogen ion concentration of the adjacent cerebrospinal fluid, rather than arterial P_{co_2} or pH.[3] Since carbon dioxide rapidly passes into the cerebrospinal fluid, the medullary chemoreceptors are readily stimulated by respiratory acidosis. On the other hand, the ventilatory response of the medullary chemoreceptors to acute metabolic acidosis is limited because hydrogen and bicarbonate ions in arterial blood are not rapidly transmitted into cerebrospinal fluid. In chronic acid-base disturbances, the pH of cerebrospinal fluid surrounding the medullary chemoreceptors is generally maintained within normal limits, probably due to active transport mechanism.[4,5] Ventilatory responses under these circumstances become dependent mainly on the activity of peripheral chemoreceptors.

Carotid and aortic bodies or the peripheral chemoreceptors are primarily responsive to changes in arterial P_{o_2}. Moderate to severe hypoxemia ($P_{ao_2} < 50$ mm. Hg) results in a significant increase in ventilation in all ages except in premature infants, whose ventilation is decreased.[6-8] Inhalation of oxygen, on the other hand, produces a transient decrease in ventilation; in the full-term and premature infants this response is enhanced. Hypoxemia potentiates ventilatory response to hypercapnia or acidosis in a multiplicative, rather than an additive, fashion.[9] In chronic hypoxemia associated with cardiopulmonary diseases or occurring at high altitude, the carotid and aortic bodies, which exhibit little adaptation to a chronic hypoxic state, are responsible for hyperventilation. They are also in part responsible for hyperventilation in hypotensive patients. Absence of respiratory stimulation in hypoxemic states such as severe anemia and carbon monoxide poisoning is due to the fact that P_{aO_2} under these conditions, in spite of a decrease in O_2 content, is maintained at normal levels, and the chemoreceptors are therefore not stimulated.

As indicated, in patients with *chronic* respiratory insufficiency and *chronic* hypercapnia, hypoxemic stimulation of the peripheral chemoreceptors provides the primary impulse to the respiratory center. If these patients are given supplemental oxygen, the stimulus of hypoxemia is removed, ventilation is decreased or ceases, P_{CO_2} is further increased, patients become comatous (CO_2 narcosis), and death may follow unless artificial ventilation is instituted immediately. Rather than oxygen therapy alone, such patients need their effective ventilation increased. This can be done by assisting their respiration mechanically; in some cases a tracheostomy will decrease the dead space and may increase the effective ventilation to the alveoli.

Barbiturates, narcotics, and general anesthetics depress the medullary chemoreceptors either directly or through inhibition of the brain stem reticular formation. Tachypnea and hyperpnea observed during inhalation of certain anesthetics, such as diethyl-ether and trichlorethylene, are caused by stimulation of sensory receptors in the lungs, which in turn send impulses to the medullary respiratory center via the vagal afferents.[10]

Occlusion of the upper airway at the end of expiration strengthens and deepens the inspiratory effort, while a sudden inflation of the lung inhibits inspiratory effort (inflation reflex of Hering-Breuer). Rhythmicity of respiration is thus modified by impulses transmitted via vagal afferents from pulmonary stretch receptors probably located in the bronchi and bronchioles. In man, the inflation reflex is most prominent at birth, but after 6 days of life it becomes very weak unless inflation of the lungs is extreme.[11]

When the conduction of the vagi is partially blocked, inflation of lungs produces prolonged contraction of the diaphgram instead of inspiratory inhibition from the inflation reflex. This reflex, the paradoxical reflex of Head, may be related to the complimentary cycle of respiration or "sigh mechanism," which functions to aerate parts of lungs that have been collapsed during normal respiration.[12] In the newborn babies, inflation of the lungs initiates grasping. Cross and associates[11] postulated that this mechanism is analogous to the paradoxical reflex and may help to inflate unaerated portions of the lungs of newborn infants.

Deflation of the lungs in animals increases the force and frequency of inspiratory effort (the deflation reflex of Hering-Breuer). This reflex, if it exists in humans, would account in part for increased respiratory effort when the lung volume is abnormally decreased as in chest compression and pneumothorax.

In addition, respiration is influenced by other factors such as thermal, emotional, and tactile stimuli. Finally, central nervous system injury, infection, increased intracranial pressure, or the direct expansion of an intracranial mass, as well as spinal or peripheral failure of nerve conduction (e.g., poliomyelitis, muscle relaxants) and muscles (e.g., amyotonia congenita, muscle dystrophy), may all interfere with the proper function of the controlling mechanisms.

With this as a general background to the control of respiration, what peculiarities and differences have been noted in infants and children?

In the first place, there is obviously some inhibitory mechanism present in utero that prevents continuous or, in fact, anything more than occasional respiratory movements. Burns[13] has shown the dependence of the rhythmicity of the medullary respiratory center on other neural systems; in the fetus the lack of the sensory impulses must in part be responsible for its apnea.

The principal factor responsible for the onset of respiration at birth seems to be chemical.[14] Parenthetically it is apparent that fetal and newborn organisms (presumably including the human fetus) have a resistance to hypoxia that is gradually lost during the first few hours and days of life. Once respiration has begun, ventilation is adjusted to achieve a lower P_{co_2} (Table 3-1) than is found in older children and adults. The basis of this difference remains to be elucidated but most likely represents a respiratory compensation for metabolic acidosis. The P_{co_2} of the infant approximates the adult level within 1 to 2 weeks after birth.

Another difference in the control of respiration between newborn and especially premature infants on the one hand and older individuals on the other is shown by their tendency to breathe irregularly (Fig. 3-1). The pH of arterialized capillary blood during irregular breathing is slightly alkalotic and the end-tidal CO_2 slightly lower than that of regular breathers.[15] Oxygen administration usually abolishes the periodic respiration, and a regular rhythm is established. A possible basis for this phenomenon is that the central respiratory mechanism in these newborn infants has not yet matured. Cross and Oppé[8] suggested that "among the many factors which may be responsible for this 'immaturity,' the inability of the respiratory center of the infant to withstand oxygen lack plays a major part." They demonstrated that newborn infants and adults respond to hypoxia similarly but that the least mature infant on the average has the least relative increase in ventilation.

The effect of age on the respiratory responses of the newborn infant has been studied by Miller and Behrle.[16] They presented data showing that when 10 to 12% O_2 is administered, the ventilation of the newborn infant on the first day of life decreases, whereas that of infants 16 to 48 days old increases. These different responses of the newborn and young organism are important but do not explain the irregular respiration noted more frequently during anesthesia in infants and young children than under similar circumstances in older persons.

The response of infants to inspired CO_2 has been studied. Avery and her associates[17] found that the ventilation of infants at a given alveolar P_{co_2}, was greater than that of adults; but the rate of change in ventilation per unit body weight was not different. The greater ventilation at a given P_{co_2} is probably related to the higher CO_2 production and a limited buffering capacity of infants.

Much further information, especially concerning the respiratory responses of anesthetized infants and children, is necessary for a complete understanding of the control of respiration in this age group. Nevertheless, with the physiologic infor-

Table 3-1. *Normal blood gas values**

	P_{o2} (mm. Hg)	S_{o2} (%)	P_{co2} (mm. Hg)	pH
Pregnant women at term (artery)	88†	96	32	7.40
Umbilical vein‡	31	72†	42	7.35
Umbilical artery‡	19	38†	51	7.29
1 hour of life (artery)	92	96	28	7.36
24 hours of life (artery)	89	97	29	7.37
Child and adult (artery)	99	97	41	7.40

*Compiled from data from Crawford, J. S.: Amer. J. Obstet. Gynec. **93:**37, 1965; Quilligan, E. H., et al.: Amer. J. Obstet. Gynec. **90:**1343, 1964; Oh, W., et al.: Acta Paediat. Scand. **55:**593, 1966.
†Estimated values.
‡Taken during labor and delivery.

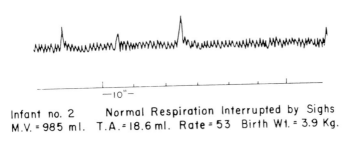

Infant no. 2   Normal Respiration Interrupted by Sighs
M.V. = 985 ml.   T.A. = 18.6 ml.   Rate = 53   Birth Wt. = 3.9 Kg.

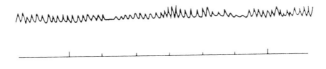

Infant no. 30   Periodic Respiration without Apnea
M.V. = 517 ml.   T.A. = 13.7 ml.   Rate = 37   Birth Wt. = 2.4 Kg.

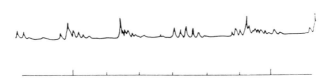

Infant no. 33   Periodic Respiration with Apneic Intervals
M.V. = 314 ml.   T.A. = 13.1 ml.   Rate = 24   Birth Wt. = 1.3 Kg.

Fig. 3-1. Body plethysmograph-spirometer tracings illustrating types of respiration in normal newborn infants: **MV,** minute volume; **T.A.,** tidal air. (From Cook, C. D. In Gordon, B. L., editor: Clinical cardiopulmonary physiology, ed. 2, New York, 1960, Grune & Stratton, Inc., p. 507. By permission.)

mation presently available, it is possible to regulate respiration in the anesthetized patient with a degree of accuracy that in most cases is adequate. If a patient with a normal cardiopulmonary system is not cyanotic while breathing room air, it is most probable that the blood P_{CO_2} is not significantly increased. However, the patient may have an excessive ventilation, which may lead to an increased elimination of carbon dioxide from the lungs and a respiratory alkalosis. This may occur more often than is realized when artificial respiration is maintained in an anesthetized patient for long periods of time and may contribute to operative and postoperative morbidity and mortality. Contrariwise, a patient breathing an oxygen-enriched atmosphere may remain acyanotic even when hypoventilating. In this situation carbon dioxide will increase and respiratory acidosis will result, and it, too, may increase the operative risk. The potential danger of respiratory acid-base imbalance would appear to be particularly critical in the management

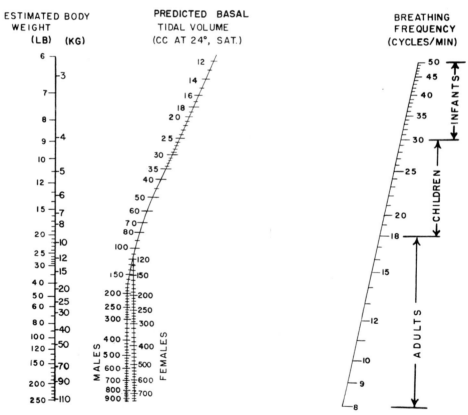

Fig. 3-2. Nomogram for predicted basal tidal volume. Corrections to be applied: add 10% if subject is awake; add 9% for each degree centigrade of fever; add 8% for each 1,000 meters of altitude above sea level; calculate the required tidal volume. If a tracheostomy is in use, subtract one half the patient's estimated physiologic dead space (i.e., subtract 1 ml. per kilogram body weight). Add the dead space of the anesthetic apparatus. (From Radford, E. P., Jr., Ferris, B. G., Jr., and Kriete, B. C.: New Eng. J. Med. **251:**877, 1954.)

of the very small or very sick infant because of his limited homeostatic mechanisms.

What techniques are available for aiding in the proper control of respiration during anesthesia and the postsurgical period? One may estimate patient's ventilatory requirements from his size. This has been done by Radford, Ferris, and Kriete,[18] and their nomogram (Fig. 3-2) has proved most useful provided that the patient has a normal cardiopulmonary system and that there is no increase in physiologic dead space and/or shunting of blood. Since anesthetized patients tend to develop atelectasis and shunting due to the absence of "sigh mechanism," it is necessary to hyperinflate the lungs periodically. One should also take the mechanical dead space of anesthetic equipment into consideration for the proper estimation of the ventilatory requirement of the patient. With the use of this estimation one still must know the tidal volume as well as the respiratory rate. A low-resistance spirometer as shown in Fig. 3-3 in the expiratory circuit of the anesthetic system will allow the anesthesiologist to gauge more accurately his efforts in relation to the patient's needs; however, no such suitable apparatus is available for small infants.

As will be apparent from the sections that follow, the ventilatory requirements are influenced not only by the patient's basic requirements and the volume of the dead space of the anesthetic apparatus, but also by the patient's temperature, the tidal volume, the altitude, and other factors. It is obvious that for a given error in the estimation of ventilatory needs, the smaller the patient, the greater will be the deviation from correct oxygenation and acid-base balance.

A more accurate method of evaluating the adequacy of ventilatory control involves the measurement of blood gas tensions. Until recently these have been

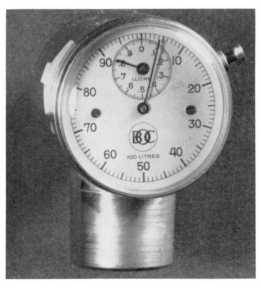

Fig. 3-3. Wright Respirometer, which can be used for measuring tidal and minute volume both in a spontaneously breathing and a manually ventilated patient. (Courtesy British Oxygen Co., Ltd., London, England.)

impractical except for research purposes, but now equipment is available for the ready measurement in the operating room of arterial P_{O_2}, P_{CO_2}, and pH.[20,21] Undoubtedly these techniques should be available and used in prolonged or complicated surgical procedures, especially those involving the heart and lungs. However, even when the equipment and personnel for blood gas measurements are available, only spot checks can be carried out. A simpler and frequently supplemental approach is based on the fact that, when no shunts are present and when the distribution of gas in the lungs is relatively even, the blood gases in the pulmonary vein have approximately the same P_{CO_2} as does end tidal air. End-expiratory air can be sampled and analyzed by rapidly responding gas analyzers (mass spectrometer, infrared analyzer), and it is therefore possible to measure indirectly but quite accurately the arterial P_{CO_2}. Such analyzers have in fact been incorporated into anesthesia machines for the automatic control of ventilation and maintenance of normal P_{CO_2}. Undoubtedly they should be used more in the cases that are, from the anesthesiologist's point of view, complicated.

Summary. Although the control (and inhibition) of the respiratory center during prenatal and neonatal life is still poorly understood, it is apparent that in most respects the control of respiration in infants and children is similar to its control in adults. However, newborn infants regulate gas exchange to effect a lower arterial CO_2 tension probably as an adjustment to metabolic acidosis. In addition, infants and small children have a tendency toward irregular breathing, which may be based on "immaturity" of the respiratory center and an inability of the center to react to oxygen lack. Finally, a variety of methods are available to aid in the regulation of respiration of the anesthetized as well as the postoperative patient.

LUNG VOLUMES

In order to understand respiration and some of the respiratory abnormalities encountered in infants and children, it is useful to review the subdivisions of the lung as shown in Fig. 3-4. In the normal person these lung volumes are related to the person's size, especially his height[22] (Table 3-2 and Figs. 3-5 and 3-6). Although the data on newborn and small infants are incomplete, it appears that in most instances the relative sizes of the lung compartments are approximately constant from shortly after birth through young adulthood. In the immediate postnatal period, however, the functional residual volume is relatively low, gradually increasing during the 24 to 48 hours of life. In the premature infant with marginal amounts of surface active phopholipids in the alveolar surface lining layer (discussed later), there is a tendency for areas of atelectasis to persist for a few days to a few weeks.

The limits of these lung volumes are imposed by both the thorax and the lungs themselves. The total lung capacity is the largest lung volume allowed by the strength of the respiratory muscles stretching the thorax and lungs, and the residual volume is the amount of air remaining after forced expiration. In open chest surgery or pneumothorax the lungs may collapse still farther, particularly if high concentrations of oxygen have been used and the trapped oxygen is taken up by the pulmonary circulation.

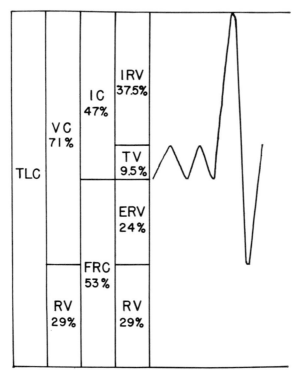

Fig. 3-4. Lung subdivisions: **TLC,** total lung capacity; **VC,** vital capacity; **FRC,** functional residual capacity; **IC,** inspiratory capacity; **IRV,** inspiratory reserve volume; **RV,** residual volume; **ERV,** expiratory reserve volume; **TV,** tidal volume. (Adapted from Comroe, J. H., Jr., et al.: The lung, Chicago, 1962, Year Book Medical Publishers, Inc.)

As can be seen from Fig. 3-4, in the person with a normal respiratory system the reserve is great. However, in the patients with abnormalities the range between tidal volume needed for metabolic requirements and the vital capacity may be very limited.

The resting lung volume (functional residual capacity) is determined by the balance between a number of different forces: the thoracic structures tend to expand the lungs while the lungs themselves tend to collapse. For the upright position the balance point in the resting state (the FRC or end-expiratory position) is reached in older children and adults when the pressure in the interpleural space is approximately −5 cm. H_2O. (In newborn infants the end-expiratory pressure is apparently −1 or −2 cm. H_2O.) In this connection it is worth noting that negative pressure outside of the lungs is the same, in respect to lung expansion, as positive pressure within the lungs; thus the net *transpulmonary* pressure represents the force expanding or contracting the lungs. On the other hand, in respect to the pulmonary circulation, negative intrathoracic pressure has quite a different effect from positive airway pressure (discussed in sections on pulmonary circulation and ventilation-perfusion relationships).

Table 3-2. *Normal values for lung functions for persons of various ages**

Age	1 wk.	1 yr.	3 yr.	5 yr.	8 yr.	12 yr.	♂ 15 yr.	♂ 21 yr.	♀ 21 yr.
Height (cm.)	48	75	96	109	130	150	170	174	162
Weight (lb.)	6.5	22	32	40	58	85	125	160	125
FRC (ml.)	75†	(263)	(532)	660	1,174	1,855	2,800	3,030	2,350
VC (ml.)	100‡	(475)	(910)	1,100	1,855	2,830	4,300	4,620	3,380
$\dot{V}_E$ (ml./min.)	550	(1,775)	(2,460)	(2,600)	(3,240)	(4,150)	5,030	6,000	5,030
V_T (ml.)	17	(78)	(112)	(130)	(180)	(260)	360	500	420
f (frequency)	30	(24)	(22)	(20)	(18)	16	14	12	12
$\dot{V}_A$ (ml./min.)	385	(1,245)	(1,760)	(1,800)	(2,195)	(2,790)	3,070	4,140	3,530
V_D (ml.)	7.5	21	37	49	75	105	141	150	126
C_l (ml./cm. H_2O)	5	(16)	(32)	44	71	91	130	150	130
Peak flow rates (L./min.)	10			136	231	325	437	457	365
R (cm. H_2O/L/sec.)	29§	(13)	(10)	8	6	5	3	2	2
D_{Lco} (ml./mm. Hg./min.)‖				11	15	20	27	28	24
Cardiac output (L./min.)	(0.9)	1.9	2.7	3.2	4.4	5.7	(7.0)	(7.6)	(7.2)
Lung weight (gram)	49	120	166	211	290	470	640	730	

*Compiled from data in Cook, C. D., et al.: J. Clin. Invest. **34**:975, 1955 and **36**:440, 1957; Comroe, J. H., Jr., et al.: The lung, Chicago, 1962, Year Book Medical Publishers, Inc.; Bucci, G., et al.: J. Pediat. **58**:820, 1961; Murray, A. B., and Cook, C. D.: J. Pediat. **62**:186, 1963; Cook, C. D., and Hamann, J. F.: J. Pediat. **59**:710, 1961; and Long, E. C., and Hull, W. E.: Pediatrics **27**:373, 1961.

†Supine.   ‡Crying vital capacity.   §Nose breathing.   ‖Single breath technique.   Parentheses = Interpolated values.

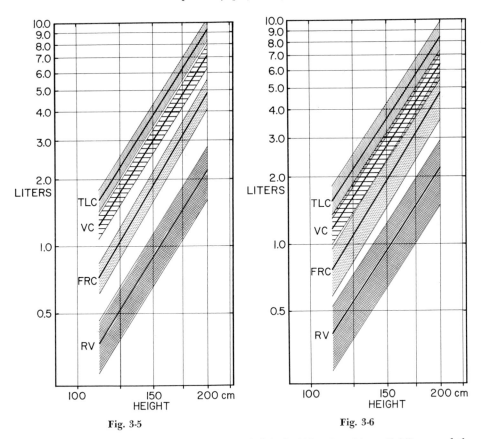

Fig. 3-5

Fig. 3-6

Fig. 3-5. Regression lines for lung volumes versus height in 106 male subjects (1 S.D. around the arithmetic mean is shown). (From Cook, C. D., and Hamann, J. F.: J. Pediat. **59:**713, 1961.)

Fig. 3-6. Regression lines for lung volumes versus height in 65 female subjects (1 S.D. around the arithmetic mean is shown). (From Cook, C. D., and Hamann, J. F.: J. Pediat. **59:**713, 1961.)

Anesthesia, surgery, abdominal distention, and disease may all alter the lung volumes. Because the abdominal contents shift, the prone or supine patient has a smaller functional residual capacity (FRC) than the standing or sitting patient. In certain conditions, such as the respiratory distress syndrome of the newborn infant, in which the lung resists expansion, the FRC may be reduced. On the other hand, when air passages are narrowed as in asthma or cystic fibrosis of the pancreas, there will be air trapping on expiration and the FRC will be increased.

The importance of the air that remains in the lungs at the end of normal expiration is often overlooked. This FRC serves as a buffer that minimizes changes in the P_{CO_2} and P_{O_2} of the blood with each respiration. In addition, the fact that air normally remains in the lungs throughout the respiratory cycle means that relatively few of the alveoli collapse. If air were completely exhaled with each expiration, all alveoli would collapse, have to be reexpanded again with inspiration, and large surface forces would have to be overcome with each breath. Although collapse does not occur during normal respiration, with the initiation of respiration at birth and with open chest surgery unusually large pressures are necessary for expansion of the lung to its normal volume. Transpulmonary pressure of 4 to 6 cm. H_2O is, under normal conditions, enough to effect an adequate tidal volume, but 15 to 25 cm. H_2O (and occasionally even more) is necessary for initial expansion or reexpansion of collapsed lungs.

Summary. It is apparent that the lung volumes of normal infants and children are comparable on the basis of body size to those of older persons. These volumes are the result of a balance between the elastic forces of thoracic structures and the elastic characteristics of the lung. A variety of conditions, including anesthesia, may influence these factors and alter the lung volumes. The air remaining in the lungs at the end of expiration minimizes the changes in blood gases during the respiratory cycle; this remaining air also reduces the surface forces that must be overcome during respiration.

MECHANICS OF RESPIRATION

In ventilating the lungs the muscles of respiration must overcome certain opposing forces within the lungs themselves. These forces can best be considered under two main headings, elastic and resistive.*

When the lungs are stretched, elastic recoil, as in a spring, must be overcome. This elastic force is fairly constant over the range of normal tidal volume but increases at the extremes of deflation or inflation (Fig. 3-7). Elastic properties of the lungs are measured and expressed as lung compliance (C_1) in units of volume change per units of pressure change. Thus $C_1 = \dfrac{\Delta V}{\Delta P}$, where ΔV is usually the tidal volume and ΔP the change in interpleural pressure necessary to obtain the V_T. These measurements are made at points of no flow, i.e., at the extremes of tidal volume when there is no flow-resistive component. Lung compliance may change with changes in the midposition of respiration without any changes in the inherent elastic characteristics of the lungs. Therefore a more accurate description of the elastic behavior of the lungs is provided by the measurement of the volume-pressure relation over the entire range of total lung capacity.

In normal individuals lung compliance measured during the respiratory cycle (i.e., the dynamic compliance) is approximately the same during quiet breathing as the static compliance. When there is airway obstruction, however, the ventilation of some of the lung units may be functionally decreased, resulting in a decreased dynamic lung compliance, particularly in comparison with the relatively little or absent change in the static measurement.

When the lungs are stretched, energy is stored up and is recovered when the lungs return to their original size. In this way, quiet, normal expiration is the result of the elastic recoil of the lungs and chest wall and involves little or no additional work. The situation in the infant and the anesthetized patient may be

---

*The term "resistive" is used to include tissue viscosity and air flow resistive factors. Since these cannot easily be separated and since air flow resistance is clinically the most important, the term "flow resistance" will be used throughout.

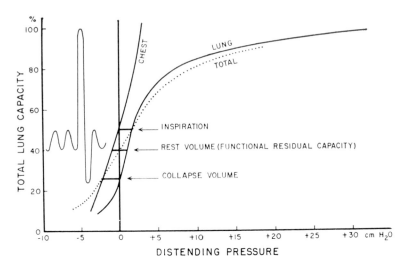

Fig. 3-7. Static pressure-volume diagram of the neonatal respiratory system. A normal spirogram is shown for volume orientation. Distending pressure on the abscissa represents transpulmonary pressure or the difference between atmospheric and interpleural pressures. Note: (1) the chest wall is extremely compliant (high slope); (2) the lung compliance decreases (low slope) at extremes of lung volume; and (3) the functional residual capacity is relatively low. (From Nelson, N. M.: Pediat. Clin. N. Amer. 13:769, 1966.)

somewhat different as there may then be an active phase to expiration, as discussed in the following paragraphs.

Lung compliance in normal persons of different sizes is, in general, directly proportional to the size of the lungs (Table 3-2). When compliance for persons of different sizes is compared per unit of lung volume (e.g., functional residual capacity, vital capacity, or total lung capacity), lung compliance is similar for all sizes.

To consider volume-pressure relations from another point of view, it is apparent that a normal tidal volume may be obtained by using *transpulmonary* pressures of approximately 4 to 6 cm. H_2O in persons of all sizes, provided the lungs are normal and normally expanded initially. The *total* transthoracic pressure necessary to ventilate the lungs in a closed chest is, in the adult, approximately twice the required transpulmonary pressure since the thoracic structures must also be expanded. In the newborn infant, however, the chest wall appears to be extremely compliant and therefore requires by itself almost no force for expansion (Fig. 3-7). The combined compliance of chest wall and lungs ($C_{(l + w)}$) may be expressed as follows:

$$1/C_{(l + w)} = 1/C_l + 1/C_w$$

Lung compliance is reduced in most situations in which lung volume is decreased (e.g., removal of lung tissue, intrapulmonary tumors). It is also decreased when surface forces are increased (as in atelectasis or the respiratory distress syndrome). Idiopathic emphysema of adults is associated with a loss of elasticity and

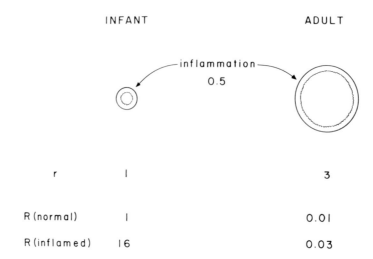

Fig. 3-8. Effect of inflammation on airway resistance in infants and adults. **r**, Radius of an air passage. **R**, Flow resistance.

therefore an increase in C_1. Chest wall compliance decreases with age and with such conditions as ankylosing spondylitis involving the thoracic structures.

Besides the lungs and chest wall, the air passages themselves have a compliance that may be important. With deep inspiration the air passages of normal persons increase in size, whereas on forced expiration they decrease to a point at which air trapping may take place. If the lungs are abnormal or if obstruction is present, considerable change in the airway size can be noted on bronchoscopy. Occasionally such findings may lead to the incorrect diagnosis of deficient cartilaginous rings in the trachea and bronchi.

The flow resistance of the lungs includes tissue viscous resistance (resistance of the tissues themselves to deformation) and resistance to the flow of air within the air passages. In contrast to compliance that can be measured only at points of no flow (e.g., at the extremes of tidal volume or during interrupted respiration), flow resistance is present only when the lungs (or air within them) are in motion.

Airflow resistance (R) is expressed as a unit pressure (P) per unit flow ($\dot{V}$) (cm. H_2O/L./sec.) and is related to the length (l) and radius (r) of a tube and the viscosity of the gas (η) as shown in Poiseuille's law: $R = \dfrac{8l\eta}{\pi r^4}$. It is apparent from the equation that the most important factor influencing flow resistance is the changes in the radius of air passages since it is inversely proportional to r^4.* Therefore it is reasonable that infants with their small air passages have higher resistances than do larger children and adults (Table 3-2). From this relationship it also might be expected that relatively small amounts of bronchiolar inflammation or secretions would lead to relatively greater degrees of obstruction in infants than in older persons (Fig. 3-8). Unfortunately, a number of other factors

---

*Air flow resistance is related to $1/r^5$ when turbulence is present.

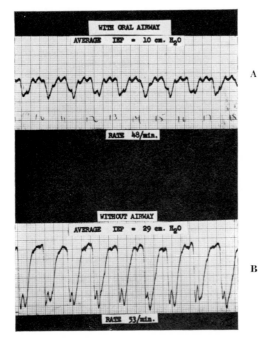

Fig. 3-9. Intraesophageal pressure measurements, **IEP,** indicating minor airway resistance with proper use of oral airway, **A,** and increased resistance due to inadequate neck and mandible extension, **B.**

such as length, shape, and turbulence are presently impossible to assess, and these factors make the exact relationship between resistance and body measurements in persons of various sizes difficult to define. It can only be said that as a person's lungs and air passages grow, flow resistance decreases.

Resistance may be increased when air passages are narrowed from bronchospasm (e.g., asthma), from secretions or inflammations (e.g., bronchiolitis and croup), from foreign bodies, or from pressure (e.g., vascular rings, mediastinal tumors, or tuberculous nodes). Resistance may also be increased during anesthesia due to improper maintenance of the airway (Fig. 3-9) or high resistance of the external apparatus. All of these factors will increase the work of breathing. Under such circumstances a relatively large tidal volume and low respiratory rate will be most efficient in relation to the work of breathing as well as to ventilation itself.

The flow resistance of individual parts of the lung will influence their ventilation. If extreme narrowing exists, only small amounts of new air will enter with each respiratory cycle and result in ventilation-perfusion imbalance, as discussed later.

Lung compliance and flow resistance can be measured by simultaneously measuring volume changes and interpleural pressure changes (Fig. 3-10). Fortunately intraesophageal pressure changes are good indices of interpleural pressure

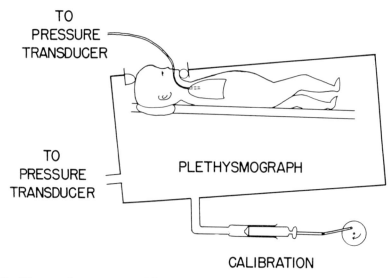

TO
PRESSURE
TRANSDUCER

TO
PRESSURE
TRANSDUCER

PLETHYSMOGRAPH

CALIBRATION

Fig. 3-10. Diagram of apparatus used for measurement of compliance and resistance in newborn infants. Intraesophageal catheter shown in place. Pressure changes in body-plethysmograph were used to measure tidal volume changes.

changes, although in the supine position the weight of the mediastinum on the esophagus produces artifacts that are difficult to evaluate. The compliance of the chest wall may be measured in the anesthetized and paralyzed patient or trained person by measuring the compliance of the entire respiratory system and subtracting that of the lungs alone.[23]

Summary. Lung compliance in the tidal range or the distensibility of lungs for a given transpulmonary pressure is directly related to body or lung size. Lung compliance is reduced at both extremes of lung volume, i.e., at very small and very large volumes. Thus collapsed lungs require much larger pressures for inflation than do previously expanded lungs. The artificial ventilation of a patient with a closed chest requires the expansion of both lungs and chest. Flow resistance is largest in persons with the smallest air passages. It may be increased by various anesthetic apparatus and, particularly in infants, by relaxation of laryngeal structures and a number of conditions affecting the size of air passages.

VENTILATION

Ventilation involves the movement of air in and out of the lungs. The diaphragm is the most important muscle for normal inspiration, although the intercostal and accessory respiratory muscles aid in a maximal inspiratory effort. Quiet expiration results from the elastic recoil of the lungs and chest wall and relaxation of the diaphragm. The exhalation of a newborn infant, even when resting or asleep, is active rather than passive as in the older child and adult.[24] A similar active expiration has been observed in anesthetized children[24] and adults,[25] but the mechanism is unknown. Forced expiration is accomplished with the aid of spinal flexors, the intercostals, and especially the abdominal muscles.

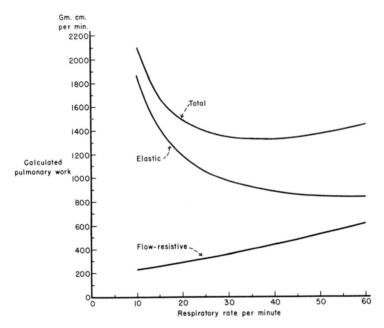

Fig. 3-11. Calculated pulmonary work in newborn infants versus respiratory rate. The theoretical minimum work of respiration occurs at a rate of 37 per minute. Observed resting respiratory rates were 38. (From Cook, C. D., et al.: J. Clin. Invest. 36:440, 1957.)

Tidal volume (V_T) is the amount of air moved into or out of the lungs with each breath. Minute volume $(\dot{V}_E)$ is the amount of air breathed in or out in a minute, i.e., $\dot{V}_E = V_T \times f$ (frequency).

Frequency of quiet respiration decreases as a person increases in age. The exact basis for this change in the rate of breathing with age is not known but may be related to the work of breathing. It has been suggested that individuals often tend to adjust their respiratory rate and tidal volumes so that their ventilatory needs are accomplished with a minimum of work.[26] The relatively high rate for newborn infants (average, 34 breaths per minute) compared to adults (average, 12 per minute) at least is consistent with this minimum work concept[27] (Fig. 3-11). However, more recently Mead[28] presented data indicating that respiration in the normal resting state is adjusted so that there is a minimum average force required of the respiratory muscles; he postulated that the principal site of the sensory end of the control mechanism may be in the lungs. In certain situations the minimum work of breathing and minimum average force required would occur at the same frequency of respiration, but this would not invariably be true.

Only part of the minute volume is effective in gas exchange, i.e., the alveolar ventilation $(\dot{V}_A)$, whereas part merely ventilates the respiratory dead space. If the minute noneffective ventilation $(V_E\text{-}V_A)$ is divided by the frequency, one obtains the calculated physiologic respiratory dead space. In the normal person the physiologic and anatomic dead spaces are approximately the same. Since the air passages are compliant structures, the size of the dead space correlates closely with the degree of lung expansion. When airway obstruction and emphysema are present, therefore, dead space increases. However, physiologic dead space is also influenced by the evenness of distribution of gas within the lungs and by the perfusion of the alveoli. Thus, when there is uneven ventilation of the lungs (as in emphysema or cystic fibrosis) or the blood supply to various areas of the lung decreases (as with pulmonary emboli), there will be increases in the physiologic dead space.

Although the dead space represents an inefficient part of the respiratory tract in respect to gas exchange, it does have several important functions: on inspiration gas is humidified and warmed in the respiratory dead space. These functions are compromised when patients are intubated or tracheotomized.

A useful approximation of the dead space in a normal person results from the fact that it can be expressed as 1 ml. for each pound of normal body weight.[18] A more exact estimate of the anatomic dead space may be obtained in children and

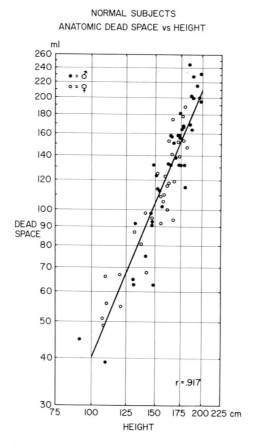

Fig. 3-12. Relation between anatomic dead space and height in 73 subjects with regression line. Values are plotted on a double logarithmic scale. (From Hart, M. C., Orzalesi, M. M., and Cook, C. D.: J. Appl. Physiol. **18:**519, 1963.)

Table 3-3. *Calculated adjustments in a 2.5-kg. infant secondary to changes in respiratory dead space*

	5 ml.	10 ml.	10 ml.
Dead space	5 ml.	10 ml.	10 ml.
Tidal volume	15 ml.	15 ml.	19.7 ml.
Minute volume	500 ml.	990 ml.	670 ml.
Rate per minute	34	66	34
Alveolar ventilation	330 ml.	330 ml.*	330 ml.*

*These calculations are based on the assumption that gas would not diffuse from the dead space to the alveoli. Actually some diffusion does occur so that with very rapid respiration patients can survive even when their dead space approaches their tidal volume or vice versa.

young adults from its relation to body height[29] (Fig. 3-12). Apparently the extra-polation of this relation to the newborn period provides a more accurate estimate of the dead space of infants than is possible if weight is used as the basis of the estimation. The importance of changes in respiratory dead space is illustrated in Table 3-3. Although the assumption that there is no diffusion of gas from dead space to alveoli is not entirely accurate, the figures illustrate the importance of the dead space. They also suggest that, from the ventilatory point of view, it is in-efficient to increase total ventilation by increases in rate; it is most effective to in-crease tidal volume to compensate for dead space changes or increased ventilatory requirements.

The V_D/V_T ratio appears to be approximately constant (0.3) from infancy to adulthood (Table 3-2). However, an *absolute* increase in dead space, whether due to respiratory abnormalities or to external apparatus, is much more critical to the infant than to the adult because of the infant's small tidal volume and the *rela-tively* larger volume of dead space added.

Alveolar ventilation $(\dot{V}_A)$ or the minute effective ventilation may be expressed in the terms of the CO_2 excretion in relation to the partial pressure of CO_2 in the peripheral arterial blood. Thus we have the equation:

$$\dot{V}_A = \frac{\dot{V}_{CO_2}}{\dfrac{P_{aCO_2}}{P_{B-47}}} = \frac{\dot{V}_{CO_2}}{F_{aCO_2}}$$

where

$\dot{V}_{CO_2}$ = CO_2 production per minute
P_{aCO_2} = Arterial CO_2 tension
P_{B}-47 = Barometric pressure minus water vapor tension at 37° C.
F_{aCO_2} = Fraction of CO_2 in the arterial blood

Perhaps the concept of $\dot{V}_A$ is easier to understand if one considers it similar in some ways to the renal clearance of a substance; in the lungs CO_2 is the substance being cleared. It can be seen that if $\dot{V}_{CO_2}$ remains constant when $\dot{V}_A$ is halved, P_{aCO_2} will double. As is apparent is Table 3-3, the measurement of $\dot{V}_A$ provides a far better index of the efficacy of ventilation than measurement of $\dot{V}_E$. $\dot{V}_E$ may be very large, but, if it is composed mostly of ineffective ventilation, $\dot{V}_A$ may not be adequate.

Alveolar ventilation is considerably higher per unit of lung volume in the normal infant than in the adult; this would be expected since the oxygen consumption is also higher per unit of lung volume or body weight.[30]

Ventilation in any area of the lungs is influenced by the flow resistance (R, expressed as $P/\dot{V}$, cm. H_2O/ml./sec.) and compliance (C, expressed as V/P, ml./cm. H_2O) of that particular area. The product of resistance and compliance (RC), or the time constant (expressed as a unit of time), is similar for the various areas of a normal lung. In diseased lungs, such as cystic fibrosis with emphysema, the time constant becomes abnormal in affected areas and is associated with uneven distribution of ventilation. The distribution of ventilation may be studied by measuring the nitrogen washout curve; this involves breathing 100% O_2 and measuring the decline of the concentration of alveolar N_2, an inert gas, in successive expirations. Nitrogen concentration for both normal children and adults is less than 2.5% after 7 minutes of oxygen breathing. This value is increased in the patient with an uneven distribution of ventilation since the elimination of nitrogen from poorly ventilated areas is prolonged.

Summary. Ventilation is made up of effective and dead space ventilation. It is very similar for all ages when compared on the basis of lung or body size. Absolute changes in dead space or ventilation are relatively more critical in smaller persons. In monitoring respiration the measurement of alveolar ventilation is more useful than total ventilation. Changes in P_{aCO_2} reflect changes in alveolar ventilation. Regional ventilation in the lung is influenced by both resistance and compliance. Changes in the regional time constants (RC) in diseased lungs are associated with uneven ventilation. Nitrogen washout curve has been used as one standard test for uneven ventilation.

GAS DIFFUSION

The ultimate purpose of pulmonary ventilation is to allow diffusion of O_2 through the alveolar epithelial lining, basement membrane, and capillary endothelial wall into the plasma and red cells, and the diffusion of CO_2 in the opposite direction. As shown on electron micrographs of lung tissue (Fig. 3-18), the distance for gases to diffuse is as low as 0.2 micron. Since these processes apparently follow the physical laws of diffusion without any active participation on the part of the lung tissue, pressure gradients must exist or gas exchange will not occur. On the other hand, if the gradient is increased because of changes of gas tensions either within the alveoli or in the blood, the exchange of gas will be more rapid. Furthermore, since the blood P_{O_2} affects the blood P_{CO_2}, changes in one moiety will produce changes in the diffusion of the other. Carbon dioxide diffuses approximately 20 times faster than oxygen in a gas-liquid environment. Therefore, the impairment of CO_2 diffusions does not take place in clinical situations.

Pulmonary gas diffusion is another example of the similarities between pediatric and adult respiratory physiology since it is relatively constant for all ages when size is taken into consideration.[31,32]

Although diffusion of gases within the lung is necessary for survival, relatively few conditions occurring in children affect diffusion per se. Diffusing capacity is decreased in the "alveolar capillary block syndrome."[33] This decrease was considered to be primarily due to increased thickness of alveolar-capillary membranes, but it is now believed that uneven distribution of ventilation with resulting ventilation-perfusion imbalance is the more important cause of arterial oxygen desaturation.[34] Anemia is also associated with a decreased diffusing capacity. This is in part explained by the decrease in the ability of blood to carry the respiratory gases. Patients with congenital heart disease and left-to-right shunts frequently have an increased diffusing capacity secondary to increased blood volume in the lungs.[35] Conversely, diffusing capacity may be reduced when blood flow through the lungs is markedly decreased as in pulmonic stenosis.

The diffusing capacity of the lungs may be measured with a foreign gas, carbon monoxide, used in small concentrations (0.3% or less), or by varying the concentration of inspired oxygen.[36] In general, these techniques are useful for research and, in a few instances of respiratory insufficiency, as diagnostic aids.

PULMONARY CIRCULATION

In prenatal life, pulmonary vascular resistance is high, and the major portion of right ventricular output runs *parallel* to the left ventricular outflow, bypassing the lungs and flowing into the descending aorta through the ductus arteriosus. With the onset of ventilation at birth, there is a sudden drastic fall in the pulmonary vascular resistance and an increase in the blood flow through the lungs that enables the organism to exchange oxygen and carbon dioxide and sustain independent existence. The principal factors that control this vital adjustment in vascular resistance are the chemical changes (i.e., changes in P_{O_2} and P_{CO_2} or pH) in the environment of the pulmonary vessels.[37] An increase in P_{O_2} also produces constriction and subsequent closure of the ductus arteriosus. The pulmonary arterial pressure, which is slightly higher than the pressure in the ascending aorta in the fetus,[38] shows some decrease at birth and continues to decrease with a concomitant rise in systemic blood pressure until it approaches the adult level within the first year of life (Fig. 3-13).[39] If the lungs do not expand adequately (as in the respiratory distress syndrome) and P_{O_2} remains low, the pulmonary vascular resistance and pressure may remain high—there will be prolonged patency of the ductus and persistent right-to-left shunting of blood.[40]

Under normal postneonatal conditions, the systemic and pulmonary vascular beds are connected in *series* to form a continuous circuit. While the systemic circulation has a high vascular resistance with a large pressure gradient between the arteries and veins, the pulmonary circulation presents a low resistance to flow.

Both hypoxemia and hypercapnia constrict the pulmonary vascular bed and increase resistance to flow. Chronic hypoxemia at a high altitude or in diseases such as severe cystic fibrosis or asthma with emphysema is associated with a pulmonary hypertension that returns to or toward normal when hypoxemia is corrected.[41] Pulmonary hypertension present for months or more frequently years results in cor pulmonale, which then further complicates the existing pulmonary insufficiency.

Under normal circumstances the arterial blood from the left ventricle contains up to 5% unsaturated blood (venous admixture). This comes mainly from the

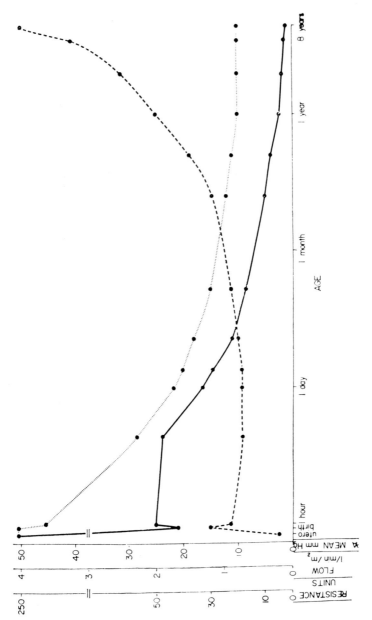

Fig. 3-13. Changes in pulmonary arterial pressure, pulmonary blood flow, and pulmonary vascular resistance with age: —, resistance; ---, flow; ......, pressure. (From Rudolph, A. M.: Pulmonary circulation. In Fomon, S. J., editor: Normal and abnormal respiration in children. Report of the Thirty-seventh Ross Conference on Pediatric Research, Columbus, Ohio, 1961, Ross Laboratories, p. 65.)

bronchial circulation but also partly from blood in the pulmonary circulation bypassing the alveoli and from blood flowing through the thebesian veins. It results in a depression of the arterial P_{O_2} from approximately 102 to 97 mm. Hg. In certain conditions, such as ventilation-perfusion imbalance (including decreased diffusing capacity), the amount of the right-to-left shunt through the lungs increases sufficiently enough to cause significant arterial hypoxemia. Intrapulmonary shunting also occurs in such entities as pulmonary A-V fistula, pulmonary hemangiomas, and increased collateral (bronchial) circulation as in bronchiectasis. In addition, shunting may occur at the cardiac level when there is congenital heart disease with right-to-left shunts.

Pulmonary hemodynamics vary significantly during the respiratory cycle. Small vessels and capillaries in the alveolar wall are apparently exposed to the pressure in the alveoli. These vessels may, therefore, be compressed or even collapsed during positive pressure breathing. On the other hand, pressure surrounding larger vessels outside of alveoli would reflect the pleural pressure and tend to distend these vessels during inflation.[42]

VENTILATION-PERFUSION RELATIONSHIPS

In order to achieve normal gas exchange in the lung, the regional distribution of ventilation and perfusion must be balanced. Without this balance, respiratory function would be impaired even though the over-all levels of ventilation and perfusion might be adequate. The normal value for the ventilation-perfusion $(\dot{V}_A/\dot{Q})$ ratio is about 0.8.

Recent studies with radioactive gases have shown that the elastic and resistive properties of various parts of the lung as well as the pulmonary blood flow are influenced by gravity. Thus, both components of the $\dot{V}_A/\dot{Q}$ ratio are affected by changes in the position of the patient.[43,44]

In the upright position, the blood flow and ventilation are both less in the apex than in the base of the lungs. Since the difference in blood flow between apex and base is relatively greater than that for ventilation, the $\dot{V}_A/\dot{Q}$ ratio increases from the bottom to the top of the lung as shown in Fig. 3-14. Thus, the apical regions $(\dot{V}_A/\dot{Q}, \text{high})$ have higher alveolar P_{O_2} and lower P_{CO_2} and P_{N_2} while the basal areas $(\dot{V}_A/\dot{Q}, \text{low})$ have lower P_{O_2} and higher P_{CO_2} and P_{N_2}. Gravity has a greater effect on the $\dot{V}_A/\dot{Q}$ ratio in hypotensive and hypovolemic patients and may be exaggerated with positive pressure breathing. In the supine position, similar differences exist between the anterior and posterior parts of the lung but are of smaller magnitude. During exercise, pulmonary arterial pressure and blood flow as well as ventilation are increased and are distributed more evenly. In infants and children, the distribution of pulmonary blood flow is more uniform since the pulmonary arterial pressure is relatively high and the gravity effect in the lungs is less.

In diseased lungs changes in $\dot{V}_A/\dot{Q}$ ratio occur as the result of uneven ventilation and/or perfusion; e.g., compression of pulmonary vessels or occlusion, reduced pulmonary vascular bed, or intrapulmonary anatomic right-to-left shunt may all contribute to nonuniform perfusion. In congenital heart conditions with increased pulmonary blood flow due to left-to-right shunting, the $\dot{V}_A/\dot{Q}$ ratio is

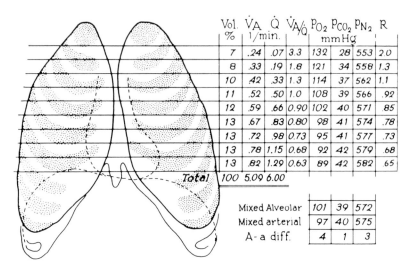

Vol. %	$\dot{V}_A$ l/min.	$\dot{Q}$	$\dot{V}_A/\dot{Q}$	P_{O_2}	P_{CO_2} mmHg	P_{N_2}	R
7	.24	.07	3.3	132	28	553	2.0
8	.33	.19	1.8	121	34	558	1.3
10	.42	.33	1.3	114	37	562	1.1
11	.52	.50	1.0	108	39	566	.92
12	.59	.66	0.90	102	40	571	.85
13	.67	.83	0.80	98	41	574	.78
13	.72	.98	0.73	95	41	577	.73
13	.78	1.15	0.68	92	42	579	.68
13	.82	1.29	0.63	89	42	582	.65
Total	100	5.09	6.00				

	P_{O_2}	P_{CO_2}	P_{N_2}
Mixed Alveolar	101	39	572
Mixed arterial	97	40	575
A-a diff.	4	1	3

Fig. 3-14. Effect of distribution of ventilation and perfusion on regional gas tensions in erect man. The lung is divided into 9 horizontal slices, and the position of each slice is shown by its anterior rib markings. **Vol %**, Relative lung volume. $\dot{V}_A$, Regional alveolar ventilation. $\dot{Q}$, Regional perfusion. $\dot{V}_A/\dot{Q}$, Ventilation-perfusion ratio. **R**, Respiratory exchange ratio. (From West, J. B.: J. Appl. Physiol. 17:893, 1962.)

decreased while it is increased when perfusion is diminished as in cases of tricuspid atresia or pulmonic stenosis.

There may be an intrinsic regulatory mechanism in the lung that, to a limited extent, functions to preserve normal $\dot{V}_A/\dot{Q}$ ratio. In areas in which $\dot{V}_A/\dot{Q}$ ratios are high, a low P_{CO_2} tends to constrict airways and dilate pulmonary vessels, and the opposite occurs in areas in which regional $\dot{V}_A/\dot{Q}$ ratios are low. In the latter case, low P_{O_2} also contributes to the vascular constriction.

Several methods are available to assess ventilation-perfusion relations. The difference between physiologic and anatomic dead spaces may be used an an index of uneven perfusion since this difference (alveolar dead space) would increase when ventilated areas are not well perfused.[45]

Uneven $\dot{V}_A/\dot{Q}$ ratios in various parts of the lungs cause an increase gradient between gas tensions of mixed alveolar air and arterial or, more specifically, mixed pulmonary venous blood. However, an increased A-a P_{O_2} gradient may also be the result of alterations in diffusion and/or direct venous admixture. Differential diagnosis of these factors can be made by changing the inspired P_{O_2}.[46] If the A-a P_{O_2} gradient is relatively unchanged by changes in inspired P_{O_2}, the most likely cause of the increased gradient is $\dot{V}_A/\dot{Q}$ imbalance. When the A-a P_{O_2} gradient increases with low inspired oxygen tensions ($P_{O_2} < 50$ mm. Hg), an impairment of diffusing capacity is the most probable cause. If, on the other hand, the A-a P_{O_2} gradient increases with high inspired oxygen tensions, the underlying pathology is most likely to be due to direct venous admixture. Nelson and his associates[47] reported higher A-a P_{O_2} gradients in newborn infants than in adults and attributed their findings to increased venous admixture, rather than to uneven $\dot{V}_A/\dot{Q}$ ratios.

Nonuniform $\dot{V}_A/\dot{Q}$ ratios throughout the lungs will also cause an increased A-a gradient of P_{N_2}. Utilization of the P_{N_2} gradient has certain advantages over P_{O_2} since the former is only slightly affected by diffusion and is not influenced by venous admixture. Since nitrogen is inert and P_{N_2} during the steady state is essentially the same in the body fluids, P_{N_2} in the urine may be used as an index of arterial P_{N_2}. The normal value for A-a P_{N_2} gradient thus obtained is below 10 mm. Hg (mean:3-5).[48] Urinary-alveolar P_{N_2} difference during the first 24 hours of life is significantly elevated ($\triangle P_{N_2} > 20$ mm. Hg).[46] This indicates that the pulmonary ventilation is not properly matched with increased pulmonary perfusion (a low $\dot{V}_A/\dot{Q}$ ratio) during the neonatal period. The P_{N_2} difference decreases rapidly toward normal values within a few days of life. In severe $\dot{V}_A/\dot{Q}$

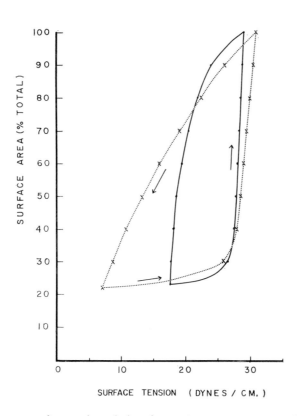

Fig. 3-15. Surface area–surface tension relations for two lung extracts measured on the Wilhelmy balance. $\bar{S}$ (stability index)[50] equals (the maximum surface tension minus the minimum surface tension) times 2 divided by (the maximum surface tension plus the minimum surface tension). $\bar{S}$ above approximately 0.85 is normal and below is abnormal. The minimum surface tension below 15 dynes/cm. is normal and above is abnormal. The lung extract for a stillborn infant had normal surface activity whereas that of the patient dying following cardiac surgery with a bypass pump did not.

imbalance, such as occurs in severe cystic fibrosis, P_{N_2} gradients may be significantly increased.

SURFACE ACTIVITY AND LUNG FUNCTION

Recent investigations have demonstrated that the alveolar lining layer contains surface active materials with unusual properties that are responsible for the stability of air spaces. These materials, which are now known to consist of specific phospholipids (discussed later), are collectively called pulmonary surfactant. The relation between pressure (P), surface tension (T), and radius (r) of a sphere is expressed by the LaPlace equation $P = \dfrac{2T}{r}$.

It can be seen from this equation that if surface tension were constant, when a number of spheres are connected, the smallest sphere would have the highest pressure. Thus, the spheres with the smaller radii would empty into the larger ones. If lung units are substituted for spheres in this concept, the lung would be unstable, with collapse of most of the units into several large ones, as in cases of the respiratory distress syndrome. This instability does not take place in the normal lungs. As Clement and his associates[49] first demonstrated with a modified Wilhelmy balance, saline extract of normal lungs exhibits an extremely low level of surface tension (0-5 dynes/cm.) during dynamic compression of the surface area while the tension increases (30-50 dynes/cm.) during expansion of surface area (Fig. 3-15). Their findings indicate that in normal lungs, as the radius of alveoli decreases so does the surface tension, and thus the stability of the lung is maintained regardless of the size of each lung unit (Fig. 3-16).

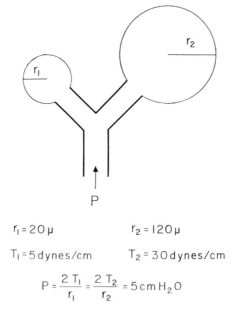

$r_1 = 20\,\mu$ $r_2 = 120\,\mu$

$T_1 = 5\,dynes/cm$ $T_2 = 30\,dynes/cm$

$$P = \frac{2\,T_1}{r_1} = \frac{2\,T_2}{r_2} = 5\,cm\,H_2O$$

Fig. 3-16. Schematic drawing of stable alveoli of different sizes.

The principal materials responsible for the unique surface activity of the alveolar lining layer have been identified as a number of saturated lecithins that are synthesized in the lung tissue.[51] These substances or their precursors are apparently produced by the type II alveolar cells (granular pneumonocytes), stored in the osmiophilic lamellar inclusions within these cells, and excreted into the air space to form surface active lining layers[52] (Figs. 3-17 and 3-18).

Not only are the surface properties of the lung lining important in normal

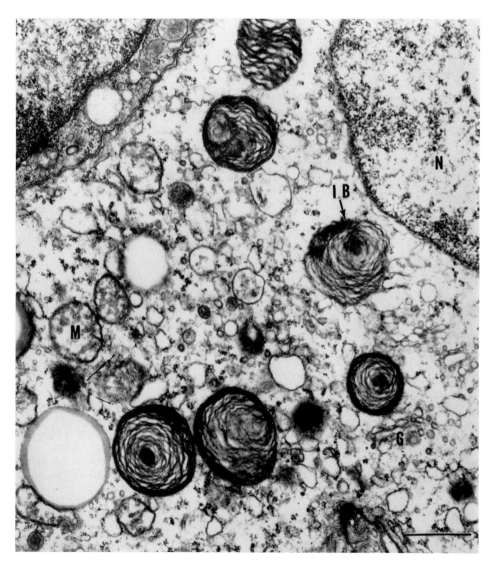

Fig. 3-17. Electron micrograph of a type II alveolar cell from the lung of an adult dog. Osmiophilic inclusion bodies, **IB**, are considered to be the source of pulmonary surfactant. **G**, Golgi apparatus. **M**, Mitochondrion. **N**, Nucleus. The scale represents one micron. (Courtesy Dr. Y. Kikkawa, Albert Einstein College of Medicine, New York, N. Y.)

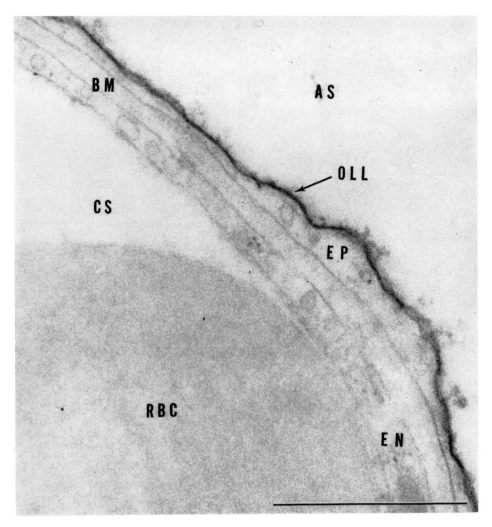

Fig. 3-18. Electron micrograph of alveolar membrane from the lung of a newborn lamb. Note the short distance between alveolar space, **AS,** and capillary space, **CS,** for gas exchange. Osmiophilic alveolar lining layer, **OLL** (dark stained), is covering the attenuated portion of type I cell. This layer most likely represents the surface-active lining layer that stabilizes the air spaces. **BM,** Basement membrane. **EN,** Capillary endothelial cell. **EP,** Type I alveolar epithelial cell. **RBC,** Erythrocyte. The scale indicates 1 micron. (From Motoyama, E. K., and Kikkawa, Y.: Unpublished material.)

pulmonary function providing the basis for lung stability, but decreases in the surface activity have been shown to be important in several clinical conditions. Avery and Mead[53] showed that the minimum surface tension of lung extracts from infants dying of the respiratory distress syndrome (hyaline membrane disease) was unusually high when measured on the Wilhelmy balance. There is a marked decrease or absence of surface active lecithins of the alveolar linings in these lungs.[54] These findings, at least in part, explain the atelectasis and low compliance of the lungs from infants with this syndrome.

A second condition with decreased surface activity of lung extracts is the "postperfusion lung syndrome" seen in some patients following prolonged cardiopulmonary bypass procedures (Fig. 3-15). In this condition, there is increased venous admixture, decreased pulmonary compliance, atelectasis, and decreased surface activity of the lung extract. A similar condition occurs after prolonged inhalation of high concentrations of oxygen.[55] The pulmonary pathology includes thickening of alveolar membranes, interstitial and intra-alveolar edema, capillary congestion, and atelectasis. Surface activity is also decreased. Whether or not the decrease in surface activity of the lung is a primary or secondary factor in the pathogenesis of these conditions remains to be elucidated.

CILIARY ACTIVITY

The cilia in the respiratory tract play an important role in the removal of mucosal secretions and harmful material. At least in animals (and presumably in human beings) these cilia move in a whiplike fashion at the rate of about 1,300 times per minute and are able to move mucus toward the upper part of the respiratory tract at the rate of about 1.5 cm. per minute. Air with a relative humidity below 50%, certain air pollutants, cigarette smoke, anesthetic gases, and increased viscosity of the secretions are among the factors reducing the function of these cilia. In addition, electrolytes, particularly hydrogen and potassium ions, are known to have a profound effect on ciliary activity, and cocaine produces paralysis. In tissue culture certain virus infections reduce ciliary motion by as much as 50%, and repeated infections in vivo can destroy the cilia entirely.[56]

Most recently it has been shown by Spock and co-workers[57] that serum from heterozygotes as well as hemozygotes with cystic fibrosis inhibits cilia in tissue culture. The relation of this to the clinical status of cystic fibrosis patients remains to be established, but it is obvious that further knowledge about cilia of the respiratory tract should help in the management of airway secretions in various respiratory diseases as well as during and after anesthesia.

NEONATAL RESPIRATORY ADAPTATION

A review of the onset of respiration of the newly born infant provides background information for a consideration of neonatal respiratory physiology as well as for an understanding of the commoner causes of respiratory failure encountered in this age period.

Maturation of the lungs is necessary before they are capable of sustaining life. Thus, flattening of the cuboidal epithelium at the terminal air sacs must take place to form alveoli, and the pulmonary vasculature must develop until the capillarization of the alveoli is adequate for gas exchange (approximately 28 weeks). At the same time the biochemical development of the lungs must proceed to the point where adequate amounts of surface active phospholipids are produced to form the normal alveolar lining layer and thereby to allow stability of the lung.[58] In the normal infant this also occurs at approximately 28 weeks' gestation, although marginal amounts of these surface-active substances may be present in the type II alveolar cells and even alveoli for weeks or months earlier.[54,59]

In utero there are normally only rare respiratory-like movements; fluid is slowly excreted from the lungs, and little if any is aspirated during intrauterine existence. At birth sudden chemical changes (in P_{O_2} and P_{CO_2} or pH) apparently initiate respiration,[14] although it is well established that profound changes in any of these depress the respiratory center. Peripheral sensory stimuli (thermal and tactile, especially) contribute also to the onset of respiration.

With the first breath large surface forces must be overcome (usually up to 25-30 cm. H_2O, but occasionally up to 70 cm. H_2O), as air enters the fluid-filled lungs. In addition, fluid must be removed rapidly from the air passages and lungs if gas exchange is to be adequate. Some of this fluid is drained from the trachea and some is absorbed by the pulmonary vascular and lymphatic systems. It would appear that this fluid removal is less efficient in the immature organism.[60] Not only fluid but also any debris in the airways must be removed for adequate ventilation.

Once expansion occurs, the pulmonary vascular resistance is reduced and the cardiopulmonary system approaches adult levels of V_A/Q balance within a few days.

This very brief review should emphasize that adequate maturation of the lungs is necessary as preparation for the alveolar gas exchange and that multiple changes must occur in the lungs with the onset of respiration if the organism is to survive separation from the functioning placenta. In spite of the fact that the

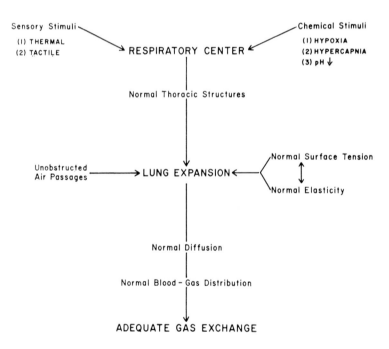

Fig. 3-19. Schematic representation of the onset of respiration.

lungs in utero have had no contributory function, the adjustments to extrauterine existence must occur within a few moments after birth (Fig. 3-19). Failure to adjust may be the result of immaturity, depression of the respiratory center (drugs, asphyxia, or trauma), or peripheral cardiopulmonary disease or anomalies.

Once birth has occurred, it is useful to realize that the minimal energy requirement exists at the neutral temperature[61] of the infant (usually about 36.5° to 37.5° C.). Above and below this temperature energy expenditure increases.

MEASUREMENT OF PULMONARY FUNCTION IN CHILDREN

Ventilatory function tests provide a quantitative or semiquantitative evaluation of the function of the lungs but rarely help in making specific diagnoses. However, the measurement of pulmonary function may be helpful by providing an objective evaluation of the general type of disability, the extent of the impairment, and the efficacy of various forms of treatment, either medical or surgical. From the practical point of view most of the simple, clinically applicable tests require the understanding of the patient and his active participation. Therefore, most of the tests cannot be used with children under 5 or 6 years of age.

The most frequent types of pulmonary disability may be classified under the general headings of (1) constrictive diseases and (2) obstructive diseases, although there is considerable overlap between the two groups. Constrictive disorders, whether due to neuromuscular defects, skeletal changes, or intrathoracic compression of the lung, result in a reduction in the patient's vital capacity. Useful rough formulas for predicting the vital capacity of both males and females of various sizes and ages have been proposed by Ferris, Whittenberger, and Affeldt[62] (Table 3-4).

In postoperative patients, especially in those who have been given muscle relaxants, their vital capacity will be a practical guide to muscle strength. The measurement of maximum static airway pressures will provide additional information but requires consideration of the concomitant lung volume for accurate interpretation.

It is usually not possible with pulmonary function tests to localize the disease process. However, the absolute and relative ventilation, vital capacity, and O_2 uptake of the right and left sides may be examined with a Carlens divided catheter and two spirometers. Because of the small size of the internal diameters of the tubes, this technique cannot be used safely in a child younger than 12 years of age.

Obstructive disability may be measured by a number of simple, indirect

Table 3-4. *Vital capacity predictions at various ages**

	5 to 15 yr. of age	*16 + yr. of age*
Males	250 ml./yr. of age	25 ml./cm. Ht.
Females	200 ml./yr. of age	20 ml./cm. Ht.

*Based on data from Ferris, B. G., Jr., Whittenberger, J. L., and Affeldt, J. E.: New Eng. J. Med. **246**:919, 1952.

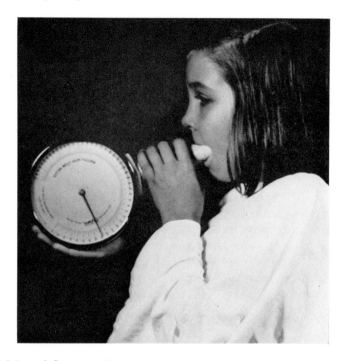

Fig. 3-20. Wright peak flow meter.*

methods that allow an estimate of the degree of airway resistance of patients. All of these depend on the measurement of the speed at which gas can be moved out of the lungs.

The relation between flow ($\dot{V}$), pressure (P), and resistance (R) is shown by the following equation:

$$R = \frac{P}{\dot{V}}$$

It is apparent that if the patient is cooperative and has normal respiratory muscle strength (or pressure), the measurement of peak flow rates will provide an index of airway resistance. Peak expiratory flow rates may be measured easily with the meter of Wright* (Fig. 3-20) in children 5 years of age or older. Graphs allowing prediction of normal values on the basis of height are shown in Figs. 3-21 and 3-22.

Serial measurements in a given patient are particularly useful in evaluating the progression or regression of obstructive disease. Another technique for indirectly estimating the degree of airway obstruction is provided by the measurement of the forced expiratory volume (FEV_t) or "timed vital capacity." With a Vitalometer† one can measure the volume of gas exhaled starting at maximal

*Air-Med, Ltd., Harlow, Essex, England.
†W. E. Collins, Inc., Braintree, Mass.

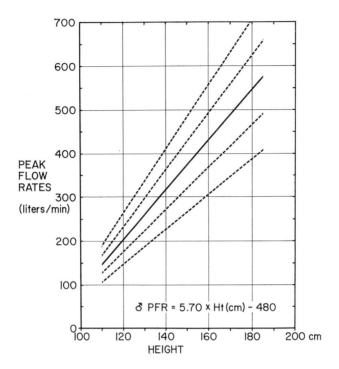

Fig. 3-21. The regression line for peak expiratory flow rate versus height for boys, One and 2 standard deviations around the line are shown. (From Murray, A. B., and Cook, C. D.: J. Pediat. **62:**187, 1963.)

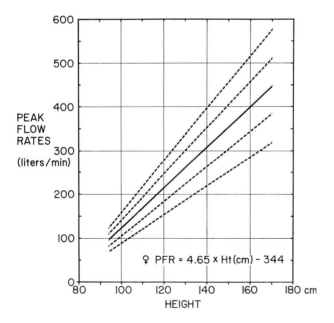

Fig. 3-22. The regression line for peak expiratory flow rate versus height for girls. One and 2 standard deviations around the line are shown. (From Murray, A. B., and Cook, C. D.: J. Pediat. **62:**188, 1963.)

inspiration, in either one or two seconds of forced expiration. In order to eliminate the factor of patient size or lung size, the results can be expressed as percent of vital capacity. A normal child should be able to exhale approximately 85% of his vital capacity in 1 second $(FEV_{1.0})$ and 95% in 2 seconds $(FEV_{2.0})$.

Diffusion studies and evaluation of pulmonary circulation require specialized equipment and personnel. However, the end result in terms of oxygen and carbon dioxide balances of any pulmonary disability should be quantitated by the measurement of arterial blood gases and pH. Finally, the patient's exercise tolerance[63] may be useful in quantitating his over-all capacity for various degrees of activity. A defect in exercise tolerance will provide an indirect estimate of the lungs' function provided cardiac or other disease can be ruled out.

LUNG BIOPSY

Although most conditions involving the lungs may be diagnosed by means of an adequate history together with physical and radiologic examinations and suitable cultures, it may occasionally be necessary to do an open lung biopsy for more direct examination of the lung tissue. Tumor masses should of course be examined and if possible removed, but in cases of diffuse, unexplained disease, biopsies, if done early in the course of the disease, may be useful (e.g., pulmonary hemosiderosis). Microscopic examination as well as cultures can then be obtained and may provide definitive answers.

EXAMPLES OF RESPIRATORY ABNORMALITIES IN INFANTS AND CHILDREN

There are a number of conditions associated with impairment of respiratory function that are seen frequently or exclusively in the pediatric age group. Brief discussion of some of these respiratory diseases follows.

The *idiopathic respiratory distress syndrome of newborn infants* is associated almost invariably with prematurity and apparently is seen more frequently following intrauterine distress. The incidence possibly may be greater in infants born to diabetic mothers but is immeasurably so when prematurity and distress are taken into account. It is apparently present at birth and is manifested by progressive respiratory difficulty. At first only slight retraction and tachypnea are present; these signs may progress until, at 1 to 2 days of age, marked sternal retraction, cyanosis, and retention of CO_2 and severe acidosis occur; finally in 10% to 20% of the cases death may ensue. Spontaneous improvement may begin at 2 to 3 days of age; if recovery takes place, no residua are usually found. However, recent reports[64] suggest that chronic pulmonary disease may result from prolonged artificial ventilation and/or prolonged administration of high concentrations of O_2 to those infants.

We currently recommend giving sodium bicarbonate, $NaHCO_3$, or THAM, tris(hydroxymethyl)aminomethane, therapy when an infant with respiratory distress syndrome has a pH < 7.25 and either a $P_{CO_2} > 55$ mm. Hg or a $P_{O_2} < 100$ mm. Hg when breathing 100% O_2 by mask for at least 15 minutes. Bicarbonate is usually used for the milder cases and when an umbilical vein is not available. When $NaHCO_3$ is used, if the pH is between 7.15 and 7.25, 3 to 4 mEq./kg. body weight are given by rapid intravenous injection and 100 mEq./L. in 10% dextrose are infused in drip at the rate of 3 ml./kg./hr. If the pH is 7.15 or less, 4-5 mEq./kg. NaHCO$_3$ are given by rapid injection and 150 mEq./L. in 10% dextrose is infused at 3 ml./kg./hr. When THAM is used (only in an umbilical vein), it is given as a 0.3 M solution in 5% dextrose. The initial dose is 1.0 to 1.5 mM (3.3 to 5.0 ml.)/kg. body weight given intravenously in 15 minutes followed by 4 mM/kg./24 hr. (14 ml./kg./24 hr.). Repeat checks of blood gases and pH every 2 to 8 hours should be done, and repeat injections of 1.0 to 1.5 mM/kg. are used as needed with the total dose not exceeding 12 mM/kg./24 hr.

The advantages of THAM over NaHCO$_3$ are as follows:
1. Rapidity of action.
2. Ability to buffer intracellularly rapidly.
3. Does not add to the total CO$_2$ content of the body.
4. Low Na content.
5. Does not depend on liver for metabolism.
6. Small volume needed.

The disadvantages of THAM are the following:
1. Instability 48 hours after dilution.
2. Rapidity of buffering action may cause respiratory depression per se (rarely seen).
3. Excretion limited by renal function.
4. Sclerosing of vessels and liver damage.
5. Hypoglycemia (may be averted by diluting in 5% dextrose).
6. Toxicity: cardiovascular collapse at high doses.

The disease can be diagnosed definitely only at autopsy by finding the characteristic lesions in the lungs. A chest x-ray film may often be helpful, however, if it shows the characteristic diffuse reticulogranular appearance of the lungs described by Peterson and Pendleton.[65] No specific treatment is currently known for this condition, although the supportive therapy as just described, together with the maintenance of the neutral body temperature, may improve the condition of these infants.

Supportive therapy with O$_2$ is useful but should never be prolonged more than necessary because of the danger of retrolental fibroplasia. It also seems probable that assisting respiration with positive pressure to the airway or negative pressure around the chest can improve oxygenation, reduce the respiratory acidosis, and also tide an occasional infant over until spontaneous regression of the disease process occurs (see preceding discussion for dangers of prolonged artificial ventilation).

The pathologic examination of the lungs indicates that these infants have severe atelectasis in association with decreased surface activity. In addition, the alveolar ducts are plugged with the hyaline membranes, which have been shown to be primarily fibrin. Consequently, these infants' lungs are reduced in effective volume and are difficult to expand. Thus, their compliance is very low, and the work of breathing is markedly increased. There is significant right-to-left shunting in many of the infants with the respiratory distress syndrome as a result of an increase in pulmonary vascular resistance. This shunt by itself results in oxygen unsaturation. In addition, as a consequence of the low tidal volume and an increased physiologic dead space, the alveolar ventilation is reduced and hypercapnia occurs, as well as further hypoxemia.

From the point of view of management of any of these infants who might require surgery, it is apparent that all major procedures should be postponed if possible until spontaneous improvement has taken place.

Cystic fibrosis of the pancreas is a hereditary disease associated with thick tenacious secretions from the pancreas and the mucous glands of the respiratory tract and results in nutritional disturbances and chronic respiratory disease. In the newborn period, meconium ileus with intestinal obstruction may occur, whereas later, nutritional failure and respiratory complications are the important factors in survival. The thick tenacious secretions of the respiratory tract lead to chronic infection, especially with the *Staphylococcus aureus* and *Pseudomonas aeruginosa* organisms, and to secondary bronchiectasis. The chronic partial obstruction and secondary chronic infection of the respiratory passages result in increased resistance to the flow of air and to air trapping, lung tissue destruction (emphysema), and limitation of vital capacity. In the very severe cases the effective volume of the lung may be reduced to such an extent that the lung compliance is markedly decreased. Clubbing, cyanosis, hypercapnia, and occasionally cor pulmonale result. Long-term antibiotic therapy is an important factor in reducing the progression of the respiratory signs and symptoms. Although the disease process invariably involves all parts of the lung, in rare instances there may be so much more extensive disease in one lobe that surgical resection is indicated. Such a procedure is probably justified only when the lobe is essentially functionless and when the remaining lung tissue shows only mild to moderate changes. These patients are poor operative risks and postoperatively tend to develop atelectasis and further progression of their pulmonary insufficiency.

Poliomyelitis with involvement of the respiratory muscles is still an important pediatric condition in many parts of the world. When respiratory failure is severe enough to necessitate mechanical assistance, the various guides (end tidal CO_2, blood gas analyses, and ventilation nomogram) will facilitate management. In the chronic phase of respiratory muscle paralysis, techniques for the measurement of lung function will be of value. Studies have shown that lung compliance gradually decreases unless there are occasional deep breaths.[66] This suggests that some means of intermittent lung stretching is necessary for the maintenance of normal lung elasticity. In addition, it has been shown that chest wall compliance is diminished in patients with severe respiratory muscle failure. Finally, the drainage of secretions by simulated coughs, by gravity, and by liquefaction all become important considerations in the management of these patients.

It is apparent that *postoperative patients* show many of the same features of respiratory difficulty exhibited by poliomyelitis patients. They have secretions that are difficult to remove, limitation of their cough reflex, reduction in their respiratory excursion, especially with chest or abdominal surgery, and frequently poor position for optimal drainage. Postoperative care of the chest should involve, when possible, the prone position with the head and chest down, humidification for liquefaction of secretions, and, if necessary, artificial stretching of the lungs to reduce the areas of atelectasis.

Patients with severe *kyphoscoliosis* represent a particular risk during and after general anesthesia. Even before surgery they frequently have a reduced vital capacity, a weak cough, and a tendency toward poor drainage and poor ventilation of certain sections of the lungs. Following surgery, secretions may be increased, coughings decreased due to pain or narcotics, and respiration still further compromised by extensive body casts. Particular attention to the maintenance of the patency of both large and small air passages and of adequate ventilation is necessary. In the later stages of severe kyphoscoliosis (usually in young adults), hypoventilation and respiratory failure occur and are frequently complicated by cor pulmonale.[67]

Interstitial fibrosis of the lungs is relatively rare in infants and children but may occur as the result of infections or bleeding into the lung tissue (e.g., idiopathic pulmonary hemosiderosis). In other instances the pathogenesis is more obscure. When present, pulmonary capillaries are obliterated by the fibrotic process; this in turn results in a significant decrease in the total diffusing capacity

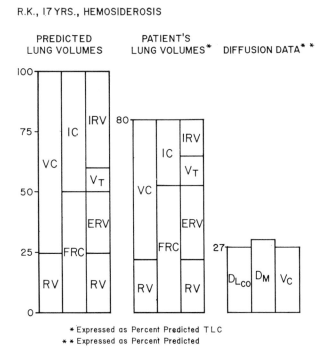

R.K., 17 YRS., HEMOSIDEROSIS

* Expressed as Percent Predicted TLC
** Expressed as Percent Predicted

Fig. 3-23. The pulmonary function changes in a disease (idiopathic pulmonary hemosiderosis) characterized by pulmonary fibrosis. The changes in lung volumes are only moderate; the decreases in total lung diffusing capacity ($D_{L_{CO}}$), diffusing capacity of the membrane (D_M), and pulmonary capillary blood volume (V_c) are striking. These are all approximately 27% of the predicted values.[81]

of the lungs and $\dot{V}_A/\dot{Q}$ imbalance, and consequently arterial oxygen desaturation (Fig. 3-23).

Bronchiectasis frequently begins in childhood and may be the result of infection secondary to structural or immunologic (hypogammaglobulinemia) defects or may follow the aspiration of foreign bodies, especially nuts. Bronchiectasis may also result from the combination of asthma and recurrent infection. With the widespread use of antibiotics the incidence of bronchiectasis following pneumonia and pertussis has been greatly reduced. In most cases of early bronchiectasis, medical management stabilizes the disease and obviates the necessity for surgery. When surgery is indicated, it should be realized that there is currently no evidence that regeneration or replacement of lung tissue takes place except possibly in small infants and that, if obstructive disease is present in the remaining lung tissue, dilation with emphysematous changes of the remaining lung may be aggravated by excision.

REFERENCES

1. Mitchell, R. A.: Cerebrospinal fluid and the regulation of respiration. In Caro, C. G., editor: Advances in respiratory physiology, Baltimore, 1966, The Williams & Wilkins Co., pp. 1-47.
2. Comroe, J. H., Jr.: Physiology of respiration, Chicago, 1965, Year Book Medical Publishers, Inc.
3. Pappenheimer, J. R., Fencl, V., Heisey, S. R., and Held, D.: Role of cerebral fluids in control of respiration as studied in unanesthetized goats, Amer. J. Physiol. 208:436-450, 1965.
4. Mitchell, R. A., Carman, C. T., Severinghaus, J. W., Richards, B. W., Singer, M. M., and Shnider, S.: Stability of cerebrospinal fluid pH in chronic acid-base disturbances in blood, J. Appl. Physiol. 20:443-452, 1965.
5. Fencl, V., Miller, T. B., and Pappenheimer, J. R.: Studies on the respiratory response to disturbances of acid-base balance, with deductions concerning the ionic composition of cerebral interstitial fluid, Amer. J. Physiol. 210:459-472, 1966.
6. Dripps, R. D., and Comroe, J. H., Jr.: The effect of the inhalation of high and low oxygen concentrations on respiration, pulse rate, ballistocardiogram and arterial oxygen saturation (oximeter) of normal individuals, Amer. J. Physiol. 149:277-291, 1947.
7. Cross, K. W., and Warner, P.: The effect of inhalation of high and low oxygen concentrations on the respiration of the newborn infant, J. Physiol. 114:283-295, 1951.
8. Cross, K. W., and Oppé, T. E.: The effect of inhalation of high and low concentrations of oxygen in the respiration of premature infants, J. Physiol. 117:38-55, 1952.
9. Cunningham, D. J. C., Shaw, D. G., Lahiri, S., and Lloyd, B. B.: The effect of maintained ammonium chloride acidosis on the relation between pulmonary ventilation and alveolar oxygen and carbon dioxide in man, Quart. J. Exp. Physiol. 46:323-334, 1961.
10. Katz, R. L., and Ngai, S. H.: Respiratory effects of diethyl ether in the cat, J. Pharmacol. Exp. Therap. 138:329-336, 1962.
11. Cross, K. W., Klaus, M., Tooley, W. H., and Weisser, K.: The response of the newborn baby to inflation of the lungs, J. Physiol. 151:551-565, 1960.
12. Mead, J., and Collier, C.: Relation of volume history of lungs to respiratory mechanics in anesthetized dogs, J. Appl. Physiol. 14:669-678, 1959.
13. Burns, B. D.: The central control of respiratory movements, Brit. Med. Bull. 19:7-9, 1963.
14. Harned, H. S., Jr., Rowshan, G., MacKinney, L. G., and Sugioka, K.: Relationships of P_{O_2}, P_{CO_2}, and pH to onset of breathing of the term lamb as studied by a flow-through cuvette electrode assembly, Pediatrics 33:672-681, 1964.
15. Avery, M. E.: The lung and its disorders in the newborn infant, Philadelphia, 1964, W. B. Saunders Co., p. 37.
16. Miller, H. C., and Behrle, F. C.: The effects of hypoxia on the respiration of newborn infants, Pediatrics 14:93-103, 1954.

17. Avery, M. E., Chernick, V., Dutton, R. E., and Permutt, S.: Ventilatory response to inspired carbon dioxide in infants and adults, J. Appl. Physiol. **18:**895-903, 1963.
18. Radford, E. P., Jr., Ferris, B. G., Jr., and Kriete, B. C.: Clinical use of a nomogram to estimate proper ventilation during artificial respiration, New Eng. J. Med. **251:**877-884, 1954.
19. Bendixen, H. H., Hedley-Whyte, J., and Laver, M. B.: Impaired oxygenation in surgical patients during general anesthesia with controlled ventilation, New Eng. J. Med. **269:**991-996, 1963.
20. Severinghaus, J. W.: Methods of measurement of blood and gas carbon dioxide during anesthesia, Anesthesiology **21:**717-726, 1960.
21. Laver, M. B., and Seifen, A.: Measurement of blood oxygen tension in anesthesia, Anesthesiology **26:**73-101, 1965.
22. Cook, C. D., and Hamann, J. F.: Relation of lung volumes to height in healthy persons between the ages of 5 and 38 years, J. Pediat. **59:**710-714, 1961.
23. Butler, J., and Smith, B. H.: Pressure-volume relationships of the chest in the completely relaxed anaesthetised patient, Clin. Sci. **16:**125-146, 1957.
24. Motoyama, E. K., and Cook, C. D.: Unpublished data.
25. Freund, F., Roos, A., and Dodd, R. B.: Expiratory activity of the abdominal muscles in man during general anesthesia, J. Appl. Physiol. **19:**693-697, 1964.
26. McIlroy, M. B., Marshall, R., and Christie, R. V.: The work of breathing in normal subjects, Clin. Sci. **13:**127-136, 1954.
27. Cook, C. D., Sutherland, J. M., Segal, S., Cherry, R. B., Mead, J., McIlroy, M. B., and Smith, C. A.: Studies of respiratory physiology in the newborn infant. III. Measurements of mechanics of respiration, J. Clin. Invest. **36:**440-448, 1957.
28. Mead, J.: Control of respiratory frequency, J. Appl. Physiol. **15:**325-336, 1960.
29. Hart, M. C., Orzalesi, M. M., and Cook, C. D.: Relation between anatomic respiratory dead space and body size and lung volume, J. Appl. Physiol. **18:**519-522, 1963.
30. Cook, C. D., Cherry, R. B., O'Brien, D., Karlberg, P., and Smith, C. A: Studies of respiratory physiology in the newborn infant. I. Observations on the normal premature and full-term infants, J. Clin. Invest. **34:**975-982, 1955.
31. Bucci, G., Cook, C. D., and Barrie, H.: Studies of respiratory physiology in children. V. Total lung diffusion, diffusing capacity of pulmonary membrane and pulmonary capillary blood volume in normal subjects from 7 to 40 years of age, J. Pediat. **58:**820-828, 1961.
32. Stahlman, M. T., and Meece, N. J.: Pulmonary ventilation and diffusion in the human newborn infant, J. Clin. Invest. **36:**1081-1091, 1957.
33. Bates, D. V.: Respiratory disorders associated with impairment of gas diffusion, Ann. Rev. Med. **13:**301-318, 1962.
34. Finley, T. N., Swenson, E. W., and Comroe, J. H., Jr.: The cause of arterial hypoxemia at rest in patients with "alveolar-capillary block syndrome," J. Clin. Invest. **41:**618-622, 1962.
35. Bucci, G., and Cook, C. D.: Studies of respiratory physiology in children. VI. Lung diffusing capacity, diffusing capacity of the pulmonary membrane and pulmonary capillary blood volume in congenital heart disease, J. Clin. Invest. **40:**1431-1441, 1961.
36. Forster, R. E.: Exchange of gases between alveolar air and pulmonary capillary blood: pulmonary diffusing capacity, Physiol. Rev. **37:**391-452, 1957.
37. Cook, C. D., Drinker, P. A., Jacobson, H. N., Levison, H., and Strang, L. B.: Control of pulmonary blood flow in the foetal and newly born lamb, J. Physiol. **169:**10-29, 1963.
38. Assali, N. S., and Morris, J. A.: Maternal and fetal circulations and their interrelationships, Obstet. Gynec. Survey **19:**923-948, 1964.
39. Rudolph, A. M.: Pulmonary circulation. In Fomon, S. J., editor: Normal and abnormal respiration in children. Report of the 37th Ross Conference on Pediatric Research, Columbus, Ohio, 1961, Ross Laboratories, pp. 65-73.
40. Strang, L. B., and MacLeish, M. H.: Ventilatory failure and right-to-left shunt in newborn infants with respiratory distress, Pediatrics **28:**17-27, 1961.
41. Goldring, R. M., Fishman, A. P., Turino, G. M., Cohen, H. I., Denning, C. R., and Andersen, D. H.: Pulmonary hypertension and cor pulmonale in cystic fibrosis of the pancreas, J. Pediat. **65:**501-524, 1964.

42. West, J. B., Dollery, C. T., and Naimark, A.: Distribution of blood flow in isolated lung; relation to vascular and alveolar pressures, J. Appl. Physiol. **19:**713-724, 1964.

43. Bates, D. V.: Measurement of regional ventilation and blood flow distribution. In Fenn, W. O., and Rahn, H., editors: Handbook of physiology, Section 3: Respiration, Washington, D. C., 1965, American Physiological Society, vol. 2, chap. 57, pp. 1425-1436.

44. West, J. B.: Topographical distribution of blood flow in the lung. In Fenn, W. O., and Rahn, H., editor: Handbook of physiology, Section 3: Respiration, Washington, D. C., 1965, American Physiological Society, vol. 2, chap. 58, pp. 1437-1451.

45. Severinghaus, J. W., and Stupfel, M.: Alveolar dead space as an index of distribution of blood flow in pulmonary capillaries, J. Appl. Physiol. **10:**335-348, 1957.

46. Rahn, H., and Farhi, L. E.: Ventilation, perfusion, and gas exchange—the $\dot{V}_A/\dot{Q}$ concept. In Fenn, W. O., and Rahn, H., editors: Handbook of physiology. Section 3: Respiration, Washington, D. C., 1964, American Physiological Society, vol. 1, chap. 30, pp. 735-766.

47. Nelson, N. M., Prod'hom, L. S., Cherry, R. B., Lipsitz, P. J., and Smith, C. A.: Pulmonary function in the newborn infant: the alveolar-arterial oxygen gradient. J. Appl. Physiol. **18:**534-538, 1963.

48. Fahri, L. E.: Atmospheric nitrogen and its role in modern medicine, J.A.M.A. **188:**984-993, 1964.

49. Clements, J. A., Brown, E. S., and Johnson, R. P.: Pulmonary surface tension and mucus lining of the lungs: some theoretical considerations, J. Appl. Physiol. **12:**262-268, 1958.

50. Gruenwald, P., Johnson, R. P., Hustead, R. F., and Clements, J. A.: Correlation of mechanical properties of infant lungs with surface activity of extracts, Proc. Soc. Exp. Biol. Med. **109:**369-371, 1962.

51. Gluck, L., Motoyama, E. K., Smits, H. L., and Kulovich, M. V.: The biochemical development of surface activity in mammalian lung. I. The surface active phospholipids; the separation and distribution of surface active lecithin in the lung of the developing rabbit fetus, Pediat. Res. **1:**237-246, 1967.

52. Kikkawa, Y., Motoyama, E. K., and Cook, C. D.: The ultrastructure of the lungs of lambs: the relation of osmiophilic inclusions and alveolar lining layers to fetal maturation and experimentally produced respiratory distress, Amer. J. Path. **47:**877-903, 1965.

53. Avery, M. E., and Mead, J.: Surface properties in relation to atelectasis and hyaline membrane disease, Amer. J. Dis. Child. **97:**517-523, 1959.

54. Gluck, L., Kulovich, M. V., Eidelman, A. I., Khazin, A. F., and Motoyama, E. K.: The biochemical development of surface activity in mammalian lung. IV. The synthesis of lecithin in the alveolar layer of the developing human and the biochemical basis for the respiratory distress syndrome, Pediat. Res. To be published.

55. Caldwell, P. R. B, Giammona, S. T., Lee, W. L., Jr., and Bondurnat, S.: Effect of oxygen breathing at one atmosphere on the surface activity of lung extracts in dogs, Ann. N. Y. Acad. Sci. **121:**823-828, 1965.

56. Kilburn, K. H., and Salzano, J. V., editor: Symposium on structure, function and measurement of respiratory cilia, Amer. Rev. Resp. Dis. **93:**1-184, 1966.

57. Spock, A., Heick, H., Cress, H., and Logan, W.: In vivo study of ciliary motility: asymmetrical ciliary beat associated with sera of patients with cystic fibrosis. In 4th International Conference on Cystic Fibrosis, Berne, Switzerland, September, 1966.

58. Orzalesi, M. M., Motoyama, E. K., Jacobson, H. N., Kikkawa, Y., Reynolds, E. O. R., and Cook, C. D.: The development of the lungs of lambs, Pediatrics **35:**373-381, 1965.

59. Gruenwald, P.: Pulmonary surfactant and stability of aeration in young human fetuses, Pediatrics **38:**912-913, 1966.

60. Boston, R. W., Humphreys, P. W., Reynolds, E. O. R., and Strang, L. B.: Lymph-flow and clearance of liquid from the lungs of the foetal lamb, Lancet **2:**473-474, 1965.

61. Brück, K., Parmelee, H., Jr., and Brück, M.: Neutral temperature range and range of "thermal comfort" in premature infants, Biol. Neonat. **4:**32-51, 1962.

62. Ferris, B. G., Jr., Whittenberger, J. L., and Affeldt, J. E.: Pulmonary function in convalescent poliomyelitic patients. I. Pulmonary subdivisions and maximum breathing capacity, New Eng. J. Med. **246:**919-923, 1952.

63. Bengtsson, E.: The working capacity in normal children, evaluated by submaximal exercise on the bicycle ergometer and compared with adults, Acta Med. Scand. 154:91-109, 1956.
64. Northway, W. H., Jr., Rosan, R. C., and Porter, D. Y.: Pulmonary disease following respirator therapy of hyaline-membrane disease, New Eng. J. Med. 276:357-368, 1967.
65. Peterson, H. G., and Pendleton, M. E.: Contrasting roentgenographic pulmonary patterns of the hyaline membrane and fetal aspiration syndrome, Amer. J. Roentgen. 74:800-813, 1955.
66. Ferris, B. G., Jr., and Pollard, D. S.: Effect of deep and quiet breathing on pulmonary compliance in man, J. Clin. Invest. 39:143-149, 1960.
67. Bergofsky, E. H., Turino, G. M., and Fishman, A. P.: Cardiorespiratory failure in kyphoscoliosis, Medicine 38:263-317, 1959.

Chapter 4

Preparing children for operation

Home preparation and hospital admission
Examination of data
    The chart
Meeting the child
    Physical examination
Preoperative orders
    Restriction of oral intake
    Enema
    Laboratory
    Cross match for transfusion
    Preoperative medication

HOME PREPARATION AND HOSPITAL ADMISSION

A carefully planned approach is necessary if a child is to be well prepared for anesthesia and operation. Naturally the *physical condition* of infants and children of any age must be studied, and the patients should be brought to optimum status in the time available before operation.

In children old enough to have fear or apprehension the *emotional factor* may be an even greater source of concern than the child's physical condition;[1,2] in fact, the greatest problem of the child's entire operative course is often the fear he experiences prior to operation. Unfortunately the degree of apprehension has no relation to the magnitude of the operation, and one small boy can be as terrified at the prospect of losing a tooth as another who is about to have an amputation. Regardless of the type of the expected procedure, every child requires the benefit of full preparation.

Psychic preparation is considered first because, when possible, this is started before the child enters the hospital. It seems reasonable to say that any normal child should be forewarned if he is going to the hospital and that he should be told why he is going there. The parents can do most to prepare the child before hospitalization; however, the pediatrician and the surgeon should assist in this project.[3] Without dwelling on unpleasant details, the parents can break the news gently that the child is to stay at the hospital for a short time to have a lump taken out or to have his heart fixed or his tooth pulled. Whatever the problem may be, it is better to avoid use of words that are ominous, misleading, or difficult to understand. A major procedure described in simple terms will be accepted lightly. Various procedures that the child will experience should be mentioned in addition to the operation. Several booklets have been prepared to assist parents in telling their children about the experiences they are to have in the hospital.[4-6] These may be quite helpful, and it is recommended that pediatricians and surgeons encourage their use by parents.

One of the best ways to ensure a successful preparation of a child is to admit him to the hospital a day prior to operation. This will enable him to have his necessary workup and will give him a chance to settle down to his new surroundings. If a number of roentgen-ray films and tiring examinations are necessary, additional time should be allowed.

After the child's admission to the hospital, the control of fear continues to be a matter of primary concern if a smooth course is to be expected. In most cases it is helpful if the mother can stay with the child while he is undressed and put into bed. The mother can be of further assistance by telling the nurse of individual eating and play habits. Often a small child has his own vocabulary for toilet habits, and the nurse should be informed of these.

Usually it is better for the parents to step outside during any diagnostic or therapeutic procedures since the child will often be far less upset if his family is not present at such times.

For many children hospitalization means their first separation from their parents. Psychiatrists place considerable importance on this factor, and some believe that it may be the most upsetting of all the phases of hospitalization.[7,8] For this reason there is increasing acceptance of the practice of having the mother sleep in the room with the child.[9-12] This would interfere excessively when children are to undergo neurosurgical or similar extensive procedures and might curtail teaching in certain situations, but in most instances involving relatively simple operations there certainly are many advantages to be gained.[13-16]

When parents are not to stay with the child to help him face the many new and disturbing experiences, it would seem reasonable to give him a mild sedative shortly after hospital admission. Barbiturates and tranquilizing agents have been tried, but the results have not been encouraging as yet. The dosage of agents for mere relief of apprehension is difficult to estimate for children, and inadequate or excessive effect often occurs. Further trial appears indicated.

Although some children do suffer emotional stress during hospitalization, most normal children seem to tolerate it remarkably well. Essential factors in enabling a child to meet this experience successfully are a normal mental makeup, plus the presence of environmental aids among which parents, other children, and television are easily the most important. Surprisingly enough, the illness and pain of the child's neighbor have very little effect upon his own spirit, and needles that puncture his friends are seldom disturbing until they are turned toward him.[17]

EXAMINATION OF DATA

It is a well-established principle that patients should be visited by the anesthetist at least once prior to operation.[18-20] This is especially important when dealing with children. Because of the varied nature of their problems and the great difference in their sizes and mental attitudes, children can be evaluated properly only by firsthand inspection. Furthermore, the preoperative visit can do much for the child, who may be greatly relieved by a few words of explanation and reassurance.

The chart. Before speaking to the patient or his parents, the anesthetist should learn as much as possible from the hospital chart. This will enable him to analyze the problem, know what to look for in the child, and avoid repetition of unnecessary questions or examination.

From the chart one should get the *child's first name,* for this will promote friendly personal relations. His *age* and *weight* are noted because both must be considered in choosing preoperative sedation and anesthesia. The *history* provides essential information concerning *symptoms, diagnosis,* and *intended operation,* and in addition a number of lesser details. *Birth history* is reviewed to see if the child had a normal delivery, whether there was any delay in crying, or if there was cyanosis or any other sign suggestive of birth injury, congenital disease, or hypoxia. Subsequent *growth* and *development* are noted, for retarded growth may accompany serious organic diseases. Special attention must be paid to warnings concerning *sensitivity* to penicillin or other drugs the child may have received. The history of *severe* or *recurrent infection* is important and may suggest decreased resistance from such causes as anemia or agammaglobulinemia or the existence of complicating lesions such as otitis, rheumatic fever, or low-grade renal infections. History of poliomyelitis demands thorough investigation for signs of residual respiratory limitation.

Regardless of the child's age, one should look for history of *previous operation.* An infant 1 month old may already have undergone several major procedures. The anesthetist should know the reason for previous operations, the type of anesthesia used, and the child's emotional and physical reaction to the experience. It is especially important to recognize any danger signals. Unexplained fever or jaundice following use of halogenated anesthetic agents should be regarded as a warning against further use at subsequent operations. Similarly, symptoms of emotional strain are significant. A hyperirritable child must be accorded special preoperative care in order to prevent development of protracted psychic disturbances.

The *system history* should not be overlooked. Briefly, the following may be of special significance:

Central nervous system. History of hydrocephalus, mental retardation, or convulsions should be noted. Etiology of convulsions should be investigated, since they may be due to epilepsy, infection, trauma, or other causes. When children have been receiving anticonvulsant therapy, this should not be discontinued prior to operation. Additional preoperative medication usually should be reduced, however, to prevent excessive depression.

Cardiovascular system. Cyanosis, fainting, poor physical development, clubbed fingers, weakness, or history of murmur should be noted.

Respiratory system. Recurrent infections, stridor, cough, respiratory obstruction, croup, and cyanosis are important. Children are more frequently subject to asthma and to tracheitis than are older patients.

Gastrointestinal system. Recurrent vomiting associated with the presenting lesion will suggest dehydration and electrolyte depletion. History of poor nutritional habits may also be of significance. Anderson[21] reported six children who died following standard 80 mg. per kilogram doses of Avertin. All were found to have been "feeding problems," and nutritional deficiency with depletion of liver glycogen was thought responsible. Decreased tolerance to divinyl ether following hepatitis has been encountered in our neighborhood.

A number of medical diseases are now treated with *therapeutic agents that complicate anesthesia.* Failure to notice use of such agents may result in serious trouble during or after operation. Children receive *cortisone* for a variety of conditions, including ivy poisoning, asthma, rheumatic fever, and thrombocytopenic purpura. Whatever the reason for its use, one of its effects is depression of adrenal cortical activity.[22] It was formerly believed that any patient who had received cortisone during the preceding 6 months should be given the drug prior to operation in order to prevent hypotension. Although such hypotension has been reported several times,[23-25] routine use of cortisone is not advised unless it had been administered recently or in relative large dosage.[26,27] The anesthetist should certainly be aware of the fact if patients have received such drugs, in order to evaluate various intraoperative or postoperative reactions.

If cortisone has recently been discontinued, it is advisable to reestablish it during the period of stress. One milligram per kilogram of body weight, started 24 hours before operation and given twice daily for 3 days, may be used as an average dosage.[28] If such therapy is not started until the time of operation, hydrocortisone may be given intravenously in dosage of 2 mg. per kilogram. Following operation, intramuscular cortisone may then be used to complete the 3-day course. If children have been on continuous cortisone therapy prior to operation, it is wise to increase the dose by 50% to 100% on the day of operation. Incidentally, administration of ACTH does not cause adrenal cortical depression and so is not an indication for cortisone therapy at time of operation.

Although less frequently encountered, other therapeutic agents offer individual problems. Chlorpromazine,[29] also used for a variety of conditions including malignancy, prolonged vomiting, hiccoughs, etc., will greatly potentiate the depressant effect of anesthetics. Agents such as Rauwolfia or reserpine (Serpasil)[30] used for reduction of hypertension may involve sudden, unexpected fall in blood pressure during anesthesia. Because of the marked instability of the vasomotor system, it has been thought safer to discontinue reserpine 24 to 48 hours before operation. This feeling has given way to the belief that these drugs should be continued, but that the anesthetist should remain alert to their presence and possible effect.

Reviewing the findings of the physical examination as listed in the chart is important. Although the anesthetist should evaluate the child's general physical condition himself and perform essential details of the physical examination, he can learn much from the chart and save the child unnecessary poking and prodding. In the report of the physical examination one can gain valuable assistance if detailed examination of the nervous system, muscle strength, or cardiac lesions has been performed. Reports from special studies such as pneumoencephalograms, cardiac catheterization, and respiratory functions tests are invaluable in assessing patients with specific disorders. Any reports of consultations should be read carefully, since these usually contain the essential of the patient's problem presented in the chief resident's most concise and carefully worded terms. The consultant's reply, if legible, may be of further assistance.

Laboratory reports are examined next. Determination of hemoglobin, hematocrit, or red blood cell count and urinalysis is required in all children prior to general anesthesia.

A question that frequently arises is whether one should set minimal acceptable levels for hematocrit and hemoglobin for children coming to operation, and if so what they should be. In dealing with adults, minimal acceptable levels for red cells have been established, usually consisting of 10 Gm.% of hemoglobin, 4 million red cells per cubic millimeter, or 32% hematocrit. During infancy, red cells and their contents show wide variation (Fig. 2-11), the hemoglobin averaging over 17 Gm.% at birth, then falling to approximately 11 Gm.%, and remaining there until children are about 2 years of age. Under such circumstances many argue that the acceptable level should be altered and lowered to 9 grams during the period in which the average is 11. Since it is not certain whether the low level denotes a normal or abnormal situation, it seems preferable to maintain 10 grams as the minimum standard. Individual consideration should be allowed patients with borderline blood levels. *It is certainly more reasonable to take steps to discover the cause of the low hemoglobin than simply to cancel the operation.* If operation can be postponed, simple anemias may be corrected by administration of ferrous sulfate, 1 tsp. 2 to 3 times daily in an elixir containing 7½ grains (370 mg.) per teaspoon. If operation is imperative, a transfusion should be given and the hemoglobin determination reported before the operation is started.

Nonprotein nitrogen determination is indicated before operations on children with genitourinary disease, whereas blood pH and CO_2 may be indicated in the presence of metabolic imbalance. In order to reduce unnecessary pain, blood loss, and expense, it is preferable to learn to judge the child's condition by clinical signs rather than to become dependent upon extensive laboratory studies.

Urinalysis is essential, and findings are judged by the same standard as those of the adult. Children who are dehydrated or have fever often show acetonuria and a concentrated urine. Glucosuria is occasionally seen, but before becoming alarmed, one should see if the child has been receiving intravenous glucose.

The chart may be checked further to note the *temperature* over a period of several days prior to operation, for it may be found that a child whose temperature is normal immediately before operation has previously been running a spiking temperature.

The nurse's bedside notes may also prove valuable, since one may find details here not noted elsewhere. Frequently the nurse will observe coughing, hoarseness, or vomiting that the doctor has either missed or regarded as unimportant. The fluid intake and output is of special significance in small children who may be upset by hospitalization and become dehydrated quite rapidly even when facing nothing more extensive than a herniorrhaphy.

In conditions in which roentgen-ray films give significant information, as in pulmonary or cardiac lesions, the anesthetist will profit by viewing these for himself. If there is still uncertainty concerning the diagnosis, the anesthetist should make his own attempt to analyze the situation and be able to add his opinion to those of the other physicians.

In most instances reviewing the patient's chart and other data need not take more than a few moments. However, if the patient is seriously ill, or if the situation is a complicated one, the anesthetist is obligated to spend considerable time in pursuing all the evidence and, if necessary, request any additional information that he believes essential.

MEETING THE CHILD

Once satisfied that he has the pertinent facts in mind, the anesthetist is ready to see the patient and his parent. It should be emphasized that not only is this a responsibility of the anesthetist but also that it is an important opportunity for him, since by personal contact he can learn much that he would miss if he confined himself to the operating room. In addition he has a chance to win the confidence of the patient and the gratitude of the parents, if they are present (Fig. 4-1).

Sincere interest in patients before and after their trip to the operating room will be rewarded not only by greater clinical success with the patients but also by increased respect on the part of one's professional associates. Lack of interest may naturally lead in the opposite direction.

The actual interview with the child may have its problems. Rather than being in his own bed, the patient is more likely to be three rooms down the hall watching a neighbor's television program. This may put the anesthetist at a disadvantage; however, it is essential that he should see the child alone for a few minutes.

Before making any statements about the operation, the anesthetist must find out if the child knows there is to be one. Many parents make the mistake of hiding the truth from the children, bringing them to the hospital with tales that they are merely to be examined or to have their picture taken. Here, the unexpected announcement of an operation can throw both patient and parent into a frenzy. Probably the safest way to bring up the business at hand is to ask the child why he is in the hospital. If the answer shows some comprehension of the situation and the parents remain calm, it will be safe to go ahead. However, if a child is old enough to understand but obviously has no idea of the coming operation and the parents suddenly start to interrupt, it is evident that the child has not been told.

It is usually best to take the parents aside and convince them that their child

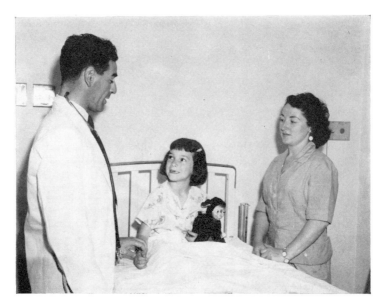

Fig. 4-1. Child, parent, and anesthetist all profit by talking things over before the operation.

should know of the operation. Sometimes the parents are obdurate in their refusal. To comply with their wishes is unfair to the child and is also unsafe, for it invites the increased risk that sudden fear and excitement impose upon the hazards of induction. While sedation can do much to obtund preoperative anxiety, it must be borne in mind that the child who awakens with a painful tube pulling at his chest, casts on his legs, or both eyes covered by bandages will be badly shocked if his only warning was that he was going to the hospital "to have his picture taken."

It is always advisable to take pains to explain to the parents that putting their child to sleep will not entail any force or mishandling. Fears are often carried over from unpleasant memories of the parents' early experiences.

Often solicitous parents merely want someone else to break the news to the child. Children frequently accept the truth more calmly than the parents had anticipated, and all are relieved after the feeling of uncertainty is cleared.

After the child has come to an understanding that he is going to go to sleep and have something fixed, the need for further discussion of the operation depends mainly upon the individual child. If he has been happily engrossed in a television program, or comic books, or his parents, it seems unwise to show him ether masks and to describe all the details of the operating room.

It is possible that with moderate sedation he will doze through his trip to the operating room and remember little of it. It seems far better to get the child's attention back to his interests and not to upset him.

On the other hand, if a boy or girl of reasoning age is crying or evidently upset, if he has been given false impressions about his hospital course, or remembers previous difficulty, it may be necessary to devote considerable time and

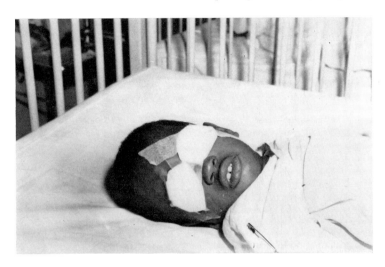

Fig. 4-2. A child who is to awaken with painful dressings or bandaged eyes should be allowed some previous word of preparation.

skill to getting this child into a more optimistic frame of mind. The direct approach often is not the best way to do this. By shifting the conversation to subjects in which the child is interested, his games, pets, or favorite gunmen, he will be more likely to relax and allow one to enter his circle. Then other children's problems can be discussed and finally his own. At last the situation is well in hand and he knows all about it. Since these situations do not occur frequently, it should be possible to give them this attention.

It is especially important that the anesthetist should try in his talks with the patient and his parents to get an idea of the emotional status of the child. It is believed that children who have shown evidence of psychic trauma during hospitalization usually have given signs of emotional instability beforehand.[17] It is extremely important that these children be recognized before operation so that they may be given special attention. Sometimes intelligent parents can inform the anesthetist of the situation, but often it is the parents or lack of parents that causes the problem, and the anesthetist must find out for himself. Excessive fear may be suggested by obvious tears and wild resistance, by passive silent cooperation, or by boisterous, bullying overactivity. Most commonly it is seen in the quiet child who stares mutely ahead and refuses to eat. First experiences may be difficult, but such problems often are compounded when repeated operations are necessary.

Physical examination. The extent of the physical examination that the anesthetist performs will depend upon the circumstances. If the patient who is scheduled for a minor operation is a small infant, and if he has been crying all afternoon and has finally dropped off to sleep, it seems wiser not to waken him. One can observe from the bedside the child's general nutritional state, skin color, character of respiration, and presence of nasal discharge. The surgeon's notes may be relied upon for the rest of the examination, and these may be rechecked in the morning prior to operation.

With older children, the anesthetist should evaluate the child's general state of health while talking with him and his parents, and then perform any procedure indicated. It seems desirable for the anesthetist to examine the heart, lungs, nose, mouth, and throat of all patients he is to anesthetize.

In the examination of a child one should look for somewhat different signs than in the adult. There is always danger of rapid onset of an upper respiratory infection with cough, running nose, and red throat. Children must be checked for this repeatedly. If an infant has a runny nose, it may be hard to tell whether it is due to an infection or is simply the result of crying. Enlarged cervical nodes also occur rather frequently with respiratory infection. Infants develop fever rapidly, and their temperatures must be observed closely. Dehydration, as evidenced by sunken fontanels, loose, dry skin, and acidotic breath may also appear unexpectedly.

Respiratory obstruction of all types is common in children and may be due to infection, anatomic anomalies, or tumors. Exact diagnosis should be made before anesthesia is started.

When a child is scheduled for procedures such as repair of lacerations, removal of a tumor, or excision of a nevus, the anesthetist should see for himself where the lesion is and how large it is (Fig. 4-3). A tumor may be the size of a

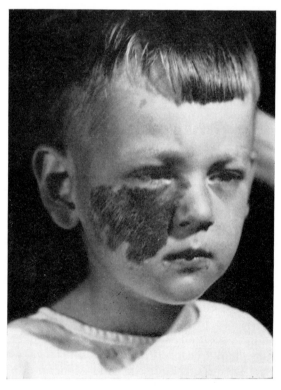

Fig. 4-3. Operation was scheduled as "excision of nevus." Only by firsthand inspection can the anesthetist evaluate his problems.

pea or a pumpkin, whereas a nevus may be a spot on a child's elbow or may cover half of his head. The anesthesia cannot be planned intelligently without knowledge of these points.

PREOPERATIVE ORDERS

After the interview and physical examination have been completed the preoperative orders may be written.

Restriction of oral intake. Whereas it is extremely important that a child's stomach is free of solids prior to anesthesia, it is also important that his fluid intake is interrupted no longer than necessary. Consequently small infants are given sugar and water feedings until 4 hours before operation and are listed for an early place in the day's operating schedule.

The following regimen is suggested:

1. *From birth to 6 months of age:* No solids or milk after midnight; clear fluids until 4 hours before operation
2. *From 6 months to 3 years of age:* No solids or milk after midnight; clear fluids until 2 A.M.
3. *Three years or older:* Nothing by mouth after midnight
4. *Children to be operated upon in afternoon:* Sweetened, clear fluids until 4 hours before operation. Grape juice, apple juice, and cola drinks offer fluid and calories. Milk and orange juice are not permitted.[31]

Enema. Although the soapsuds enema has been traditional for many years, it is tiring and upsetting to most patients, and its value is questionable. It may be indicated occasionally, but it is a routine procedure only when surgery on the lower bowel is planned.

Laboratory. Red blood cell count or hematocrit and urinalysis are to be repeated if they were performed more than 48 hours before operation.

Cross match for transfusion. If there is probability that the patient will receive blood during the operation, the blood should be ordered and prepared the day before.

Preoperative medication. This phase of preparation brings up one of the most controversial problems in pediatric anesthesia. Since there are many sides to the question, it will be discussed in detail in Chapter 5.

REFERENCES

1. Potts, W. J.: The heart of a child, J.A.M.A. **161**:487-490, 1956.
2. Gofman, H., Buckman, W., and Schade, G. H.: The child's emotional response to hospitalization, Amer. J. Dis. Child. **93**:157-164, 1957.
3. Rogers, K. D., and Wishik, S. M.: The pediatrician's responsibility when his patient is anesthetized, Pediatrics **11**:549-553, 1953.
4. Sever, J. A.: Johnny goes to the hosptal, Cambridge, Mass., 1953, The Riverside Press.
5. When a child goes to the hospital, Chicago, 1957, Pamphlet prepared by the American Society of Anesthesiologists.
6. Skeie, H. G.: Dede has her tonsils out, New York, 1956, Pageant Press.
7. Francis, L., and Cutler, R. P.: Psychological preparation and premedication for pediatric anesthesia, Anesthesiology **18**:106-109, 1957.
8. Bierman, G.: Kind und Operationstrauma, Anaesthetist **5**:184-189, 1956.
9. Kennell, J. H., and Bergen, M. E.: Early childhood separations, Pediatrics **37**:291-296, 1966

10. Bowlby, J.: Some pathological processes engendered by early mother-child separation. In Senn, M. F. E., editor: Infancy and childhood, Transaction of Seventh Conference, March 23-24, 1953, New York, Josaiah Macy, Jr. Foundation.

11. Ainsworth, M. D., and Boston, M.: Psychodiagnostic assessments of a child after prolonged separation in early childhood, Brit. Med. Psychol. 25:169-176, 1952.

12. Robertson, J.: Young children in hospitals, New York, 1958, Basic Books, Inc.

13. Jersild, A. T.: Child psychology, ed. 5, Englewood Cliffs, N. J., 1960, Prentice-Hall, Inc.

14. Jackson, K.: Psychological preparation as a method of reducing emotional trauma of anesthesia in children, Anesthesiology 12:293-300, 1951.

15. Eckenhoff, J. E.: Relationship of anesthesia to postoperative personality changes in children, Amer. J. Dis. Child. 86:587-591, 1953.

16. Pickerill, C. M., and Pickerill, H. P.: Keeping mother and baby together, Brit. Med. J. 2:337, 1946.

17. Smith, R. M.: Children, hospitals and parents, Anesthesiology 25:461-465, 1964.

18. Nicholson, M. J., and Crehan, J. P.: Preoperative preparation. In Hale, D. E., editor: Anesthesiology, ed. 2, Philadelphia, 1963, F. A. Davis Co., pp. 179-208.

19. Karp, M.: The importance of preoperative rounds, Anesth. Analg. 36:36-41, 1952.

20. Egbert, L. D., Lamdin, S. J., and Hackett, T. P.: Psychological problems of surgical patients. In Eckenhoff, J. E., editor: Science and practice in anesthesia, Philadelphia, 1965, J. B. Lippincott Co.

21. Anderson, D. H.: Avertin poisoning with acute yellow atrophy of the liver and toxic nephrosis, Anesthesiology 6:284-301, 1945.

22. Lundy, J. S.: Cortisone problems involving anesthesia, Anesthesiology 14:376-381, 1953.

23. Root, B.: Postoperative adrenal insufficiency, a review, Anesth. Analg. 34:78-95, 1955.

24. Salossa, R. M., Bennett, W. A., Keating, F. R., Jr., and Sprague, R. G.: Postoperative adrenal cortical insufficiency. Occurrence in patients previously treated with cortisone, J.A.M.A. 152:1509-1515, 1953.

25. Lewis, L., Robinson, R. F., Yee, J., Hacker, L. A., and Eisen, G.: Fatal adrenal cortical insufficiency precipitated by surgery during prolonged continuous cortisone treatment, Ann. Intern. Med. 39:116-126, 1953.

26. Alper, M. H., Flacke, W., and Krayer, O.: Pharmacology of reserpine and its implications for anesthesia, Anesthesiology 24:524-542, 1963.

27. Vandam, L. D.: Effects of prior drug therapy on the course of anesthesia. In Eckenhoff, J. E., editor: Science and practice of anesthesia, Philadelphia, 1962, J. B. Lippincott Co.

28. Gillies, A. J.: Cortisone therapy prior to surgical intervention, Anesth. Analg. 37:47-51, 1958.

29. Bourgeois-Gavardin, M., Nowill, W. K., Margolis, G., and Stephen, C. R.: Chlorpromazine; a laboratory and clinical investigation, Anesthesiology 16:829-847, 1955.

30. Coakley, C. S., Alpert, S., and Boling, J. S.: Circulatory responses during anesthesia of patients on rauwolfia therapy, J.A.M.A. 161:1143-1144, 1956.

31. Woodbridge, P. D.: Preanesthetic breakfast, Anesthesiology 4:81, 1943.

Chapter 5

Preoperative medication

ADVANTAGES AND DISADVANTAGES OF PREOPERATIVE MEDICATION

Preoperative medication has long been an active area of interest in pediatric anesthesia. This is due not only to the fact that the problem arises in every child who comes to anesthesia, but also because new drugs are continually being produced, they lend themselves easily to clinical trial, and as yet few, if any, are truly satisfactory.

In general, medication has been required in order to (1) replace fear and anxiety with calmness, (2) prevent secretions, and (3) control vagal stimulation. With decreased use of ether, the problem of secretions has largely been eradicated, but that of vagal stimulation has increased. Although methods differ, the great majority of anesthetists agree that preanesthetic medication is indicated for children.

On the other hand, there have always been those who believed that such medication was undesirable. Robson,[1] a pioneer in pediatric anesthesia, stated that belladonna agents should be avoided because of the possibility of heat retention. This will be discussed later. The danger of respiratory depression is often stressed in criticism of barbiturates and narcotics.

Jackson[2] wrote that sedation was unnecessary in older children because they could be persuaded to cooperate. In general there is a slight over-all tendency to decrease the dosages of preanesthetic agents and to rely more upon personal persuasion. In our experience, however, even though a great many older children can be persuaded to summon enough self-control to submit to anesthesia, the experience may remain quite unpleasant for them. This is occasionally evident in children who restrain themselves nicely until they are about to lose consciousness—then they are released from their inhibitions and suddenly fight like demons.

A factor of secondary importance is the large expenditure of time involved in attempting verbal control of all children. This time would be invested gladly were it not possible to do the job more effectively by medication. For both safety and simplicity, the use of sedation seems definitely indicated, provided that care is taken to avoid overdosage and depression.

SUGGESTED AGENTS AND DOSAGES

Problems in selection of drugs. The agents for preoperative medication include a wide and rapidly increasing variety. Usually a belladonna agent is given to prevent secretions and vagal activity, and a hypnotic is ordered to decrease fear and excitement and bring amnesia. Barbiturates have been the most widely used hypnotics. Drugs of the opiate class may be added to increase the hypnotic effect and allay pain if present.

In addition to these standard agents, many alternatives exist. Some use is made of paraldehyde and chloral hydrate, but their popularity has never been widespread. Basal anesthesia by rectal administration of tribromoethanol (Avertin) has been used since 1926, and more recently use of thiobarbiturates and methohexital by rectum has been popular.

The problem of preoperative sedation became increasingly confusing by the introduction of numerous central nervous system depressants loosely classified as tranquilizing or ataractic agents. Typical of these are meprobamate (Equanil), glutethimide (Doriden), and hydroxyzine hydrochloride (Vistaril).

The wide variety of sedatives from which to choose is further complicated by other variables. The effectiveness of all drugs will depend upon optimum dosage, the proper route of administration, and the correct time of administration. Until these factors have been assessed more adequately, choice must rest largely upon individual preferences.

Specific drugs and dosages. In 1938 Waters[3] published a classical paper recommending preanesthetic medication for children. Since that time a variety of different schedules of medication have been proposed,[4-6] most of which are basically alike and produce relatively similar and not quite satisfactory results.

Both the sedative and the dosage that are chosen will vary with the effect that one hopes to produce, some anesthetists preferring considerably more sedation than others. The ideal agent or combination of agents would seem to be one that can be given to an excited, frightened child on the ward and transform him into a drowsy, unconcerned person who is not comatose or depressed but who simply appears relaxed and completely relieved of the cares of the world (Fig.

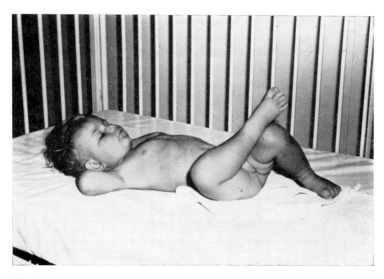

Fig. 5-1. Sedation without depression. Such evident relaxation decreases the risk of major operation. This little boy was about to undergo repair of ventricular septal defect.

5-1). This is what most anesthetists mean by the phrase "sedation without depression," the ultimate goal in pediatric premedication.

Anesthetic induction. It should be recognized that successful induction of anesthesia depends upon three factors—the sedative agents, the anesthetist's approach, and the technique of induction. Some have relied upon the sedative to do all the work, at the expense of depression and side effects of the drugs. With greater attention devoted to gaining the child's confidence and to skillful use of a pleasant induction method, the importance of the sedative will be greatly reduced.

The standard upon which our medication has been based for a number of years is shown in Table 5-1. This has given us better results than have other combinations in popular use, but it still leaves room for improvement, since the desired effect is attained in only about 75% of cases.

Anticholinergic agents. Twenty years ago atropine and scopolamine were the only anticholinergic agents used, and there was continual debate as to which was superior. Between 1950 and 1960 there was much interest in other derivatives and synthetic substitutes including l-hyoscyamine (Bellafoline),[7] oxyphenonium (Antrenyl),[8] and methantheline (Banthine),[9] each of which was thought to improve upon the action of the original agents in duration or dependability. The sudden interest appears to have been fleeting, for atropine and scopolamine now are back in popular use and the "new" agents are rarely seen.

In choosing between atropine and scopolamine, it is now well established that scopolamine has superior drying action.[10-12] However, this is of less importance since the use of ether has decreased. Scopolamine is chosen approximately 25% of the time for pediatric anesthesia, largely because of its sedative effect. Atropine is chosen in the majority of cases because of its superior effect in block-

ing vagal activity. Our own choice of atropine is based on this factor. The sedation that scopolamine provides can be obtained by hypnotics.

The value of atropine has become much more evident because of the increasing use of such vagotonic agents as cyclopropane, halothane, and succinylcholine.[13] Numerous instances of severe bradycardia or asystole have occurred,
which might have been prevented by proper use of atropine.[14] It should be emphasized that dosage and timing are equally important in atropine administration. The drug is definitely tachyphylactic, and repeated administration bears no
danger of cumulative action.[15] A schedule is given showing comparable dosages
of several anticholinergic agents (Table 5-2).

It has been reported that atropine increases respiratory dead space and that
it causes dangerous arrhythmias. The increase in dead space is too slight to be
of any significance. The arrhythmias may be of consequence, but it should be
emphasized that these rarely occur if atropine is used prophylactically. Such
cardiac irregularities are most frequently seen if severe vagal action occurs, and
atropine is *then* given to correct it.[15] It is unquestionably true that the drying
effect is unpleasant to the patient, as is the needle. For this reason we often

Table 5-1. *Standard premedication form at the Children's Medical Center,
Boston—directions for preoperative medication for infants and children*

Age	Average weight (lb.)	Pentobarbital (Nembutal) (mg.)	(grains)	Morphine (mg.)	(grains)	Atropine or scopolamine (mg.)	(grains)
Newborn	7	—	—	—	—	0.2	1/300
6 mo.	16	30 p.r.	½	—	—	0.2	1/300
1 yr.	21	50 p.r.	¾	1.0	1/60	0.2	1/300
2 yr.	27	60 p.r.	1	1.5	1/40	0.3	1/200
4 yr.	35	90 p.r.	1½	3.0	1/20	0.3	1/200
6 yr.	45	100 p.r.	1½	4.0	1/15	0.4	1/150
8 yr.	55	100 p.o.	1½	5.0	1/12	0.4	1/150
10 yr.	65	100 p.o.	1½	5.0	1/10	0.4	1/150
12 yr.	85	100 p.o.	1½	6.0	1/8	0.6	1/100

1. This table is a guide to be followed only for average, well-developed patients. Reductions
must be made in medication for subnormal patients.
2. Atropine is to be given to all patients who are to receive anesthesia.
3. Patients receiving Avertin should have atropine, but *no morphine or barbiturate.*
4. No morphine or barbiturate is to be given to patients under 6 months of age.
5. Nembutal is to be given by rectum to children under 8 years of age.
6. For rectal use Nembutal is to be dissolved in 10 ml. water and injected with syringe and
catheter, at least *90 minutes* before operation. It may also be used in the form of a suppository.
7. Demerol, or morphine, and atropine are to be given hypodermically 45 minutes before operation.
8. Before ether, cyclopropane, or Pentothal anesthesia, give Nembutal, morphine, and atropine,
as suggested by table.
9. Approximate dosage:
    Under 8 years: pentobarbital, 2.5 mg./lb. by rectum; morphine, 0.75 mg./yr. of age.
    8 years and over: pentobarbital, 100 mg. by mouth; morphine, 0.5 mg./yr. of age up to 8
    mg.

delay administration until induction of anesthesia has provided analgesia. If an infusion is already running, atropine is given by this route.

Dosage of scopolamine is customarily less than that of atropine. This may result in a satisfactory drying effect, but the vagolytic action of scopolamine will be inadequate unless the dosage is equal to or more than that of atropine.

Fears about belladonna toxicity have been voiced but seldom realized. Actually there appears to be a wide margin of safety in the use of this type of agent. Our British colleagues use larger doses than we do and still encounter little trouble.[16,17] The most common side effect seen with belladonna drugs is a blotchy rash that actually has no significance. Heat retention with resultant elevation of temperature may occur in hot environments or when patients are dehydrated or ill. In such cases one should correct the underlying cause by cooling the patient and giving fluids. In addition it may be wise to reduce the dose of atropine or, better yet, to delay its administration until immediately before operation and then give it intravenously. Under usual circumstances atropine is given subcutaneously or intramuscularly 45 minutes before operation.

Actual toxicity from atropine and related agents has been reported in infants and in adults, but usually as a result of gross overdosage.[18] Joos[19] reported the case of a 7-week-old infant who recovered after receiving more than 40 mg. of atropine in 24 hours, where as Alexander, Morris and Eslick[20] reported the recovery of an adult who had ingested 1 Gm. (1,000 mg.) by mouth.

Hypnotic agents. Among the agents used as hypnotics for children the barbiturates have been most popular, and of the barbiturates secobarbital (Seconal) and pentobarbital (Nembutal) have been most frequently used. Although secobarbital is stated to have more rapid action, it is difficult to distinguish between the two drugs in clinical use.

Choice of dosage and route of administration differ considerably. If an exact amount must be given, the parenteral route is preferable. However, the dosage of preoperative sedation is subject to so many variables that the accuracy afforded by parenteral injection does not seem to be of enough value to justify the added discomfort, expense, and time involved.

Table 5-2. *Comparable dosages of anticholinergic drugs for pediatric use*

Age	Average weight (lb.)	Atropine sulfate (mg.)	Scopola-mine (mg.)	l-Hyoscyamine (Bellafoline) (mg.)	Oxyphenonium (Antrenyl) (mg.)	Methantheline (Banthine) (mg.)
Newborn	7	0.2	0.2	0.2	0.10	1.0
6 mo.	16	0.2	0.2	0.2	0.10	1.0
1 yr.	21	0.2	0.2	0.2	0.10	1.0
2 yr.	27	0.3	0.3	0.3	0.15	2.0
4 yr.	35	0.3	0.3	0.3	0.15	4.0
6 yr.	45	0.4	0.4	0.4	0.20	6.0
8 yr.	55	0.4	0.4	0.4	0.20	8.0
10 yr.	65	0.4	0.4	0.4	0.20	10.0
12 yr.	80	0.6	0.6	0.6	0.30	10.0

For children under 10 years of age, rectal administration has proved as successful as the parenteral route in our experience, provided the barbiturates are administered properly. Capsules should not be inserted in the rectum, for, even if perforated, their contents rarely will be absorbed, and usually the entire capsule will be expelled. When barbiturates are to be given by rectum, they should be given either in the form of a suppository, or, if provided in capsule form, the contents of the capsule should be removed, dissolved in 10 ml. of water, and injected with catheter and syringe. Dosage of barbiturates when given by rectum is approximately 2.5 mg. per pound of body weight for normal robust children.

The dosages shown in any sedative schedule are to be used only as a rough guide and must be altered according to each individual. Fat children and obviously ill children will require relatively less per pound of body weight, whereas hyperactive children may require more. Most of the present methods of premedication have an obvious fallacy. The sedation required by two normal children of the same age, weight, and outward appearance may differ widely. As long as we try to produce sedation by administration of a single predetermined dose of any agent, our results will never attain the accuracy we need.

In order to gain the desired level of sedation with agents now available, it would be necessary to give small individual doses at repeated intervals until the desired end point is reached. Such an approach was suggested by Poe and Karp,[21] and certainly is preferable, but unfortunately it is too time-consuming for practical use. Perhaps a sweetened chloral hydrate lollipop could be invented that could act as a simple servomechanism. The child would suck on it as long as he was awake, and, when his individual requirement had been taken, he would drop the lollipop and go to sleep.

Criticism of barbiturates usually concerns respiratory depression and excitement. Actually pentobarbital causes remarkably little respiratory depression when compared to its hypnotic effect, and children tolerate it in relatively large amounts. Of more concern is the excitement seen in children who may fall into a disturbed type of sleep when left alone but who will scream and thrash about if they are moved or awakened. Usually they remember nothing about it later, but the experience is not a desirable one, especially for nearby children and anyone attending these excited patients.

The time at which hypnotics are administered is important. The usual custom is to give barbiturates 90 minutes before operations. With this method children who are not scheduled for operation until 10 or 11 o'clock must remain hungry and apprehensive until mid-morning. However, if all children who are scheduled for operation before noon are given their barbiturate at 6 A.M., they will be spared this ordeal and can doze comfortably through the morning hours until their turns arise. This plan has been very successful in our experience.

Children to be operated upon in the afternoon are allowed clear fluids by mouth until 6 A.M. and are given their barbiturate at 8 or 9 A.M. so that they, too, may have a peaceful morning.

Narcotics. The use of narcotics as routine preoperative medication has been justly criticized[22]; nevertheless morphine has proved singularly effective as a

Table 5-3. *Comparable dosages of narcotics for pediatric use*

Age (yr.)	Average weight (lb.)	Morphine (mg.)	Morphine (grains)	Meperidine (Demerol) (mg.)	Alphaprodine (Nisentil) (mg.)	Phenazocine (Prinadol) (mg.)
1	21	1.0	1/60	10	4.0	0.1
2	27	1.5	1/40	20	8.0	0.2
4	35	3.0	1/20	30	12.0	0.3
6	45	4.0	1/15	40	15.0	0.4
8	55	4.0	1/15	40	15.0	0.4
10	65	5.0	1/12	50	20.0	0.5
12	85	6.0	1/10	60	25.0	0.6

sedative for small children and, in addition, helps to prevent rapid, jerky respiration during thoracic surgery.

After an adequate dose of morphine, a child lies awake but calm and unafraid, in contrast to a child under barbiturate sedation, who lies in a troubled, enforced sleep, to waken in excitement and confusion when disturbed. Morphine, if used alone in dosage sufficient for sedation, would carry the danger of respiratory depression; consequently, a combination of barbiturate and morphine is used.

Because of difficulty in estimating fractional dosages and the danger of respiratory depression, it seems better to avoid use of opiates until children are 1 year old. However, small infants with severe cardiac lesions often are benefited by morphine, and it may be necessary to prescribe it in doses up to 1 mg. per 10 pounds merely to enable them to reach the operating table.

The choice of morphine from comparable narcotics is open to question. Morphine probably causes more nausea and vomiting than meperidine (Demerol) and alphaprodine[23] (Nisentil), but, as just noted, it has been proved especially valuable in children with congenital heart disease and, in addition, has been associated with less dizziness than is noted with meperidine and less respiratory depression than that seen with alphaprodine. Use of any of these narcotics seems justified, and a table of comparable doses is provided. Dosage by the metric system is more practical for accuracy in small amounts (Table 5-3).

Narcotics are given subcutaneously 45 minutes before operation. This time is chosen because it gives the narcotic time to act, it enables the nurse to give it in the same syringe as the atropine, and it also gives time to note the action of the previously administered barbiturate. If the child has already fallen fast asleep, it is preferable to withhold the narcotic in order to avoid depression.

LIMITATIONS TO MEDICATION SCHEDULE

Any medication schedule will require modification, as already pointed out. In addition, there are many situations in which the condition of the patient or the type of surgery requires departure from the schedule completely. For minor surgical procedures and emergency surgery, special considerations are involved, and adapted sedation is described (Chapter 24). For neurosurgery, tonsillectomy, and cardiac catheterization other sedatives are used as described in special sections on these topics.

ALTERNATIVE SEDATIVES AND DOSAGE

Many types of sedatives have been suggested for pediatric sedation. Actually our most reliable agent for induction of sleep without side effects or complication has been tribromoethanol (Avertin). This will be discussed in Chapter 8.

Alcohol in the form of brandy or whisky has been popular for use in small infants. This may be given by mixing 10 ml. of brandy with 30 ml. of sweetened water, administering it by gavage. An initial dose of 3 ml. per pound of body weight may be tried, and if after 15 minutes the infant is not quiet and relaxed, an additional 1.5 ml. per pound can be added.

Instead of using alcohol to pacify infants during operations under local anesthesia, we find it preferable merely to withhold the baby's feeding and then give it to him during operation. This approach has been useful during reduction of depressed skull fracture in newborn infants. It is not advised during abdominal surgery.

Paraldehyde was long believed to be safer than barbiturates, and for this reason was occasionally used, especially for patients with renal disease, in spite of its unpleasant taste and odor. The dose for rectal instillation was 0.25 ml. per pound of body weight. Now it is no longer believed to have any greater safety and consequently is rarely used.

Chloral hydrate is still thought to be safe, and is inexpensive. In a nonalcoholic elixir, Stetson and Jessup[24] reported a dose of 22 mg. per 5 pounds to be effective. It has a rather bitter aftertaste but is usually accepted by children of all ages.

Ataractic and tranquilizing agents. An apparently endless number of sedatives are being introduced to challenge the long-standing monopoly of the barbiturates. Each pharmaceutical company champions a slightly different formula with a slightly more soporific name; Nytol, Placidyl, Harmonyl, and Suavitil are but a few of these. Most are advertised with the claim that they are "nonbarbiturates," that they bring calmness and tranquility without depression, and that they have a wide margin of safety.

Actually these drugs represent considerable variation both in chemical structure and in effect. Dobkin[25] has made an excellent survey of the ataractic agents and divide them into five different structural groups that include Rauwolfia alkaloids, phenothiazine derivatives (chlorpromazine, etc.), benzohydrol derivatives, hydroxypropane derivatives (meprobamate, etc.), and a group of miscellaneous unrelated sedatives such as glutethimide and ethinamate.

Several of these agents have been used for preoperative sedation in children, the phenothiazine derivatives having received the most attention. Although the usefulness of chlorpromazine is decidedly limited because of its prolonged effect and tendency to cause hypotension, the less potent promethazine is used occasionally. When subjected to close scrutiny,[26] the tranquilizing agents have been quite unimpressive. Many have either been withdrawn from production or have fallen into disuse. In this country hydroxyzine (Vistaril, adult dose 100 mg.) is being used, while the British seem to favor trimeprazine.[27]

In our hands phenothiazine derivatives and other tranquilizing agents have all been disappointing, giving a barely appreciable effect unless the dosage was increased to several times the suggested amount. In general the effect of these drugs seems comparable to that of phenobarbital.

Neuroleptic drugs used for premedication. Recent interest in psychoactive agents of the butyrophenone class has led to their trial in pediatric anesthesia for preoperative sedation. Werry and Davenport[28] evaluated droperidol for pediatric premedication, comparing its psychologic effects with those of morphine. Although neuroleptic agents had been reported to sedate without depressing cortical function, this was not borne out by the study. Postoperative motor disturbances further complicate and make questionable the use of droperidol in children.

EVALUATION OF PREOPERATIVE SEDATIVES

It is obvious that the problem of sedation is a confusing one. This is due not only to the large variety of sedatives available but also to the inadequate methods by which most of these sedatives have been evaluated. *The purpose in using preoperative sedatives is to eliminate apprehension without causing cardiorespiratory depression or other side effects.* Many of the studies on pediatric premedication have consisted of administration of a predetermined dose of known agent in an uncontrolled series of children.

In assessing the merits of these reports numerous shortcomings have been apparent. Among those most frequently encountered are (1) failure to define desired effect of sedative, (2) failure to determine most effective dose of sedative, (3) failure to evaluate patient prior to sedation, (4) inadequate method of evaluating effect of drug, and (5) omission of considering side effects, cost, method of administration, taste, size of pill, and other contributing factors. Freeman and Bachman[29] and Root[30] have met many of these criticisms in their studies of sedation. Smith and Jeffries[31] suggested that new agents be compared to a standard sedative, such as pentobarbital, as local anesthetics are compared to procaine; they also developed a method of evaluating the sedative and depressing effects of different agents. By plotting the effect of a sedative in units of sedation versus units of depression, it is easily determined not only whether depression outweighs sedation but it is also indicated when an unsatisfactory result may be explained by either inadequate or excessive dosage.

The study by Rackow and Salanitre[32] is one of the few that attempts to trace dose-response relationships of sedatives used in children.

REFERENCES

1. Robson, C. H.: Anesthesia in children, Amer. J. Surg. 34:468-473, 1936.
2. Jackson, K.: Psychological preparation as a method of reducing the emotional trauma of anesthesia in children, Anesthesiology 12:293-300, 1951.
3. Waters, R. M.: Pain relief for children, Amer. J. Surg. 39:470-475, 1938.
4. Leigh, M. D., and Belton, M. K.: Premediction in infants and children, Anesthesiology 7:611-615, 1946.
5. Anderson, S. M.: Principles and practice of paediatric anaesthesia. In Evans, F. T., and Gray, T. C., editors: General anaesthesia, London, 1959, Butterworth & Co. (Publishers), Ltd.

6. Smith, R. M.: Method of induction in pediatric anesthesia, New Eng. J. Med. 240:761-765, 1949.
7. Stephen, C. R., Bowers, M. A., Nowill, W. K., and Martin, R. C.: Anticholinergic drugs in preanesthetic medication, Anesthesiology 17:303-313, 1956.
8. Mushin, W. W., and Adams, A. S.: The antisialogogue effect of Antrenyl (oxyphenonium bromide), Brit. J. Anaesth. 27:519-524, 1955.
9. Alver, E. C., and Vanderwood, J. M.: The use of Banthine as a drying agent in pediatric anesthesia, Anesthesiology 17:73-81, 1956.
10. Wyant, G. M., and Dobkin, A. B.: Antisialogogue drugs in man, Anaesthesia 12:203-214, 1957.
11. Galloon, S.: A comparison of the antisialogogue action of atropine and hyoscyamine, Brit. J. Anaesth. 28:113-117, 1956.
12. Burstein, C. L.: Pediatric preanesthetic preparation, Anesthesiology 14:567-571, 1953.
13. Eger, E. I.: Atropine, scopolamine, and related compounds, Anesthesiology 23:365-383, 1962.
14. Leigh, M. D., McCoy, D. D., Belton, M. K., and Lewis, G. B.: Bradycardia following intravenous administration of succinylcholine to infants and children, Anesthesiology 18:698-702, 1957.
15. Sagarminiga, J., and Wygands, J. E.: Atropine and the electrical activity of the heart during induction of anesthesia in children, Canad. Anaesth. Soc. J. 10:328-342, 1963.
16. Gaviotaki, A., and Smith, R. M.: Use of atropine in pediatric anesthesia, Internat. Anesth. Clin. 1:97-113, 1962.
17. Rees, J. G.: Anaesthesia in the newborn, Brit. Med. J. 2:1419-1426, 1950.
18. Morton, H. G.: Atropine intoxication; its manifestations in infants and children, J. Pediat. 14:755-760, 1939.
19. Joos, H. A.: Atropine intoxication in infancy, Amer. J. Dis. Child. 79:855-861, 1950.
20. Alexander, E., Jr., Morris, D. R., and Eslick, R. H.: Atropine poisoning, New Eng. J. Med. 234:258-259, 1946.
21. Poe, M. F., and Karp, M.: Seconal as a basal anesthetic for children, Anesth. Analg. 27:88-91, 1948.
22. Cohen, E. N., and Beecher, H. K.: Narcotics in preanesthetic medication, J.A.M.A. 147:1664-1668, 1951.
23. Eckenhoff, J. E., and Helrich, M. H.: Study of narcotics and sedatives for use in preanesthetic medication, J.A.M.A. 167:415-422, 1958.
24. Stetson, J. B., and Jessup, G. V. S.: Use of chloral hydrate mixtures for pediatric premedication, Anesth. Analg. 41:203-214, 1962.
25. Dobkin, A. B.: Efficacy of ataractic drugs in clinical anaesthesia; a review, Canad. Anaesth. Soc. J. 5:177-209, 1958.
26. Dickel, H. A., and Dixon, H. H.: Inherent dangers in the use of tranquilizing drugs in anxiety state, J.A.M.A. 163:422-426, 1957.
27. Cope, R. W., and Glover, W. J.: Trimeprazine tartrate for premedication in children, Lancet 1:858-860, 1959.
28. Werry, J. S., and Davenport, H. T.: The psychological effects of premedication for paediatric anaesthesia, New Zeal. Med. J. 64:641-646, 1965; abstract in Survey Anesth. 10:477-478, 1966.
29. Freeman, A., and Bachman, L.: Pediatric anesthesia: an evaluation of preoperative medication, Anesth. Analg. 38:429-437, 1959.
30. Root, B.: Problems of evaluating effects of premedication in children, Presentation of a key-sort card, Anesth. Analg. 41:180-193, 1962.
31. Smith, R. M., and Jeffries, M.: The evaluation of sedative agents for preoperative use in children, Anesth. Analg. 38:166-172, 1959.
32. Rackow, H., and Salanitre, E.: A dose-effect study of preoperative medication in children, Anesthesiology 23:747-754, 1962.

Chapter 6

Equipment

Many serious complications in pediatric anesthesia are due to the failure to have proper equipment at hand. Sufficient apparatus is now available for most needs in this field, and there is little excuse for inadequate preparation.

There are actually so many different sizes, shapes, and types of anesthetic and supportive equipment that this in itself creates a problem in properly equipped services. When planning a new department this should be kept in mind, and maximum space should be allowed for placing equipment where it is visible and immediately accessible (Figs. 6-1 and 6-2), thus providing a tremendous asset in managing busy schedules and caring for emergencies.

ESSENTIAL APPARATUS

Many procedures can be performed with very simple equipment. However, general anesthesia should never be started without the following items:

    1. A suction apparatus, within reach and in working condition and with adequate catheters

Fig. 6-1

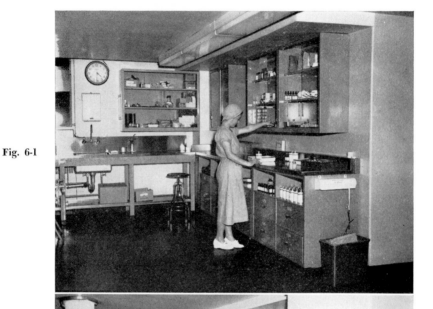

Fig. 6-2

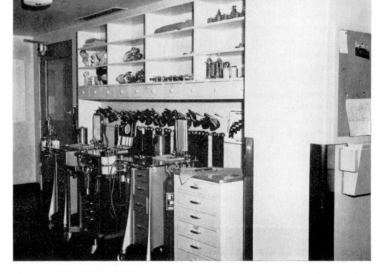

Figs. 6-1 and 6-2. The anesthesia department should be planned to provide ready accessibility of equipment.

2. Oxygen, for maintenance or resuscitation
3. Oropharyngeal airways of correct size
4. Laryngoscope of proper size
5. Endotracheal tubes in a variety of sizes
6. Stethoscope

To this probably should be added succinylcholine, a syringe, and a needle for the management of laryngeal spasm. These items are shown in Fig. 6-3.

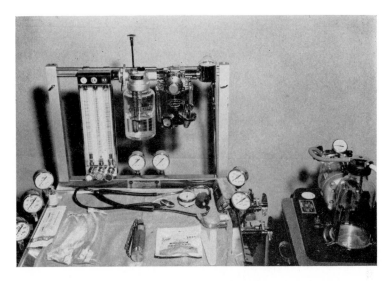

Fig. 6-3. Essential apparatus for general anesthesia includes complete suction equipment, oxygen, airways, stethoscope, tongue blades, laryngoscope, endotracheal tubes, syringes, needles, and succinylcholine.

EQUIPMENT FOR INHALATION ANESTHESIA

The choice of equipment for the administration of anesthesia depends to a considerable extent upon personal preference. Underlying factors must guide this choice, however. Equipment is suited to the individual patient, with especial care to avoid resistance, dead space, fatigue, and trauma, since all of these insults are easily imposed upon small patients.

Masks. Masks for *open-drop anesthesia* should be carefully chosen and prepared. For infants it is important to use a small mask, such as the infant Yankauer, or one of the modifications having a nipple for oxygen insufflation (Fig. 6-4). These masks should be covered with not more than four layers of loosely woven gauze. High-peaked masks covered with heavy cloth are definitely to be avoided. For children between 1 and 3 years of age a regular Yankauer mask is satisfactory if covered with not more than four layers of gauze. In children over 3 years of age the regulation Yankauer mask may be covered with eight layers of gauze.

Suitable infant masks for nonrebreathing or closed-system techniques are now available for most sizes and shapes. The Ohio premature and newborn masks* have the advantage of being soft and easily molded to the face. With these an airtight fit can be maintained even when a Levin tube is being used. The Rendell-Baker masks are designed to fit the facial contours more closely and to reduce dead space, but being of firmer rubber they are less adaptable.

---

*Ohio Chemical and Surgical Equipment Co., Madison, Wis.

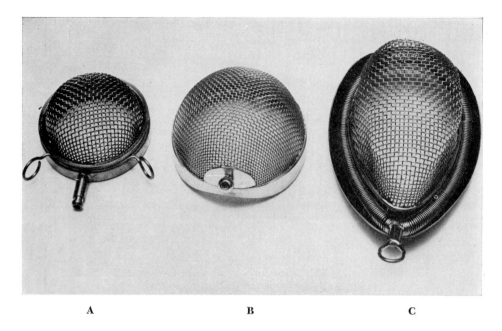

A   B   C

Fig. 6-4. Wire masks for open-drop anesthesia. **A,** Hawks. **B,** Infant Yankauer. **C,** Yankauer.

Much importance has been placed upon the amount of dead space in infant masks. At present masks are seldom used for maintenance of general anesthesia in infants, since most of these very small patients require intubation. Masks are used for brief periods during induction and recovery, and occasionally for resuscitation in nonsurgical patients. In these situations a tight fit is of greater importance than reduction of dead space. A few measurements of apparatus dead space as reported by Brown and Hustead[1] are listed in Table 6-1.

For larger infants and children the Rendell-Baker,* MIE Everseal,† Warne anatomical,‡ and Ohio Trimar§ masks are all useful, and each will prove valuable under varying conditions (Fig. 6-5). It is to be noted that except for the Rendell-Baker type most infant masks fit across the eyes and forehead and should not have an indentation for the bridge of the nose. In older children, however, masks do fit across the nose. Then it is desirable to have a wide nasal notch, as in the Trimar mask.

Oropharyngeal airways. Oropharyngeal airways of plastic, rubber, or metal are commonly used (Fig. 6-6). None is distinctly superior, but our preference is for the plastic Guedel type airway with an inner plastic or metal strut. These airways appear to be strong and relatively atraumatic (Fig. 6-7). The most important factor here is that a sufficient variety of sizes be stocked. To be ready for

---

*Anesthesia Associates, Inc., Hudson, N. Y.
†Anesthesia Specialties Co., Bridgeport, Conn.
‡Air-Shields, Inc., Hatboro, Pa.
§Ohio Chemical and Surgical Equipment Co., Madison, Wis.

Table 6-1. *External dead space in infant breathing apparatus**

Apparatus	External dead space
Bennett No. 3 mask	13.0 ml.
Rendell-Baker Soucek No. 1 mask	8.7 ml.
Ohio newborn mask	7.4 ml.
Bennett No. 3 mask with Stephen-Slater, Leigh, or Sierra valves plus 90° elbow or Ohio swivel-Y valve	19.0 ml.

*From Brown, E. S., and Hustead, R. F.: Anesthesiology **28:**241, 1967.

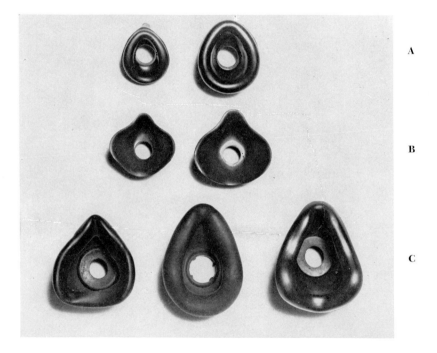

Fig. 6-5. Rubber masks for closed-system anesthesia. **A,** Ohio premature and newborn sizes. **B,** Rendell-Baker premature and infant sizes. **C,** MIE, Warne, and Ohio Trimar child-sized masks.

all contingencies one must have at least five sizes of airways (sizes 00, 0, 1, 2, and 3).

Endotracheal tubes. Endotracheal tubes may be of rubber or plastic material. It is important to use tubes that are thin walled and that give maximum lumina but retain enough firmness so that they do not kink or collapse. All sizes between 12 and 34 Fr. (2.5 and 8.5 mm. internal diameter) may be needed and should be maintained in readiness.

If a cuffed tube is used, the cuff takes up space, and it will be necessary to use a tube with a smaller lumen than when no cuff is used. Consequently, in children

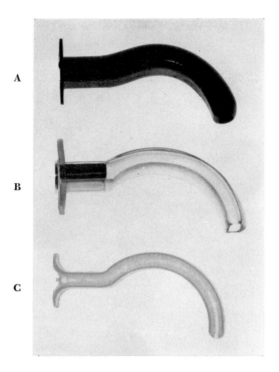

Fig. 6-6. Oropharyngeal airways. **A,** Rubber Guedel. **B,** Plastic and metal Guedel. **C,** Plastic Berman.

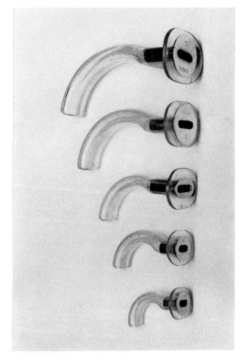

Fig. 6-7. Oropharyngeal airways, plastic with metal strut, sizes 00, 0, 1, 2, and 3.

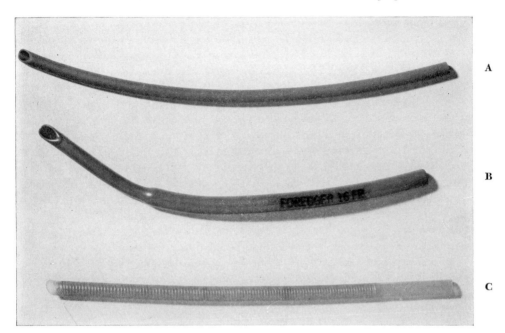

Fig. 6-8. Endotracheal tubes used in pediatric anesthesia. **A,** Magill, **B,** Cole, and, **C,** wire inlaid (armored) tubes.

under 8 to 10 years of age (80 to 100 pounds) in whom maximal airway lumina are of primary importance, cuffed tubes are not advised.

The Magill uniform-bore endotracheal tube is the standard form that can be used for most purposes. However, several modifications of the Magill tube have been introduced (Fig. 6-8). The Cole tube[2,3] is so designed that only the terminal portion is narrow enough to pass through the vocal cords. This prevents the passage of the tube into one of the bronchi. Latex tubes reinforced by coiled wire are popular in England and are extremely valuable when the head is to be sharply flexed during operation, as during a craniotomy in the prone or sitting positions.

Laryngoscopes. There are several important features in the design of a laryngoscope. Although the length is of obvious importance, so also are the width and shape of the tip, the bore, curvature, and metallic finish. The large number of variations show that opinions differ widely in each. A straight blade should give the greatest exposure in children but will require slightly greater relaxation than a curved blade. The downward deflection of the tip, as in the Miller infant blade, will enable one to retract the epiglottis, as with a Macintosh blade, rather than lift it. The wider tip of the infant Wis-Hipple is better adapted to lifting the epiglottis. With infants the wider bore or aperture of the Wis-Hipple and Flagg blades enable one to see and to pass a tube (especially the Cole tube) more easily than the flattened aperture of the Miller blades. In older children the flatter Miller No. 2 blade becomes more advantageous since it is less likely to chip large new incisor teeth. For teen-age children with stronger jaws and larger mouths a cuffed tube will often be chosen. Then it is usually easier to employ the Macintosh curved blade, which allows more room to pass the bulky cuff. The small curved blade (No. 2 Macintosh) is occasionally useful in special situations, as in a small child with an ankylosed jaw, or in burn contractures of the neck.

The light bulb is most important and deserves special attention. For small patients it is important to have the bulb near the tip of the blade. One finds considerable variation in this feature. If the bulb is more than ½ inch from the tip, the soft tissues of the infant's pharynx will close in around it and obstruct the light. The larger bulb will carry more light and will be more durable. In some laryngoscopes the bulb is recessed so that it is difficult to change or clean. Conversely, many British blades are built with the bulb on an independent carrier. This is slightly clumsy in use but is great for maintenance (Fig. 6-11).

The lighter penlight handle is easier to manipulate, but the batteries become exhausted so quickly that we find the medium-sized handle more reliable. It should be emphasized that in testing a laryngoscope, one should be sure that the light is white. One is tempted to accept any bulb that lights, but a yellow or orange color denotes a failing battery or poor connection, and the light obtained may prove quite inadequate. The metal finish of the blade, if shiny, may cause excess reflection; thus a dull finish is preferable.

It is advisable to have laryngoscopes of several different sizes for pediatric patients because of the wide variation in age, size, and underlying disease (Fig. 6-9). Recommendations for choice of suitable laryngoscopes are given in Table 6-2. For those who engage in pediatric anesthesia only occasionally, it is suggested

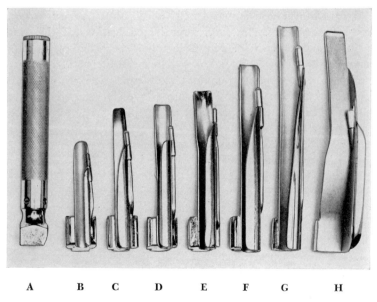

A   B   C   D   E   F   G   H

Fig. 6-9. Laryngoscopes for pediatric use. **A,** Penlite handle. **B,** Miller premature. **C,** Wis-Hipple. **D-F,** Flagg, Nos. 1, 2, and 3. **G,** Wis-Foregger No. 3. **H,** Macintosh No. 4 blades.

that the combination of a Wis-Hipple infant blade and a Miller No. 2 blade will prove the most versatile two-blade set (Fig. 6-10). One may start with these and add to them as the need arises (Fig. 6-9). When possible, a choice should be available, and one will find that the smallest blade that can be used easily will result in the least trauma. In addition to this equipment, bronchoscopic apparatus should be available at all times for use by the anesthesia service.

Nonrebreathing apparatus. Nonrebreathing techniques are essential in pediatric anesthesia. Two methods are popular at present: the valveless technique introduced by Ayre,[4,5] employing a T or a Y tube, and the nonrebreathing valve method, introduced by Leigh and Belton[6] and subsequently modified by Stephen and Slater,[7] Fink,[8] and others.[9,10]

Equipment for the Ayre method consisted originally of a specially constructed metal T tube (Fig. 6-12). Although this still is popular and effective, a number of

Table 6-2. *Laryngoscopes recommended for use in infants and children*

Age	Type of laryngoscope blade	Length (mm.)
Premature and newborn	Miller premature	75
Newborn to 1 mo.	Wis-Hipple	100
1 mo. to 1 yr.	No. 1 Flagg	102
1 to 3 yr.	No. 2 Flagg	110
3 to 10 yr.	No. 2 Miller	154
10 to 16 yr.	Wis-Foregger No. 3	162
16 yr. and over	Macintosh No. 4	158

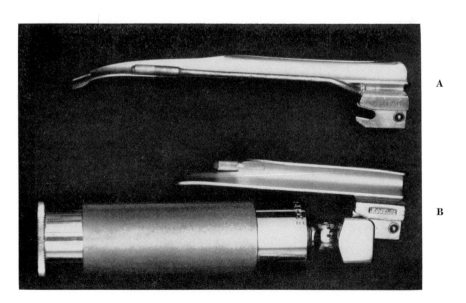

Fig. 6-10. Recommended basic combination of laryngoscope blades for pediatric use. **A,** Miller No. 2 blade. **B,** Wis-Hipple infant blade.

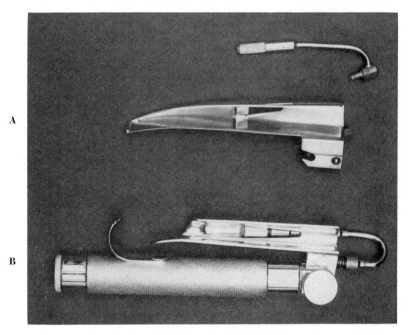

Fig. 6-11.   English laryngoscopes. **A,** Robertshaw. **B,** Anderson.

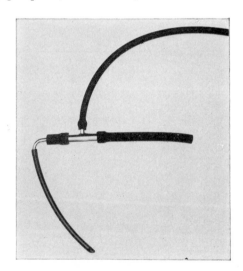

Fig. 6-12.   Original Ayre T-tube nonrebreathing system.

modifications have been introduced to fit different conditions. Plastic T tubes and Y-shaped tubes of metal or plastic are all useful provided that the lumen of all such adapters is not smaller than that of the endotracheal tube. For infants under 1 year of age a ¼-inch lumen usually is adequate (Fig. 6-13). Children more than 1 year of age require a Y tube with a larger lumen. A Y tube with a ½-inch bore may be purchased as a standard piece of anesthetic apparatus.

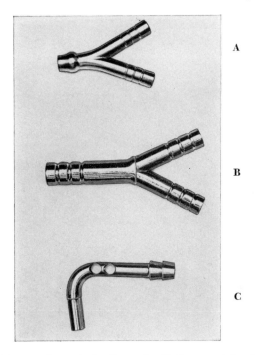

Fig. 6-13. Variations of Ayre τ pieces. **A**, Small γ tube. **B**, Large γ tube. **C**, Turnbull harelip adapter.

As demonstrated by Lewis and Spoerel[11] the simplest type of nonrebreathing system consists merely of providing a generous hole in the adapter of the endotracheal tube. This can be made by cutting a hole in the rubber inflow tubing or by using a perforated metal adapter. Slocum and Allen,[12] Turnbull,[13] and others have used various modifications of this principle (Fig. 6-14).

The British have consistently favored valveless nonrebreathing systems. Rees[14] introduced the concept of extending the expiratory limb of the Ayre system and providing it with an open-tailed 500-ml. breathing bag. A sufficient volume of fresh gas (2 to 3 times minute volume) is administered to prevent rebreathing, and respiration is assisted or controlled by closing the tail of the bag with the fingers and squeezing the bag. Several variations of this modification have naturally occurred. Rees uses a thick, straight tube, while many use a corrugated tube to allow better manipulation (Fig. 6-15). The Montreal version adds an adjustable valve at the tail of the bag and a rubber venting valve on the bag, so placed that the thumb will close it with each manual assist on the bag. Keats has designed an adapter to replace the τ piece (Fig. 6-16). This more conveniently conducts inflow and outflow gases in parallel; it also reduces dead space by bringing inflow gases right up to the mask, rather than mixing them in the adapter or τ piece (Fig. 6-17).

The Hustead τ-piece adapter (Fig. 6-16) goes one step further. By special construction of inlet and escape outlet, any flow of 4 L. or more will guarantee CO_2 elimination and adequate release of pressure. A proposed "standard" pe-

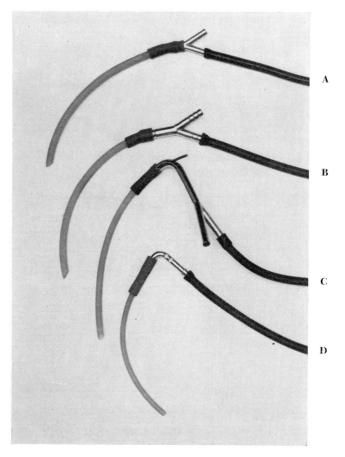

Fig. 6-14. Assembled apparatus for Ayre systems. **A,** Small Y. **B,** Large Y. **C,** Meade. **D,** Turnbull adapters. Probe at angle of Meade adapter indicates orifice for suction.

diatric apparatus has also been suggested, consisting of a sequence of one-way adapting units (Fig. 6-18). This assembly carries the danger of falling apart.

Nonrebreathing valves. Leigh and Belton's[6] original nonrebreathing valve consisted of a metal casing fitted with two metal one-way valves, the first allowing ingress of gases from the anesthetic machine and reservoir bag, the second providing exit for expired air (Figs. 6-19 and 6-20). Stephen and Slater[7] modified this by replacing the metal valves with light rubber valves but retaining the same basic design. A disadvantage of this system is that both hands must be used if assisted or controlled respiration is desired. To meet this difficulty Fink[8] constructed a valve with a vent connecting the reservoir bag to the exhalation orifice, which enables the anesthetist to assist or control respiration using only one hand. By squeezing the bag, the bag contents are forced through the inspiratory valve and at the same time through the vent, thus closing the exhalation valve and forcing gases into the patient. For expiration, release of pressure on the bag

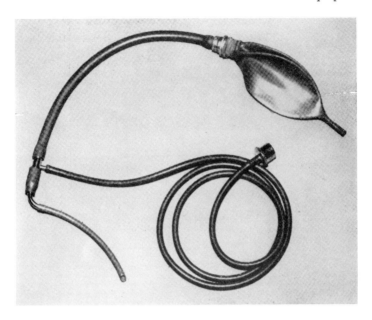

Fig. 6-15. Nonrebreathing system: Rees modification of Ayre's ⊤-piece apparatus. (From Wilton, T. N. P., and Wilson, F.: Neonatal anaesthesia, Philadelphia, 1965, F. A. Davis Co.)

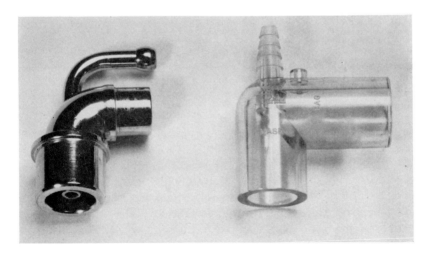

Fig. 6-16. Keats and Hustead ⊤-piece elbow adapters.

allows unobstructed escape of gas through the expiratory valve. Subsequently Frumin, Lee, and Papper,[15] Ruben,[10] and Rudolph have all introduced nonrebreathing valves of varying patterns, but all are designed for one-hand use. Most of the nonrebreathing techniques can be used with success by careful anesthesiologists. In general, however, the valveless systems have appeared less subject to such human errors as accumulation of dirt with consequent sticking of valves, improper assembling, and faulty manipulation. If a valve is to be used, it is

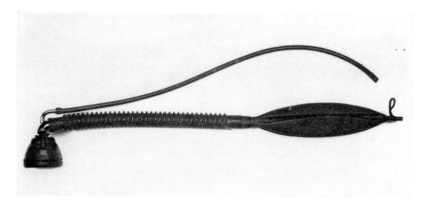

Fig. 6-17. Nonrebreathing system with Keats elbow adapter.

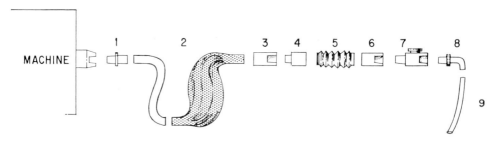

Fig. 6-18. Diagram of "standard" nonrebreathing system with noninterchangeable fittings: **1,** 15-mm. endotracheal tube connector; **2,** breathing bag; **3,** bag and breathing tube bushing, female; **4,** bag and breathing tube bushing, male; **5,** breathing tube, corrugated; **6,** bag and breathing tube bushing, female; **7,** expiratory or nonrebreathing valve; **8,** 15-mm. curved endotracheal tube adapter; **9,** endotracheal tube.

preferable for one person to retain the valve for his own use so that it will not be subject to the abuse and neglect of most common property.

The nonrebreathing valves have been designed and used almost exclusively in America, while the T-tube and its modifications have been British. The British have deservedly won this skirmish, for the valves are seldom encountered, and the more reliable T-system has become the most widely used of all pediatric techniques.

Vaporizing apparatus and humidifying devices. For vaporization of ether, a moderate degree of accuracy has been satisfactory, but for continued efficiency it has been essential to prevent excessive cooling. Glass containers have been inadequate in this respect, especially with high flows of gases.

In pediatric anesthesia a device known as the Richardson bottle served as an effective ether vaporizer for many years. This consists of a Mason jar with a metal top so constructed that a variable flow of oxygen or air could be blown over the surface of the liquid anesthetic and then carried to the patient (Fig. 6-21). Cooling is prevented by placing the ether bottle in a pan of warm water.

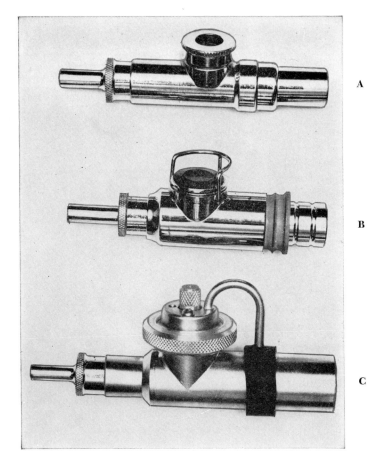

Fig. 6-19. Nonrebreathing valves. **A,** Leigh, **B,** Stephen-Slater, and, **C,** Fink valves.

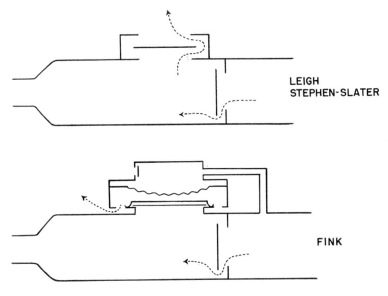

LEIGH
STEPHEN-SLATER

FINK

Fig. 6-20. Diagrams of the mechanism of nonrebreathing valves.

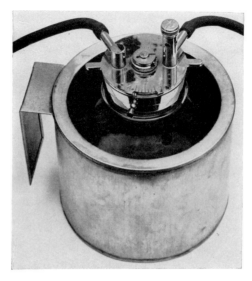

Fig. 6-21. Richardson bottle vaporizer with pan for warm-water bath.

With the introduction of halothane, which is potent and rapidly effective, it became necessary to develop more accurate anesthetic vaporizers. With the greater use of nonrebreathing systems and with the use of large gas flows, it was necessary to have vaporizers that did not cool rapidly and, when used in circle system, to have a vaporizer placed outside of the circle. The "copper kettle" is satisfactory with ether but becomes clogged with halothane. For halothane, the Fluotec* vaporizer has proved fairly satisfactory. Standard ether vaporizers may be used for methoxyflurane and fluroxene, but the Pentec* is more accurate for methoxyflurane.

Humidifiers have been badly neglected. Rashad and associates[16] showed that rapid cooling and drying are caused when unhumidified and unwarmed nonrebreathing systems are employed, and they make it obvious that the use of an effective humidifying device is definitely indicated in procedures lasting more than 30 minutes. In our hands the Bennett warming and humidifying device[17] has proved useful (Fig. 6-22). Allan mounts a halothane vaporizer on an Engström ventilator, humidifying the gases with the Engström humidifier.

Closed-system apparatus. Equipment is now available for both to-and-fro and circle absorption techniques for patients of all ages.

To-and-fro systems. The to-and-fro technique, once favored for both adult and pediatric anesthesia, is virtually extinct in adult use and is rarely seen in pediatric work. Its virtues include complete elimination of valves and retention of warmth and moisture. The undesirable features that caused its disappearance are its clumsiness, the problem of particles and "dust" of soda lime that may be blown into the patient's face and respiratory tract, and the fact that as the soda lime is used, the dead space increases.

On the other hand, the to-and-fro system is portable and more easily as-

*Ayerst Laboratories.

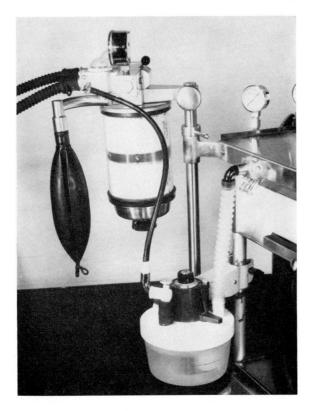

Fig. 6-22. Bennett humidifier in position in inflow line.

sembled for such cases than are the circle systems. If the to-and-fro system is to be used, equipment must be adapted to the size of each child (Fig. 6-23):

1. For infants under 5 pounds a very satisfactory apparatus may be assembled using a one-piece conductive rubber premature-sized mask, a curved metal chimney adapter with nipple, a 90-ml. canister, a straight metal adapter, and a 500-ml. conductive bag. The mask is fitted with a four-pronged head strap retainer for use with an infant four-tailed head strap (Fig. 6-24). For endotracheal anesthesia a curved or right-angled adapter is used (Fig. 6-25).

2. For infants of 5 to 10 pounds a newborn-sized mask and a 1-L. double-ended bag with escape valve are substituted in the original assembly.

3. For children of 10 to 20 pounds a change is made to the child-sized mask, a 180-ml. canister, and 3-L. bag. The infant head strap will be too small and is replaced by an adult head strap (Fig. 6-24).

4. For children of 20 to 35 pounds a 250-ml. canister and 3-L. bag may be used. For children over 35 pounds the adult circle system seems preferable.

Circle system. Circle absorption apparatus has enjoyed considerable popularity for pediatric use in America but is seldom used in Britain. Its use in this country apparently reached its peak in the years between 1960 and 1965; since this time the nonrebreathing systems have largely replaced it.

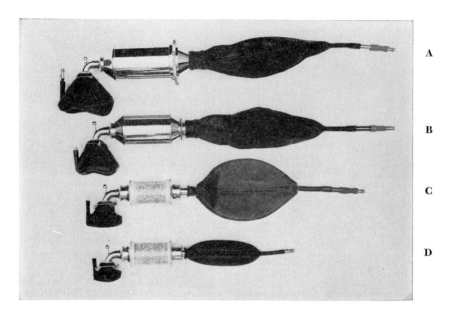

Fig. 6-23. To-and-fro apparatus. **A,** Small adult-sized mask, 250-ml. canister, 3-L. bag. **B,** Child-sized mask, 180-ml. canister, 3-L. bag. **C,** Newborn-sized mask, 90-ml. canister, 1-L. bag. **D,** Premature-sized mask, 90-ml. canister, 500-ml. bag.

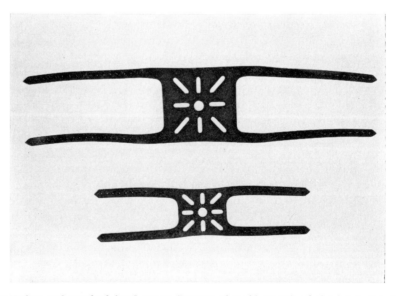

Fig. 6-24. Infant and standard head straps. Because of rapid growth of the head, the standard head strap is suitable for most patients more than 1 or 2 months of age.

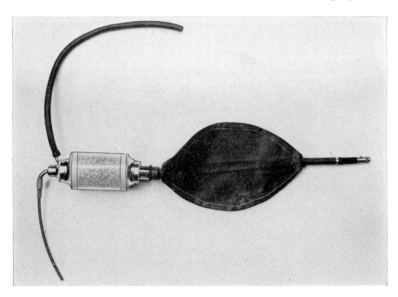

Fig. 6-25. Infant to-and-fro apparatus adapted for endotracheal anesthesia.

The advantages of the circle system are that it enables one to use an explosive gas such as cyclopropane with minimal danger (and with maximal economy). It also conserves body heat and moisture, as in to-and-fro apparatus; but dead space does not increase as soda lime is exhausted, and there is less chance that absorber "dust" will be blown into the patient's mouth and lungs.

Several different types of circle absorption apparatus have been designed. Leigh and Belton[6] introduced an early model using a 90-ml. canister and incorporating valves in the chimney adapter. Adriani, Griggs, and Berson[18,19] introduced an apparatus using normal adult canisters, a divided chimney piece to reduce dead space, and a rubber bulb with which to help circulate gases in the system. Hay of the Ohio Chemical Company fashioned a more compact unit, using the divided chimney, and added a sensitive pressure gauge (Fig. 6-26). Next came the Bloomquist[20] version, which was basically similar to the original Leigh model except that a 350-ml. canister was used and fixed in a vertical position on a mobile arm attached to the anesthesia machine (Fig. 6-27).

A combination of adult absorber and half-sized breathing tubes includes advantages of both small and large systems (Fig. 6-28).

Two faults exist in the circle system. The main disadvantage lies in the fact that any circle apparatus must depend upon valves, and valves always introduce the hazard of increased resistance due to sticking and faulty action. Many unnecessary complications have already been caused by the use of various types of valves, and their use does not seem justified with small or weak infants. A second and minor disadvantage consists of the fact that most of the infant circle systems do not have the vaporizer incorporated in the circle.

Mention should be made of the concept of the valveless circulator pump conceived by Revell and associates,[21,22] which in many respects more nearly ap-

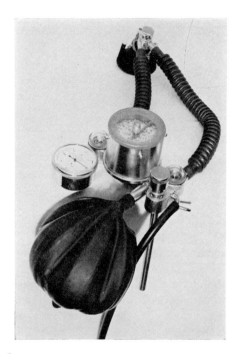

Fig. 6-26. Ohio infant circle apparatus.

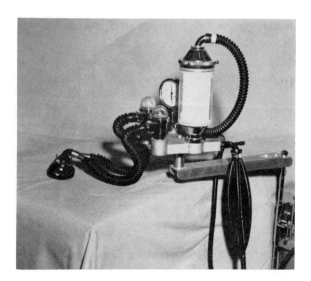

Fig. 6-27. Bloomquist infant circle apparatus.

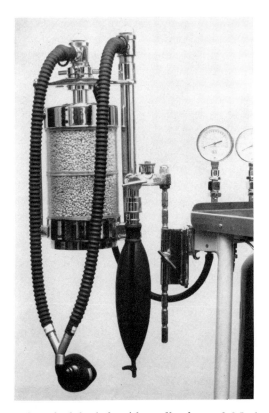

Fig. 6-28. Dundas adaptation of adult circle with small tubes and 1-L. bag.

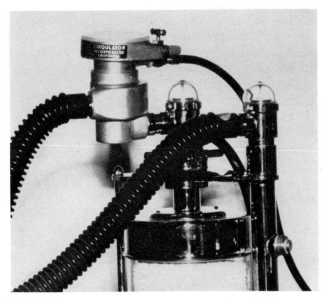

Fig. 6-29. Revell circulator.

proaches the ideal than do any of our current methods (Fig. 6-29). A small pump or fan powered by suction apparatus creates a constant circulation of gases through the circle, thus eliminating both resistance and dead space.

It should not be assumed that all parts of infant apparatus must be smaller than equivalent parts of adult equipment. If corrugated breathing tubes are too narrow, there will be excessive turbulence; if breathing bags contain less than 20 to 25 times the patient's tidal volume, a small leak will cause an empty bag, and a tight system will bring too much pressure. Valves, especially, must not be reduced in area, for large anesthesia valves open more easily than small ones. Graff, Holzman, and Benson[23] have brought many false assumptions to light in evaluating the use of adult circle apparatus for infants. If adequate flow is used, the adult circle proves acceptable for use in small infants.

Anesthesia machines. Because of frequent improvements in anesthesia machines of different makes, it is not possible to specify which one is best suited to pediatric use. There are certain specifications that should be required, however. These include accurately and finely calibrated gauges that are distinctly marked, floats that are visible at all times, fail-safe and pin-index systems, an oxygen flush valve that cannot drive oxygen or gases through a vaporizer, ready adaptability to circle or nonrebreathing systems, efficient vaporizers for ether and halothane, and a humidifying device for nonrebreathing technique. At present it seems advisable to construct machines for use with two oxygen, two nitrous oxide, and one cyclopropane attachment.

MONITORING DEVICES

For most pediatric anesthesia, relatively simple apparatus is preferable for observation of the patient. Essential equipment consists of the following items:
1. *Stethoscopes:* A stethoscope should be used throughout every procedure in pediatric anesthesia.
    (a) The *standard binaural stethoscope* is of primary importance since it is the most valuable type to use with small infants (Fig. 6-30).
    (b) The *Ploss monaural stethoscope*[24] is more comfortable and may be substituted in larger patients.
    (c) For teaching purposes, a precordial or esophageal stethoscope with two sets of earpieces is often helpful (Fig. 6-31).
    (d) An esophageal stethoscope will prove useful in many thoracic procedures, as well as in children with burns of the upper thorax (Fig. 6-32).
2. *Blood pressure equipment:* Blood pressure cuffs suitable for all ages should be available (Figs. 6-33 and 6-34). The following sizes are recommended:
    (a) Newborn infant size (inflatable cuff $5\frac{1}{4}$ by $1\frac{1}{4}$ inches)*
    (b) Large infant size (inflatable cuff 6 by $2\frac{1}{4}$ inches)*
    (c) Child size (inflatable cuff 6 by 3 inches)†
    (d) Small adult size (inflatable cuff 9 by 4 inches)†

---

*Davol Rubber Co., Providence, R. I.
†W. A. Baum Co., Copiague, N. Y.

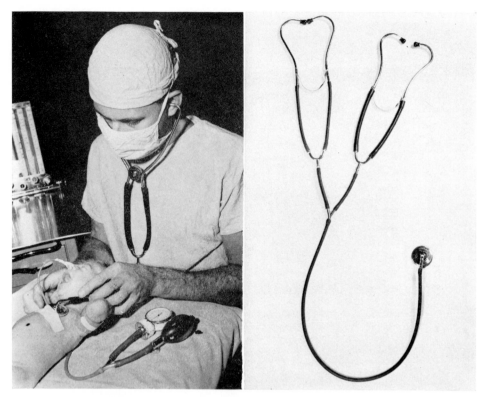

Fig. 6-30   Fig. 6-31

Fig. 6-30. Standard binaural stethoscope is most reliable for use in infants. (From Smith, R. M.: Internat. Anesth. Clin. 1:153, 1962.)

Fig. 6-31. Stethoscope with two headpieces for teaching purposes.

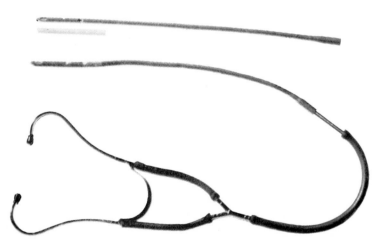

Fig. 6-32. Esophageal stethoscope, made by cutting additional holes toward the end of a urethral catheter and covering them with a thin tubular rubber dam. The catheter is then joined to an earpiece. (From Smith, R. M.: In Benson, C. D., Mustard, W. T., Ravitch, M. M., Snyder, W. H., and Welch, K. J.: Pediatric surgery, Chicago, 1962, Year Book Medical Publishers, Inc.)

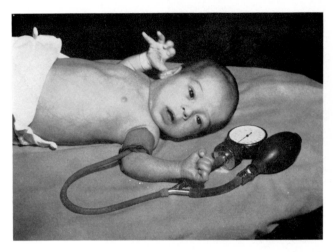

Fig. 6-33. Satisfactory blood pressure apparatus is now available for patients of all sizes. (From Smith, R. M.: Internat. Anesth. Clin. 1:153, 1962.)

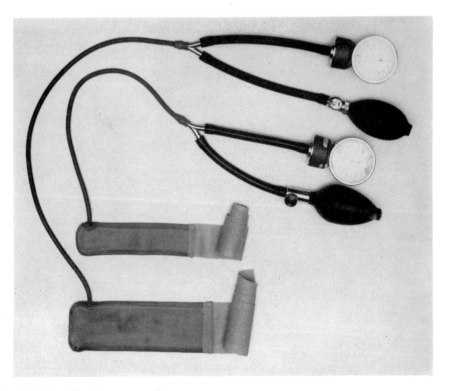

Fig. 6-34. Infant blood pressure cuffs.

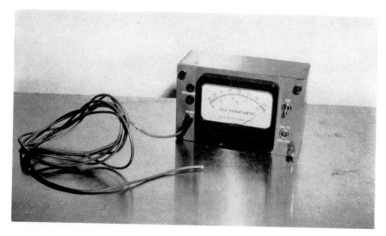

Fig. 6-35. Thermometer with esophageal or rectal probe for continuous registration of temperature. (From Smith, R. M.: Internat. Anesth. Clin. 1:153, 1962.)

3. *The chart:* Actually the anesthesia chart is one of the most valuable monitoring devices if used rationally. Visible continuing recording of vital signs makes an invaluable aid in evaluation of the patient's response to anesthesia and operation.

4. *Thermometer:* Continuous temperature indicator with rectal and esophageal probes* (Fig. 6-35).

5. *Water mattress to control body temperature:* Though not a monitoring device, it is a necessity and may be included here.

6. *Wright spirometer:* Measurement of respiratory exchange and pressure is not yet carried out as a routine procedure; however, the Wright spirometer is of practical value in many situations. It is also useful to incorporate a pressure-registering device into apparatus used for infant anesthesia.

7. *Venous pressure determination* is of special importance in patients undergoing open heart procedures, or in any operation involving extensive blood replacement, especially when the patient has an enlarged or weakened heart.

Additional equipment may be useful for a particular situation. The electrocardiograph, though not necessary as a routine, certainly should always be available, and should be used for any patients in critical condition, for those with cardiac arrhythmias, and for patients undergoing extensive surgical procedures. Oximeters, carbon dioxide analyzers, and the electroencephalograph have occasional use for special operations and for investigational purposes.

CARE OF EQUIPMENT

It is naturally essential that anesthetic equipment must be kept in good working order, must be cleaned thoroughly after use, and many items must be steril-

---

*Yellow Springs Instrument Co., Yellow Springs, Ohio.

ized. Scrubbing with soap and water is adequate for articles that do not enter a patient's mouth. Sterilization with ethylene oxide may be used for breathing tubes, masks, breathing bags, and airways as an effective method of cleaning all types of equipment without damaging the material. Although routine sterilization of endotracheal tubes by ethylene oxide has been widely employed, there is danger of chemical irritation of cords and trachea unless tubes have been thoroughly aired for a prolonged time (48 hours or more). An intelligent cleansing routine might prove more practical for general use.

VENTILATING DEVICES AND RESUSCITATORS

Most of the mechanical ventilating devices may be adapted for use in the operating room, and several have been designed specifically for this purpose. They may be used for larger children during extensive procedures such as spinal fusion, laminectomy, or various orthopedic or general surgical operations. Usually it seems preferable to avoid the use of these devices for most pediatric anesthesia and to retain the use of manual bag management. This is especially desirable during thoracic procedures in which manual inflation of the lungs can easily be timed to give the surgeon optimal opportunity for a quiet field.

Devices such as the Kreiselman unit may be used to revive newborn infants in the delivery room, but otherwise mechanical resuscitators are rarely needed in operating rooms where standard anesthetic apparatus is available.

For postoperative assistance of apneic or depressed patients, mechanical ventilators may be of great service. Standard tank respirators (iron lungs) are satisfactory for children with brain damage following neurosurgery, but following thoracic operations ventilators that do not enclose the body are mandatory. A machine for this purpose should be designed so that air may be mixed with oxygen and the mixture may be humidified and warmed. Simplicity in design is important because constantly shifting teams of residents and nurses may have to manage the apparatus. The ultimate ventilator should be adaptable to the smallest infant, as well as to a large adult, with respiratory rate, sensitivity, and pressures varying accordingly. Furthermore, it should be dependable for continuous effective ventilation in spite of slight changes in patient compliance or respiratory effort. To date, no single ventilator appears to fill this need. Bennett, Emerson, Bird, and Engström ventilators all are adaptable to small infants. Further improvements are developing in this rapidly progressing area (Chapter 29).

Apparatus should be available throughout every hospital for ventilating patients who suddenly develop respiratory depression or apnea. Each of our nursing wards is equipped with a large tackle box labeled "Resuscitation Apparatus," and each of these kits has standard equipment consisting of an Ambu self-inflating ventilating bag with assorted masks, laryngoscopes, endotracheal tubes, and adapters, suction catheters, and narcotic antagonists. If a patient shows ventilatory insufficiency, the airway is cleared and ventilatory assistance is immediately provided by abdominal compression, mouth-to-mouth, or bag-and-mask resuscitation. If necessary, an endotracheal tube is passed, and direct inflation of the lungs is carried out.

ACCESSORY APPARATUS

There are numerous items invaluable to the pediatric anesthetist that he may not appreciate until he has to work in a hospital where they are not provided. It is certainly easier for the team if the operating table is narrower than usually employed for adults. It is even more important to have special ether screens, arm boards, and such table accessories.

Several different sizes of the regulation ether screen should be available. A small adjustable screen has been of great service in our experience. This is a homemade device constructed of brass and having a broad base that may be slipped under the mattress of the operating table for stabilization (Fig. 6-36). The adjustable crossbar may be raised or rotated to the position needed. This is especially useful to support the drapes during mastoid or facial surgery where standard screens are inadequate.

Padded arm boards for intravenous work will be needed in several sizes (6 by 2 inches, 8 by 3 inches, 12 by 3 inches, and 18 by 4 inches). Special infusion apparatus is of much importance and will be described in Chapter 26.

Padded head rings or "doughnuts" to facilitate endotracheal intubation or for support during neurosurgery and other procedures are useful and may be prepared by wrapping sponge rubber rings with sheet wadding. For infants a ring 5 inches in diameter is adequate, whereas larger rings 8 and 10 inches in diameter are better for older children.

Two metal arm supports were designed for specific purposes. The first is a two-tiered adjustable support for patients in the lateral position (Fig. 6-37). The lower plate is fixed, but the upper plate may be raised or rotated as desired.

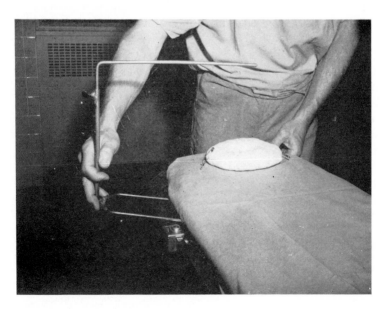

Fig. 6-36. Adjustable pediatric ether screen.

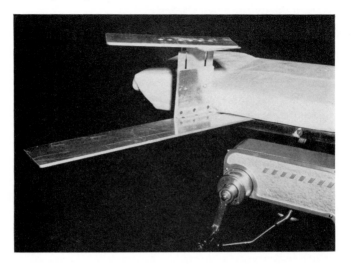

Fig. 6-37. Two-tiered adjustable arm support for maintaining patients in lateral position.

The second device was made to support the arms of patients during spinal fusion. Each arm support consists of two metal plates with an adjustable joint to allow the arms to rest in flexion.

TOYS AND MORALE BUILDERS

Usually children must wait near the operating room until anesthesia is started. A room should be provided where they can be watched by specially trained personnel. Toys, books, and well-chosen music will promote relaxation. The walls and even ceilings may be painted or decorated to interest and comfort the children.

Toys must be soft and have no sharp edges or detachable or edible parts. Balloons are popular and meet these requirements. There seems to be an ever-increasing number of children who are devoted to a "security blanket" or some disheveled rag doll that gives them great comfort. These are not taken from the child, for they often play an important part in keeping up his morale. Similarly, infants who are kept happy by constantly sucking on rubber nipples are allowed to retain them.

Several specially constructed toys have been designed to induce children to accept anesthesia. Nitrous oxide or cyclopropane may be blown at unsuspecting children through tubes concealed in telephones or toy animals. Although these have considerable popular appeal, in our experience a music box has been the most effective device to help the anesthetist lull a small child to sleep.

REFERENCES

1. Brown, E. S., and Hustead, R. F.: Rebreathing in pediatric anesthesia systems, Anesthesiology **28**:241-242, 1967.
2. Cole, F.: A new endotracheal tube for infants, Anesthesiology **6**:87-88, 1945.
3. Cole, F.: An endotracheal tube for babies, Anesthesiology **6**:627-628, 1945.

4. Ayre, P.: Anesthesia for harelip and cleft palate in babies, Brit. J. Surg. **25**:131-132, 1937.
5. Ayre, P.: Endotracheal anesthesia for babies: with special reference to harelip and cleft palate operations, Anesth. Analg. **16**:330-333, 1937.
6. Leigh, M. D., and Belton, M. K.: Pediatric anesthesia, ed. 2, New York, 1960, The Macmillan Co.
7. Stephen, C. R., and Slater, H. M.: Nonresisting, nonbreathing valve, Anesthesiology **9**:550-552, 1948.
8. Fink, B. R.: A nonrebreathing valve of new design, Anesthesiology **15**:471-474, 1954.
9. Lewis, G. B., and Leigh, M. D.: Lewis-Leigh nonrebreathing valve, Anesthesiology **17**:618, 1956.
10. Ruben, H.: A new nonrebreathing valve, Anesthesiology **16**:643-645, 1955.
11. Lewis, A., and Spoerel, W. E.: A modification of Ayre's technique, Canad. Anaesth. Soc. J. **8**:501-511, 1961.
12. Slocum, H. C., and Allen, C. R.: Orotracheal anesthesia for cheiloplasty, Anesthesiology **6**:355-358, 1945.
13. Turnbull, L. F.: Pediatric endotracheal connectors, Anesthesiology **16**:1034-1035, 1955.
14. Rees, J. G.: The child as a subject for anaesthesia. In Evans, F. T., and Gray, T. C., editors: Modern trends in anaesthesia, New York, 1958, Paul B. Hoeber, Inc., Medical Book Department of Harper & Row, Publishers.
15. Frumin, M. J., Lee, A. S. J., and Papper, E. M.: New valve for nonrebreathing systems, Anesthesiology **20**:383-385, 1959.
16. Rashad, K., Wilson, K., Hurt, H. H., Jr., Graff, T. D., and Benson, D. W.: Effect of humidification of anesthetic gases on static compliance, Anesth. Analg. **46**:127-133, 1967.
16a. Allan, D.: Personal communication.
17. Wynands, J. E.: A simple method of humidifying gases, Canad. Anaesth. Soc. J. **13**:403-405, 1966.
18. Adriani, J., and Griggs, T.: Rebreathing in pediatric anesthesia: recommendations and descriptions of improvements in apparatus, Anesthesiology **14**:337-347, 1953.
19. Griggs, T., Adriani, J., and Berson, W.: Aids to pediatric anesthesia, Anesth. Analg. **32**:340-349, 1953.
20. Bloomquist, E. R.: Pediatric circle absorber, Anesthesiology **18**:787-789, 1957.
21. Revell, D. G.: Circulator to eliminate mechanical dead space in circle absorption systems, Canad. Anaesth. Soc. J. **6**:98-103, 1959.
22. Roffey, P. J., Revell, D. G., and Morris, L. E.: An assessment of the Revell circulator, Anesthesiology **22**:583-590, 1961.
23. Graff, T. D., Holzman, R. S., and Benson, D. W.: Acid-base balance in infants during halothane anesthesia with use of an adult circle-absorption system, Anesth. Analg. **43**:583-589, 1964.
24. Ploss, R. E.: A simple constant monitor system, Anesthesiology **16**:466-467, 1955.
25. Winchell, S. W., and Davis, G.: Sterilization and care of equipment. In Safar, P., editor: Respiratory therapy, Philadelphia, 1965, F. A. Davis Co.

AVAILABLE METHODS AND STANDARD PROCEDURES

Most of the agents employed in adult anesthesia may be used for infants and children,[1] and there are proponents of spinal, epidural, intravenous, intramuscular, and rectal routes of administration (Table 7-1). From the standpoint of safety and practicality, however, the field can be narrowed down considerably.

The inhalation technique is the most widely used method in pediatric anesthesia. This technique is simple, versatile, effective, and easily controlled. Among the various agents ether long remained the undisputed prototype for children. Reliance was placed upon ether for several reasons, among which were minimal respiratory depression, reliable anesthetic signs, gradual change of anesthetic depth,[2] good relaxation, compatibility with catecholamines, and vagolytic action. In spite of these attributes, ether has been completely discarded by many pediatric anesthetists, while others retain its use either for teaching purposes or because of economic restrictions. This has come about because of the general preference for nonexplosive agents in all situations, plus the irritative effect of ether on respiratory and gastrointestinal systems. Secretions are excessive with ether, and

Table 7-1. *Agents and techniques available for pediatric anesthesia*

Agents	Techniques
For use with local techniques	Local
Procaine (Novocain)	Topical
Tetracaine (Pontocaine)	Infiltration
Lidocaine (Xylocaine)	Regional
Dyclonine (Dyclone)	
Prilocaine (Citanest)	
For inhalation anesthesia	Inhalation
Divinyl ether (Vinethene)	Open-drop
Diethyl ether	Insufflation
Ethyl chloride	Nonrebreathing methods
Chloroform	Ayre tube
Trichlorethylene (Trilene)	Nonrebreathing valves
Halothane (Fluothane)	Semiopen
Methoxyflurane (Penthrane)	Semiclosed
Fluroxene (Fluoromar)	Closed
Nitrous oxide	To-and-fro absorption
Ethylene	Circle
Cyclopropane	Endotracheal
	Oral
	Nasal
For rectal administration	Rectal
Tribromoethanol (Avertin)	
Thiobarbiturates	
Thiopental (Pentothal)	
Thiamylal (Surital)	
Methohexital (Brevital)	
For intravenous and intramuscular use	Intravenous
Barbiturates	
Propanidid	
Relaxants	Intramuscular
d-Tubocurarine	
Gallamine (Flaxedil)	
Succinylcholine (Anectine, Scoline)	
Decamethonium (Syncurine)	
Neuroleptanalgesia	
Droperidol	
Fentanyl	
CI-581	
Combinations of above	Combinations of above

postoperative nausea and vomiting, though numerically not always excessive, appear much more distasteful to the patient.

One of the great underlying factors in the changing attitude toward ether lies in the fact that this agent is no longer the old standby familiar to all. A customary reason for using ether in children formerly was that in unusual situations it would be wisest to use the agent one knew best. Anesthetists no longer know ether best

—some know it hardly at all; consequently in approaching the occasional pediatric patient ether is as strange to them as is the child, and they are more confident with their favorite halogenated agents or relaxants.

In the displacement of ether, cyclopropane was the first to assume any importance. In small infants, children with cardiac lesions, and many poor-risk patients, the rapid smooth induction, ease of control, and prompt return of all functions gave cyclopropane preference in a large number of cases. Only its explosibility prevented it from being widely used throughout all pediatric anesthesia.

Shortly after its introduction for use in adults in 1956, halothane (Fluothane) was tried in pediatric anesthesia and promptly gained wide favor. Initially there was considerable apprehension concerning halogen toxicity, myocardial depression, and the absence of suitable signs of anesthetic depth. Following meticulous investigative study and caution in its early clinical use, application of the agent was gradually expanded to all aspects of pediatric anesthesia. Although small infants appeared to show appreciable cardiovascular depression, older children tolerated it better than adults. Clinical signs, though meager, proved sufficient for adequate control, and no cases of hepatic toxicity were reported. In many respects halothane was considered especially adaptable to pediatric anesthesia and has been employed by several as the standard agent for most pediatric operations.

Outstanding advantages of halothane were nonflammability, decreased irritant quality, and rapid awakening. Although such minor disadvantages as respiratory depression and incomplete relaxation prevented its acceptance as the ideal anesthetic, halothane, by 1963, had become a close rival to ether in most parts of the world and in many had completely displaced it. Related halogenated agents, methoxyflurane (Penthrane) and fluroxene (Fluoromar), also enjoyed increasing usage, although these agents showed less versatility. After halothane had become generally accepted, reports of hepatic necrosis in 1963 caused serious concern,[3-6] but this was quieted in 1966 by the appearance of the report of the Subcommittee on the National Halothane Study,[7] and use of halothane became more widespread than ever. During 1967 one death in our hospital and news of several other cases of massive liver necrosis[8] greatly reduced our enthusiasm for halogenated agents; however, their use continues to increase throughout the world.

More recent additions to the field of pediatric anesthesia have been the combination of droperidol and fentanyl, known as neuroleptanalgesia, and a short-acting drug thus far termed CI-581. Droperidol is a long-acting (8-12 hr.) dissociative sedative that may show pyramidal tract twitching late in the recovery phase, while fentanyl is a potent, very short-acting narcotic. Although this particular combination seems of restricted value in children,[9] the intravenous use of a hypnotic and potent narcotic shows increasing value. Morphine and propiomazine have been employed successfully in older children. CI-581 acts as a heavy sedative with marked analgesic powers and may prove useful for pneumoencephalography, burn dressings, and similar procedures.[10]

Propanidid, a drug basically similar to eugenol, has gained favorable reports as a truly rapidly metabolized agent especially suited to short outpatient procedures. It is used intravenously in 5% solution and is less irritative than the earlier eugenol.

CONSIDERATIONS DETERMINING CHOICE

In assessing the merits of both drugs and techniques, it is important to consider many individual factors of the patient and the situation rather than to limit attention to the relative merits of methods to be employed. Among the most important variables are the following:

1. Age of the child
2. Operative considerations (operation, position, use of cautery)
3. Disease and general condition of the patient
4. Experience of the anesthetist
5. Preference of the surgeon
6. Preference of the patient
7. Local factors

Age. The age of the child does not set strict rules but limits the choice considerably and suggests the following generalizations:

1. The very premature or weak infant needs little anesthesia, and often local infiltration serves best for other than intrathoracic procedures. Cyclopropane, halothane, or d-tubocurarine each has advantages for use in the newborn. Small infants resist ether strenuously, and inductions may be prolonged and associated with cyanosis and depression. Halothane has the advantage of being nonirritative, but cardiorespiratory depression may occur with little warning.
2. Healthy infants will tolerate most agents, but cardiorespiratory reflexes are active, obstruction by secretions or spasm is easily stimulated, and slow induction may be associated with crying and excitement. Halothane appears least irritative of the inhalation agents. A previously established infusion or easily available vein may be used to avoid induction hazards. Relaxation is not a major problem in this age, and use of deep anesthesia or relaxants is not usually necessary.
3. Valves offer resistance and are best avoided in smaller infants. A general principal not to use any respiratory valves in patients weighing less than 10 pounds has been observed locally with satisfaction. Our local custom has been to use valveless systems in patients under 10 pounds, an infant circle or T system in infants 10 to 35 pounds, and an adult circle system for children over 35 pounds.
4. It seems preferable not to use intravenous agents for maintenance of anesthesia in children under 6 or 8 years of age for fear of immediate and/or prolonged respiratory depression.
5. Many children tolerate local anesthesia and brachial block surprisingly well, but their reactions are difficult to predict. To employ spinal anesthesia in children under 10 or 12 years of age or to expect them to undergo any prolonged or extensive procedure under local anesthesia seems to be asking too much of them.

Operative considerations. The type of operation to be undertaken, its duration, the relaxation required, the position of the patient, and the expected use of cautery or x-ray are factors to take into account.

Disease and general condition of patient. The major surgical pathology is of primary importance in determining the type of anesthesia. The presence of a brain tumor demands a smooth induction and avoidance of elevation of cerebral fluid pressure; liver and renal diseases rule against the use of agents that are broken down or excreted by these organs; and poliomyelitis usually rules out the use of spinal anesthesia. Many other specific lesions will deserve consideration.

In such generalized conditions as malnourishment, toxicity, or metabolic imbalance it is better to avoid ether and to employ agents that have little metabolic effect and that are rapidly excreted, such as cyclopropane or nitrous oxide and short-acting relaxants.

Experience of anesthetist. Regardless of his experience with adults, an anesthetist who has had limited experience in pediatric anesthesia will do well to use conservative methods with children. Errors will be few and they will be forgiven. Relaxants and intravenous and block anesthesia have advantages, but only when used by qualified individuals. This does not mean that special techniques should be restricted to personnel in teaching or specialized hospitals. It implies that an anesthetist should refrain from using complicated approaches until he has had considerable experience in the use of standard inhalation techniques and unless he can use the more exacting techniques often enough to maintain proficiency in these methods.

Preference of surgeon. Although the opinion of the surgeon should not be the predominating factor, his wishes certainly should be given due consideration. Compromises must often be made by both anesthetist and surgeon, and the fear of losing face must be put aside when considering the best way to get a job done. Usually there are several alternative methods that are suitable, and if one of them makes the surgeon's task less difficult, it is only reasonable to use that one.

Preference of patient. On similar grounds, even the patient has a right to say which agent he likes best. Some children who have been anesthetized several times prefer an induction by intravenous methods rather than by inhalation, whereas with others the situation is reversed.

Local factors. Several additional influences may alter the normal choice of anesthetic or technique. In hot climates, especially when the humidity is great, the natural tendency will be to avoid the use of ether unless operating rooms are air-conditioned. Many hospitals are still without modern conductive equipment, and in these it is not uncommon to find that the use of cyclopropane has been officially banned. Although alternative methods may be used with equally good results, it is unfortunate to have the choice of anesthetic limited by restrictions that are unnecessary or are easily overcome.

RECOMMENDED AGENTS AND TECHNIQUES

In general, certain broad policies can be recommended on the basis of experience. Inhalation anesthesia is recommended as first choice for most cases because of its simplicity, controllability, and effectiveness. Unless an infusion has already been established, a nicely prepared child usually can be anesthetized more gently by blowing a nonirritant gas over his face than by use of intravenous injection. Maintenance then is merely a matter of administration of the same anesthetic by means of mask or endotracheal tube. There is a definite tendency to abandon all explosive agents, and although it appears that the possibility of explosion has been greatly overestimated by commercial exploitation, there are definite advantages in the actual elimination of any hazard of such magnitude. For these reasons, halothane today seems the agent of choice in about 75% of pediatric anesthesia. Intravenous barbiturates with nitrous oxide and narcotics make useful combinations for orthopedic operations in older children, while relaxants are especially valuable for intubation and for patients needing additional relaxation.

Endotracheal intubation is used not as a standard routine but is reserved for situations in which intubation will be definitely advantageous for the patient. When nonrebreathing systems are employed, the Ayre T-tube method usually is given priority. Many of the reasons for such preferences will be given in discussions of individual procedures in later chapters.

SIGNIFICANT FEATURES OF GENERAL ANESTHETIC AGENTS AND RELAXANTS

For complete information concerning anesthetic agents, one should consult the standard texts of pharmacology and current literature.[11,12] Brief information is presented in Table 7-2 to point out the important advantages and disadvantages of various anesthetics when used for children.

INHALATION TECHNIQUES

Since inhalation techniques used in children differ considerably from those commonly employed for adults, they deserve special discussion.

Open-drop anesthesia. Open-drop anesthesia has the advantage of being extremely simple and available under widely varying circumstances. Since respiration cannot be assisted, only anesthetics that stimulate respiration, such as divinyl ether and ether, should be given by this method.

In a teaching program the open-drop technique forms an excellent basic approach since it enables the anesthetist to visualize the details of the anesthetic process most clearly. With practice the method becomes a skill that can be applied successfully to many situations.

During open-drop anesthesia one should try to keep a steady, slow rate of administration rather than to soak the mask and then rest. Oxygen is introduced under the mask at 500 ml. per minute. The eyes are covered with a dry cloth, and the anesthetist is careful not to allow ether to get into the child's eyes. At intervals the mask is raised so that the child's face can be examined for skin irritation or pressure marks.

Insufflation. Insufflation is not employed frequently but may serve a purpose for minor procedures, especially those performed near the face and mouth. If a mole is to be removed from a child's cheek or an eyebrow is to be sutured, anesthesia can be maintained by attaching the rubber anesthesia tubing to an airway having a nipple or to a large catheter inserted into nostril or pharynx, thus avoiding necessity of endotracheal intubation in a child soon to be discharged.

Since one cannot assist respiration, here again one is limited to the choice of nondepressing agents. Obviously resuscitation is not readily carried out by this method.

Table 7-2. *Important advantages and disadvantages of various anesthetics*

Advantages	Disadvantages
Chloroform[13,14]	
1. Nonirritating	1. Toxic to liver
2. Rapid induction and recovery	2. Myocardial depression
3. Good relaxation	3. Limitations: generally discarded as too toxic to heart and liver
4. Nonexplosive	
Cyclopropane	
1. Pleasant, generally nonirritating	1. Explosive
2. Rapid induction and recovery	2. Sensitizes myocardium
3. Controllable	3. Bronchoconstrictor
4. Adequate relaxation	4. Dangerous with explosive hazards and for patients with toxic thyroid or pheochromocytoma
5. No secretions	
6. 100% anesthetic	
7. Indicated in poor-risk patients, prematurity, newborn, and cardiac disease for induction and maintenance	
Divinyl ether	
1. Pleasanter than ether	1. Explosive
2. Stimulates respiration	2. Irritant, emetic
3. Rapid induction and recovery	3. Convulsive action[15]
4. Easy to administer and control	4. Toxic danger in patients with liver damage, nutritional disease
	5. Dangerous in weak patients; all use limited to 15 minutes
Ether	
1. Minimal respiratory depression	1. Irritant
2. Good relaxation	2. Explosive
3. Highly soluble	3. Emetic
4. Reliable signs of anesthetic depth	4. Potential myocardial depression[16]
5. Bronchodilator	5. Dangerous with full stomach, prematurity, uncontrolled diabetes, myasthenia gravis, and metabolic disorders
6. A 100% anesthetic	
Ethyl chloride	
1. Less irritant than ether	1. Myocardial depressant
2. Rapid induction and recovery	2. Toxic to liver
3. Easy to administer and control	3. Explosive
4. Local anesthesia by freezing (poor)	4. Limitations: generally discarded as unsafe due to myocardial effect[17]
Ethylene	
1. Analgesic	1. Explosive
2. Does not disturb metabolism	2. Unpleasant smell
	3. Poor relaxant
	4. Requires low oxygen concentration
Fluroxene (Fluoromar)	
1. Nonexplosive	1. Poor relaxant
2. Nonirritant	2. Emetic
3. Mild cardiorespiratory depressant	
4. No catecholamine sensitization	

Table 7-2. *Important advantages and disadvantages of various anesthetics—cont'd*

Advantages	Disadvantages
Halothane (Fluothane)[18-26]	
1. Nonexplosive	1. Myocardial depressant[24]
2. Pleasant	2. Sensitizes to catecholamines
3. Nonirritating	3. Awakening excitement
4. No secretions	4. Possible hepatotoxicity
5. Rapid action	
6. Nonemetic	
Methoxyflurane (Penthrane)[27,28]	
1. Nonexplosive	1. Prolonged induction and recovery
2. Good relaxant	2. Emetic
3. Very soluble in blood; great margin of safety	
4. No catecholamine sensitization	
Nitrous oxide[29]	
1. Pleasant	1. Weak, poor relaxant
2. Nonexplosive	2. Difficult to control
3. Analgesic	3. Requires low O_2 concentrations
4. Nonemetic	4. Limitations: poor agent to use alone for surgery requiring relaxation
5. No effect on metabolism	
6. Indicated for short minor surgery without relaxation, induction in open or closed system, and as supplement for thiopental and relaxant	
Trichloroethylene[30-32]	
1. Pleasant	1. Weak, poor relaxant
2. Nonirritating	2. Tachypnea
3. Analgesic	3. Cardiac irregularities
4. Nonexplosive	4. Myocardial depressant
5. Good for dental extractions, short minor procedures with nitrous oxide	5. Combines with CO_2 absorbent to form HCL and dichloracetylene
	6. Limitations: must not be used in presence of CO_2 absorbent
Intravenous barbiturates	
1. Pleasant induction if needle already in place	1. Needle undesirable to most children
2. Suitable for maintenance of older children, if supplemented	2. Poor analgesic
3. Nonexplosive	3. Poor relaxant
4. Nonemetic	4. Increased danger of laryngospasm
	5. Parasympathomimetic
	6. May have prolonged depression
	7. Total dose should be limited to 10 mg. per pound of body weight
	8. Contraindicated in patients with full stomach, or in prone position, having decreased respiratory exchange or for maintenance in children under 6 years of age

Table 7-2. *Important advantages and disadvantages of various anesthetics—cont'd*

Advantages	Disadvantages
Relaxants	
1. Rapid, complete relaxation	1. Respiratory depression, immediate or prolonged
2. Release of vocal cord spasm	
3. Indicated for:	2. Relaxation of cardiac sphincter of esophagus
(a) Muscular relaxation	
(b) Breaking vocal cord spasm	3. Contraindicated in patients with full stomach
(c) Facilitating endotracheal intubation	4. Response different in children
Neuroleptanalgesia (droperidol-fentanyl)[9]	
1. Deep analgesia	1. Poor controllability
2. Minimal cardiac depression	2. Late pyramidal tract symptoms
3. No cardiac irritability	3. Respiratory depression
CI-581[10] *(Ketalar)*	
1. Easy induction	1. Poor relaxation
2. Rapid recovery	2. Short duration
3. Nonemetic	3. Limited application

Nonrebreathing techniques. Although Ayre[33] introduced the T tube system for use with ether, and Rees[34] modified it for use with relaxants, this method today is being used most widely for administration of halothane.

T-tube nonrebreathing systems also have the advantage of being simple and valveless and afford an easy means of assisting or controlling respiration. They can be used either with a mask or an endotracheal tube.

Ayre's original T-piece, as illustrated in Fig. 6-12, consisted of a metal T-shaped tube, with incoming gases entering at midpoint, and having a 6-inch to 8-inch extension on the expiratory limb. Three basic variations of the T-piece system have been used, as pointed out by Harrison,[35] the first having no expiratory limb, the second having an expiratory limb with capacity less than the tidal volume, and the third having an expiratory limb with capacity greater than tidal volume. In all systems, the diameter of the expiratory limb should not be less than 10 mm.

For use with ether, T-piece systems with little or no expiratory limb have been useful, allowing the patient to breathe spontaneously and drawing in air if tidal volume exceeded the gases supplied. No rebreathing can occur; the system is practically foolproof except when assisted respiration is preferable—then it is awkward to use. Addition of the longer expiratory limb and the open-ended bag enable the anesthetist to assist or control respiration easily but involve a real possibility of rebreathing and require a careful estimation of rate of flow of incoming gas necessary to prevent accumulation of carbon dioxide. Mathematical relationships have been worked out in some detail by Harrison,[35] Onchi, Hayashi, and Veyanma,[36] Inkster,[37] and Mapleson.[38] Lewis and Spoerel[39] and others agree that use of the Rees type system, with prolonged expiratory tube and bag, requires a gas flow 2.5 to 3 times the child's minute volume. (Minute volume is easily calculated by multiplying dead space (1 ml. per pound) by 3 to equal tidal volume; then rate × tidal volume = minute volume.

The T-piece system is equally useful for anesthesia with ether, halothane, or nitrous oxide and curare. It is of especial value with halothane, for it facilitates accurate measurement of halothane concentration. This device is extremely useful in smaller children and in our hospital is used for most children weighing under 35 pounds.

Our preference at this time is to use a Keats type adapter, a 14-inch corrugated tube, and a 500-ml. or 750-ml. double-ended bag. It seems reasonable to clamp the open end of the bag when a mask is in use, but preferable to remove any valve or clamp if an endotracheal tube is used.

Disadvantages of all nonrebreathing systems of course include the expense of using high flows of gases and the danger that would be associated with an explosive gas such as cyclopropane.

Of perhaps greater practical importance now is the loss of heat and moisture from the patient by systems entailing use of fresh gases that are neither warmed nor humidified. In any anesthesia lasting more than one hour, it is advisable to use a warming and humidifying apparatus.

This problem is recognized, and several attempts to answer it have been reported.[40-42] The Bennett warming and humidifying unit[43] has been found to be useful for this purpose, as well as that described by Rashad and associates.[42a]

To-and-fro absorption. As described in Chapter 17, the to-and-fro system is best suited to use in small infants because of absence of valves, combined with retention of body heat and moisture. It is seldom used at present because of the combined problems of increasing dead space, clumsiness, and dust from soda lime that may be blown into the child's face and mouth.

Infant circle absorption systems. Small circle apparatus has the advantage of conserving the infant's heat and moisture and of preventing spillage of explosive gases. In contrast to the to-and-fro system, there is no problem of soda-lime dust or increasing dead space. It does contain valves, which can develop resistance. The Bloomquist infant circle with visible horizontal dome valves gives reasonable safety and appears preferable when cyclopropane is administered to infants under 30 pounds. The addition of a pressure gauge would be advantageous here.

Revell system. By incorporating a blower to circulate gases through the circle systems, it is theoretically possible to eliminate valves and dead space. The Revell circulator[44] was introduced for the purpose of making adult-sized circle apparatus applicable to infants and children. Its effectiveness has been documented,[45] but its use has not been widespread. Many prefer to use small apparatus for children because they dislike the clumsiness of large tubes and adapters.

Use of adult circle in infants and children. It has been a traditional feeling that adult circle apparatus was unphysiologic for use in small children because of dead space and resistance in tubes, valves, or canisters. Upon testing such equipment with infants, Graff, Holzman, and Benson,[46] found little evidence to support these fears, and there has been growing interest to find equipment that can be used in both adults and children.[47,48] Rackow's combination circle and nonrebreathing apparatus approaches this, and small breathing tubes are now available for use with adult circle systems.

In choosing any of these systems, it should be pointed out that there probably is less actual difference than would be expected. If, as is usually the case, gases are flowing at 2 to 4 L. per minute, all systems are virtually nonrebreathing even when circle type apparatus is employed; furthermore, inspiratory valves will offer no resistance if respiration is being assisted or controlled.

REFERENCES

1. Leigh, M. D., and Belton, M. K.: Special considerations in the selection and employment of anesthetic agents and methods in infants and children, Anesthesiology 11:592-598, 1950.
2. Harris, T. A. B.: The mode of action of anaesthetics, Edinburgh, 1951, E. & S. Livingstone, Ltd.
3. Brody, G. L., and Sweet, R. B.: Halothane anesthesia as possible cause of massive hepatic necrosis, Anesthesiology 24:29-37, 1963.
4. Lindenbaum, J., and Leifer, E.: Hepatic necrosis associated with halothane anesthesia, New Eng. J. Med. 268:525-530, 1963.
5. Bunker, J. P., and Blumenfeld, C. M.: Liver necrosis after halothane anesthesia: cause or coincidence? New Eng. J. Med. 268:531-534, 1963.
6. Abajian, J., Jr., Brazell, E. H., Dente, G. A., and Mills, E. M.: Experience with halothane (Fluothane) in more than five thousand cases, J.A.M.A. 171:535-540, 1959.
7. Subcommittee on the National Halothane Study. Possible relation between halothane anesthesia and post-operative hepatic necrosis, J.A.M.A. 197:121-136, 1966.
8. Babior, B. M., and Davidson, C. S.: Post-operative massive liver necrosis, New Eng. J. Med. 276:645-653, 1967.
9. Werry, J. S., and Davenport, H. T.: The psychological effects of premedication for paediatric anaesthesia, New Zeal. Med. J. 64:641-646, 1965; abstract in Survey Anesth. 10:477-478, 1966.
10. Corssen, G., and Domino, E. F.: Dissociative anesthesia: further pharmacologic studies and first clinical experience with the phencyclidine derivative CI-581, Anesth. Analg. 45:29-40, 1966.
11. Goodman, I. S., and Gilman, A.: The pharmacological basis of therapeutics, ed. 3, New York, 1965, The Macmillan Co.
12. Adriani, J.: The pharmacology of anesthetic drugs, ed. 3, Springfield, Ill., 1956, Charles C Thomas, Publisher.
13. Waters, R. M., editor: Chloroform; a study after 100 years, Madison, 1951, University of Wisconsin Press.
14. Siebecker, K. L., and Orth, O. S.: A report of seven administrations of chloroform for open thoracic operations, Anesthesiology 17:792-797, 1956.
15. DiGiovanni, A. J., and Dripps, R. D.: Abnormal motor movements during divinyl ether anesthesia, Anesthesiology 17:353-357, 1956.
16. Brewster, W. R., Jr., Isaacs, J. P., and Anderson, T. W.: Depressant effect of ether on the myocardium of the dog and its modification by reflex release of epinephrine and norepinephrine, Amer. J. Physiol. 175:399-414, 1953.
17. Stephen, C. R., and Slater, H. M.: Agents and techniques employed in pediatric anesthesia, Anesth. Analg. 29:254-262, 1950.
18. Raventos, J.: The action of Fluothane; a new volatile anesthetic, Brit. J. Pharmacol. 11:394-410, 1956.
19. Johnstone, M.: The human cardiovascular response to Fluothane anesthesia, Brit. J. Anaesth. 28:392, 1956.
20. Stephen, C. R., Lawrence, J. H., Fabian, L. W., Bourgeois-Gavardin, M., Dent, S., and Grosskreutz, D. C.: Clinical experience with Fluothane-1,400 cases, Anesthesiology 19:197-207, 1958.
21. Junkin, C. I., Smith, C., and Conn, A. W.: Fluothane for paediatric anesthesia, Canad. Anaesth. Soc. J. 4:259-265, 1957.

22. McGregor, M., Davenport, H. T., Jegier, W., Sekely, P., Gibbons, J. E., and Demers, P. P.: The cardiovascular effects of halothane in normal children, Brit. J. Anaesth. **30**:398-408, 1958.

23. Taylor, C., and Stoeling, V. K.: Halothane (Fluothane) anesthesia for paediatric cardiac surgery, Canad. Anaesth. Soc. J. **8**:247-256, 1961.

24. Morrow, D. H., and Morrow, A. G.: Effects of halothane on myocardial contractile force and vascular resistance, Anesthesiology **22**:537-541, 1961.

25. Bookallil, M., and Lomax, J. G.: Some observations on the use of halothane ("Fluothane") in paediatric anaesthesia, M. J. Australia **1**:666-670, 1962; abstract in Survey Anesth. **8**:40, 1964.

26. Reynolds, R. N.: Halothane in pediatric anesthesia. In Smith, R. M., editor: Pediatric anesthesia, Boston, 1962, Little, Brown & Co.

27. Artusio, J. F., Jr., Van Poznak, A., Hunt, R. R., Tiers, F. M., and Alexander, M.: Clinical evaluation of methoxyflurane in man, Anesthesiology **21**:512-517, 1960.

28. Bagwell, E. E., and Woods, E. F.: Cardiovascular effects of methoxyflurane, Anesthesiology **23**:51-57, 1962.

29. Clement, F. W.: Nitrous oxide-oxygen anesthesia, Philadelphia, 1939, Lea & Febiger .

30. Nowill, W. K., Stephen, C. R., and Searles, P. W.: The evaluation of trichloroethylene, an anesthetic and analgesic agent, Arch. Surg. **66**:35-47, 1953.

31. Dundee, J. W.: Tachypnoea during administration of trichloroethylene, Brit. J. Anaesth. **25**:3-23, 1953.

32. Norris, W., and Stuart, P.: Cardiac arrest during trichloroethylene anesthesia, Brit. Med. J. **1**:860-863, 1957.

33. Ayre, P.: Anesthesia for harelip and cleft palate in babies, Brit. J. Surg. **25**:131-132, 1937.

34. Rees, G. J.: Anaesthesia in the newborn, Brit. Med. J. **2**:1419-1426, 1950.

35. Harrison, G. A.: Ayre's T-piece: a review of its modifications, Brit. J. Anaesth. **36**:115-120, 1964.

36. Onchi, Y., Hayashi, T., and Veyama, H.: Studies on the Ayre T piece technique, Far East J. Anesth. **1**:30-40, 1947.

37. Inkster, J. S.: The T-piece technique in anaesthesia, Brit. J. Anaesth. **28**:512-519, 1956.

38. Mapleson, W. W.: Theoretical considerations of the effects of rebreathing in two semi-closed anaesthetic systems, Brit. Med. Bull. **14**:64-68, 1958.

39. Lewis, A., and Spoerel, A.: A modification of Ayre's technique, Canad. Anaesth. Soc. J. **8**:501-511, 1961.

40. Walker, J. E., Wells, R. E., Jr., and Merrill, E. W.: Heat and water exchange in the respiratory tract, Amer. J. Med. **30**:259-267, 1961.

41. Burton, T. D. K.: Effects of dry anaesthetic gases on the respiratory mucous membrane, Lancet **1**:235-238, 1962; abstract in Anesth. Analg. **41**:762-765, 1962.

42. Chase, H. F., Trotta, R., and Kilmore, M. A. Simple methods for humidifying nonrebreathing anesthetic gas systems, Anesth. Analg. **41**:249-256, 1962.

42a. Rashad, K., Wilson, K., Hurt, H. H., Graff, T. D., and Benson, D. W.: Effect of humidification of anesthetic gases on static compliance, Anesth. Analg. **46**:127-133, 1967.

43. Wynands, J. E., and Wrigley, F. R. H.: A simple method of humidifying anaesthetic gases, Canad. Anaesth. Soc. J.: **13**:403-405, 1966.

44. Revell, D. G.: Circulator to eliminate mechanical dead space in circle absorption systems, Canad. Anaesth. Soc. J. **6**:98-103, 1959.

45. Roffey, P. J., Revell, D. G., and Morris, L. E.: An assessment of the Revell circulator, Anesthesiology **22**:583-590, 1961.

46. Graff, T. D., Holzman, R. S., and Benson, D. W.: Acid-base balance in infants during halothane anesthesia with the use of an adult circle absorption system, Anesth. Analg. **43**:583-589, 1964.

47. Graff, T. D., Sewall, K., Lim, T. S., Kantt, O., Morris, R. E., Jr., and Benson, D. W.: The ventilatory response of infants to airway resistance, Anesthesiology **27**:168-175, 1966.

48. VerSteeg J., and Stevens, W. C.: A comparison of respiratory effort of infants anesthetized with several adult and pediatric systems, Anesthesiology **27**:229, 1966.

Chapter 8

Techniques for the induction of general anesthesia

Whether the operation is to be a tonsillectomy or a pneumonectomy, the induction period is loaded with potential dangers and complications. For this reason induction always is an important and fascinating challenge for the anesthetist. To take a responsive, conscious, and perhaps resistant child and convert him without mishap into a stabilized, completely controlled biologic mechanism often calls for a sympathetic heart, a variety of medical skills, and a nice sense of timing.

TECHNIQUES FOR INFANTS UNDER 1 YEAR OF AGE

Premature and other weak neonates may be operated upon under local anesthesia, in which case general anesthesia and the problems of induction will be avoided.

Healthy infants usually require general anesthesia, which may consist of halothane, cyclopropane, nitrous oxide with relaxants, or ether. Although open-drop ether is no longer considered a good agent for small infants, it can be used successfully.[1] In such cases divinyl ether may be used initially, or ethyl ether can be given from the start if a carefully graduated administration is employed.

Previous chapters have dealt with basic principles and specific details. Here at last a patient is actually about to be anesthetized. The first act at this time is *not* to reach for the mask and turn on the gases. A final stage of rechecking is important. Well before anesthetizing an infant one should check the room temperature, and preferably warm the room to 75° F. It may be advisable to turn off the air conditioning to prevent excessive air currents. A heating device should be employed for most operations on neonates. The last act of the anesthetist prior to induction is to wash his hands well. Infection is still a major cause of mortality in the neonate, and he deserves the same precautions of cleanliness in the operating room that he receives on the ward.

A final check of equipment and chart is made, tape is torn, and everything is laid out in complete readiness. One should make sure that an adequate dose of atropine has been given *within the last hour*. If any question exists, it is better to repeat the full dose. If given intravenously its vagolytic action will be effective within one minute; if given intramuscularly, it will be effective within 3 to 5 minutes.

Now the child is placed on the operating table and the clothing is loosened, exposing chest and abdomen. A blood pressure cuff is applied, but the activity of the infant usually makes it impractical to try to take a reading before he is anesthetized. The legs and arms of small infants shoud be wrapped in sheet wadding to prevent heat loss. A stethoscope is strapped to the child's chest, being careful not to impede respiration by using too much tape. The heart rate is counted and recorded. The anesthesia starting time should also be recorded at this point.

Induction by open-drop technique. If induction is to be carried out with open-drop ether or divinyl ether in a small infant, one should have two infant Yankauer masks, covered with at least 4 layers of gauze, and should have additional dry gauze to prevent splashing ether into the eyes or over the face. Under most conditions it seems preferable to avoid the use of eyedrops or ointments. The mask must be held close to the child's face, or vapors will be too highly diluted. The anesthetic should be dropped, never poured, at a rate increasing as rapidly as the child will tolerate it. If too rapid, the infant will hold his breath and become cyanotic. Then the mask must be lifted, and the process will start over again. Young infants are so resistant to the cold vapor of ether that this method is to be avoided if possible. Divinyl ether is slightly less irritating but still difficult to administer, and overdosage will cause hypoxia and convulsive activity. If one mask becomes saturated and wet, it should be set aside and the second mask used in its place. Young infants may be able to feel pain and exhibit displeasure (Chapter 2). Fear and apprehension do not appear to be major problem, however, and special precautions to avoid psychologic trauma do not seem necessary. In fact, a small baby may be quite difficult to induce by the open-drop technique unless his respiratory exchange is increased by crying. Consequently, it is actually preferable that these small babies cry and kick their legs a little during induction (Fig. 8-1).

A very important rule that must be observed at all times in dealing with small children is that they should never be left unattended on a litter or operating table or in a crib with the side lowered. This rule applies to sedated and

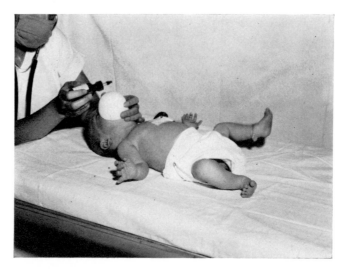

Fig. 8-1. Open-drop technique with divinyl ether. Crying and kicking will stimulate a small baby's respiration and speed induction.

anesthetized children, as well as to those who are awake. Since the anesthetist may not leave the infant, an assistant can prove very helpful. During the actual induction he stands by but does not restrain the baby's movements.

Because of the danger of overdosage, our use of divinyl ether has decreased sharply in recent years. By blowing nitrous oxide and oxygen (or cyclopropane and oxygen) over the infant's face, induction is less irritating and less hazardous. An attempt is made to envelop the child's face in a soft cloud of anesthetic gas; thus a wide-orificed breathing hose is preferable to the jet from a narrow rubber tubing. It is even better to attach the gas line to the nipple of a small Yankauer-type wire mask (covered with four layers of gauze) and hold this above the infants' face (Fig. 8-2).

At the start, flows of 8 L. of nitrous oxide to 1 L. of oxygen will be necessary for a few moments, after which the ratio is reduced to 4 to 1. Cyclopropane may be blown over the child's face with oxygen, both gases flowing at 1 L. per minute. As the infant begins to appear drowsy or shows nystagmoid ocular movement, the mask is brought down into contact with the face. Ether is dropped on the mask, very slowly at first, then accelerating as rapidly as the child will tolerate it. The anesthetic gas flows are reduced gradually, for it requires several minutes to achieve an effective blood level of ether. A flow of 500 ml. per minute of oxygen should be maintained throughout the procedure.

With the efficient vaporizers now available, one can introduce vaporized ether from the anesthesia machine, blowing it under the cloth mask, thus avoiding the disadvantages of the cold liquid ether, yet retaining the simplicity of the open system.

During induction the respiration and heart rate are monitored by stethoscope. The eye signs are of little value in infants, and the eyelids should not be

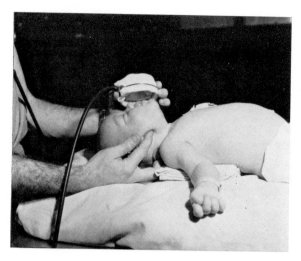

Fig. 8-2. Induction by blowing oxygen and nitrous oxide or cyclopropane under mask.

pried open for this purpose. When the infant's respiration is regular, he no longer moves his arms and legs, and he tolerates the passage of an oral airway. It is better not to induce deep anesthesia but is preferable to have the infant lightly anesthetized, with flexor tone present in his hands and arms.

Nonrebreathing and closed-system techniques. It is certainly preferable to use a method that enables the anesthetist to assist respiration (Fig. 8-3). Whether nonrebreathing or closed-system apparatus is employed, the technique of induction should be practically the same. Small infants actually require relatively strong concentrations of anesthetic drugs for induction. This has been attributed to the brown adipose tissue that neonates possess and that has a high oxygen uptake.[2,3] In any event, nitrous oxide has relatively little value for induction, and it is not used to begin induction as it is in older patients. If halothane is to be used, one may start with 1% halothane and increase this to 2.5% or 3% as the infant accepts it. After the child is asleep and relaxed, the percentage may be reduced to 1 or even 0.5 and maintained with nitrous oxide and oxygen in a 3:2 ratio.

If cyclopropane is to be employed, initial flows of cyclopropane, oxygen, and nitrous oxide, each at 1 L. per minute, should give minimal airway irritation with rapid effect.

When using halothane for induction in neonates, the main problem will be that of overdosage, with resultant flaccidity, hypotension, and eventually cardiac asystole. If adequate atropine has been given, bradycardia will not be an early sign of overdosage. Without atropine, bradycardia should be an important sign.

Cyclopropane can also cause rapid depression, but with infants a more common complication is laryngotracheal obstruction, which may become severe and cause total airway occlusion. Sometimes airway obstruction is caused by the tongue, and this is promptly relieved by inserting an airway. When the obstruc-

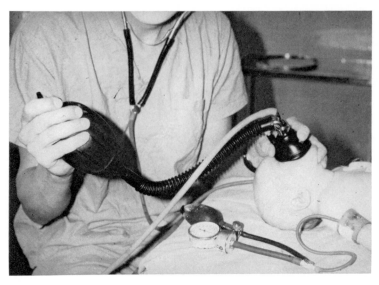

Fig. 8-3. Induction with nonrebreathing system.

tion is in the larynx, however, it is more difficult to overcome. Manual pressure on the breathing bag sometimes accentuates the condition and cannot be relied upon. Severe obstruction can best be relieved by succinylcholine, 1 mg. per pound given by intravenous or intramuscular route. Once cyclopropane has been established at the level of surgical anesthesia, airway problems are decreased but not eliminated. This, to me, is the principal disadvantage of the agent. After induction with cyclopropane, an infant usually will require a relatively high concentration (20% to 25%) to maintain adequate depth.

If endotracheal intubation is performed prior to induction and without a relaxant, oxygen is administered by mask first, then the child is intubated, apparatus is attached, and anesthesia is started. If halothane is used, a 1.5% mixture is advised. If cyclopropane is chosen for induction, a 50% concentration may be employed until the infant becomes tranquil. When induction thus follows intubation, it is usually preferable to retain spontaneous respiration and refrain from assisting or controlling ventilation until exchange is stabilized.

If a relaxant has been employed and the child is apneic, respiration will be controlled, and weaker anesthetic mixtures should be used. Here 0.5% halothane or 10% cyclopropane (100 mg. cyclopropane to 900 ml. oxygen) should suffice until respiratory activity returns.

TECHNIQUES FOR OLDER INFANTS AND CHILDREN

Techniques for induction of anesthesia in older infants and children differ from those used in small infants. In older infants and children apprehension and fear become major problems, and both for safety and kindness it is important to prevent emotional reactions. Several methods of induction are available and include the following: (1) rectal, (2) inhalation, (3) intravenous, and (4) hypnoinduction.

Basal anesthesia with rectal agents. From the child's standpoint, induction by rectal administration of thiobarbiturates (Pentothal, Surital, Neraval), methohexital (Brevital), or tribromoethanol (Avertin) has the great advantage of involving neither mask nor needle. Most children under 5 or 6 years of age have no objection to the passage of a rectal tube, and, after the solution is given, the child falls into a drowsy state and then into a deep sleep, undisturbed by retching, gagging, or excitement. For children 1 to 3 years old, who are the most excitable and at the same time the least approachable, induction by rectally administered agents is undoubtedly the most reliable method by which to gain an even, calm induction. It is also especially suited for use in children who are mentally retarded because these children often react poorly to oral or parenteral sedatives.

Tribromoethanol (Avertin). Although this anesthetic is not widely used today, it is still one of the most reliable agents for induction of anesthesia by rectum.[4,5] If used within certain limitations it is quite safe. Attention has been called to its toxic potentialities when used in excessive amounts,[6] or in the presence of liver or kidney disease or malnutrition.[7] It seems advisable to place the following *restrictions* on the use of tribromoethanol:

1. Do not use for infants under 9 months of age.
2. Do not use in dosages greater than 80 mg. per kilogram if general anesthesia is to be added or in dosages greater than 100 mg. per kilogram if used alone.
3. Barbiturates and narcotics are not to be used when tribromoethanol is given as basal anesthesia.

Table 8-1. *Tribromoethanol (Avertin) dosage scale (80 mg. per kilogram; 35 mg. per pound)*

Weight (lb.)	Avertin fluid (ml.)	Distilled water (ml.)
10	0.35	14
15	0.5	20
20	0.7	28
25	0.9	36
30	1.1	44
35	1.2	48
40	1.4	56
45	1.6	64
50	1.8	72
55	2.0	80
60	2.2	88
65	2.4	96
70	2.5	100
75	2.6	104
80	2.8	112
85	3.0	120
90	3.3	132
95	3.4	136
100	3.5	140

4. Do not use for patients who are toxic, dehydrated, malnourished, or febrile or who have liver or renal disease.
5. Tribromoethanol is not to be given to patients until they are in the operating suite. After giving tribromoethanol, the anesthetist must remain in constant attendance with the child.

DISADVANTAGES. Tribromoethanol is not universally popular for a number of reasons:

1. When not used frequently, it is bothersome to prepare, because special equipment is necessary for its preparation. When the apparatus is readily at hand, preparation actually takes about 90 seconds.
2. Tribromoethanol is slightly irritating to the rectal mucosa, and it may cause emptying of the large bowel. This tendency is decreased but not prevented if a cleansing enema is given the evening before operation. In emergencies tribromoethanol appears to give effective sedation whether an enema has been given or not.
3. For preadolescent girls and boys rectal medication may be embarrassing, especially if given in the presence of others.
4. Since children receive no other medication, they are brought to the operating suite quite alert and have no sedation until receiving tribromo-

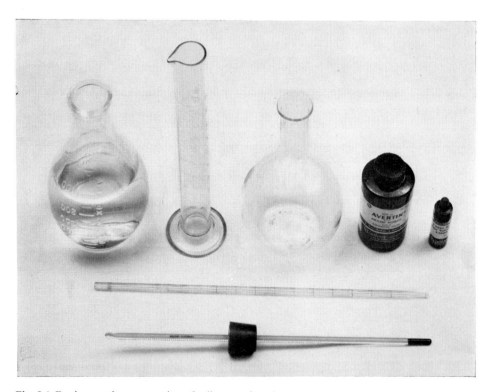

Fig. 8-4. Equipment for preparation of tribromoethanol.

ethanol immediately before operation. Often it is preferable to start medication earlier with other agents.

PREPARATION OF TRIBROMOETHANOL. As shown in Fig. 8-4, convenient equipment for preparation of tribromoethanol consists of these items:

1. 500-ml. flask of distilled water
2. 100-ml. graduate
3. 500-ml. Erlenmeyer flask
4. Avertin fluid
5. Congo red indicator
6. 1-ml. pipette, graduated to 0.1 ml.
7. Thermometer, graduated 0° to 100° C. and fitted with No. 6 rubber stopper

To prepare the solution, as for a 20-pound child, one consults the scale (Table 8-1) and then, using the graduate, measures 28 ml. of distilled water, pouring it into the Erlenmeyer flask. The water is heated to 40° C. under a hot-water tap; then 0.7 ml. of Avertin fluid is pipetted into the water, and the flask is shaken briskly. Two or three drops of Congo red are added. The appearance of a red color shows that the solution has not undergone decomposition, but a blue or purple reaction (pH less than 5) shows the presence of dibromacetic aldehyde, hydrobromic acid, and alkalis, and the solution should be discarded.

After preparation, the solution should be held at body temperature until administration. This is best done by use of a Thermos jar. The solution is administered by use of a lubricated catheter, connected by a short rubber tubing to the barrel of an Asepto syringe. The solution is poured into the syringe barrel and allowed to run into the child by gravity. If the child strains, it may be necessary to start the fluid by use of the syringe bulb. After administration of tribromoethanol, one should be sure to apply a diaper securely because evacuation may occur. Sleep may be expected within 7 to 10 minutes after administration.

Following this induction, general anesthesia is easily accomplished with either volatile or gaseous agents.

Rectal thiobarbiturates (Pentothal, Surital). There has been considerable enthusiasm for the use of thiobarbiturates by rectum.[8-10] The advantages are much the same as those of tribromoethanol, and choice between the two types of agents depends on rather small factors, the first of which probably is convenience. In most institutions it is considerably easier to prepare thiopental, which is used intravenously many times daily and is always at hand. Other comparative factors are listed in Table 8-2.

Table 8-2. *Practical factors in evaluation of rectal agents*

Tribromoethanol (Avertin)	*Thiobarbiturates (Pentothal, Surital)*
1. Sympathomimetic action, bronchodilating, no bronchospasm	1. Parasympathomimetic, bronchoconstricting, with tendency for bronchospasm
2. Fairly safe after eating, no vomiting	2. Contraindicated after eating; increased tendency to severe laryngospasm
3. Predictable effect, anesthesia in 7 to 10 minutes	3. Onset similar in 7 to 10 minutes
4. Prolonged recovery	4. Probably shorter acting
5. Toxicity established in ill patients	5. Less toxic to liver and kidney

It is to be noted that if thiobarbiturates are to be used for basal anesthesia, the same precautions should apply as with use of tribromoethanol, namely, that the agents should not be administered until the patients are in the operating suite and that the anesthetist is to stay with the child thereafter.

PREPARATION AND ADMINISTRATION OF RECTAL THIOPENTAL. When thiopental was first used rectally, the dosage recommended was 1 Gm. per 50 pounds of body weight in a 10% solution, or 20 mg. per pound. This often gave deep sleep with depression of respiration and some fall in blood pressure. At present the use of a 5% solution in a dosage of 15 mg. per pound is generally preferred. A suspension of thiopental is available in multidose calibrated syringes. This also is administered in doses of 15 mg. per pound.

Since thiopental is usually mixed in a 2% or 2.5% solution for intravenous use, it has been proved most convenient in our hands to mix rectal thiopental in similar strength.

After the administration of rectal thiopental the child falls asleep in 7 to 10 minutes. Inhalation anesthesia may then be undertaken by open-drop or closed methods. Due to the respiratory depression and parasympathomimetic effect of thiopental, open administration of volatile agents may be slow and irritating. Closed methods, using halothane or cyclopropane, give the best induction after rectal thiopental.

Stetson[11] has been impressed with the use of methohexital (Brevital) as an induction agent for rectal administration in children. The powder is mixed in a solution of distilled water to make a 10% solution and is given in dosage varying between 8 and 14 mg. per pound of normal body weight. The usual dose for children who have not had other sedation is 10 mg. per pound. If given as a supplement to previous but inadequate sedation, 8 mg. per pound is advised.

Sleep usually occurs in 4 to 6 minutes. Following a short general anesthesia, children can be expected to be ambulatory within 1 to 1½ hours.

Induction with open techniques. Infants 6 months of age usually are given some preanesthetic sedation to prevent excessive excitement. Thus most of the patients now under consideration will have received a barbiturate, or, after 1 year of age, a barbiturate and a narcotic. Those induced by rectal Avertin are exceptions to this policy. Sedation is expected to allay some of the unhappiness caused by hunger and strange surroundings, but it is not expected to cause sleep. A quiet, receptive child is ideal. To the anesthetist then is left the task of keeping the child's confidence and morale through induction. How this is done depends upon the child's age, whether he is quiet or resistant, healthy or sick, and other factors. The most widely employed method of induction for children at present is with nitrous oxide and halothane using either nonrebreathing or closed-system apparatus.

After rechecking apparatus and chart (and atropine administration), the pulse rate and starting time are noted *and recorded*. Nitrous oxide and oxygen are started at flows of 6 L. and 1 L. The anesthetist in the meantime is talking to the child, recalling the visit of the night before, and carrying on a running bit of "chatter" intended to reassure the child and keep his mind off his immediate problems. Small infants who cannot understand the words are consoled

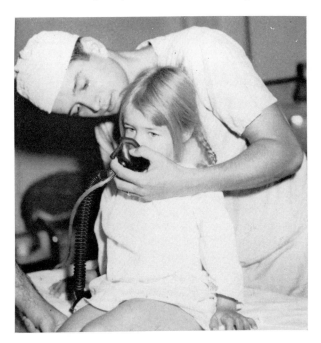

Fig. 8-5. Children who are afraid to lie down on the table often accept a mask if allowed to sit up.

by the sound of the voice. If the child has a security blanket or toy, this certainly is exploited fully. The chief goal is to keep the child from feeling scared and alone.

Naturally some children have individual fears and preferences. Many are most docile when brought into the operating room but refuse to lie down on the operating table. Such children are not forced. Induction usually is easily carried out with the child on the table supported in a sitting position, or held on the anesthetist's lap (Fig. 8-5).

The most important factor is to keep in contact with the child. The voice is most important, but the hands are useful also. An assistant should be present to render moral support—most children and many adults are comforted greatly by having a hand to hold as they go to sleep. When a child is dozing off, the anesthetist can reassure him by passing his hand across the child's forehead or cheek to remind him he is not being abandoned.

The method of reassuring patients is important. If a child is cooperative and drowsy, he should not be bombarded with questions. A few words in hypnotic repetitious monotone will smooth and hasten induction. Words suggesting discomfort, dizziness, or pain should not be mentioned in any manner. "You're a good boy, close your eyes, you're going to sleep now" makes a comforting sound and can be repeated ad infinitum to a drowsy child.

It is quite different when a child is alert or apprehensive. The alert child often may be reassured by an anesthetist who has taken the trouble to find out the child's interests or favorite television program. Television is usually the surest subject under unprepared conditions, and the adept pediatric anesthetist should always be familiar with one or two popular children's programs.

The truly apprehensive child presents the real test, for the anesthetist must seize the initiative from the start and really convince the child all is going to be fine. Here is the time for a barrage of questions, or to have the child blow up the anesthesia bag, or count backward from 10, or 100, or whatever would absorb his attention. Here is where the child must not for a moment be allowed to feel alone or sorry for himself, or all may be lost.

It is most important in such circumstances for the anesthetist to continue his verbal and manual reassurance of the child well after the child has appeared to fall asleep. There is a very critical phase when the child is quiet, but not asleep. Hearing remains intact, emotional controls are gone, and fear may overwhelm a child who suddenly loses his sense of security. At the risk of appearing overenthusiastic, one should continue to reassure the child for several minutes after he has appeared to lose consciousness.

The steps taken in the usual manner of induction (Figs. 8-7 and 8-8) consist of starting with a 6 to 1 mixture of nitrous oxide and oxygen that is made to flow over the child's face. If a child is truly apprehensive, the mask can be removed so that the gases come from a less noticeable T piece or yoke. Rather than blowing the gas straight at the child, the anesthetist can more gently direct it into the child's nose and mouth by cupping his other hand and deflecting it toward the patient.

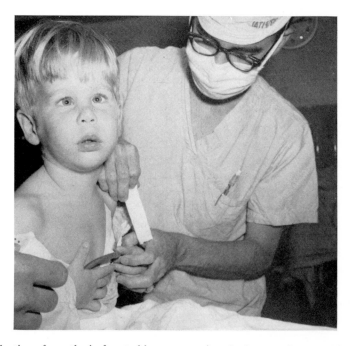

Fig. 8-6. Induction of anesthesia for strabismus correction. Stethoscope is strapped to chest.

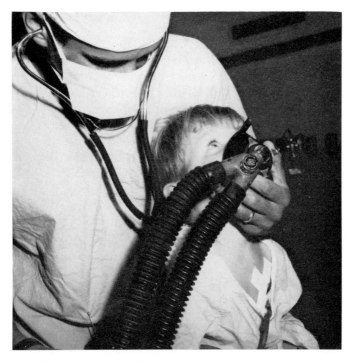

Fig. 8-7. Nitrous oxide and oxygen are given until nystagmus appears; then halothane is added.

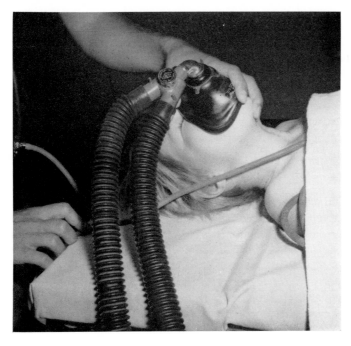

Fig. 8-8. As child relaxes, he can be placed in normal position.

The child at first appears to be unaffected, but then his eyes show nystagmus and he usually becomes quiet and cooperative. At this time, he will allow a mask to be fitted to his face (Fig. 8-7), and those who have not wanted to lie down may be lowered gently into the usual supine position.

Halothane can be started at 0.5% concentration and increased by 0.5% every 6 to 8 breaths until a 2.5% or 3% mixture is reached. Cardiorespiratory action is monitored by stethoscope and by observing chest expansion. It is a natural tendency to start correcting a patient's position as soon as he falls asleep. If all is going well and there is no airway obstruction, it is wise to allow induction to proceed and not change anything until the child is more securely stabilized. Airway obstruction must be treated promptly; however, it may be sufficient merely to elevate the chin, or an oral airway may be required. In inserting an oral airway, loose deciduous teeth may easily be dislodged if the airway is rotated or inserted roughly. It is best to depress the tongue with a wooden tongue blade and slide the airway in over the tongue without rotating it (Fig. 8-9). Cardiac action is also observed by stethoscope, and the blood pressure cuff is applied as soon as the child is asleep. In most cases a rectal thermistor is also installed. As induction with halothane proceeds, respiration may become depressed, and the anesthetist must be ready to assist or control respiration at any time. Should such respiratory depression occur, the concentration of halothane should be reduced to 0.5% or 1% to avoid overdosage.

Cyclopropane induction may begin by blowing a mixture of 500 ml. each of cyclopropane and oxygen, and gradually bringing the mask up the child's face. The rather unpleasant odor of cyclopropane makes this less acceptable to most children, although the drug, once accepted, is more rapidly effective. As with infants, laryngotracheal spasm is the chief complication in cyclopropane induction. Since the tongue very often sticks to the roof of the mouth under cyclopropane, it should be a routine practice to insert an airway as soon as possible. The hazard of explosion must not be overlooked, however, and openly flowing gases plus a moving child may set up a potentially hazardous situation.

A nitrous oxide–ether sequence can be employed using standard anesthetic machines, starting with a 6 to 1 L. nitrous–oxide oxygen mixture until nystagmus is noted, then reducing the flow to 4 to 1, and starting a minimal flow of ether that will then be graduated in very small increments every 3 to 4 breaths as tolerated. Breath-holding or irritation of any sort will call for holding to the mixture then in use, or cutting back to a weaker one until the child will tolerate the ether, and then progressing again. More gagging, phonating, and secretions are seen with ether than with halothane or cyclopropane, but when the child is finally under anesthesia there is less uncertainty than with the more smoothly acting agents.

The 4 to 1 concentration of nitrous oxide is not reduced until the child is well anesthetized and accepting 15% to 20% ether without resistance. If inducting agents are reduced prematurely, the child will gag, cough, and show other signs of awakening, and induction will have to be repeated under worsened conditions.

Intravenous methods. Induction of anesthesia by intravenous techniques is

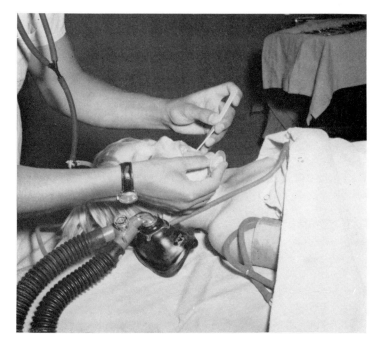

Fig. 8-9. Oral airway is inserted. Note use of tongue stick instead of fingers.

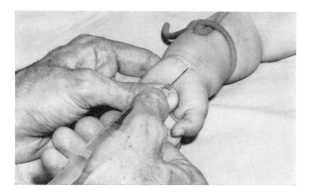

Fig. 8-10. Intravenous induction via wrist vein in small infant.

indicated rather frequently in children. Whenever any child over 2 or 3 years of age already has an intravenous infusion running, it is preferable to employ this route. At other times if a 25-gauge needle is used, venipuncture actually causes very little discomfort and need not be feared (Fig. 8-10). Many children who have undergone several anesthetic inductions will state a preference for the needle rather than the slow, confusing inhalation induction. Finally, in the case of the resistant unmanageable child, it is much more humane to perform a venipuncture than to force a mask upon the child's face.

Traditionally, there has been reluctance toward intravenous anesthesia in children. I believe any airway obstruction or question of full stomach or distention should be firm contraindications to this technique, but, in competent hands, thiopental and similar agents seem acceptable in children 2 to 3 years of age. The presence of an accessible vein is usually the critical problem. In smaller patients, the volar aspect of the wrist is generally the most likely area for a useful vein (Fig. 8-10).[12] However, the wrist contains important vessels, nerves, and tendons, and extravasation may be destructive; therefore this area should rarely if ever be employed for infusions after induction.

The dose of thiopental for a child will usually be approximately 1 mg. per pound, and should be given slowly to prevent extravascular injection or inadvertent overdosage. The standard 2.0% solution is satisfactory for patients of all ages.

Parental attendance at induction. It has long been customary to forbid parents to stay with children during induction for fear that emotions would interfere with anesthesia.

In our experience it has often been apparent, especially in outpatient procedures, that an intelligent mother can do much to reassure a frightened child, and such a parent is often invited to stand beside the child until induction is completed. Although the policy has not been extended to our major operative procedures, it is being evaluated in other institutions, and surprisingly favorable results have been reported.[13]

Induction following excessive or inadequate sedation. Occasionally a child will show more effect from the medication than was intended. Slight respiratory depression can be compensated by use of assisted or controlled respiratory technique. Depression of blood pressure, however, denotes a more critical type of depression, and should serve as ample cause for postponing or canceling operations.

If children are inadequately sedated and are still resistant and hyperexcitable, it generally is preferable to refrain from the usual inhalation methods of induction. Our usual method is to administer additional sedation in the form of rectal thiopental or methohexital (Brevital) in a dose of 10 mg. per pound.

Problem of the unmanageable child. Occasionally problems arise that require special management. A small child may appear in the induction room having had what was thought to be a proper amount of sedation yet still be highly excited and resistant. Many of these children are very easily handled by administration of a reduced dose of rectal thiopental (5 to 10 mg. per pound) or methohexital (8 to 10 mg. per pound).

The most difficult children are those who, because of mental retardation or severe personality problems, remain entirely unapproachable in spite of all attempts at sedation or persuasion. To force a mask on such a terrified, uncomprehending child is undoubtedly the most brutal method possible. An effective and much less upsetting method is to use the intravenous route. One anesthetist can grasp the child's forearm and hand securely so that a second anesthetist can make the venipuncture. There is a short jab similar to others the child has experienced but no frightening mask or gradual loss of consciousness. Induction is quickly effected, and the process is surprisingly easy for all concerned.

Hypnoinduction. Many anesthetists quite naturally employ hypnosis as they induce their patients, repeating calm, reassuring words in a sleepy monotone. The technique of hypnosis, or hypnoinduction, as described by Betcher,[14] may be carried much further than this. Children are good candidates for hypnosis, and, if the approach is varied to suit different age levels, most children from infancy through adolescence can be strongly influenced by suggestion.

To prepare for the use of hypnoinduction, Betcher emphasizes the importance of the preoperative visit to acquaint the patient with the intended approach and to set up an understanding between child and anesthetist. At the time of induction infants are best controlled by the lullaby approach, which consists of gently soothing the baby with comforting words or a simple tune and stroking or fondling him. At the same time nitrous oxide or cyclopropane is unobtrusively introduced by gravity flow, and the child dozes off.

The 3-year-old to 8-year-old group is most susceptible to the "make believe" approach and happily enters into games of pretending. Such pretending naturally centers about going to sleep or showing a pet or a friend how to go to sleep.

The 9-year-old to 14-year-old group responds best to the television technique. The anesthetist places the child under light hypnosis, then asks him to imagine that he is watching a television program, and to describe it step by step. Many children enter into this easily. Some who appear unable to take this active part will be quite receptive if a favorite program is described to them while the anesthetics are being wafted over their faces.

For adolescents the more standard hypnotic technique is used. The patient is asked to concentrate his gaze on a fixed point, and then the anesthetist repeats in quiet convincing tones: "You are feeling tired, you are getting sleepy, your eyes are heavy, you feel wonderful and relaxed, you are tired," and so on.

The technique of hypnosis has many advantages that are only beginning to be realized. It has special potentialities for children who must return time after time for esophageal dilation or other repeated treatments. Not only does hypnoinduction decrease excitement and fear but it also reduces the need of sedation and speeds recovery.

REFERENCES

1. Stephen, C. R.: Elements of pediatric anesthesia, Springfield, Ill., 1954, Charles C Thomas, Publisher.
2. Rackow, H.: Unpublished data.
3. Adamsons, K., Jr., and Towell, M.: Thermal homeostasis in the fetus and newborn, Anesthesiology 26:531-548, 1965.
4. Macon, E. B.: Clinical anesthesia in children, Anesth. Analg. 25:163-167, 1946.
5. Bourne, W.: Avertin anesthesia for crippled children, Canad. Med. Ass. J. 35:278-281, 1936.
6. Beecher, H. K.: Fatal toxic reactions associated with tribromethanol anesthesia, J.A.M.A. 111:122-129, 1938.
7. Andersen, D. H.: Avertin poisoning with acute yellow atrophy of the liver and toxic nephrosis, Anesthesiology 6:284-301, 1945.
8. Weinstein, M. L.: Rectal Pentothal sodium: a new pre- and basal anesthetic drug in the practice of surgery, Anesth. Analg. 18:221-223, 1939.
9. Burnap, R. W., Gain, E. A., and Watts, E. H.: Basal anesthesia in children using sodium Pentothal by rectum, Anesthesiology 9:524-531, 1948.

10. Mark, L. C., Fox, J. L., and Burstein, C. L.: Preanesthetic hypnosis with rectal Pentothal in children, Anesthesiology 10:401-405, 1949.
11. Stetson, J. B.: Unpublished data.
12. Wilton, T. N. P., and Wilson, F.: Neonatal anaesthesia, Philadelphia, 1965, F. A. Davis Co.
13. Shulman, J. L., Foley, J. M., Vernon, D. T. A., and Allan, D.: Effect of mother's presence at anesthesia induction, Pediatrics 39:111-114, 1967.
14. Betcher, A. M.: Hypno-induction techniques in pediatric anesthesia, Anesthesiology 19:279-281, 1958.

Chapter 9

Endotracheal intubation

Endotracheal intubation has wide application in pediatric anesthesia because of the many factors that threaten to block the child's airway or depress his respiratory effort. It must be remembered, however, that although intubation has increased value in children, the hazards are also increased, and one must weigh the odds before adopting such a practice as a standard routine.

ADVANTAGES OF ENDOTRACHEAL INTUBATION

The advantages of endotracheal intubation have been enumerated by several authors.[1-5] They include the following:

1. Prevention of aspiration of vomitus. Endotracheal intubation is the most reliable method by which to prevent fatalities in anesthetized patients with full stomach or intestinal obstruction.
2. Prevention of aspiration of blood and tissues from mouth and pharynx. This is especially important in oral, dental, and nasal surgery.

3. Control of ventilation in open-chest surgery, apneic techniques of anesthesia, and resuscitation. Complete airway control is obligatory when the anesthetist is providing total ventilation.
4. Ventilatory assistance in prone position. In the face-down position, patients, especially children, are in danger of respiratory depression, and ventilation should be assisted or controlled. Endotracheal intubation is mandatory for this purpose.
5. Removal of apparatus from the surgical field. Intubation enables the anesthetist to relinquish his position so that the surgeon can have freedom to work on the head, face, or neck.

DISADVANTAGES OF ENDOTRACHEAL INTUBATION

The undesirable features of intubation vary all the way from minor inconveniences to fatal complications.[6,7] They include the following:
1. Reduction of tracheal lumen. The presence of any endotracheal tube reduces the barely adequate lumen of the child's trachea.[8,9,9a] The radius of the trachea is reduced by the width of the wall of the tube, the diameter by twice the width of the tube wall. This may be of critical significance in the small infant.
2. More apparatus. The introduction of additional equipment usually employed with endotracheal anesthesia, including breathing valves, inflatable cuffs, or throat packs, immediately adds a new group of risks.
3. Complications at the time of intubation. Spasm, apnea, loosened and dislodged teeth, or lacerations of soft tissues must be expected to occur occasionally with oral intubation. Nasal intubation adds the danger of hemorrhage due to tearing of mucosal and adenoid tissue.[10]
4. Complications while tube is in place. Kinking of the tube, obstruction of the bronchus, and accidental extubation during operation also may raise problems.
5. Extubation spasm. This is one of the most difficult complications to prevent in children and may deal a telling blow to a child after a critical operation.[11]
6. Postoperative complications. Hoarseness, sore throat, tracheitis, and forgotten pack are a few of the postoperative complications that have been known to occur.

Listing of these disadvantages of endotracheal anesthesia does not imply that the method should be abandoned. Endotracheal tubes, like automobiles, are here to stay, but neither should be used without full realization of the possible dangers involved.

INDICATIONS FOR ENDOTRACHEAL ANESTHESIA

Having reviewed the major arguments for and against intubation, it is now possible to be more specific and point out those situations in which the advantages outweigh, balance, or are outweighed by the disadvantages and thus divide various procedures into categories in which intubation seems mandatory, preferable, optional, or not justified.[4]

Conditions in which endotracheal intubation is mandatory. There are several types of operations in which the advantages of intubation so far outweigh the disadvantages that no patient should be operated upon under general anesthesia unless intubation is employed. These include the following:

1. Operations upon patients with full stomach or intestinal obstruction
2. Intrathoracic procedures
3. Major operations in the prone position
4. Intracranial operations

Conditions in which intubation is definitely preferable. There are a number of operations that are more safely and more easily performed under endotracheal anesthesia. If a competent anesthetist is available, intubation is indicated, but operation may reasonably be undertaken without intubation. The following procedures might be included here:

1. Major operations about the mouth, face, and neck.
2. Operations in the kidney or lateral jackknife position and similar compromising positions.
3. Operations in the upper abdomen.
4. Pneumoencephalogram.
5. If tonsillectomy is to be performed while the child is in the sitting position, endotracheal anesthesia is certainly indicated. If the surgeon objects to intubation, the only solution is to place the child in the head-down position.
6. Infants with pyloric stenosis require special consideration because they frequently have been fed clear fluids shortly before operation. If a Levin tube is passed and the infant's stomach is emptied of this fluid before operation, an endotracheal tube is not mandatory; however, if curds or solids are present, one cannot be sure that these are all removed, and an endotracheal tube is necessary.

Conditions in which intubation is optional. There are some procedures in which the advantages of intubation are rather evenly balanced by the disadvantages. As a result there is heated but pointless disagreement as to whether intubation should or should not be performed. The outstanding example is tonsillectomy.[12] If the patient is in the head-down position and a reliable mouth gag such as the Brown-Davis gag is used, a clear airway may be maintained without intubation, and the use of an endotracheal tube may be justifiable but certainly is not mandatory. In this category are found the following operations:

1. Tonsillectomy in the horizontal or head-down position
2. Operations in the lower abdomen
3. Minor operations about the head, mouth, and neck

Conditions in which routine intubation seems unjustified. There is an increasing tendency among anesthetists to intubate all children during general anesthesia. Such a practice has advantages that are immediately seen, but it carries a certain amount of latent danger. Although experienced personnel may be able to carry out the practice, the occasional pediatric anesthetist may be led into serious trouble. Believing he should intubate all children for herniorrhaphy, circumcision, and such simple procedures, he may subject his patients to unnecessary trauma in repeated attempts at intubation and to other complications caused by inexperience or lack of training. In the hands of the skilled anesthetist complications will be rare, but even a dislodged tooth or a nosebleed would deserve criticism if intubation were not truly indicated, and the event of a tracheotomy or death following "routine" intubation would be inexcusable. Procedures that do not justify routine intubation include the following:

1. Short plastic and orthopedic procedures on limbs with the patient supine
2. Perineal operations (circumcision, cystoscopy) in the supine position
3. Herniorrhaphy
4. Minor surgery on body or limbs (incision and drainage, excisions, biopsies) with the patient supine

ORAL AND NASAL ROUTES FOR INTUBATION

Under most circumstances the oral route for endotracheal intubation is definitely preferable. Nasal intubation is slightly more difficult, and often causes epistaxis or pharyngeal hemorrhage due to tearing of the mucosal lining of the nose.[10] Large pieces of adenoid tissue may be torn off, and these and other scrapings may be carried down into the trachea. Furthermore, it is often necessary to use a smaller tube if the nasal route is chosen.

For prolonged postoperative ventilation of infants and children, nasal endotracheal intubation causes less gagging and is more easily tolerated. Increased familiarity with this technique has led many to use it more frequently for operative procedures in children. However, in our practice we retain this nasal route for specific situations such as repair of cleft palate and prolonged dental procedures.

PREPARATION OF EQUIPMENT FOR ENDOTRACHEAL INTUBATION

If intubation is intended, all of the necessary equipment should be fully prepared before induction of anesthesia. Forgotten items cause embarrassment under all circumstances, but if a relaxant is used and apparatus is not ready, the situation can be serious. The various types of apparatus have already been described (Chapter 6). Items for an individual case will include the following:

1. Laryngoscope
2. Endotracheal tubes (3 sizes)
3. Tape for fixation of tube
4. Adapters for connecting nonrebreathing or closed-system apparatus
5. Suction catheters that will pass through tubes easily
6. Packing (if airtight system is desired in children 1 to 8 years old) or syringe and clamp for inflatable cuff (for airtight system in older patients)
7. Lubricant (optional)
8. Long forceps (if nasal route is chosen for intubation)
9. Small basin of water to moisten catheter tip

When intubation is not intended, as in herniorrhaphy or circumcision, a suitable laryngoscope, endotracheal tube, and suction catheter should be at hand for emergency use, but additional equipment need not be prepared beforehand.

The choice of a suitable laryngoscope is not difficult in most cases. In general,

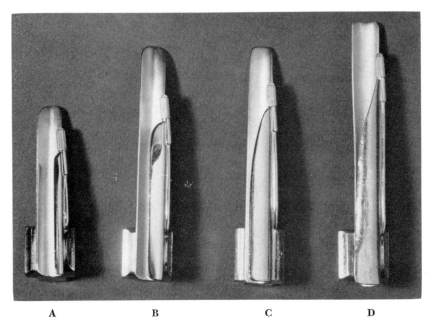

     A   **B**   **C**   **D**

Fig. 9-1. Infant laryngoscope blades vary in size and position of bulb, length and shape of tip, curvature, and over-all length. **A,** Miller premature. **B,** Miller infant. **C,** Wis-Hipple. **D,** Foregger No. 1.

the anesthetist should choose a straight blade for children and should use the smallest one that will do the job (Fig. 9-1). Thick, wide blades are especially to be avoided. A guide for the choice of apparatus is shown in Table 6-2 (p. 103). In most situations it is possible to substitute the next smaller or next larger laryngoscope for the one indicated in the guide. When a cuffed tube is used, however, it is definitely desirable to use a blade with a wide aperture. The Miller and the Macintosh blades are especially valuable here.

In choosing the endotracheal tube, the plastic Magill tubes are satisfactory for all purposes in children up to 7 or 8 years of age. If an airtight fit is desired in older children, the cuffed tube is preferable.

It is of the utmost importance that exactly the correct size of endotracheal tube is used. A tube that is too large will be traumatic; one that is small will offer excessive airway resistance, and there is little margin for error.

Formulas have been devised for predicting the size of tube that will be correct for individual patients, but none has been proved completely reliable. One scheme is to guess the size of the glottis by the lumen of the external naris. The safest method is to consult a guide based on clinical experience, such as that compiled by Slater and associates[13] or that contained in Table 9-1. One chooses the tube indicated by such a guide as being most suitable and, in addition, picks out the next larger and next smaller sizes of tubes. Of these three endotracheal tubes, one will usually be correct.

Table 9-1. *Guide to choice of endotracheal tubes*

Age	Weight (lb.)	Size Internal diameter (mm.)	Size External diameter (French)	Length (cm.)	Type
Newborn	3 to 5	3,3.5	12, 14	10	Plain Magill
Newborn	5 to 7	4.0	16	12	Plain Magill
1 mo.	7 to 10	4.5	18	13	Plain Magill
6 mo.	14	4.5	18	14	Plain Magill
1 yr.	21	5.0	20	15	Plain Magill
2 yr.	27	5.5	22	16	Plain Magill
3 yr.	31	5.5	22	16	Plain Magill
4 yr.	35	6.0	24	17	Plain Magill
5 yr.	40	6.0	24	17	Plain Magill
6 yr.	50	6.5	26	18	Plain Magill
8 yr.	65	6.5	26	18	Plain or cuffed
10 yr.	80	7.0	28	20	Plain or cuffed
12 yr.	100	7.0	28	20	Plain or cuffed
14 yr.	110	7.5	30	24	Plain or cuffed

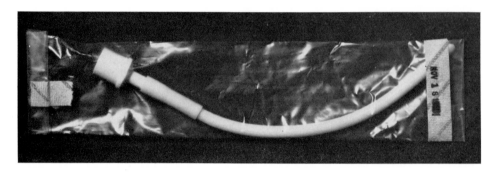

Fig. 9-2. Endotracheal tube with connector and adapter in sterile envelope.

The length of the tube must also be considered, for most endotracheal tubes are too long as manufactured and must be cut to appropriate length before use in order to reduce dead space, resistance, and the tendency to kink. For intubation by nasal route, endotracheal tubes should be about 20% longer than those used for oral intubation.

Of equal importance to using tubes of correct size is the need for using endotracheal tubes that are *clean*. Tracheitis was a frequent and often a severe complication of endotracheal intubation until the importance of clean apparatus was appreciated.[14,15] Tubes and adapters must be washed immediately after use, sterilized, and stored where they will not easily be contaminated. Jacoby[16] proved the importance of cleaning tubes immediately after use. It is now customary to sterilize endotracheal tubes by soaking in germicidal solutions such as alcohol or zephiran, by gamma radiation, or by gas sterilization with ethylene oxide. In either case much care must be taken to free the tubes from the irritant qualities of the sterilizing agents. After soaking in cleansing solutions, equipment must be rinsed thoroughly, and following gas sterilization it must be aired for 36 to 48 hours before use. Storage after cleansing is equally important, and for this individual packing of endotracheal tubes in plastic envelopes is recommended (Fig. 9-2).

When preparing to intubate a patient, the tubes should not be contaminated. The container should be opened, and the tube should be left easily available but not placed in contact with other equipment. During the process of intubation, the tube is handled only by the end that is to remain outside of the patient's mouth.

CHOOSING THE TIME TO INTUBATE

Awake intubation. The anesthetist has a choice of several methods of intubation of the newborn infant. Probably the safest method is to intubate the infant awake. Babies tolerate this extremely well and will maintain their own ventilation with very little reflex irritability and a surprising absence of complications. For very weak, nonresisting infants this technique seems clearly preferable. It is also advisable when anesthetists are relatively inexperienced and certainly is justified for any who prefer this method. The anesthetist who first attempts to intubate a small infant will find the anatomy unlike that of the adult, the epiglottis being folded and soft, the glottic chink high and anterior, and the tongue large and bulky (Fig. 9-3).

The first step should consist of oxygenating the child well with bag and mask. Then it helps to apply topical anesthesia by letting the baby suck it from a tongue blade or by spraying the hypopharynx with one hand squeeze of 4% lidocaine (total dose 0.1 ml.). Oxygen is again applied until the child is well saturated and the local anesthetic has had time to become effective.

Intubation is more easily accomplished if an assistant immobilizes the infant's head, holding it so that it is extended and at the same time depressing the shoulders so that the infant will not throw his chest forward (Fig. 9-4). The anesthetist then introduces the laryngoscope gently so that the infant continues to breathe and cry even when the glottis is exposed. If the baby chokes or becomes apneic, one should withdraw the laryngoscope, let the baby breathe, and start again. After successful intubation, closed-system apparatus is attached and rapid induction is provided with cyclopropane or halothane.

Most small infants will squirm while this is being performed, although there is no true bucking on the tube. Because of the resistance, it is never so easy to expose the glottis and the cords are never so relaxed as when the infant is anesthetized. This is important in that it often prevents one from using as large a tube as would be possible had the child been completely relaxed. Thus, although safe, the method is never quite ideal, and many anesthetists choose to anesthetize all infants prior to intubation.

By the time they are 2 weeks old most infants develop sufficient strength in their tongues and jaws to resist strenuously the introduction of the laryngoscope. From this point onward awake intubation is contraindicated, except in such situ-

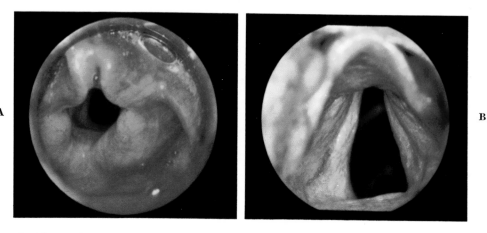

A   **B**

Fig. 9-3. A, Infant glottis, magnified ×6, and, **B,** adult glottis, ×2. Note soft, edematous appearance of infant tissues and folded gamma (Ω) shape of epiglottis. (Courtesy Dr. Paul Hollinger, Chicago, Ill.)

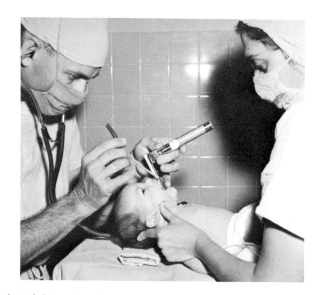

Fig. 9-4. Intubation of the awake infant requires correct positioning of the head. Baby should be held with head extended and shoulders down to prevent arching of the back. (From Psaltopoulo-Mehrez, M.: Internat. Anesth. Clin. 1:169, 1962.)

ations as when the patient has abdominal distention, is in coma, or is extremely weak.

Intubation under anesthesia. Although intubation under anesthesia can more nearly approach perfection, all methods involve potential hazards that must be appreciated. For newborn infants, ether induction is irritating and prolonged. Both cyclopropane and halothane are more rapid and smooth, but cyclopropane is likely to induce laryngospasm, and with both agents depth is difficult to evaluate—one has the tendency to attempt intubation prematurely and provoke severe vocal cord spasm, and relaxants, in turn, always bear the danger of extended apnea and anoxia.

The most important feature of intubation is judging the correct time to pass the tube. Under ether anesthesia the signs of depth are fairly reliable. Adequate relaxation for endotracheal intubation is usually associated with general muscular relaxation, including relaxation of the jaw, and regular rhythmic respiration with early dominance of diaphragmatic breathing. In children more than 1 year of age there is an additional and valuable sign, i.e., fixed pupils that are beginning to dilate.

It is usually wise to insert an oral airway prior to intubation whether it appears needed or not. This enables the anesthetist to check jaw relaxation and frequently shows him that the patient is not as well anesthetized as he expected. He can then replace the mask and take a few extra minutes to induce the child, without revealing his error or breaking the even course of the induction. Another hint often found useful is to wait until the patient appears ready for intubation and then to take one more minute before attempting to pass the tube. It is quite obvious that we all have the tendency to be too impatient!

Before attempting to intubate a patient under cyclopropane one should be sure that the patient is well relaxed and that respiration is considerably depressed. Infants require relatively high levels of cyclopropane, whether administered in a strong concentration or for prolonged periods. Slight slowing of the heart may also be taken as a sign of depth, but this is not one to be desired. Muscle tone should be tested in the arms, but it is preferable not to pry open the infant's eyes to test anesthetic level. In all patients over 6 months of age, however, *centered, fixed pupils represent the best single indication of the time to intubate.* Intubation while the eyes are still deviated often is performed easily and quickly, only to be followed by active and forceful responses. Since unsuccessful attempts to intubate under cyclopropane or halothane may lead to severe laryngospasm, it is advisable to have succinylcholine prepared for immediate use. When infants are to be induced with these agents, the signs of intubation depth are even more misleading. Invariably the beginner will start with a fine induction, continue with 5 minutes of uneventful anesthesia, and then upon attempting to pass the tube will find the patient virtually awake. If halothane is used alone, fixation of the eyes again is the most reliable sign in older patients, while jaw relaxation and toleration of an oral airway should be used as supplementary indications.

Relaxants are of considerable use for intubation in infants and children. Tracheal catheterization under oxygen and relaxants without anesthesia have real justification. When used alone or as a supplement to other anesthetics, succinylcholine may be given to infants in doses of 1 mg. per pound either by intravenous or intramuscular route. Following intramuscular injection relaxation occurs within 90 to 120 seconds. The method seems very satisfactory, especially if there is no easily available vein.

Of the several techniques in use for intubation of the newborn infant, the one I prefer is to oxygenate the infant for one or two minutes by mask and then inject succinylcholine, 1 mg. per pound, by intramuscular route. Oxygen administration is resumed, and ventilation is assisted with gradually increasing effort as the relaxant becomes effective. After 90 seconds the infant will still be breathing spontaneously, but all hyperactivity should have disappeared. The jaw will be opened without resistance, and the glottis will be easily exposed. Intubation will be greatly facilitated, but since the patient still is exchanging, there will be less danger of hypoxia than when the intravenous route is used.

One might imagine that it would be most unpleasant to have an endotracheal tube inserted without anesthesia, but it has been shown that after receiving relaxants, awake subjects tolerate intubation quite easily.

When induction of anesthesia is performed with general anesthetics, intubation may be facilitated by the use of succinylcholine, unless specifically contraindicated by airway obstruction or full stomach. Using succinylcholine by intravenous route, a dose of 0.5 mg. per pound is usually sufficient, and apnea and relaxation will occur immediately. Under such circumstances hypoxia is always to be feared, and intubation must be accomplished promptly.

There is the additional danger of severe bradycardia or asystole, especially when cyclopropane or halothane is the principal anesthetic. Bradycardia is somewhat less likely to be severe following intramuscular injection, but it still can be serious. This complication can be completely prevented by atropine, if given with proper dosage and timing. If atropine is administered during the period of active vagal stimulation, the activity will be controlled, but often rather pronounced arrhythmias will occur as the atropine takes effect.

Small infants seldom show fasciculation following administration of succinylcholine. With a standard dose of 1 mg. per pound, endotracheal intubation usually may be performed 10 seconds after intravenous injection and 90 seconds after intramuscular injection. Using other relaxants, one should follow administration

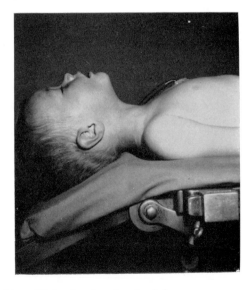

Fig. 9-5. "Classical" position with head and neck extended.

of the relaxant by assisted respiration for 2 or 3 minutes, test the jaw relaxation, and be able, by squeezing the breathing bag, to expand the patient's chest with total absence of patient resistance.

POSITION

Immediately before intubation, the child's head is positioned. Instead of the hyperextended or "classical" position[2] (Fig. 9-5), the "amended" position is pre-

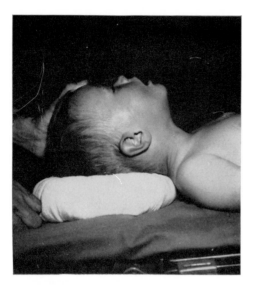

Fig. 9-6. "Amended" position: pillow under head, neck flexed, head extended.

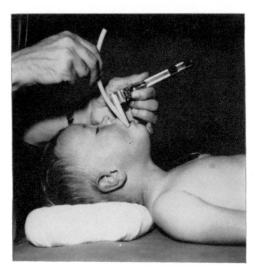

Fig. 9-7. Intubation then follows the anatomic curve of the trachea.

ferred, with the head elevated on a padded ring or pillow, the neck flexed, and the head extended in the so-called "sniffing" position (Fig. 9-6). Passage of the laryngoscope and endotracheal tube will then follow the natural anatomic curve of the trachea (Fig. 9-7).

INSERTION OF TUBE

After the head is positioned, the airway is removed, and a rapid survey is made for loose or fragmented teeth. The laryngoscope is then taken in the left hand, and the blade is inserted to the right of the midline of the mouth in order to avoid the upper incisor teeth, if present, and in order to displace the tongue toward the left. As the blade is advanced carefully the oropharynx is exposed and then the hypopharynx and upper end of the esophagus. The glottis lies anterior to this, or above it, as the patient is lying supine. To bring the glottis into view the laryngoscope blade should not be pried upward by hauling back on the handle, but the whole floor of the mouth must be raised by lifting the laryngoscope in the direction of the handle. The epiglottis will then be seen, and by elevating the tip of the epiglottis the cords and larynx are exposed.

With infants it may be helpful to depress the larynx in order to visualize the glottis, This may be performed by an assistant[16,17] but it is more to the satisfaction of the anesthetist if he can do it himself. This can be done simply by sweeping the fifth finger of the left hand under the chin while the remaining fingers are being used to hold the laryngoscope.

Only if the glottis is open should the anesthetist proceed with intubation. If the cords are in spasm or are inadequately relaxed, attempts to pass a tube will result only in coughing and more spasm. The mask should be replaced and relaxation sought with a deeper plane of anesthesia or with the aid of relaxants.

If the glottis is open, the anesthetist quickly chooses the largest tube that will pass without requiring force, moistens the tip by dipping it in water, and inserts it gently through the cords. The end of the tube should stop halfway between cords and carina. The tube is quickly taped in place,* and the necessary connections are made. Time must not be wasted here, for the patient may either be apneic and in danger of becoming hypoxic or he may be light and on the verge of awakening. As rapidly as possible the anesthetist must see that the patient is ventilating, that anesthesia is reestablished, and that the tube is secured firmly in place. It is also necessary that he check the child's chest with a stethoscope to make sure that the end of the tube has not passed beyond the carina, thus obstructing one bronchus. Absence of breath sounds on one side and unequal chest expansion call for gradual retraction of the tube until respiration is equal on both sides of the chest. The child's chest should then be inflated by way of the endotracheal tube in order to be sure the tube is still in the trachea.

If an airtight fit is desired in infants and small children, neither packing nor cuff is necessary, the round cricoid ring serving as a seal about the tube. In older children, as in adults, leaking around the tube is often a problem. In children be-

---

*One must be sure, too, that the adhesive tape used for fixation of the tube is stuck to the tube itself and not to an adapter or connecting piece. Unless the tube is secured it may separate from the connecting piece and slip down into the trachea.

tween the ages of 2 and 10, a moistened gauze pack may be inserted into the hypopharynx to control the leak. In larger children one should use a cuffed tube if an airtight fit is mandatory. Actually, especially when large gas flows are used, a slight leak around the tube may be acceptable. It shows that the tube is not too tight and also promotes CO_2 washout and elimination of dead space. If any form of packing is used, one end should be left protruding out of the mouth so that it cannot be forgotten.

ADDITIONAL APPARATUS

After insertion of the tube, it is advisable to place a rolled-up sponge between the child's teeth to prevent biting down on the tube. A soft bite block like this is less traumatic to the mouth and pharynx than is a stiff airway. Furthermore, as demonstrated by Code Smith,[18] it is preferable to have the endotracheal tube enter the center of the mouth. Then it can arch up along the roof of the mouth, and there will be less danger of kinking than if the tube were held horizontally between the jaws, to be angulated sharply as it bends to descend into the throat.

If the open-drop technique is to be used, it will not be necessary to add adapters to the endotracheal tube, but after intubation one usually employs nonrebreathing or closed techniques, and for these methods adapters will be needed (Figs. 9-8 and 9-9).

One of the most common errors seen in pediatric anesthesia is the insertion of a small adapter into the lumen of the endotracheal tube (Fig. 9-10), thus reducing the airway and greatly increasing the resistance, as shown by studies of Macon and Bruner[8] and of Orkin, Siegel, and Rovenstine.[9]

One should use an adapter that has a lumen as large as or larger than that of

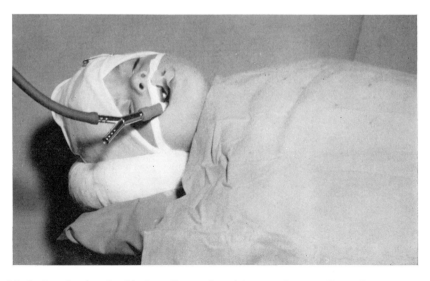

Fig. 9-8. Patient intubated with Ayre Y nonrebreathing attachment. (From Gross, R. F.: The surgery of infancy and childhood, Philadelphia, 1953, W. B. Saunders Co.)

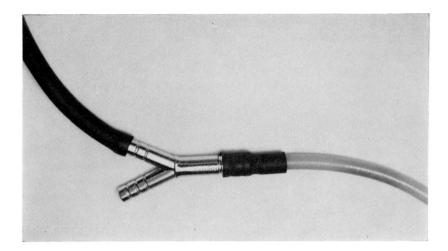

Fig. 9-9. Close up of T-tube apparatus, showing coupling of endotracheal tube and Y tube with rubber connecting piece.

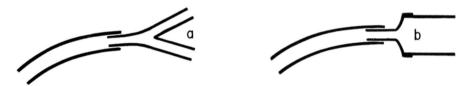

Fig. 9-10. Wrong way. Do not reduce the lumen of the airway by inserting Y tube, **a,** or adapter, **b,** inside of endotracheal tube.

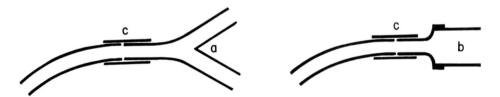

Fig. 9-11. Right way. Maintain maximal airway by using Y tube, **a,** or adapter, **b,** that has a lumen at least as large as the endotracheal tube and bridging both with a rubber connecting piece, **c.**

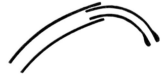

Fig. 9-12. Avoid narrow, curved adapters, which increase resistance and make the use of suction difficult.

the endotracheal tube (Fig. 9-11). This may be coupled to the tube by a rubber connector that overlaps the end of the tube and the end of the adapter. Although any pliable tubing of appropriate size may be used, the tapered, funnel-shaped ends of urethral catheters are excellent for this purpose.

Another safe method of fitting adapter to endotracheal tube is to use an adapter the bore of which is just large enough to fit *over* the endotracheal catheter.

One should avoid the use of narrow, curved adapters or sharply angulated connections that increase airway resistance and also make suctioning difficult or impossible (Fig. 9-12).

If all endotracheal tubes were made with dilated outer end, the situation would be greatly improved.

In fitting apparatus to the endotracheal tube, it must be remembered that excessive distance between the lips and the exhalation vent or canister will add to dead space and cause carbon dioxide accumulation. Consequently this distance must be reduced to a minimum.

PROBLEMS ENCOUNTERED DURING INTUBATION

Several difficulties may complicate the insertion of the endotracheal tube. A number of these may be caused by anatomic or pathologic lesions that interfere with laryngoscopy or passage of the endotracheal tube itself. Large tumors of the mouth and throat, skeletal deformities of the face or cervical spine, cervical abscesses, and tumors about the face and neck are not uncommon in children. These will be discussed in later chapters.

Reference has been made to the occasional situation in which an endotracheal tube may be inserted beyond the vocal cords but is obstructed by constriction of the trachea at the cricoid ring. In such cases a considerably smaller tube must be used than would be normal for that child. This cricoid narrowing has been reported by Eckenhoff,[19] and by Colgan and Keats.[20] In our experience several similar cases have been observed but only in children who had hydrocephalus or some other craniocerebral defect.

EXTUBATION OF THE TRACHEA

As emphasized by Hallowell,[21] extubation of the trachea may initiate serious bronchospasm and other complications that will completely upset an otherwise successful anesthesia. The management of this phase of anesthesia is described in Chapter 11.

REFERENCES
1. Gillespie, N. A.: Endotracheal anaesthesia in infants, Brit. J. Anaesth. **17**:2-12, 1939.
2. Gillespie, N. A.: Endotracheal anaesthesia, ed. 2, Madison, 1948, University of Wisconsin Press.
3. Leigh, M. D., and Belton, M. K.: Pediatric anesthesia, ed. 2, New York, 1960, The Macmillan Co.
4. Smith, R. M.: Indications for endotracheal anesthesia in pediatric anesthesia, Anesth. & Analg. **33**:107-114, 1954.
5. Pender, J. W.: Endotracheal anesthesia in children, advantages and disadvantages, Anesthesiology **15**:495-506, 1954.

6. Flagg, P. J.: Endotracheal inhalation anesthesia: special reference to postoperative reactions and suggestions for their elimination, Laryngoscope **61**:1-12, 1951.

7. Carruthers, H. C., and Graves, H. B.: The complications of endotracheal anaesthesia, Canad. Anaesth. Soc. J. **3**:244-253, 1956.

8. Macon, E. B., and Bruner, H. D.: The scientific aspect of endotracheal tubes, Anesthesiology **11**:313-320, 1950.

9. Orkin, L. K., Siegel, M., and Rovenstine, E. A.: I. Resistance to breathing by apparatus used in anesthesia, Anesth. & Analg. **33**:217-233, 1954.

9a. Glauser, E. M., Cook, C. D., and Bougas, T. P.: Pressure-flow characteristics and dead spaces of endotracheal tubes used in infants, Anesthesiology **22**:339-341, 1961.

10. Dingley, A. R.: Nasal intubation—dangers and difficulties, Brit. Med. J. **1**:693-694, 1953.

11. Shumacher, H. B., Jr., and Hampton, L. J.: Sudden death occurring immediately after operation in patients with cardiac disease, with particular reference to role of aspiration through the endotracheal tube and extubation, J. Thorac. Surg. **21**:48-56, 1951.

12. Collins, V. J., and Granatelli, A.: Anesthesia for tonsillectomy in children, J.A.M.A. **161**:5-9, 1956.

13. Slater, H. M., Sheridan, C. A., and Ferguson, R. H.: Endotracheal tube sizes for infants and children, Anesthesiology **16**:950-952, 1955.

14 Smith, R. M.: The prevention of tracheitis in children following endotracheal anesthesia, Anesth. & Analg. **32**:102-112, 1953.

15. Zindler, M., and Deming, M. V.: The anesthetic management of infants for the surgical repair of congenital atresia of the esophagus with tracheoesophageal fistula, Anesth. & Analg. **32**:180-190, 1953.

16. Jacoby, J., Ziegler, C., Macpherson, C. R., and Garvin, J.: The anesthesiologist and hospital infections, Anesth. Analg. **39**:75-80, 1960.

17. Davenport, H. T., and Rosales, J. K.: Endotracheal intubation of infants and children, Canad. Anesth. Soc. J. **6**:65-74, 1959.

18. Smith, C.: Lecture at Anesthesia Research Symposium, Bal Harbor, Fla. March, 1964.

19. Eckenhoff, J.: Some anatomic considerations of the infant larynx influencing endotracheal anesthesia, Anesthesiology **12**:401-410, 1951.

20. Colgan, F. J., and Keats, A. S.: Subglottic stenosis: a cause of difficult intubation, Anesthesiology **15**:265-269, 1957.

21. Hallowell, P.: Endotracheal intubation of infants and children, Internat. Anesth. Clin. **1**:135-151, 1962.

Chapter 10

Maintenance of anesthesia

ILLUSTRATIVE CASE

Perhaps the easiest way to show the features of the maintenance technique would be to describe a case such as that of a 2-year-old boy who is to have a herniorrhaphy under open-drop ether. This will not present all the problems but will give the simplest version of pediatric anesthesia, to which many variations may be added.

We can assume that induction has been accomplished with nitrous oxide, ethyl ether, and oxygen and that ethyl ether is now being given by open drop on a gauze-covered Yankauer mask while the anesthetist maintains continual support of the child's jaw (Fig. 10-1). The child's respirations become rhythmic, full, and even, and intercostal and diaphragmatic action are present. The boy's eyes are fixed, and the pupils that were dilated during the excitement stage are

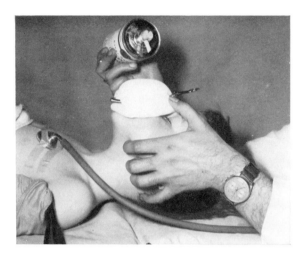

Fig. 10-1. To maintain a free airway the angle of the jaw must be supported at all times.

now small again. Through the precordial stethoscope the heart sounds are heard at about 160 per minute with regular rhythm. Breath sounds are audible through the stethoscope and are full and unobstructed. The child's body and limbs have become relaxed. There are no involuntary motions. The blood pressure cuff and stethoscope are strapped on, and the blood pressure is found to be 100/80, within normal range for this age. The data are charted. An oral airway is slipped into the mouth, the ether mask is replaced, and the administration of ether is resumed.

Ether is maintained at an even rate, usually about 40 to 60 drops per minute, and oxygen is introduced under the mask by a catheter at 500 ml. per minute. The use of supplemental oxygen is of special importance when dealing with Negro children. Care should be taken to prevent injury to the eyes from ether or pressure of the mask. Rather than put foreign material into the eyes, when possible it seems preferable to protect them by covering them with dry, folded gauze, Care should be taken to see that the lids remain closed. An additional precaution that may be taken while giving drop ether is to bring the ether can up from below the chin rather than to use the customary path directly over the eyes. As the ether can is being moved, the last drop often misses the mask, and it is better to have it fall on the neck than in an eye.

The anesthetist makes sure that eager operating room personnel do not pull the child into position or start to wash the operative site while the patient is still in a light unsteady plane. As the surgeon prepares the area of incision it is well to see that the drapes are not too heavy and that the room temperature is not over 70° F. when older children are being anesthetized.

Before the operation is started the anesthetist checks the patient for adequate depth of anesthesia. The pupils are fixed with minimal dilatation, and body musculature, including that of the jaw, is relaxed. Respiration is full and unobstructed, and the rhythm is regular. Intercostal and diaphragmatic respiration are about equal, and inspiration is slightly more forceful than expiration. Pulse and blood pressure are checked and are found to be within normal limits. The anesthetist gives the go-ahead sign to the surgeon and notes on the chart the starting time of the operation.

At the first incision the anesthetist watches the patient carefully to see if he might have been mistaken as to adequate level of anesthesia. A sharp inspiration, laryngeal crowing, or change in pulse rate would suggest that the level of anesthesia is somewhat too light and that more anesthesia is needed. No reaction to the incision suggests adequate depth.

Once an operation is begun, the anesthetist may feel that all he has to do is sit back and wait for the surgeon to complete the procedure. Within a fairly short period of time, however, he learns that there are a number of important items to take care of *during* anesthesia, and it is best to establish a systematic approach that includes broad objectives, general rules, and detailed check points.

OBJECTIVES

The principal objectives of the anesthetist during operation are (1) to provide the necessary working conditions for the surgeon and (2) to protect the patient. The surgeon usually requires immobilization and exposure of the area in which he is operating. If the operation is a herniorrhaphy, the anesthetist can attain both of his objectives, but in many situations it is impossible to give complete satisfaction to the surgeon and at the same time provide normal physiologic conditions for the patient. During intrathoracic operations, for example, the surgeon wants the lung deflated while the anesthetist wants to provide normal expansion. In such cases a compromise is the only fair solution.

GENERAL RULES

Since a child's reactions to anesthesia and surgery are rapid and extreme, the single most important principle in maintenance technique is *constant observation*. For this reason the following rules should be followed during anesthesia:

1. The anesthetist should remain at the head of the patient and not leave him at any time. If infusions are to be started or lights are to be adjusted at the foot of the table, someone else must do it. Also, the practice of changing anesthetists during an operation should be avoided. Since fatigue may become a real hazard in extremely prolonged cases, it occasionally may be wise to allow the anesthetist time to break away to refresh himself, but routine coffee or cigarette breaks and shifting of personnel are dangerous and should be prohibited.
2. The anesthetist must monitor the patient's heart and respiration continuously by means of a stethoscope (Fig. 10-2). When possible, a finger should be kept on a palpable pulse in the face, neck, wrist, or groin, depending upon the position of patient and anesthetist.
3. The face of the patient is kept in view, except when in the face-down position in a headrest. Drapes are held away from the face, airway, and breathing apparatus to prevent obstruction or kinking of the equipment and to maintain an accessible avenue of approach for applying suction.

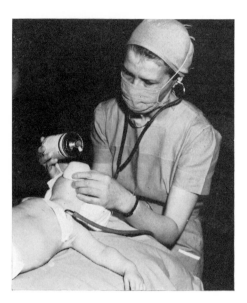

Fig. 10-2. The heart and respiration are monitored by a stethoscope during every operation. (If the left chest is to be entered, the stethoscope is fixed under the right axilla, or an esophageal stethoscope may be used.) (From Smith, R. M.: J. Amer. A. Nurse Anesth. **24:**9, 1956.)

4. An accurate chart is to be prepared and maintained for all cases (Fig. 10-3). The data concerning preoperative evaluation, history of illness and medications, and details of anesthetic and supportive management form documentation of direct value in the correct treatment of the patient (and are also of considerable legal value to the anesthetist). As usual, blood pressure, pulse, and respiration are recorded every 5 minutes. It has been of considerable benefit in our experience to designate columns for serial charting of both fluids and temperature. Pertinent data are also added concerning medication, application and release of tourniquets, or repositioning of the patient. Any complications are described at once. The full value of a chart is realized only when items are entered in detail.

SPECIFIC SIGNS AND CHECK POINTS

Attention must be kept upon the patient continually, but must not be fixed on one detail to the exclusion of others. While the overmeticulous anesthetist is charting carefully, the patient might wake up or the infusion might run dry. All of the following items should be given frequent attention:

1. Signs of anesthetic level
2. Ventilation
3. Circulation and blood pressure
4. Fluid therapy
5. Body temperature
6. Position
7. Progress of the operation
8. Gastric distention
9. Apparatus
10. Planned system

Signs of anesthetic level. The term "depth of anesthesia" was coined when ether was the principal agent employed. By the use of the classic signs of ether

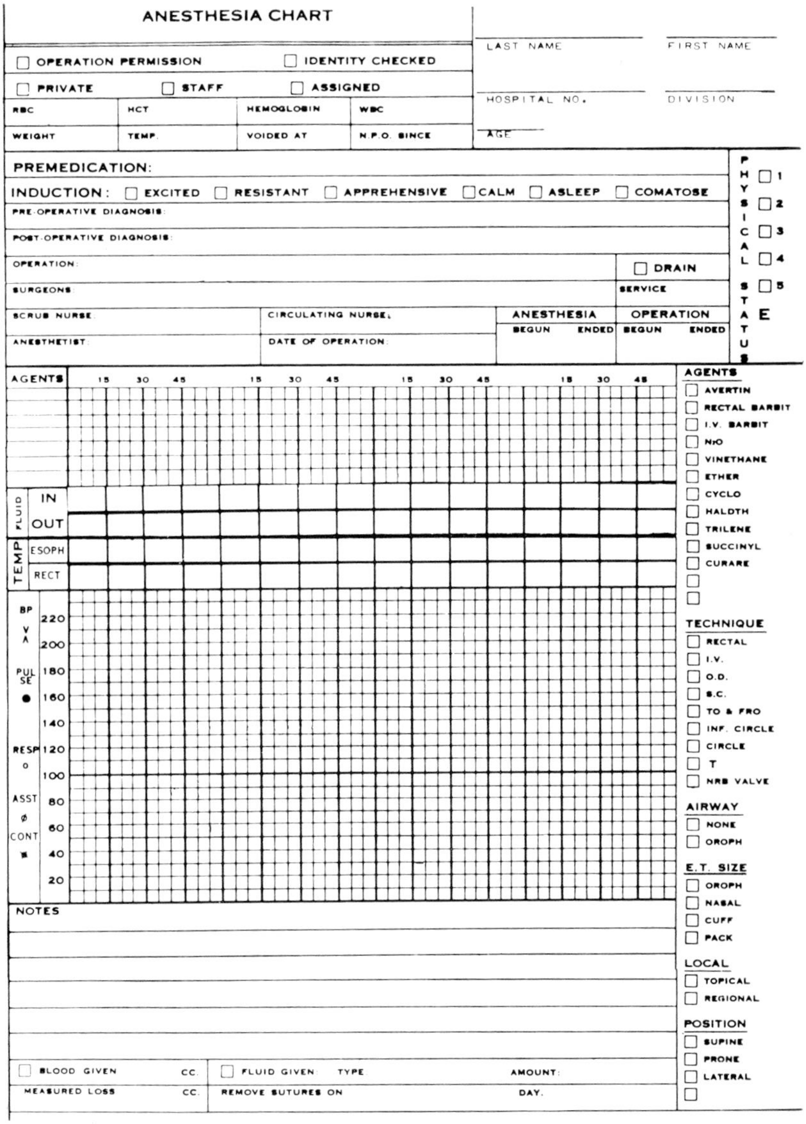

ANESTHESIA CHART

LAST NAME FIRST NAME

HOSPITAL NO. DIVISION

AGE

☐ OPERATION PERMISSION ☐ IDENTITY CHECKED

☐ PRIVATE ☐ STAFF ☐ ASSIGNED

RBC HCT HEMOGLOBIN WBC

WEIGHT TEMP. VOIDED AT N.P.O. SINCE

PREMEDICATION:

INDUCTION: ☐ EXCITED ☐ RESISTANT ☐ APPREHENSIVE ☐ CALM ☐ ASLEEP ☐ COMATOSE

PRE-OPERATIVE DIAGNOSIS:

POST-OPERATIVE DIAGNOSIS:

OPERATION: ☐ DRAIN

SURGEONS: SERVICE

SCRUB NURSE: CIRCULATING NURSE: ANESTHESIA BEGUN ENDED OPERATION BEGUN ENDED

ANESTHETIST: DATE OF OPERATION:

PHYSICAL STATUS ☐ 1 ☐ 2 ☐ 3 ☐ 4 ☐ 5 E

AGENTS 15 30 45 15 30 45 15 30 45 15 30 45

FLUID IN OUT

TEMP. ESOPH RECT

BP V Λ PULSE ● RESP O ASST Ø CONT ✱

220 200 180 160 140 120 100 80 60 40 20

NOTES

☐ BLOOD GIVEN CC. ☐ FLUID GIVEN TYPE AMOUNT:

MEASURED LOSS CC. REMOVE SUTURES ON DAY.

AGENTS: ☐ AVERTIN ☐ RECTAL BARBIT ☐ I.V. BARBIT ☐ N₂O ☐ VINETHANE ☐ ETHER ☐ CYCLO ☐ HALOTH ☐ TRILENE ☐ SUCCINYL ☐ CURARE ☐ ☐

TECHNIQUE: ☐ RECTAL ☐ I.V. ☐ O.D. ☐ S.C. ☐ TO & FRO ☐ INF. CIRCLE ☐ CIRCLE ☐ T ☐ NRB VALVE

AIRWAY: ☐ NONE ☐ OROPH

E.T. SIZE: ☐ OROPH ☐ NASAL ☐ CUFF ☐ PACK

LOCAL: ☐ TOPICAL ☐ REGIONAL

POSITION: ☐ SUPINE ☐ PRONE ☐ LATERAL ☐

Fig. 10-3. Anesthesia chart. For pediatric use specific columns for recording fluid exchange and temperature are recommended.

anesthesia, which were first described by Snow[1] and subsequently developed by Guedel,[2] the degree of anesthesia can be judged by pupillary reflexes, respiratory activity, and muscular relaxation (Fig. 10-4).

Since the introduction of cyclopropane, thiopental, halothane and relaxants, the phrase "depth of anesthesia" has lost its former meaning. As emphasized by Woodbridge,[3] anesthetic agents have four principal effects—those of analgesia, relaxation, blocking of reflexes, and hypnosis. Each agent affects the various re-

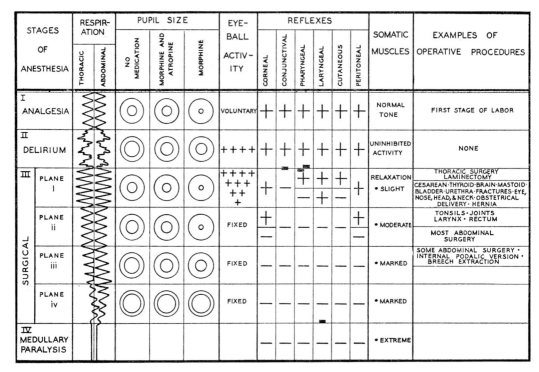

Fig. 10-4. Stages and planes of anesthesia. (From Goodman, L. S., and Gilman, A.: The pharmacological basis of therapeutics, ed. 2, New York, 1955, The Macmillan Co.)

ELEMENTS OF "ANESTHESIA" (NERVOUS DEPRESSION)

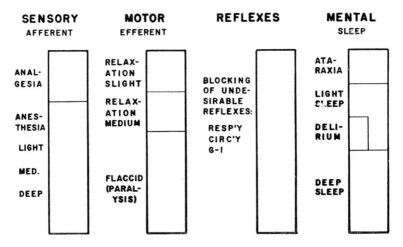

Fig. 10-5. Four components of general anesthesia. (From Woodbridge, P. D.: Anesthesiology **18:**536, 1957.)

sponses differently, thiopental causing deep hypnosis with little relaxation, the relaxants having exactly the opposite effects. Consequently, to estimate the degree of anesthesia, all four factors actually should be considered separately (Fig. 10-5).

Children show less definite signs of anesthesia than do adults, but those elicited during ether anesthesia are more reliable than when other agents are used. Probably the most valuable guides are character of respiration, degree of relaxation, and the eye signs.[4]

Character of respiration in ether anesthetic. When ether is being used by open-drop method or insufflation, the type of respiration gives the anesthetist considerable information about the child's level of anesthesia and about his physiologic condition in general. A well-oxygenated child in the first or the upper second plane of ether anesthesia breathes with regular rhythm, with intercostal activity definitely present. The duration of inspiration is equal to that of expiration and, although there is no gasping or tugging, inspiration has an element of force, whereas expiration is entirely passive and relaxed. If expiration is more forceful than inspiration, this suggests greater depth than is desirable. If an even, physiologic respiration is maintained under ether, one can be relatively sure that the patient has adequate analgesia, is relaxed, has reflex obtundation, and is asleep. As the plane of anesthesia of the patient becomes lighter, the rhythm of respiration may be interrupted by sighing, phonation, swallowing, and/or retching. Inspiration may become more full, but it loses the forceful, regular, pulling quality. Crowing may occur with either light or deep planes of anesthesia.

As the child passes from second into third plane, diaphragmatic breathing becomes more marked. Diaphragmatic respiration is evident in children in lighter planes than in adults.[5] Similarly, during entrotracheal anesthesia and during intrathoracic operations, diaphragmatic respiration is seen to be more pronounced.

Gasping respiration and grossly irregular rhythms are seen most frequently in infants and children under 2 years of age and may result from a stormy induction with much excitement or may be due to excessive depth, hypoxia, obstruction, or carbon dioxide accumulation during anesthesia. Tugging respiration, or "tracheal tug,"[6] with a downward jerking jaw may be regarded as a sign of inadequate ventilation, whether due to excessive depth, obstruction, or carbon dioxide excess. Tracheal tug and retraction of intercostal and suprasternal spaces may both be present together, or either may exist separately. Retraction when associated with rhythmic respiration is more often a sign of airway obstruction. The treatment of all of these respiratory abnormalities consists of clearing the airway, regaining a light, even plane of anesthesia, and improving the oxygenation of the child by hyperventilation with oxygen.

Muscular relaxation. In very small infants the degree of muscle tone is a valuable sign during anesthesia. Under general anesthesia the infant's plane may be kept light enough to allow flexor tone in elbows and fingers (Fig. 10-6). Some anesthetists hold a finger in a baby's mouth and have the plane of anesthesia light enough so that the infant will bite on the finger during the operation. In a 2-year-old child this it not desirable. Furthermore, during ether

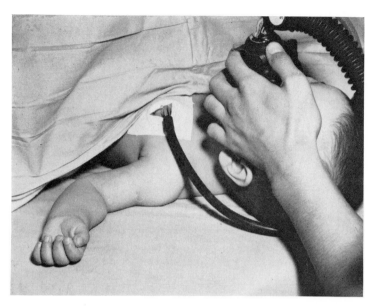

Fig. 10-6. Under general anesthesia the infant may be allowed to retain flexor tone in biceps and fingers.

anesthesia for herniorrhaphy a 2-year-old child's limbs and jaw should be relaxed.

General signs. One should not attempt to watch eye signs in infants. The eyelids are held closed during light anesthesia, and to force them open causes swelling of the lids and face. Furthermore, the irides of the baby's eyes are so dark that it is difficult to tell how large the pupil is.

When children are 2 or 3 years old, their eyes are less easily traumatized, and it becomes reasonable to follow the eye signs. Rolling eyes denote that a patient is in the first plane of surgical anesthesia. When the eyes stop moving but remain uncentered, one may assume that the patient has reached mid-first plane, and as the eyes become centered the patient passes into the second plane of surgical anesthesia.[7] It is rarely necessary to carry a child into a deeper plane of anesthesia since this level is adequate for most pediatric surgery.

The size and shape of the pupils have less definite meaning. Pupils are large during the excitement stage, become normal in the first plane, and then gradually dilate with greater anesthetic depth. Dilated pupils also may be caused by atropine, epinephrine, hypoxia, carbon dioxide accumulation, and cardiac defibrillation. Most causes of dilated pupils are harmful; consequently dilated pupils should be regarded as a danger sign. Unequal pupils (anisocoria) are seen fairly often during ether anesthesia and usually have little significance. One should bear this phenomenon in mind, however, and observe both eyes rather than either one alone. If one uses pupillary size as a sign, it is more important to note the change in size of the pupils of the individual patient than to judge by the absolute size at any one time. Irregularly shaped pupils are less often seen, but when seen, they have been associated with shock or hypoxia.

A useful sign is observed by holding the chin with one hand and keeping the fifth finger of this hand resting on the patient's larynx. As the anesthetized patient approaches the excitement stage, the larynx may be felt to move prior to swallowing and retching. If this is noted promptly, the deeper anesthesia usually can be gained in time to prevent complications.

CYCLOPROPANE. Under cyclopropane anesthesia children show definitely different signs than when ether is employed. Respiration does not have the forcefulness seen with ether but becomes depressed in a relatively light plane of surgical anesthesia. Infants and children, however, do not appear to become apneic under cyclopropane as readily as adults do. Children may develop an obstructed respiration with retraction of suprasternal and subcostal areas, but they usually continue to make respiratory efforts.

The pulse rate is a useful guide to cyclopropane anesthesia. In patients who have received adequate atropinization, the pulse remains regular and slightly faster than the preanesthetic rate. With deeper surgical anesthesia the heart may become slow or irregular, with runs of extraventricular beats. Eye signs are useful, and a roving eye means a light plane, as in ether. Dilatation of pupils occurs in the third plane, usually at a deeper level than with ether.

Obviously muscular relaxation is a useful sign of cyclopropane level. With infants, muscular tone may be retained in order to ensure a light plane and rapid return of activity.

HALOTHANE. The signs of anesthesia in children receiving halothane are even more difficult to determine than those of cyclopropane. The hazards of unexpected awakening during operation, however, do not appear to be as great as with ether, and the less obvious signs have not created as much difficulty as was originally expected. Much importance has been placed on knowing exactly what concentration was being administered—hence the necessity for using calibrated vaporizers and nonrebreathing systems.[8] Although these features seem justified, many rely on clinical signs rather than numbered dials.

For anesthetic induction of normal children, halothane may be increased to 2.5% or 3.0% until the child is relaxed and the pupils are fixed and centered. In contrast to ether, halothane makes the pupils more constricted with greater depth. Usually the child should not require enough halothane to cause more than minimal pupillary constriction.

Pulse and blood pressure give especially important information during halothane anesthesia.[9] The pulse slows very perceptibly with depth.[10] Even when atropine has been employed, induction of anesthesia usually brings a decrease in heart rate of 10 to 20 beats per minute. Blood pressure is not affected in lighter planes, but as the patient is carried down into surgical anesthesia an early fall is noted.[11] This will be more marked in weak patients, especially small infants and patients with cyanotic heart disease involving large central shunts.

Arrhythmias are frequently encountered during both cyclopropane and halothane anesthesia. Correction of hypoxia, excessive anesthetic depth, and hypercarbia are the first steps to be taken. Use of agents such as the beta adrenergic blocker propranolol involves possible further complications, and should be undertaken only with full understanding of these complications[12] (Chapter 29).

Shortly after the introduction of halothane, it became evident that ventricular arrhythmias often occurred upon additional use of epinephrine. There was much subsequent discussion as to whether epinephrine should be prohibited completely, might be allowed in specific instances, or should be limited to a certain amount. After conservative trial, our practice is to allow use of epinephrine with halothane, with particular care when used in the pharynx, and to use a 1/100,000 solution, employing 0.002 mg./lb. as the maximum dose of epinephrine in any 15-minute period.

METHOXYFLURANE. Methoxyflurane (Penthrane) is roughly similar to halothane in regard to clinical signs.[13] Being slower in action, signs change more gradually, but full abdominal relaxation is obtained without supplemental agents. If the Pentec vaporizer is used, the concentration must be advanced to 3% during induction. Unless other more rapid agents are used, induction with nitrous oxide and methoxyflurane will require 10 to 15 minutes. After induction, the concentration may be reduced to 0.3% to 0.8% depending upon the procedure in hand.

FLUROXENE. Fluroxene (Fluoromar) may be vaporized by means of the FNS vaporizer. In general it behaves more like halothane than like methoxyflurane, giving somewhat less relaxation but slightly more analgesia.

With all of the agents that are respiratory depressants it must always be borne in mind that assisted and especially controlled respiration will have a strong tendency to introduce large amounts of the agent into the patients with resultant increase in the depth and duration of anesthesia. Consequently, one should repeatedly reduce the agent to the point at which the patient is obviously showing return of respiratory activity.

Ventilation. Respiratory function must be watched not only to judge the depth of anesthesia but also to ensure optimal oxygenation and carbon dioxide excretion. The rate of respiration is customarily noted, but this tells little about alveolar ventilation unless either the tidal exchange or the minute volume is taken into consideration. When judging the adequacy of a child's respiration, it is impossible to set up rules concerning the desired rate or rhythm; however, one must judge the over-all picture as to whether enough air is being moved by the patient per minute. The most practical method of following respiratory ventilation is by use of a stethoscope, the beauty of which lies in its easy application and direct usefulness. The color of the skin and that of the blood in the operative wound may be observed as a further check, but cyanosis is known to be a delayed and crude sign of hypoxia.[14]

Circulation and blood pressure. The state of the child's cardiovascular system is checked by palpation of pulse strength, pulse rate, blood pressure, color, capillary refill, lips, conjunctivae, and stethoscopic heart sounds. Although the pulse is charted only every 5 minutes, the heart should be monitored beat by beat.

Fluid therapy. When an infusion is being administered, the anesthetist must check it repeatedly to make sure that it continues to run and still be equally sure that the child does not become overinfused (Chapter 26).

Body temperature. It is easy to forget about a child's temperature, but it may invite a costly error. Temperature elevation may lead to hypoxia and convulsions and must be prevented. If a child's temperature rises above 100° F., corrective steps should be taken as needed. These include cooling the room, the use of water mattresses and cooling devices, and the application of ice packs to exposed areas. If hyperthermia occurs unexpectedly during operation, probably the most effective method of controlling it is to pass a Levin tube and rinse the stomach with iced saline solution. If the thoracic or abdominal cavity is open, rapid cooling may be obtained by pouring cold saline solution into the chest or the abdomen.

Heat loss in small infants is very frequently encountered in the air-conditioned operating rooms now in standard use. Merely exposing an infant on the operating table and preparing the skin with cold solutions may be enough to drop the temperature to 92° or 93° F. Such excessive temperature loss should be prevented by raising the room temperature and by the use of warming mattresses and similar devices (p. 250). It is advisable not to allow a child's temperature to fall below 95° F. during operation, and it is important to have it approximately normal on the child's recovery from anesthesia, so that there will be neither hypothermic depression nor shivering (Chapter 17).

Position. The anesthetist must check repeatedly to see that the patient's position is satisfactory, that he is lying in a natural posture, and that neither arms

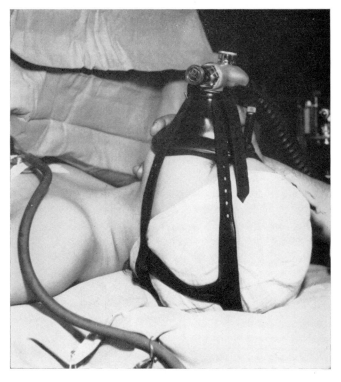

Fig. 10-7. Pressure from a tight mask may traumatize the face during long operations unless the mask is removed and the face is massaged at intervals.

nor legs have become twisted or press against any hard part of the table or ether screen. Anesthetic masks must not be strapped too tightly to the patient's face or left in place for long periods of time (Fig. 10-7). In order to prevent pressure sores, masks should be loosened and the face massaged at 15-minute intervals. In the face-down position, much care must be observed to lift the child's head frequently to prevent development of pressure areas. When the patient is small, it is especially important for the anesthetist to run his hand under the drapes from time to time in order to free them over the child's chest and abdomen as much as possible and to make sure that no instruments or hands are interfering with the child's respiration.

Progress of the operation. It appears to be customary for some anesthetists to retire behind the anesthesia screen, with little concern about the operation. If the anesthetist does not always know what the surgeon is doing, he is not taking proper care of the child. He certainly should be aware at all times of the adequacy of relaxation, the amount of bleeding, and the structures that are being dissected, and he should note as well when any undue traction or other stimulation occurs.

Furthermore, simply following the progress of operation is not enough, for the anesthetist should anticipate the needs of the surgeon and the patient and should be ready when the chest is opened, the hilum retracted, or the aorta cross-clamped. Toward the end of operation preparation for recovery should be attended to. When patients are receiving halothane, it is often wise at this time to administer a narcotic in order to prevent emergence excitement. It is also customary for an alert anesthetist to bring his patient up to a light plane toward the end of the operation, so that he will awaken promptly. It creates a rather poor impression when the surgeon pulls away the drapes to find the anesthetist still pumping anesthetics into a flaccid child.

Gastric distention. The stomach may be distended before anesthesia is started or may become distended during the course of operation. This will increase nausea and postoperative discomfort and, if marked, may decrease respiratory exchange. When encountered, such distention must be relieved immediately by manual pressure on the abdomen and by gastric suction. Routine use of a Levin tube will reduce this complication to a minimum.

Apparatus. Throughout an operation, a competent anesthetist makes a practice of checking his apparatus and equipment regularly. This means going over the suction system and catheters, oxygen supply and reserves, and resuscitation equipment, including the laryngoscope and endotracheal tubes. When an anesthesia machine is used, not only the flowmeters are checked, but the tank gauges also are inspected repeatedly lest they run low during long procedures. Soda lime should be watched; if it is in enclosed canisters, these should be opened to visualize the state of the absorber rather than to guess on the basis of elapsed time. Freedom of valve action is also a point to be checked repeatedly.

Planned system. Finally, it is an excellent idea if each anesthetist works out a plan of his own for maximum patient supervision. Short operations or those on poor-risk patients rarely give the anesthetist a chance to let his mind wander from the case, but in a long procedure on a fairly strong patient it may become difficult for the anesthetist to keep his attention on the patient. This is one of the great dangers in anesthesia, and in this situation the anesthetist should set himself a strict plan of action to keep in touch with the patient. Approaches that may be used are as follows:

1. Review in detail the advantages, disadvantages, and potential hazards of the agents and technique being used
2. Charting assiduously, though not to the point of neglecting the patient
3. Trying variations in technique and agents
4. Using monitoring devices that may not be necessary but that are harmless and give additional information
5. Setting up and carrying out clinical problems

USE OF MONITORING DEVICES

To aid the anesthetist in evaluating the condition of the patient a number of monitoring devices are available. These fall into several types in relation to the functions they monitor. It might almost be said that their value for routine procedures varies in inverse proportion to their expense. For simple cases, such as the herniorrhaphy under consideration, the stethoscope, sphygmomanometer, and thermometer are adequate.

Modifications of the stethoscope have been described previously (p. 117). Although the monaural type is more comfortable for continuous use, when dealing with small infants in whom signs may be difficult to determine, I am convinced that a standard binaural stethoscope is more reliable.

The esophageal stethoscope is useful for any patient with a large heavy chest and during thoracic procedures or operations on patients who have burns of the upper thorax.

When teaching residents infant anesthesia, it has been extremely helpful to attach two head sets to the same precordial bell; then the instructor can know what the resident is or is not hearing and can give him intelligent advice.

Use of a blood pressure cuff is required in most cases and is especially useful in long operations on newborn infants. Although a number of special sensing devices have been suggested to determine when blood flows past the cuff, none of the newer methods has given evidence of reliability or increased usefulness. For infants under a year old we use the cuff without a stethoscope and determine systolic pressure by active fluctuation of the needle on the aneroid gauge. This may be difficult to see at times, but it is present and informative more often than other methods. In older children, especially those undergoing extensive procedures, the stethoscope will allow more exact determination of blood pressure, and it should be used. Occasionally, as when patients have lesions on both arms, it will be necessary to use the thigh for blood pressure determination. In larger children the stethoscope may be placed in the popliteal space.

The measurement of venous pressure is of great value in major procedures in which extensive blood loss occurs, especially in the presence of a weak heart. Should hypotension occur in such a case, venous pressure determination will be the best way to distinguish between inadequate blood replacement (low venous pressure) and myocardial failure (high venous pressure).

There is real need for greater clinical use of devices to monitor respiration. The Wright respirometer is probably the best one presently available, and although one does not use it as a standard routine, it is an excellent teaching device and valuable for use in patients whose ventilation appears abnormal.

The electrocardiograph has use in specific cases in which children have preoperative arrhythmias, and it is also useful as a guide for administration of calcium during massive infusion of blood (Chapter 26). In cardiac procedures, especially involving extracorporeal circulation, the electrocardiograph is also useful in showing heart block. In order to reduce the amount of confusion in the operating room, the signal may be transmitted by transistor to a telemetric recorder in an adjoining room.

Electronic devices for counting pulse rate seem in no way superior to a stethoscope. The electroencephalograph, though recommended by some for use in open-heart procedures, appears to be of little practical value in pediatric anesthesia. Monitoring devices with computer recording, analyzing, and read-out now show considerable promise in more critical cases.

Use of the oximeter and the pH electrode is becoming of increasing importance with the realization that acidosis is a large factor in cardiac depression following extracorporeal circulation, as well as in patients who have received large amounts of bank blood and in any patients who have suffered surgical shock.

The carbon dioxide analyzer enjoyed popularity as one of the early electronic monitors, but its use has not continued to increase, partly because of the necessity for frequent calibration and partly because of problems of interpretation.

A nerve stimulator is of considerable aid during anesthesia with muscle relaxants. This can be used to tell the type and degree of muscle block. It can be used to indicate when additional doses are needed and to aid in the diagnosis of postrelaxant apnea.

USE OF VENTILATING DEVICES DURING ANESTHESIA

There has been less enthusiasm for use of ventilating apparatus during surgical procedures in children than in adults; however, some anesthetists feel that ventilating apparatus ensures a predictable degree of ventilation as well as a more exact and stable level of anesthesia. Either volume-limited or pressure-limited apparatus may be used for this purpose.

OPERATING ROOM ETIQUETTE

In some operating rooms silence is golden, and the voice is used only when absolutely necessary. In others it is customary for conversations to be carried on without restriction. Even here, however, it seems better to refrain from carrying on conversations with associates unless it is definitely related to the patient or indicated for teaching. Loud and distracting conversations not only are poor manners and bother the surgeons but also of necessity interfere with the care of the patient.

REFERENCES

1. Snow, J.: On chloroform and other anaesthetics, London, 1858, John Churchill, reprinted Chicago, 1950, by The American Society of Anesthesiologists, Inc.

2. Guedel, A.: Inhalation anesthesia, New York, 1937, The Macmillan Co.

3. Woodbridge, P. D.: Changing concepts concerning depth of anesthesia, Anesthesiology **19**:536-550, 1957.

4. Smith, R. M.: Signs of depth and danger, Internat. Clin. Anesth. **1**:153-167, 1962.

5. Leigh, M. D., and Belton, M. K.: Pediatric anesthesia, ed. 2, New York, 1960, The Macmillan Co.

6. Harris, T. A. B.: The mode of action of anaesthetics, Edinburgh, 1951, E. & S. Livingstone, Ltd.

7. Mushin, W. W.: Signs of anesthesia. In Evans, F. T., and Gray, T. C., editors: General anaesthesia, London, 1959, Butterworth & Co.

8. Abajian, J., Jr., Brazell, E. H., Dente, G. A., and Mills, E. L.: Experience with halothane (Fluothane) in more than five thousand cases, J.A.M.A. **171**:535-540, 1959.

9. Reynolds, R. N.: Halothane in pediatric anesthesia, Internat. Anesth. Clin. **1**:209-227, 1962.

10. McGregor, M., Davenport, H. T., Jegier, W., Sekely, P., Gibbons, J. E., and Demers, P. P.: The cardiovascular effects of halothane in normal children, Brit. J. Anaesth. **30**:398-408, 1958.

11. Stephen, C. R.: Clinical use of halothane, Clin. Anesth. **1**:81-102, 1962.

12. Craythorne, N. W. B., and Huffington, P. E.: Effects of propranolol on the cardiovascular response to cyclopropane and halothane, Anesthesiology **27**:580-583, 1966.

13. Van Posnak, A.: Clinical administration of methoxyflurane, Clin. Anesth. **1**:103-120, 1962.

14. Comroe, J. H., and Botelho, S.: Unreliability of cyanosis in the recognition of arterial anoxemia, Amer. J. Med. Sci. **214**:1-6, 1947.

Chapter 11

Normal recovery

CHECKING THE PATIENT'S CONDITION

Recovery does not begin in the recovery ward but on the operating table. As soon as the anesthetist stops active administration of anesthetic agents, the patient starts the hazardous ascent from apnea and areflexia upward through stages of gagging, gasping, and excitement toward the normal state of conscious control. The most important part of the recovery period occurs in the operating room, and the best way to prevent later difficulties is to make sure that this phase is attended with extreme care. To be certain that the child is in optimal condition at the end of the procedure, the anesthetist must see to it that respiratory function is restored, circulation is stabilized, blood volume is replenished, fluid and electrolyte balance is restored, the temperature is controlled, and the stomach is empty.

Several aspects require special attention at this time. It is obvious that the child's color should be good and that the blood pressure and pulse should be within normal limits.

Respiration must be even and full and the airway clear. It is always essential to make sure that no secretions remain to block the pharynx, trachea, or bronchi. Gross sounds may be heard without assistance, but a stethoscope should be used to check the chest at the end of all operations. Depressed or irregular respiration indicates inadequate return of function and makes it imperative that the anesthetist assist ventilation until normal exchange is restored. If apneic techniques have been employed, there is a natural tendency to watch the patient carefully until respiration first returns and then turn one's attention to other things. This is a dangerous error, because the mere presence of respiration gives no assurance that exchange will be adequate. Usually there is a period of 5 to 10 minutes, and often considerably more, when the patient's shallow respiratory efforts are definitely insufficient. Careful attention is necessary throughout this entire period.

EXTUBATION OF THE TRACHEA

When endotracheal anesthesia has been used, extubation must be performed with care in order to avoid such complications as vocal cord spasm, apnea, aspiration of vomitus, and cardiac arrhythmias. The best time to extubate should be considered, as well as the details of the actual extubation.

Time to extubate. Extubation of small infants who are still under anesthesia often is followed by apnea, which may lead to bradycardia and cyanosis. However, if the tube is left in place, they show very little reaction to it. Therefore, in infants less than 2 or 3 months of age, extubation is delayed until the baby is fully awake and is moving his arms and legs. The younger the infant, the more important this becomes.

Older infants and children show less tendency toward sudden depression and show greater irritation from the tube when extubation is delayed. Consequently, older children who are exchanging normally are extubated as soon as they begin to show the return of reflexes, with one important exception—the child with the full stomach. Such a child is allowed to awaken completely before extubation in order to give evidence of the full return of the gag reflex (Chapter 24).

Technique of extubation. The removal of the endotracheal tube must be carried out with as much attention to detail as was needed for intubation. Several steps are of importance (Figs. 11-1 to 11-4).

First, a suction catheter is passed down through the endotracheal catheter to clear the trachea and major bronchi. The suction catheter must be small enough to allow air to pass around it so that respiration will not be obstructed. Furthermore, it must be borne in mind that using suction in the trachea reduces oxygen tension rapidly[1] and for this reason should not be continued for more than 10 seconds without interruption. Five or six full respirations should be provided before suctioning is repeated.

Next, the upper airway is cleared. The most important item to remember here is the removal of any packing that may have been used by anesthetist or operator. Large quantities of thick mucus may accumulate in the nose during anesthesia, and these should be completely removed. When clearing the mouth and pharynx, if the patient is sufficiently relaxed, it is preferable to take a laryngoscope and inspect the area under direct vision while the endotracheal tube is still in place. This gives assurance that secretions, packs, and other material have been removed and saves the patient the traumatic effect of being jabbed blindly and ineffectively with the suction catheter. On withdrawal of the laryngoscope, an oral airway is inserted so that the patient cannot clamp his teeth together on the endotracheal tube.

If necessary, suction is applied in the trachea once again, using a clean cath-

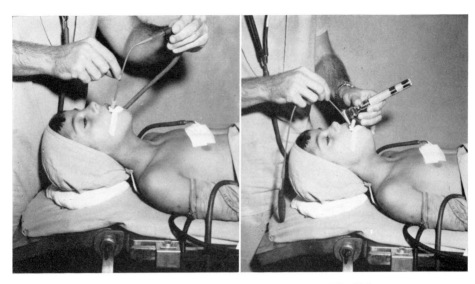

Fig. 11-1   Fig. 11-2

Fig. 11-1. The endotracheal tube and trachea are cleared with a small suction tube.
Fig. 11-2. If possible, the mouth and pharynx are exposed with a laryngoscope so that suction can be applied under direct vision.

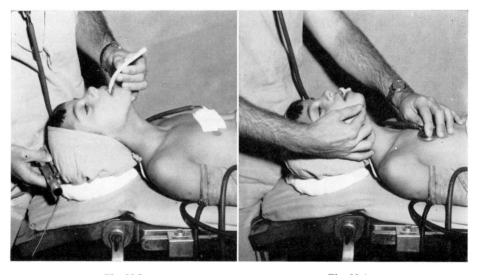

Fig. 11-3   Fig. 11-4

Fig. 11-3. Extubation is performed without simultaneous suction.
Fig. 11-4. The heart and lungs are checked immediately.

eter that has not been used in the nose. It is especially important that the catheter be withdrawn, that the patient be oxygenated, and that he regain his normal, rhythmic respiration before extubation. At this point the anesthetist should extend the head and place the fingers under the angle of the jaw, elevating it forcibly. By thus establishing and maintaining excellent anatomic position prior to extubation, one has the best chance of avoiding initiation of obstruction and spasm.[2] Finally, when all has been prepared, the endotracheal tube is slipped out, simply and unceremoniously, and *without simultaneous suction*. This point is emphasized because suction at the time of extubation reduces oxygen tension and stimulates laryngotracheal reflexes at the same time—a situation that has lead to a number of deaths.[3]

The first moments following extubation are critical, especially in infants. Even with the greatest precautions, spasm may occur with extubation. One must forget all else and, with the aid of the stethoscope, concentrate only on the child's exchange, for spasm, hypoxia, and bradycardia may occur in rapid succession. If respiration is not resumed at once, preparation to take active steps must be made. If apnea is caused by momentary depression, this may be overcome simply by pressing on the child's abdomen a few times. If spasm is not present, exchange will occur easily, and the patient usually will resume spontaneous respiration promptly. In case of spasm, oxygen can often be forced past the vocal cords by use of a bag and a mask. In severe laryngeal spasm this maneuver may not be effective. Consequently, as soon as spasm occurs it is wise to have an *assistant* prepare succinylcholine for immediate use while the anesthetist continues to attempt oxygenation. Five to ten milligrams of succinylcholine will be adequate to relieve spasm in a newborn infant at once if given intravenously and will be effective in 30 to 60 seconds if injected intramuscularly. If an intravenous infusion is not already in place, the intramuscular route may prove quicker than the intravenous route when time is taken for venipuncture.

After ventilation has been established, persistent rhonchi may be an indication for further aspiration before the patient is ready to be moved. If the patient objects to the presence of an oral airway but still has pharyngeal obstruction, a nasal catheter may be preferable.

Postoperative vomiting can occur at any moment during recovery. The hazard of inhaling vomitus is decreased if a Levin tube is passed during or at the completion of operation. The routine use of a Levin tube during operations is advisable. When the stomach is distended or if there is any question of retained gastric contents, it becomes mandatory to employ such a tube in addition to taking further precautions (Chapter 24). Occasionally a child's stomach becomes distended during operation. Recognition and prompt relief of this situation will be a large factor in safeguarding recovery.

TIME OF AWAKENING

Early awakening has definite advantages. If the postoperative nursing care is limited either by number or experience of personnel, it may be dangerous to return the child to his bed until his reflexes have fully returned and he is practically awake. Prompt awakening in general speeds recovery and the return to normal eating and activity. When there is adequate nursing care available, however, immediate awakening is not obligatory. In such circumstances it is better to have the child sleep an extra 5 or 10 minutes rather than to have him wake up while a complicated head bandage is being applied or during application of an important cast. Following many operations the patients awaken only to be in severe pain. If these children can sleep safely for an hour or two after operation, it seems more humane to let them do so.

MOVING THE PATIENT TO THE RECOVERY ROOM OR WARD

If a rapid return of consciousness is expected, as after use of cyclopropane or halothane anesthesia, it is wise to keep the child on the operating table until he awakens.

After it is evident that the patient is breathing normally, that color, circulation, and general condition are satisfactory, it is usually safe to move the child to the recovery room or ward. However, following the more critical procedures, such as intrathoracic operations, spinal fusion, or any operations during which shock or severe depression may have occurred, it is often wise to keep the child on the operating table for additional observation before moving.[4]

During transportation the airway must be maintained carefully. Following tonsillectomy and similar operations it is important to place the child face down on the litter with a sandbag supporting one shoulder (Fig. 11-5).

It is preferable for children to be cared for in a recovery room following operation if it is suitably staffed and equipped.[5,6] In hospitals where children are less frequently treated, the best nursing care and equipment for children may be

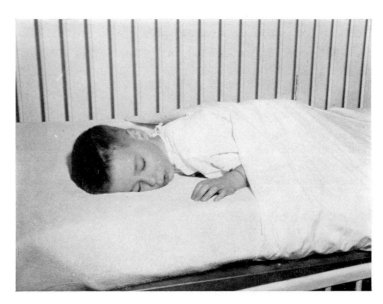

Fig. 11-5. After operation the child lies face down with shoulder supported and one arm and leg flexed.

concentrated in a single pediatric ward. In such circumstances it is better to return the children directly to their own ward, provided it is not too far from the operating room.[7]

On arrival in the recovery room or ward, the child is carefully placed in bed, in a position that will ensure an unobstructed airway and ready drainage of oral secretions. The child should not be wrapped in blankets unless he is cold. The traditional "ether bed" has been the cause of many postoperative temperature elevations.

Before leaving the child, the anesthetist must be sure his patient is in good condition and that a nurse or attendant is present who understands the problems involved. She should know what type of operation was performed and should be told if any complication such as shock, depression, or hypoxia has occurred during operation.

The anesthetist checks the bedside equipment, which must always include suction apparatus (in working order) and suction catheters of appropriate size. Tongue blades, blood pressure equipment, etc. should be standard equipment at the bedsides. In a well-equipped pediatric ward laryngoscopes and endotracheal tubes should be kept available so that it will not be necessary to race off to the anesthesia department when emergencies arise.

POSTOPERATIVE ORDERS

The orders for postoperative care may be written by the surgeon or the anesthetist. It has proved an excellent practice to have the anesthetist read the orders aloud to the nurse before leaving the patient. This will make it imperative for the anesthetist to recheck the orders and will help the nurse to decipher and understand them. These orders will provide for general routine care as well as the special needs of individual patients.[8]

Orders for general care include the following:

1. *Position*   Usually on side, or face down with shoulder support; position should be changed every 30 minutes.
2. *Vital signs*   Check pulse and respiration every 15 minutes for the first hour, every 30 minutes for the second hour, every hour for the following 4 hours, and every 4 hours thereafter; blood pressure is checked at similar intervals.
3. *Temperature*   Taken every hour for 4 hours or until stable and then every 4 hours.
4. *Oral intake*   Nothing by mouth if on gastric suction; otherwise liquids are allowed, progressing to semisolids and solids if the child is not nauseated.
5. Intravenous blood is ordered to complete replacement of estimated loss; following this it is usually advisable to order enough 5% dextrose in water to allow for half the daily water requirement (Chapter 26); to prevent drowning the patient by rapid infusion, the amount of fluid left in the container should not total more than 10 ml. per pound of the patient's weight; with infants the rate of administration in drops per minute (usually 8 to 10) is specified.

6. *Sedation*[8]   Small infants are denied sedation for fear of depression; from 6 months to 1 year of age healthy infants may be given phenobarbital, 15 to 30 mg., if the drug is dissolved and administered rectally; morphine or meperidine may be ordered for children at the age of 1 year; the first postoperative dose should be cut to half the regular dose; the regular dosage of morphine may be reckoned at 0.75 mg. per year of age (up to 12 years), and meperidine at 0.5 mg. per pound; the individual dosage must be altered to conform to the child's condition; narcotics should never be ordered "by the clock" but should be given only if needed.

Special orders to provide for additional needs of individual patients include the following:

1. *Oxygen*   Infants and poor-risk patients receive oxygen postoperatively; the type of apparatus, the liter flow per minute, and the percent concentration should be specified; small infants should not be exposed to oxygen concentration in excess of 60% unless it is specifically indicated.

2. *Humidification*   Cold vapor is ordered if there has been appreciable instrumentation of the airway, as in bronchoscopy, or if the child shows signs of stridor, hoarseness, or airway obstruction on awakening. If these signs do not abate promptly, it is advisable to administer a steroid such as dexamethasone, 0.3 mg. per pound up to 15 mg., I.V. or I.M., and repeat every 4 hours until improved.

3. *Gastric suction*   A Levin tube connected to an intermittent or Bell suction is used following intestinal operations.

4. *Temperature regulation*   Infants are usually cold after operation in air-conditioned operating rooms and require warming with blankets or carefully prepared and wrapped hot-water bottles (water not over 105° F.).

Many older patients will also require similar treatment, but specific orders need not be written.

For postoperative hyperthermia immediate steps should be taken; the bedclothes should be removed, and the patient may be sponged with alcohol or ice water if he is unconscious; aspirin is administered by rectum in dosages varying from 50 mg. in small infants to 600 mg. in older children.

5. *Antibiotics*   When infection is present or threatened, the following combination is often indicated:
   (a) Procaine penicillin, 100,000 units twice daily if infants are less than 2 months old; 300,000, if more than 2 months old.
   (b) Streptomycin, 10 mg. per pound of body weight twice daily; not more than 1 Gm. total per day.

POSTOPERATIVE RESPONSIBILITIES OF THE ANESTHETIST

It is the privilege, as well as the obligation, for the anesthetist to take part in the postoperative care of his patients. Regular ward visits are made to all children, and those who are in critical condition may require inhalation therapy or other attention.

During daily ward visits, the anesthetist checks the child's recovery from anesthesia, the time of awakening, and his general activity and also looks for specific postanesthetic responses. The lungs are examined, and the mouth and pharynx are inspected for loosened teeth, soft tissue lacerations, and evidence of tracheitis.

The child's food and fluid intake are investigated, as well as the clinical and laboratory reports, and the floor nurse is asked for details concerning his degree of discomfort and his general morale. After a satisfactory appraisal of the situation, the anesthetist should enter a note on the chart, stating briefly the child's mental and physical reaction to anesthesia and surgery.

The personal relationship between patient and anesthetist is especially important in the postoperative phase, for it is then that the anesthetist can do most to give the child a reasonable understanding of the whole hospital stay and to prevent his leaving with a distorted, unpleasant picture in his mind. The careful preoperative preparation is a poor investment if the patient is allowed to struggle through a harrowing recovery with no word of explanation or encouragement.

REFERENCES

1. Stephen, C. R., Slater, H. M., Johnson, A. L., and Sekelj, P.: The oximeter—a technical aid for anesthesiologist, Anesthesiology **12:**541-555, 1951.
2. Stetson, J. B.: The pediatric airway, Internat. Anesth. Clin. **1:**115-134, 1962.
3. Schumacher, H. B., and Hampton, L. J.: Sudden death occurring immediately after operation in patients with cardiac disease, with particular reference to the role of aspiration through the endotracheal tube and extubation, J. Thorac. Surg. **21:**48-56, 1951.
4. Dripps, R. D.: Hazards of the immediate postoperative period, J.A.M.A. **165:**795-799, 1957.
5. Beal, J. M., editor: Manual of recovery room care, New York, 1956, The Macmillan Co.
6. Sadove, M. S., and Cross, J. H.: The recovery room, Philadelphia, 1956, W. B. Saunders Co.
7. Adriani, J., and Parmley, J. B.: The recovery room. A symposium, Springfield, Ill., 1958, Charles C Thomas, Publisher.
8. Kieswetter, W. B.: Pre- and post-operative care in the pediatric surgical patient, Chicago, 1956, Year Book Medical Publishers, Inc.

Chapter 12

Local and regional anesthesia

Topical anesthesia
Local infiltration
Regional block
    Spinal anesthesia
    Epidural and caudal block
    Brachial plexus block
Intravenous regional anesthesia
Diagnostic and therapeutic blocks

The applications of local anesthesia in pediatric surgery are somewhat different from those for adult work. The need of patient cooperation and the possibility of frightening children have influenced some anesthetists to discard this approach. However, local anesthesia includes many techniques and may serve a wide variety of purposes. Any pediatric anesthetist must be conversant with these techniques and be ready to apply them when the indication arises.

TOPICAL ANESTHESIA

Diagnostic and operative procedures about the upper respiratory tract have served as the most frequent indication for topical anesthesia in adults and children alike. Application of cocaine in concentrations varying from 2% to 20% has been the anesthetic of choice for examination of nose, throat, and trachea, as well as for such operative procedures as correction of deviated nasal septum, excision of nasal or laryngeal polyps, and dilatation of laryngeal stenoses. Cocaine in 4% solution has long been used for operative procedures on the eye.

Over many years the search for a safer agent led to the trial of scores of newer anesthetics. Tetracaine (Pontocaine) and lidocaine (Xylocaine) have appeared the most popular of the modern agents, although dyclonine (Dyclone),[1] a recent addition to the field, gives promise of being effective and remarkably safe and prilocaine (Citanest) and others are constantly being introduced.

The pediatric anesthetist may use topical anesthesia in the nose and nasopharynx prior to the passage of nasotracheal tubes, in the pharynx to decrease

192

reflex responses to oral airways, or in the larynx and trachea prior to the passage of endotracheal tubes or bronchoscope. The same considerations obtain here as in choosing agents for adult anesthesia. A 4% spray of lidocaine or a 5% lidocaine aqueous ointment has been our choice in view of the relative safety, effectiveness, and bacteriostatic quality of this agent. The rapid absorption of topical anesthetics from the respiratory tract has been emphasized by Moore and Tolan,[2] and added care must be taken to use minimal doses in small patients. When possible, an ointment is chosen in preference to a spray, first, because of decreased chance of overdosage, and, second, because spraying the cords prior to intubation may in itself cause reflex stimulation if the patient is in a light plane at the moment.

As will be noted later, a topical anesthetic is of great assistance during operative diagnostic bronchoscopy. For this purpose the agent may be applied by spray or by application with a pledget. If sprays are used, the atomizer should contain only the amount that is to be used and should deliver a finely divided spray rather than coarse droplets.

Topical anesthesia may also be useful in cystoscopic procedures. An aqueous jelly applied to the urethra often enables the anesthetist to use very light supplemental anesthesia.

LOCAL INFILTRATION

Whether employed by surgeon or anesthetist, local infiltration anesthesia probably has wider use in pediatric anesthesia than in adult work. In addition to its usefulness for suturing lacerations and for other minor procedures, local anesthesia may be the best technique for extensive abdominal and neurosurgical operations in premature and weak newborn infants. In such cases the child is held in position by well-padded restraints, and 0.5% procaine is infiltrated along the line of incision. A sugar nipple may help to pacify the baby, or in some cases his regular feeding may be given during the procedure. For more resistant infants a solution of brandy (or vodka) and sugar may be used, or nitrous oxide and oxygen may be blown over the infant's face.

During abdominal procedures under local anesthesia it often is helpful to instill 4 or 5 ml. of 0.5% procaine into the abdominal cavity.[3] This provides appreciable relaxation and facilitates closure of the peritoneum. The amount of solution to be given in this way is calculated by using 1 ml. of 0.5% procaine per pound of body weight. The total dose of local agent that is safe for small infants has not been definitely determined. It appears reasonable to assume a limit of 5 mg. (1 ml. of 0.5% solution) of procaine per pound of body weight for use in entering the abdomen, to be followed by the same amount used within the abdomen for closure. Under this policy signs of toxicity have not been observed in our experience. Wilton[4] gives 3.5 mg. per pound as the limit for lidocaine.

When operating under local anesthesia, one should remember to infiltrate the areas where towel clips are to be placed.

REGIONAL BLOCK

A variety of regional blocks may be used in children for operative or therapeutic purposes. In general, such blocks are relatively easy to perform in children. Except for the longer extension of the spinal cord within the dural sac, the anatomic relationships are similar in child and adult. The spine of the child is more flexible, and lumbar puncture is more easily performed. At birth the tip of the spinal cord is at the level of the third lumbar vertebra, but by the time the child is 1 year old the cord is in its permanent position, ending at the first lumbar interspace.[5]

The use of regional blocks for pediatric surgery has been advocated for the following reasons:

1. Less danger of aspirating vomitus, especially in emergency procedures
2. Safer in the presence of head injury or recent coma
3. Less danger of respiratory spasm
4. Less metabolic disturbance in presence of chronic disease
5. Preferable in the presence of upper respiratory disease

These reasons seem logical. An additional claim is also made that I believe is false and dangerous—that is, that regional anesthesia is indicated in toxic patients such as those with peritonitis and dehydration.[6] I am convinced that the use of regional anesthesia in sick patients with high fever and rapid pulse is dangerous and illadvised. Such patients show decreased tolerance to local as well as general anesthesia. Several experiences have confirmed this belief. Any patient who is dehydrated, acidotic, or otherwise critically ill should be fully prepared before receiving either regional or general anesthesia.

Spinal anesthesia. All types of regional blocks are applicable to children, but only a few have received very much attention. Following an early report by Gray[7] in 1909, spinal anesthesia was used for children, especially in Canada,[8-11] where there has even been enthusiasm for performing intrathoracic operations under spinal block. This technique became less popular with the advent of better methods in general anesthesia.

Under favorable conditions spinal anesthesia has been proved to be a safe and effective technique for children.[11,12] Patients are evaluated carefully, and only those who appear reasonably cooperative are chosen. The procedure is explained to those old enough to understand, and adequate premedication is ordered to prevent apprehension and resistance.

Although hypobaric solutions have been recommended,[10,14] hyperbaric solutions have been more widely accepted for pediatric use. Berkowitz and Greene[12] have been staunch advocates of spinal anesthesia in children. They advise routine intramuscular injection of a preanesthetic vasopressor drug, and they favor Neo-Synephrine (0.1 ml. of 1% solution per 25 pounds). For the anesthetic agent they recommend hyperbaric procaine, Pontocaine, or Nupercaine, as outlined in Table 12-1.

At present spinal anesthesia for adults has been somewhat simplified inasmuch as a single agent may be used and its duration may be prolonged by addition of a vasoconstricting drug. This technique is adaptable to children as well.

If 1% tetracaine (Pontocaine) is used in dosage of 0.1 mg. per pound of body weight and is diluted in twice its volume of 10% dextrose, the mixture will allow 45 to 90 minutes of anesthesia. When additional duration is required, phenyl-

Table 12-1. *Recommended dosages for spinal anesthesia in children**

Expected duration of operation	Agent	Dose
Under 45 minutes	5% Procaine	1 mg. per pound
45 to 90 minutes	1% Pontocaine	0.1 mg. per pound
More than 90 minutes	0.5% Nupercaine	0.01 mg. per pound

*Compiled from Berkowitz, S., and Greene, B. A.: Anesthesiology **12:**376-387, 1951.

ephrine (Neo-Synephrine) is added to the solution. For use in adults, 2 mg. of phenylephrine is sufficient for the purpose.

A comparable amount of vasoconstrictor for an infant or child might be difficult to measure; however, this problem may be simplified by mixing 3 mg. (0.3 ml.) of 1% phenylephrine in 3 ml. of 10% dextrose prior to preparation of the anesthetic solution. Subsequently, when the tetracaine and dextrose are mixed in correct proportions for any patient, a suitable dosage of phenylephrine will be present. Thus, for prolonged-action spinal anesthetic for an 8-year-old boy weighing 80 pounds, the steps would be as follows:

1. Open ampules of tetracaine and dextrose.
2. Add 0.3 ml. (3 mg.) of phenylephrine to ampule containing 3 ml. of dextrose and mix.
3. Draw up 0.8 ml. (8 mg.) of tetracaine and 1.6 ml. of dextrose-phenylephrine mixture in 5-ml. syringe.
4. Inject solution via spinal needle in third lumbar interspace.

Children often accept spinal anesthesia with surprising cooperation, and some even enjoy the experience of being awake during their operation. Others become apprehensive or openly resistant, especially if they become nauseated or experience unpleasant sensations during traction on the viscera. For this reason the anesthetist should have an infusion ready for supplemental intravenous anesthesia at a moment's notice. The administration of oxygen is always indicated, as in adult techniques.

In our practice spinal anesthesia is used occasionally, but rarely. The smallest child who was given spinal anesthesia was 1 month old and weighed 9 pounds. He had a strangulated hernia and also was recovering from pneumonia, still having multiple miliary lung abscesses. Lidocaine, 0.9 mg. in 1.8 ml. of 10% glucose, produced anesthesia to the rib margin, and the operation was successful. Other indications for spinal anesthesia in children have been compound fractured leg with skull fracture and appendectomies in the presence of a full stomach. Epidural and caudal anesthesia appear to offer somewhat less advantage than spinal anesthesia and require more skill on the part of the anesthetist and more cooperation on the part of the patient. The indications seem rare, unless one wishes to make a specialty of such techniques and the surgeon has plenty of time.

Epidural and caudal block. Ruston[13] revived interest in the use of epidural block in infants and children, pointing to its ease of administration and its wide application for intraabdominal and perineal operations, as well as such procedures as hip fusion and excision of a meningocele. Children are given relatively heavy premedication so that they may sleep through the procedure and thus avoid emotional trauma.

The child is held in the sitting position by an assistant, and, after preparation of the back and injection of a local anesthetic, a 22-gauge needle is introduced at the second or preferably the third lumbar interspace. After the needle has pierced the intraspinous ligament, the stylus is withdrawn and the needle hub is filled with anesthetic solution. The needle is then advanced carefully so that a drop is left hanging from the hub until entrance into the epidural sac is denoted by negative pressure, which partially sucks up the hanging drop.

One per cent lidocaine with 1:200,000 epinephrine is suggested as the anesthetic. Ruston calculates the amount of lidocaine by the formula:

$$\text{Dosage in milliliters of 1\% lidocaine} = 0.5 + \frac{\text{Weight in pounds}}{2}$$

As soon as the solution is injected, the child is placed in the supine position and is observed carefully for evidence of anesthetic effect. This type of block may be expected to last 3 to 4 hours.

Spiegel[15] reported successful experience with caudal anesthesia in a series of 124 infants and children, in which he used lidocaine or mixtures of tetracaine and lidocaine, the dosage and concentration of which he varied in relation to the patients' ages. He stressed the importance of adequate preoperative medication, and restraint if necessary, and stated that caudal anesthesia is the regional anesthesia of choice for surgery of the abdomen, perineum, and lower extremities for children 2 years of age or younger. Using approximately 0.1% lidocaine or tetracaine, he calculated the total dosage by the formula $V = 4 + \dfrac{D - 15}{2}$, where V is the total volume of anesthetic in milliliters and D is the distance between C_7 and the sacral hiatus.

Brachial plexus block. Fractured arms, lacerated tendons, and amputated fingers are all commonplace in pediatric surgery, and such patients rarely have empty stomachs. For these children and for others facing elective surgery, brachial block offers the advantages previously listed, including prevention of aspiration of vomitus and early ambulation for those who are to be discharged after treatment.

In earlier use of brachial plexus block in children the *supraclavicular* approach was generally employed. Small[16] reported a series of 150 children ranging from 15 months to 12 years in which this technique was used as follows: The child lies supine, the head turned away from the affected side and the shoulder slightly depressed. The area is prepared and draped and a skin wheal is made one-half inch above the midline of the clavicle (Fig. 12-1). A 23-gauge needle is inserted through the wheal and slightly medially, downward, and forward until it strikes the first rib just lateral to the subclavian artery. Although some children can report paresthesias, many will not, and this guide cannot be relied upon. A syringe holding 0.2% tetracaine or 1.5% lidocaine with 1:200,000

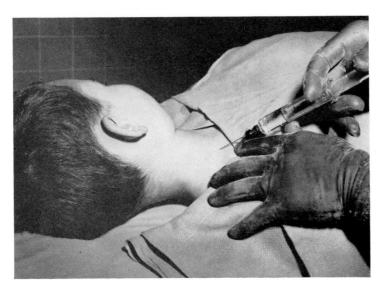

Fig. 12-1. Brachial plexus block has many indications in children.

epinephrine is then attached to the needle, and aspiration is attempted to make sure that the needle has not entered the chest or pierced a vessel.

Injection of one third of the solution is then made while the needle is gradually retracted toward the skin. The anesthetist inserts the needle two more times, each time directing it approximately 1 cm. farther backward along the first rib and inserting more anesthetic. The needle is then withdrawn and the area massaged to diffuse the anesthetic. Sensory loss should occur in 10 to 15 minutes and last 2 to 3 hours.

The amount of solution required varies between 5 ml. for a 1-year-old child and 20 ml. for an average 12-year-old child, with due regard for individual differences.

At present the *axillary* route (Fig. 12-2) has almost completely displaced the supraclavicular route for brachial block in children.[17,18] The advantages for the axillary approach in younger patients include greater simplicity, less needling, and elimination of danger of pneumothorax. Since many patients upon whom brachial block is performed are outpatients, it is important that pneumothorax, no matter how rarely it occurs, should be avoided if patients are to be discharged promptly. Situations in which the axillary route will be contraindicated include fractures of the humerus that do not allow abduction of the arm, and surgery of the upper arm.

Axillary block for children is performed as described by De Jong for adults, using proportionately less anesthetic.[19] A 1.5% concentration of lidocaine is satisfactory, with 1/100,000 epinephrine. A child should be given a relatively generous dosage of premedication, such as pentobarbital, 2.5 mg. per pound, plus morphine, 0.1 mg. per pound. He lies with the affected arm extended, and the elbow bent at 45°. An attendant should have him turn his head away from the scene of activity, and should distract his attention.

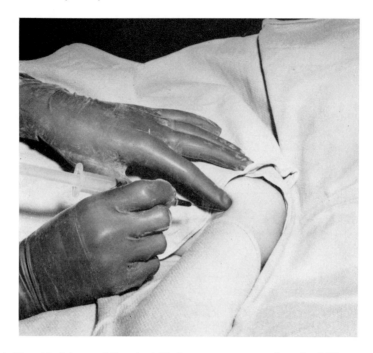

Fig. 12-2. Axillary block is especially adaptable for emergency procedures in children.

The anesthetist, properly scrubbed and gowned, prepares the axilla and upper two thirds of the arm as for operation and drapes the area. The axillary artery is then palpated at the level of the insertion of the pectoralis major muscle. Using a 10-ml. syringe with a ½-inch 25-gauge needle, a small wheal is made over the artery; the needle is then advanced through the fascia, above the artery toward the area containing median antebracheal cutaneous, median, and musculocutaneous nerves, in that order (Fig. 12-2). Aspiration is attempted as the needle is advanced, and if blood is encountered the needle is retracted and reinserted more cephalad. Paresthesias are not sought for, and one should not inject solution into these nerves. Using a total dosage of 3 mg. per pound, one half of the solution is injected above or cephalad to the artery, and the needle is then withdrawn until the lip is immediately subcutaneous; then it is advanced below the artery, where the remainder of the solution is injected to anesthetize the ulnar and radial nerves. A period of 15 to 20 minutes should be allowed for complete effect of the block.

INTRAVENOUS REGIONAL ANESTHESIA

The use of regional block established by intravenous injection of local anesthetics has been promoted enthusiastically for adults[20] and may be applied to children in a number of situations. It is especially useful for operations on hand and arm. The basic technique consists first of exsanguination of the arm by elevation and Esmarch bandage, and application of a double pneumatic tourniquet.

The upper or proximal tourniquet is inflated and the anesthetic injected intravenously. For this we recommend lidocaine 0.5% (without epinephrine) using a total dose of 1.5 mg. per pound. Ten minutes is allowed for fixation of anesthesia; then the lower tourniquet is inflated and the proximal one released.

DIAGNOSTIC AND THERAPEUTIC BLOCKS

Although seldom used for treatment of vascular disease, as in older patients, sympathetic nerve blocks may be used following fractures of arms or legs, extensive soft tissue damage, as in "wringer arm," or following injury to major vessels. After extensive surgical procedures on the limbs, stellate or lumbar sympathetic blocks may be performed to promote circulation and reduce edema formation. Techniques are similar to those used in adults.[21,22]

Inoperable tumors are seen all too frequently in children, and here therapeutic blocks can be used with good effect. Ample sedation should be used prior to performing the block, and light nitrous oxide or cyclopropane anesthesia may be used as well. As recommended by Bonica,[21] a preliminary block with procaine should precede destructive blocks with alcohol or phenol.

In actuality, it often is much more practical to perform a low spinal anesthesia on a small child than it is to perform a lumbar sympathetic block. It entails far less needling, and the resultant block is more predictable and more rapidly effective.

For the upper extremity a stellate block is not difficult, but here again an axillary brachial block will prove as effective and probably entails fewer hazards.

REFERENCES

1. Harris, L. C., Jr., Parry, J. C., and Greifenstein, F. E.: Dyclonine—a new local anesthetic agent: clinical evaluation, Anesthesiology **17:**648-652, 1956.
2. Moore, D. C., and Tolan, J. F.: Anesthesia for surgery of the nose, pharynx, larynx, and trachea, Arch. Otolaryng. **63:**275-288, 1956.
3. Bohne, M. T.: Personal communication.
4. Wilton, T. N. P., and Wilson, F.: Neonatal anaesthesia, Philadelphia, 1965, F. A. Davis Co.
5. Gray, Henry: Anatomy of the human body, ed. 22, revised and re-edited by W. H. Lewis, Philadelphia, 1930, Lea & Febiger.
6. Amster, J. L.: Spinal anesthesia for poor pediatric surgical risks, Med. Rec. Ann. **144:**213-216, 1956.
7. Gray, T.: Study of spinal anesthesia in infants and children, Lancet **2:**913-917, 1909.
8. Robson, C. H.: Anesthesia in children, Amer. J. Surg. **34:**468-473, 1936.
9. Junkin, C. I.: Spinal anesthesia in children, Canad. Med. Ass. J. **28:**51-53, 1953.
10. Slater, H. M., and Stephen, C. R.: Hypobaric Pontocaine spinal anesthesia in children, Anesthesiology **11:**709-715, 1950.
11. Leigh, M. D., and Belton, M. K.: Pediatric anesthesia, ed. 2, New York, 1960, The Macmillan Co.
12. Berkowitz, S., and Greene, B. A.: Spinal anesthesia in children; report based on 350 patients under 13 years of age, Anesthesiology **12:**376-387, 1951.
13. Ruston, F. G.: Epidural anesthesia in pediatric surgery, Anesth. Analg. **36:**76-82, 1957.
14. Lund, P. C., and Rumball, A. C.: Hypobaric Pontocaine spinal anesthesia, 1640 cases, Anesthesiology **8:**181-199, 1947.
15. Spiegel, P.: Caudal anesthesia in pediatric surgery, Anesth. Analg. **41:**218-221, 1962.
16. Small, G. A.: Brachial plexus block anesthesia in children, J.A.M.A. **147:**1648-1651, 1951.
17. Clayton, M. L., and Turner, D. A.: Upper arm block in children with fractures, J.A.M.A. **169:**327-329, 1959.

18. Eather, K. E.: Axillary brachial plexus block, Anesthesiology **19:**683-684, 1958.
19. DeJong, R. H.: Axillary block of the brachial plexus, Anesthesiology **22:**215-225, 1961.
20. Atkinson, D. I., Modell, J., and Moya, F.: Intravenous regional anesthesia, Anesth. Analg. **44:**313-317, 1965.
21. Bonica, J. J.: The management of pain, Philadelphia, 1953, Lea & Febiger.
22. Moore, D. C.: Regional block, ed. 2, Springfield, Ill., 1957, Charles C Thomas, Publisher.

Chapter 13

Intravenous anesthesia

Advantages and disadvantages
Age limit to use of intravenous anesthesia
Indications
　　For induction of anesthesia
　　For maintenance of anesthesia
　　Treatment of convulsive disorders
Agents, techniques, and maintenance for intravenous anesthesia
Complications

The use of intravenous anesthesia in children has been somewhat controversial. In the United States the use of intravenous anesthesia for infants and small children is relatively unusual,[1-3] whereas in Great Britain thiopental–relaxant–nitrous oxide anesthesia is the routine approach in several large pediatric hospitals.[4-6]

ADVANTAGES AND DISADVANTAGES

Intravenous anesthesia provides the same advantages when used in children as when used in adults—pleasant, rapid induction, noninflammability, relative freedom from metabolic disturbance, and decreased postoperative nausea.

The disadvantages are slightly magnified in children. Venipuncture may be considerably more difficult and children may object strenuously, even when venipuncture is easy. Of greater importance is the possibility of overdosage of intravenous agents with respiratory depression and delayed recovery unless definite limits are placed on the amount of agent used.

In the past, inhalation agents have been considered to be more controllable and to ensure more prompt awakening. This difference is less obvious now, and recovery following intravenous anesthesia usually is quieter than that following halothane and more prompt than that following methoxyflurane.

When compared to the ease of administration of halothane, intravenous anesthesia is relatively cumbersome. However, due to growing concern over possible toxicity following halogenated agents, our use of intravenous anesthesia is rapidly increasing.

AGE LIMIT TO USE OF INTRAVENOUS ANESTHESIA

The question is often raised as to how young a patient may be safely anesthetized with intravenous agents. Actually there seems to be no definite restriction. The difficulty and delay involved in venipuncture reduce the popularity of the method for induction in children under 3 or 4 years of age; however, some use the technique for small infants. Obviously this can be done safely only if full preparations are made to support respiration and cope with laryngeal obstruction.

Children over 6 or 7 years of age can tolerate almost any anesthetic combination that is employed for adults. Consequently intravenous agents and nitrous oxide, supplemented when necessary by a relaxant, can be suited to almost any procedure.

INDICATIONS

For induction of anesthesia. One cannot specify each type of situation in which the intravenous technique of induction is indicated, but there are several that offer special advantages:

1. Prior to thiopental–nitrous oxide anesthesia in older children
2. Prior to cyclopropane anesthesia
3. For induction of retarded or unmanageable children (p. 150)

If an infusion has been established previously or if a large vein is available, the advantages of this method will naturally be increased. In the absence of a ready or promising vein, however, it may be better to change plans and spare the child an unpleasant and unprofitable experience.

For maintenance of anesthesia. Among the procedures for which intravenous anesthesia is most useful are the following:

1. Orthopedic operations in children over 6 or 8 years of age if they are lying in supine or lateral position
2. Neurosurgical procedures in older children in supine, lateral, or sitting position
3. Cystoscopy in female patients
4. Operations on body or limbs in children in supine position

Treatment of convulsive disorders. In the event of an anesthetic convulsion during ether or local anesthetic, administration of barbiturates has long been advocated to bring the patient under control. However, there is real danger of direct cardiac depression if larger doses of barbiturates are administered rapidly; consequently this approach has been modified considerably (Chapter 27). Anesthetists may also be called upon to manage children convulsing because of acute infections, tetanus, or epileptic seizures. If these seizures are severe enough to cause hypoxia, they should be controlled at once. Minor seizures that do not interfere with respiratory exchange do not need heroic treatment, and care should be taken not to complicate the picture by excess therapy.

If seizures are severe and continuous, they should be controlled promptly.

Ultimately the treatment must be guided by the diagnosis, but the initial therapy will be directed simply toward gaining sufficient control of the patient to provide adequate ventilatory exchange. For patients in the prolonged convulsive condition seen in status epilepticus, initial relaxation may be attained by intravenous injection of succinylcholine followed by endotracheal intubation and artificial ventilation. For long-range control of such patients diazepam (Valium)[7] has recently been found to have especial value.

For severe convulsions of short duration intravenous thiopental may be used in children 3 or 4 or more years of age, while open-drop ether probably is safer for infants.

For children with tetanus a long-range organized approach is necessary. Tracheostomy is performed at once, and convulsions are controlled by the use of relaxants and ventilatory assistance,[8] by a long-acting sedative such as tribromo-ethanol, or by combinations of barbiturate, chlorpromazine, and mephenesin or zoxazolamine.[9,10] Although early attempts to treat tetanus in hyperbaric oxygen tanks were encouraging,[11,12] further investigation showed this form of therapy to be ineffective.

AGENTS, TECHNIQUES, AND MAINTENANCE
FOR INTRAVENOUS ANESTHESIA

Of the anesthetics available for intravenous administration, hexobarbital (Evipal) was the first one to have wide use in adults, but thiopental (Pentothal) subsequently proved far more popular and was the first agent to be used to any extent in pediatric anesthesia. Subsequently several competing barbiturates have been developed, each boasting more rapid recovery and freedom from respiratory spasm and depression. Thiamylal (Surital)[13] proved to be almost identical to thiopental clinically. Methitural (Neraval) was shown to be metabolized more rapidly and to afford more rapid return of consciousness than thiopental. Induction with methitural is definitely slower than with other thiobarbiturates, however, unless given rapidly, in which case it causes severe sneezing and coughing.[14] Methohexital (Brevital), more closely resembling the original evipal than the barbiturate, claimed more rapid metabolic breakdown and consequently more prompt recovery, as well as freedom from side effects.[15] The actual advantage in the saving of time has not been impressive, and there has been some concern over hiccups that occur with rapid induction with the agent.

In 1964 propanidid* (Epontol)[16] appeared as an even more rapidly acting intravenous agent. This drug is basically similar to eugenol, previously discarded because it caused venous thrombosis. Propanidid in 5% concentration is less irritant than eugenol and has been employed for a variety of short procedures in children in dosage of 10 mg./kg. Although it has caused minimal respiratory spasm, the vascular irritation is still sufficient to limit its usefulness.

For several years the combination of a potent narcotic (fentanyl) and a dissociative hypnotic (droperidol) has been employed in adults under the name of

*3-methoxy-4- (N,N-diethylcarbamoyl-methoxy)-phenylacetic acid-n-propylester.

neurolept analgesia.[16a] The prolonged effect and delayed postoperative extrapyramidal responses following droperidol have been disturbing, although Foldes[16b] believes that these may be eliminated by reducing droperidol dosage to 150 μg./kg. Other combinations, especially that of morphine and the mild ataractic propiomazine (Largon) have been remarkably effective in our hands. Induction is accomplished with thiopental or halothane plus nitrous oxide. If endotracheal intubation is required, this is accomplished with the aid of succinylcholine. Then, using a mixture of 10 mg. morphine and 20 mg. propiomazine diluted to 10 ml., an initial dose of 1 ml. per 10 kg. is injected and the halothane discontinued. Supplemental doses are used to eliminate response to pain or other stimuli.

Prior to the use of intravenous anesthetics children should receive adequate medication with a belladonna agent, barbiturate, and narcotic as previously indicated in Table 5-1.

Thiobarbiturates may be used by intermittent injection or by drip infusion. Drip infusion, which is allowed to run continuously, always involves greater risk of anesthetic overdosage. Also, in order to give the desired amount of anesthetic, it may be necessary to give an excess quantity of fluid. In order to avoid these dangers it seem preferable to use a 2% or 2.5% solution by intermittent injection.

Usually a regular infusion is started by either the cut-down or the percutaneous method. After this is established, the anesthetic is added by the side-arm or a threeway stopcock attachment. If the child is resistant and rapid induction is necessary, a needle and syringe may be used. Thiopental is injected directly into the vein, the infusion system being connected after the child has become quieted. In small children or when venipuncture is difficult, the initial injection may be performed with a 25-gauge or 26-gauge needle that will hardly be felt and that can be used in the smallest of vessels. After the child is asleep a larger needle may be used for maintenance of the infusion.

When children are cooperative, intravenous induction should be performed gradually to prevent unnecessary overdosage and depression. A small initial dose is given, the effect is watched, and additional amounts are given at 30-second intervals until the eyelids cease to flutter on stimulation and the pupils become centered. Suggested dosages are shown in Table 13-1. As the child becomes sleepy the chin is supported, the mask is applied, and supplemental anesthesia is started.

Regardless of the duration of thiopental anesthesia, oxygen must be supplied and respiration must be assisted at all times. In addition it should be the general plan to rely on the barbiturate as little as possible for the anesthesia and to use

Table 13-1. *Approximate dosages for induction and maintenance of thiopental anesthesia (2.0%)*

Age (yr.)	Weight (lb.)	Induction dose (ml.)	Induction dose (mg.)	Intermittent fractional dose (mg.)	Total dose (mg.)
3	30	1.5	30	20	300
6	60	3	60	40	600
9	75	4	80	40	750
12	100	5	100	40	1,000

nitrous oxide or other analgesic agents for the anesthetic effect. Naturally, barbiturates must not be expected to provide any relaxation.

At present nonrebreathing techniques are favored in small children. With larger children, circle apparatus may be employed using reduced gas flows.[17]

The signs of most value[18] are the motility of the eyes, respiration, and motor activity. As a patient becomes more deeply anesthetized with thiopental, as with other agents, his eyes will become centered and fixed. Since a child's eyes may be centered before anesthesia, this neutral position will not be a definite sign that the child is well anesthetized. A moving or uncentered eye, however, is a reliable sign that the patient is in a light plane.

Respiration may be markedly depressed during light anesthesia, and it, too, is a poor measure of depth. During the course of anesthesia, however, the relative degree of resistance to manual compression of the breathing bag is a useful guide.

Movement of the body or limbs usually means that the patient is reacting to stimulation, although rarely is the patient conscious of pain. More anesthetic is usually indicated, but one must not be led into the error of giving excessive doses of barbiturate to control such activity. After reasonable or expected doses have been given, other agents may be added in place of more barbiturates.

The question of total dose is important. It is necessary to set a definite limit to the amount of thiopental to be used or prolonged depression may occur in the postoperative period. If this limit is set at *10 mg. per pound of body weight,* patients may recover consciousness quite readily after prolonged operations.

If the thiopental is inadequate, or if the dose limit is reached before completion of the operation, a supplementary agent should be used rather than adding more thiopental. Meperidine (1 mg./15 lb.) will add much to the analgesic potency of the anesthetic. Halothane, of course, can be used to replace the thiopental, as can any of the general anesthetic agents.

In intracranial procedures in older children thiopental is useful for an induction agent as well as for maintenance. These patients require endotracheal intubation, for which relaxation should be provided by use of either an inhalation or a curarizing agent. If anesthesia is to be maintained by thiopental and nitrous oxide, it will be helpful to use a local anesthetic spray or an analgesic catheter lubricant to decrease stimulation of the pharynx and the lower respiratory tract.

COMPLICATIONS

When employing intravenous anesthetics, one must always be prepared to deal with acute respiratory depression by assisting respiration with a bag and mask or occasionally by intubation. Laryngeal spasm is a great potential hazard that always must be kept in mind. Manipulation about the airway, such as passing a suction catheter into the nose or placing an oral airway in the mouth, can initiate considerable irritation and laryngospasm. If an airway is used, one does well to spray the pharynx with a topical anesthetic. If vocal cord spasm occurs, it is best treated by positive-pressure oxygen and by use of succinylcholine to break the spasm of the vocal cords. Fortunately this complication rarely occurs in children.

Prolonged respiratory depression may follow overdosage or increased susceptibility. Numerous agents have been proposed to stimulate respiration or counteract the barbiturate. These include the analeptic agents nikethamide (Coramine), pentylenetetrazol (Metrazol), picrotoxin,[19] and β,β-methylethyl glutarimide (Megimide),[20,21] as well as sodium succinate,[22] methylphenidate (Ritalin),[23] and ethamivan (Emivan). As yet these have not been found reliable, and efforts at treatment still should be concentrated on maintaining the airway and providing ventilation until the child recovers full spontaneous activity.[24-28]

Doxapram hydrochloride (Dopram) has more recently stimulated some enthusiasm for treatment of postoperative respiratory depression. Stephen and Talton[29] and Noe[30] report brief but significant improvement in artificial oxygen and reduction of carbon dioxide concentration. Drugs used previously for respiratory stimulation frequently led to convulsive phenomena, but with doxapram there is a much greater margin of safety.

Shivering following thiopental often occurs during recovery.[31] This is harmless in healthy patients, but the associated increase in oxygen demand may be dangerous in patients with cardiac disease. This complication is described in Chapter 27.

Sensitivity to thiobarbiturates is rare, but death has been known to occur following administration of as little as 50 mg. of thiopental to an adult. Dundee and associates[32,33] drew attention to the fact that patients with porphyria could not metabolize thiobarbiturates. This established a very definite contraindication to the use of these agents and probably explained some of the earlier cases of apparent sensitivity.

The use of intravenous anesthetics may be contraindicated either because of potential danger due to respiratory depression and laryngospasm or due to problems of pharmacologic breakdown and possible toxicity. It would certainly seem unwise to use intravenous agents for patients with any airway abnormality or inflammatory condition, operation about the nose or throat, or in patients with respiratory disease or muscular weakness.

If patients have diseases such as myocardial failure, hepatic disease, burns, or shock, minute doses may be given for induction, but then only with great caution, and further use of the agent should be avoided. In the specific disease porphyria, intravenous barbiturates should not be used at all.

REFERENCES

1: Webster, C. F., and Van Bergen, F. H.: Pentothal-curare mixture with endotracheal N_2O and O_2 in infants, Bull. Univ. Minnesota Hosp. & Minnesota M. Found. **20**:525-533, 1949.
2. Wasmuth, C. E., and Hale, D. E.: Thiopental sodium anesthesia in infants and children, J.A.M.A. **156**:1321-1323, 1954.
3. Egan, C. F.: Pentothal-curare-nitrous oxide anaesthesia for children and infants: a technique and dosage scales for rapid intubation and maintenance, Canad. Anaesth. Soc. J. **2**:41-63, 1955.
4. Rees, G. J.: The anaesthetist in the paediatric unit. In Evans, F. T., and Gray, T. C., editors: Modern trends in anesthesia, London, 1958, Paul B. Hoeber, Inc., Medical Book Department of Harper & Row, Publishers.
5. Rees, G. J.: Neonatal anaesthesia, Brit. Med. Bull. **1**:38, 1958.
6. Anderson, S. M.: Anaesthesia for children, Practitioner **189**:180-186, 1962.
7. Prensky, A. L., Raff, M. C., Moore, M. J., and Schwab, R. S.: Intravenous diazepam in treatment of prolonged seizure activity, New Eng. J. Med. **276**:779-784, 1967.
8. Van Bergen, F, and Buckley, J. J.: Management of severe tetanus, Anesthesiology **13**:599-604, 1952.

9. Jenkins, M. T., and Luhn, N. R.: Review: active management of tetanus based on experience of an anesthesia department, Anesthesiology 23:690-709, 1962.

10. Lawrence, D. R., Berman, E., and Scragg, J. N.: Clinical trial of chlorpromazine against barbiturates in tetanus, Lancet 1:987-991, 1958.

11. Trapp, W. G.: The therapeutic use of high-pressure oxygen, Canad. Med. Ass. J. 88:356-359, 1963.

12. Boerema, I.: An operating room with high atmospheric pressure, Surgery 49:291-298, 1963.

13. Tovell, R. M., Anderson, C. C., Sadove, M. S., Artusio, J. F., Papper, E. M., Coakley, C. C., Hudon, F., Smith, S. M., and Thomas, G. F.: A comparative clinical and statistical study of thiopental and thiamylal in human anesthesia, Anesthesiology 16:910-926, 1955.

14. Smith, C.: Methitural sodium for the induction of paediatric anaesthesia, Canad. Anaesth. Soc. J. 4:378-384, 1957.

15. Taylor, C., and Stoelting, V. K.: Methohexital sodium—a new ultrashort acting barbiturate, Anesthesiology 21:29-34, 1960.

16. Zindler, M., editor: Intravenous anaesthesia for out-patients, Acta Anaesth. Scand., supp. 17, Sept. 20, 1964.

16a. Corsson, G., and Domino, E. F.: Dissociative anesthesia: further pharmacologic studies and first clinical experience with the phencyclidine derivative CI-581, Anesth. Analg. 45:29-40, 1966.

16b. Foldes, F. F.: Personal communication.

17. Foldes, F. F., Ceravelo, A. J., and Carpenter, S. L.: The administration of nitrous oxide-oxygen anesthesia in closed systems, Ann. Surg. 136:978-981, 1952.

18. Etsten, B., and Himwich, H. E.: Stages and signs of Pentothal anesthesia: physiologic basis, Anesthesiology 7:536-548, 1946.

19. Goodman, L. S., and Gilman, A.: The pharmacological basis of therapeutics, New York, 1955, The Macmillan Co.

20. Shaw, F. H.: Further experience with Megimide, a barbiturate antagonist, Med. J. Aust. 2:889-891, 1955.

21. Boyan, C. P., and Howland, W. S.: Beta, beta-methylethyl-glutarimide (Megimide) in treatment of barbiturate poisoning, J.A.M.A. 163:835-837, 1957.

22. Barrett, R. H.: The analeptic effect of sodium succinate on barbiturate depression in man. I, Anesth. Analg. 26:74-81, 1947; II, Anesth. Analg. 26:105-113, 1947.

23. Gale, A. S.: Intravenous Ritalin: a barbiturate and meperidine antagonist, Anesthesiology 19:101-102, 1958.

24. Macris, S. G., Kadoglou, O. N., Cacouri, A. N., and Macris, G. J.: A clinical comparison of the effectiveness of nikethamide, ethamivan, methylphenidate and bemegride in postanesthetic arousal, Anesth. Analg. 41:593-598, 1962.

25. Schmidt, C. F.: Recent developments in respiratory physiology related to anesthesia, Anesthesiology 6:113-123, 1945.

26. Giarman, N. J., Rowe, R. P., and Young, J. F.: The effect of sodium succinate and some of its derivatives on thiopental anesthesia, Anesthesiology 15:122-125, 1954.

27. Dillon, J. B.: The management of patients with acute barbiturate poisoning, Anesth. Analg. 33:381-385, 1954.

28. Plum, F., and Swanson, A. G.: Barbiturate poisoning treated by physiological methods, with observations on effects of β,β-methylethylglutarimide and electrical stimulation, J.A.M.A. 163:827-835, 1957.

29. Stephen, C. R., and Talton, I.: Investigation of doxapram as a postanesthetic respiratory stimulant, Anesth. Analg. 43:628-640, 1964.

30. Noe, F. E.: Respiratory stimulation with doxapram hydrochloride during the anesthesia recovery period, Anesth. Analg. 45:479-483, 1966.

31. Smith, R. M., Bachman, L., and Bougas, T.: Shivering following thiopental sodium and other anesthetic agents, Anesthesiology 16:655-664, 1955.

32. Dundee, J. W., and Riding, J. E.: Barbiturate narcosis in porphyria, Anaesthesia 10:55-58, 1955.

33. Dundee, J. W., McCleery, W. N., and McLoughlin, G.: The hazard of thiopental anaesthesia in porphyria, Anesth. Analg. 41:567-574, 1962.

Chapter 14

Use of muscle relaxants

BACKGROUND

Muscle relaxants, whether used in the jungle or in the operating room, have always seemed highly dramatic and uniquely interesting. The pharmacologic nature of these drugs invites investigation, their sudden effectiveness commands respect, and their clinical application arouses continuing debate.

Although disagreement has been more intense concerning use of relaxants in adults,[1,2] there has been wide divergence of opinion in pediatric circles and considerable changing of minds as more experience and information have accumulated. This dynamic state of affairs still exists.

DEVELOPMENT OF CONCEPTS

In 1942 Griffith and Johnson[3] introduced curare into the field of anesthesia, and the next year Cullen[4] extended its use to infants. Soon afterward many others in America and England followed—it was adopted more readily in areas in which cautery was regarded as necessary for surgery.

With the first use of relaxants in children the practice evolved of operating on infants under curare and oxygen alone, without an anesthetic agent. To test the rationale of this technique, Scott Smith[5] allowed himself to be deeply curarized while conscious and proved that curare had no appreciable anesthetic effect. After this demonstration, curarization without anesthesia was generally abandoned.

All the relaxants have been used in children, and various techniques have been employed. In 1949 Webster and Van Bergen[6] reported the use of a thiopental-curare mixture with endotracheal nitrous oxide on twenty-seven infants, and in 1951 Anderson[7] described her use of *d*-tubocurarine and gallamine in a considerably larger series of pediatric procedures. It was generally believed that curare was an acceptable agent for children of all ages.

As other relaxants were introduced, each was tried on children. Succinylcholine, because of its short duration of action, was assumed to be safest, and for a time it was the relaxant of choice for pediatric patients. With increased use, however, succinylcholine showed evidence of such disadvantages as prolonged apnea and severe bradycardia, and it superiority was questioned.

RESPONSE OF INFANTS AND CHILDREN TO RELAXANTS

Much of the uncertainty about clinical use of relaxants in children has been due to the fact that the response of infants and children to both depolarizing and nondepolarizing agents has been thought to be different from that of adults. Confusion still exists concerning the reason for this change, its degree, its duration, and, in fact, the actual existence of such altered response.

In 1955, the first news of the child's different reaction to relaxants came from the Jackson Rees school in Liverpool, when Stead[8] noted that infants showed

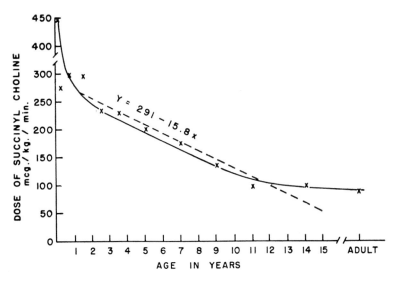

Fig. 14-1. Relationship of age to dosage of succinylcholine necessary to maintain apnea. The formula $Y = 291 - 15.8X$ represents the regression equation. The regression coefficient for the equation was $p < 0.01$, a significant figure. (From Telford, J., and Keats, A. S.: Anesthesiology 18:841, 1957.)

increased tolerance to succinylcholine, but were more sensitive to d-tubocurarine than were older patients.

Stead and Rees[9-11] also showed that the infant's reaction to d-tubocurarine was much like that of a myasthenic patient. Several others reported similar findings and enlarged upon them. Telford and Keats[12] analyzed the quantity of succinylcholine required by patients of different ages during cardiovascular operations and found that the newborn infant required 447 mg./kg./min. as compared to the adult's need of 92 mg./kg./min., an unexpected fivefold differ-

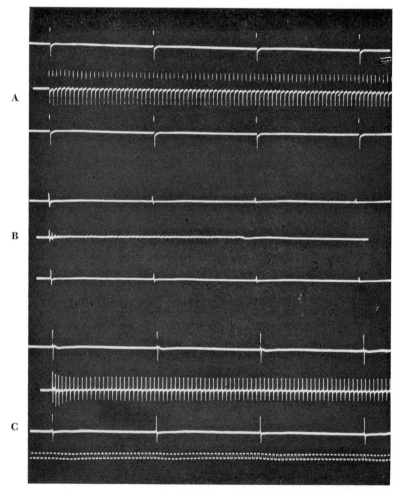

Fig. 14-2. Effect of d-tubocurarine and neostigmine in a neonate (M.U.) **A,** Control showing the effect of twitch rates of nerve stimulation (2.5/sec.) before and after tetanic stimulation (50/sec.). **B,** Same after administration of 600 μg. d-tubocurarine; photograph taken at ninth minute. **C,** Same 4 minutes after administration of 0.148 mg. neostigmine methyl sulfate; photograph taken at fourteenth minute. Time base = 0.01 second. (From Churchill-Davidson, H. C., and Wise, R. P.: Canad. Anaesth. Soc. J. 11:1, 1964.)

ence. The relationship of age to dosage of succinylcholine was shown to be an inverse linear curve extending from birth to 10 years (Fig. 14-1).

Churchill-Davidson and Wise,[13] using electromyographic techniques, were able to delineate the situation further. They found that the neonate's response to the depolarizing relaxant decamethonium was indeed much like that of a myasthenic, exhibiting poor maintenance of tetanic contraction, followed by posttetanic exhaustion. This differs from the adult in such a way as to suggest a biphasic type of neuromuscular block that may be prolonged and that is not reliably reversible. It was also found that the infant required three times the equivalent adult dose of decamethonium (Fig. 14-2).

In subsequent investigation of d-tubocurarine Churchill-Davidson and Wise[14] found that the average dose required for paralysis of hand muscles in the infant corresponded closely with the equivalent dose for an adult, but that the infant's respiration was considerably more depressed. The reversal of d-tubocurarine in the neonate was found to be prompt with either neostigmine or edrophonium (Tensilon) but often was only temporary with edrophonium.

Bush and Stead[15] reported on further observations, pointing to the dangers of suxamethonium (repeated administration, uneven muscle relaxation, and phase II block), at the same time attesting the reliability of d-tubocurarine. They found that the infant at birth requires only half the normal dose by weight but that this sensitivity decreases and disappears in the first month of life. Based on the greater reliability of d-tubocurarine, these authors, as well as Churchill-Davidson and Wise, recommended it for infants in preference to succinylcholine. Adding to the confusion, Lim, Davenport, and Robson[16] evaluated relaxant activity by measuring mean CO_2 expiration. They found that the younger children metabolized succinylcholine more rapidly but that the drug produced deeper relaxation in infants under 1 year than in older patients.

Further electromyographic investigation carried out by Nightingale, Glass, and Bachman[17] gave evidence of tolerance of the young child to succinylcholine when given in a dosage of 0.3 mg./kg. but not when given in a dosage of 0.5 mg./kg. The intensity and duration of action of a 0.3 mg./kg. dose, as measured by action potentials, was found to increase steadily in patients studied between 4 months and 13 years of age.

The reason for the infant's altered response to relaxants is not understood. Since the increased tolerance to succinylcholine and depolarizing agents extends through childhood, while the sensitivity to d-tubocurarine is limited to early infancy, it appears unlikely that there is any single factor that could explain both responses.

Theories advanced include altered uptake of drugs,[18] difference in transport and distribution among neuromuscular end plates,[19] difference in anatomic structure of end plates,[20] variations in enzymatic activity,[11,21-24] and elimination of the compounds. Thus far few of these areas have been studied. Anatomic development of the end plate has been worked out carefully.[25] It is known that the neonate has his full complement of muscles, nerves, and end plates, but that individual structural development may not be complete until 2 years of age. Alteration of response could be involved here. Cholinesterase activity has been demonstrated in the mid-fetal period, and Drachman[25] used *d*-tubocurarine effectively on chick embryos with predictable response even at this age. Thus, all the essential structural units certainly would appear to be present at birth.

The sensitivity to *d*-tubocurarine, if it does truly exist, appears to parallel the early physiologic changes of neonates in adapting to extrauterine life. It might be related to renal or hepatic development rather than to changes of the neuromuscular structure.

Clarification of succinylcholine tolerance should lie in other directions. The relative size of fluid compartments may play an important part in distribution of relaxants to end plates. The initial preponderance of the extracellular space at birth and the gradual shift to intracellular preponderance is in line with the gradually diminishing succinylcholine tolerance.[18]

The enzymatic breakdown of succinylcholine naturally deserves scrutiny in relation to altered succinylcholine effect. Increased tolerance to depolarizing drugs would suggest increased cholinesterase activity. Evidence appears to destroy this hypothesis, however—cholinesterase levels in infants have been found to be slightly reduced, with mean levels of 59 units for premature infants and 66 units for mature newborn infants as compared to the adult mean of 85 units.[21,23] Normal response in adults has been found with cholinesterase levels of 60 or below, hence the enzyme concentration does not appear to explain the child's altered reaction.

Zsigmond and Patterson[24] question the clinical observations of the infant's tolerance to succinylcholine. In their study of the potency of plasma cholinesterase activity, they found the absolute activity of plasma cholinesterase in infants to be only one third of that in adults. Again we are left with inconclusive and contradictory evidence, and it appears that a more satisfactory explanation will be found to be related to a gradually altering relationship between end plates, muscle mass, and body fluid compartments. Absence of fasciculation is characteristic of the myasthenic and also parallels the absence of shivering in the neonate.[26] This could demonstrate either immature or pathologic neuromuscular development. The marked cardiac slowing seems to be evidence of parasympathetic predominance thought to be peculiar to the infant.

In most respects the older child's reaction to relaxants resembles that of the adult, as described by Foldes.[31]

Advantages and indications. The advantages of relaxant agents are well known. In addition to complete relaxation unrelated to generalized depression, they include nonflammability, direct route of administration without dependence upon ventilation, rapid effect, freedom from metabolic effects or toxicity, and little if any effect on myocardium or peripheral vascular system. The same advantages exist for children as for adults, but the need for relaxants is less marked. Abdominal relaxation is usually adequate with halothane, ether, or cyclopropane without supplemental use of relaxants. Indications for relaxants in children include endotracheal intubation and other short-term use for brief periods of relaxation during abdominal closure or reduction of fracture, or for relief of laryngeal spasm or convulsion. In addition, relaxants are used for longer periods in combination with thiopental, nitrous oxide, and narcotics as noted below. Since the Liverpool school employs relaxants for practically all procedures, they obviously can be used in a wide variety of procedures. In this country, however, relaxants are usually reserved for procedures in which they have proved of significant advantage. If the use of relaxants for intubation is excluded, it is probable that these agents are used for less than 5% of procedures in infants and children in America. At the Children's Hospital Medical Center in Boston use of relaxants has been somewhat greater and has increased further since the recent incidence of hepatitis in two children following anesthesia with halogenated agents.

Additional use of relaxants is indicated in certain nonsurgical situations, such as when patients require paralyzation during treatment for seizures or tetanus.

TREATMENT OF TETANUS

In the treatment of tetanus, relaxants offer the unique advantage of controlling convulsions without depressing the central nervous system. In this respect they are definitely preferable to sedatives, which control seizures through depression of the motor cortex. Preparations of curare in oil were popular at one time but were not easily controlled and have been replaced by the use of short-acting relaxants given by intravenous drip.[27] Incidentally the use of curare in tetanus is not new. In 1899 Farquharson[28] listed a series of thirty-three cases treated by extracts of woorara.

Reports from centers treating large numbers of patients who have tetanus have shown a definite trend away from the use of curarizing agents because of the excessive amount of supervision involved. The use of combinations of barbiturates, chlorpromazine,[29] and mephenesin appears to be more practical. For treatment of occasional cases, tribromoethanol has proved remarkably effective[30] and in past years was our standard form of therapy.

AGENTS

Although all relaxants may be used for infants and children, clinical experience and investigation have been limited chiefly to *d*-tubocurarine, gallamine, succinylcholine, and decamethonium, which serve most purposes adequately. Since little information is available concerning pediatric use of other agents, discussion will be limited to these.

d-Tubocurarine,[31] as noted, is a nondepolarizing agent that shows increased potency in neonates and has questionable histaminogenic properties. Its value lies especially in the long duration of relaxation (15 to 20 minutes), its reversibility, and its freedom from toxicity and other side effects.

Gallamine (Flaxedil) is of slightly shorter duration than *d*-tubocurarine, approximately ⅕ the potency per milligram, a reversible nondepolarizing agent that also has vagolytic action. Consequently, this may be the relaxant of choice for patients with slow pulse or for supplementation of cyclopropane anesthesia.

Succinylcholine (Anectine) is rapid in action and is quickly broken down. Its vagotonic effect is blocked by atropine. It is a depolarizing agent and is not pharmacologically reversible.

Decamethonium is a more slowly acting agent like curare but acts as a depolarizing agent, is not histaminogenic, and is not pharmacologically reversible.

This agent occasionally shows an irregular action, blocking the intercostal muscles and leaving the abdomen rigid. It is seldom used at present.

DOSAGES

The dosages of relaxants recommended for pediatric use have varied widely both in quantity and in unit of measurement. Scott Smith[32] was one of the first to suggest a specific amount for use in infants. Following induction with cyclopropane, nitrous oxide, or thiopental, he recommended the use of 0.5 unit of curare per pound of body weight, or 0.25 unit per pound if used with ether.

Anderson[7] reported that 2.5 mg. of curare per 14 pounds of body weight was most satisfactory and gave 1 mg. per pound as the preferable dose for gallamine.

Theoretically it is probably not correct to base the dosage of relaxants upon weight, since the number and distribution of motor end plates are greater

Table 14-1. *Doses (mg./lb.) of d-tubocurarine and gallamine with various inhalation agents for newborn infants**

Inhalation agent	d-Tubocurarine dose (mg./lb.)		Gallamine dose (mg./lb.)	
	Initial	Fractional	Initial	Fractional
Ether	0.05	0.025	0.25	0.1
Cyclopropane	0.1	0.05	0.5	0.25
Halothane	0.1	0.05	0.5	0.25
Nitrous oxide	0.15	0.07	0.75	0.5

*For those over 3 months of age multiply by 2.

Table 14-2. *Relaxant dosage chart for pediatric use**

Lb.	d-Tubocurarine (3 mg./ml.)		Gallamine (20 mg./ml.)		Succinylcholine (20 mg./ml.) I.V.		Fractional dose
10	3 mg.	(1.0 ml.)	15 mg.	(0.75 ml.)	10 mg.	(0.5 ml.)	One fourth to
25	8 mg.	(2.5 ml.)	40 mg.	(2.0 ml.)	20 mg.	(1.0 ml.)	one half the
50	15 mg.	(5.0 ml.)	75 mg.	(3.5 ml.)	40 mg.	(2.0 ml.)	original
75	25 mg.	(8.0 ml.)	120 mg.	(6.0 ml.)	50 mg.	(2.5 ml.)	dose
100	30 mg.	(10.0 ml.)	140 mg.	(7.0 ml.)	60 mg.	(3.0 ml.)	

*Dosage is for use with nitrous oxide only; when used with ether, halothane, or cyclopropane, d-tubocurarine and gallamine dosage should be reduced by one third or one half; when used with halothane or cyclopropane, succinylcholine should be reduced by one half; when used by intramuscular route succinylcholine may be increased by one half.

Table 14-3. *Succinylcholine dosage (mg./lb.)*

Body weight	I.V.	I.M.
0-50 lb.	0.75	1.0
Over 50 lb.	0.50	1.0

determining factors in the response of the patient to the agent.[33] For practical use, however, weight is still the best guide available. If weight is used, it should be borne in mind that the dosage for an obese child should be estimated on the basis of his lean weight; otherwise gross overdosage may result. As has been noted, infants require less nondepolarizing agent than older children and adults.

Definitive and practical guides to relaxant dosages are listed in Tables 14-1 to 14-3. The recommended initial and fractional doses of *d*-tubocurarine and gallamine with various inhalation agents are listed in Table 14-1.

For quick reference, Table 14-2 may serve as a more practical guide. All dosages are comparatively high and may be altered to suit one's clinical judgment.

TECHNIQUES

The most common indication for use of muscle relaxants in children is for *endotracheal intubation.* When general anesthesia is used, supplemental relaxation is less important in pediatric patients, but it speeds and facilitates the procedure. With small infants intubation is often performed under a relaxant without anesthesia.

Succinylcholine is preferable for intubation because of its rapid action and complete effectiveness. It may be used by either intravenous or intramuscular route. In either case bradycardia may occur, and a vagolytic agent, preferably atropine, should be active when the relaxant is given. If succinylcholine is injected intravenously, a dose of 0.75 mg./lb. will cause apnea in 8 to 10 seconds. The child should be ventilated with oxygen prior to intubation.

Because of the greater danger of bradycardia with intravenous injection of succinylcholine, it seems preferable to use the intramuscular route.[34] With a dose of 1 mg./lb. the onset of action is more gradual. The child will become less active but will maintain spontaneous respiration for approximately 2 minutes. Ninety seconds after intramuscular injection, infants usually may be intubated with ease but are protected by the fact that they can still oxygenate themselves to a limited degree.

When either *d*-tubocurarine or gallamine is used for endotracheal intubation, the intravenous route is usually preferable. Then one should allow 2 to 3 minutes for full effect of the agent. It has been found, however, that when *d*-tubocurarine is given to neonates intravenously, the effect may be almost instantaneous.

There are several situations in which succinylcholine may be used for brief *periods of apnea or full relaxation.* During bronchography and angiocardiography, momentary induction of apnea is of considerable advantage in obtaining satisfactory films.[35] For removal of a foreign body from the trachea, complete relaxation of vocal cords may be necessary at the moment of delivery. This is described in Chapter 22. Apparatus must be available to maintain ventilation under such circumstances. A dose of 0.5 mg./lb. is usually adequate as a supplement to general anesthesia. This definitely should be given by intravenous route to ensure rapid onset and short duration of action. Similar use is indicated during difficult closure of the peritoneum as with meconium ileus or other forms of intestinal obstruction, or possibly for diaphragmatic hernia or omphalocele (p. 259). Here again it should be emphasized that intravenous administration is mandatory since an infant might be cold at this time, and absorption of the drug would be delayed.

Children entering the hospital with simple fractures often have eaten recently, in which case regional anesthesia should be employed as first choice. If general anesthesia is required, brief relaxation with succinylcholine may be advantageous. In such cases, it is preferable to induce anesthesia with nitrous oxide–oxygen and halothane and to pass a snugly fitting endotracheal tube before using any relaxant. When the surgeon is about to reduce the fracture, 1.0 mg. of succinylcholine/kg. body weight can be given intravenously to provide prompt relaxation of short duration.

For prolonged periods of relaxation in major surgical procedures, relaxants may be used in a variety of situations. In abdominal operations relaxants are especially helpful in upper abdominal work in which complete relaxation and control of diaphragmatic motion are desired. A relaxant–nitrous oxide technique may be employed, or a general anesthesia may be supplemented with intermittent doses of *d*-tubocurarine or gallamine.

When extensive bleeding is anticipated, relaxants are of increased value, since they have little effect on blood pressure and do not distort the signs of blood loss. It is in abdominal procedures that one encounters many of the dangers associated with relaxants. As previously emphasized, these agents should not be employed for intubation in the presence of a full stomach or intestinal distention, or when there is marked electrolyte imbalance. Ether, neomycin, and similar agents, of course, will intensify the neuromuscular blocking effect of curare, and, as in all types of surgery, children must be kept warm to prevent delayed recovery.

In my personal experience, the greatest use of relaxants in pediatric anesthesia has been in thoracic surgery. Most of our first 300 open heart procedures were performed under nitrous oxide–oxygen supplemented with thiopental and intermittent doses of succinylcholine. More recently, succinylcholine has been replaced by *d*-tubocurarine, and in other cases anesthesia was maintained without relaxants with halothane or fluroxene (Fluoromar). Because of its reversibility and lack of myocardial depressant activity, *d*-tubocurarine with nitrous oxide–oxygen seems to be preferable for the production of anesthesia for open heart surgery.

Our most crucial test of the relaxant methods has been in infants operated upon in the hyperbaric chamber for severe congenital cardiac lesions. These infants, especially those having right to left intracardiac shunts, tolerated halothane poorly and showed marked fall in blood pressure. With *d*-tubocurarine and 50% nitrous oxide–oxygen the blood pressure remained much more stable. Infants recovered well under standard reversal technique at the end of the procedures.

Use of nitrous oxide–relaxant technique. When relying upon the combination of nitrous oxide and relaxant as the major agents, one starts with generous atropinization and rather modest sedation, to guarantee prompt recovery of respiration postoperatively.

Induction of anesthesia in most children is performed using a 25-gauge or

26-gauge needle.[9] In infants the best vein is frequently found in the volar aspect of the wrist. This fine needle often can be inserted without the child's apparent knowledge. Furthermore, the lumen is so small that the needle may be left unattached to syringe or infusion set, and back-bleeding will not occur. A sleep dose of 2% thiopental is administered, and the jaw is supported as the child drops off to sleep. Nitrous oxide and oxygen are given in 3:2 ratio.

If the procedure is to be under 30 minutes in duration, succinylcholine is used. In a dosage of 1 mg./lb., the trachea is intubated, and respiration is controlled using T system in smaller patients, or semiclosed circle in those over 30 pounds. Patients are actively hyperventilated to prolong relaxation, and, if necessary, additional succinylcholine is given by vein (0.5 mg./lb.). In the neonate, thiopental is omitted, and one starts by injecting the relaxant.

If the operation is expected to be longer than 30 minutes, *d*-tubocurarine is employed as the relaxant. The Liverpool school[10,11] recommends an initial dosage of 0.15 mg./lb. for the first 3 months of life, and 0.3 mg./lb. thereafter. Endotracheal intubation is performed after 2 to 3 minutes of assisted or controlled ventilation, and then after intubation the patient is hyperventilated as with succinylcholine. Supplementary doses of *d*-tubocurarine are given as needed, using one fourth to one half of the original dose, as suits the individual case.

One disadvantage of such use of *d*-tubocurarine is that it may be difficult to foretell when the relaxant is about to wear off, and the child may become active rather suddenly. One gradually learns to sense this by a change in resistance of the breathing bag shortly before the return of action. A relaxing dose of *d*-tubocurarine should last 15 to 20 minutes, and often considerably longer when aided by premedication and hyperventilation. Each patient is slightly different, but after 2 or 3 doses the pattern of an individual can be recognized and followed.

If the relaxant wears off just before the end of the operation, one may add a fraction of the average dose, and, by ventilating the child with increased vigor, finish up in good form. If one is not a purist he can allow a bit of halothane to leak into the system.

As the surgeon is closing the skin, atropine is administered to prepare for reversal, and then, after the last suture is placed, prostigmine is added as described in the following paragraphs.

REVERSAL AND RECOVERY

Undoubtedly the greatest hazard in the use of relaxants lies in the recovery phase. Inadequate return of ventilatory strength too often goes undiagnosed and may cause hypoxia, atelectasis, or death. Usually, if a patient is completely apneic at termination of operation, he will be carefully attended. It is when the patient starts to breathe that the anesthetist may erroneously assume the exchange to be adequate and leave him unattended.

When respiration unexpectedly remains depressed after the use of either depolarizing or nondepolarizing agent, one must continue full ventilation and not attempt to stimulate respiration by inducing either hypoxia or hypercarbia. A reasonable first step is to test for muscle twitch with a nerve stimulator (Fig. 14-3).[36-38] Presence of normal nerve response will immediately show that residual

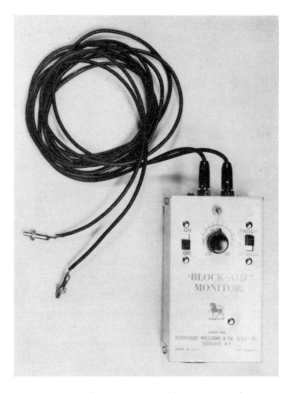

Fig. 14-3. Nerve stimulator (Block-Aid) should be used in diagnosis of prolonged apnea.

relaxants are not the cause of the apnea, and one should suspect hyperventilation, premedicant overdose, brain damage, or other causes. If muscle twitch is found to be depressed, general and definitive steps should be taken.

After the use of nondepolarizing agents (*d*-tubocurarine and gallamine), it is advisable to make a standard practice of reversing the block with neostigmine. For pediatric use, the Liverpool formula of 0.008 mg./lb. of atropine followed by 0.036 mg./lb. of neostigmine is effective.[15] It is believed to be preferable not to attempt to reverse agents too soon after their administration. If active respiration begins or if 30 minutes have passed since curarization, reversal is thought to be justified. Often, when spontaneous respiration has returned following curarization, one is tempted to omit use of reversal. Since one can rarely be certain that relaxant effect has entirely disappeared, it seems preferable to take the precaution of using the neostigmine.

The recommended dose of 0.036 mg./lb. for neostigmine is in the order of 5 mg. per 150 lb., which seems rather terrifying to Americans. Rees feels that the whole dose should be given at once for best effect, but Gray[39] and others condone the dividing of the total dose into two or three parts to be given at successive 5-minute intervals as required.

The large dosage of atropine and neostigmine has aroused concern. However, reports of arrhythmia following atropine seem to exaggerate this danger. Such arrhythmias have occurred chiefly when atropine has been given to correct vagotonic activity already aroused, such as during cyclopropane anesthesia or at the height of succinylcholine bradycardia.[40] When given prophylactically, atropine rarely causes arrhythmias.

Neostigmine may cause bradycardia if patients are not protected by vagolytic agents, but the fatal reactions to this drug earlier reported are considered to be the result of grossly mismanaged anesthesia with severe hypercarbia. We are told the salivation that may occur can be reduced if patients are properly hyperventilated. This appears to be true.

Foldes[41] described factors that may retard reversal of nondepolarizing agents in adults, and children follow the same general rules. Certainly one must be sure that the child is in optimum condition if prompt reversal is to be expected. If the child is cold,[42] hypovolemic, hypotensive, or in electrolytic imbalance, delayed recovery from relaxants may be expected whether reversing agents are used or not.

Evaluation of reversal and recovery. Numerous methods of evaluation of recovery are employed but few are reliable, and those most accurate are not often used. Most frequently the anesthetist waits until the patient can take a reasonably deep breath and then hurries away. Bendixen[43] has shown that slight obstruction can greatly reduce the ventilation of patients who are in the process of recovery, and measurement of inspiratory force, using a simple manometer fixed to a mask, will be of real assistance. This is useful for all ages but as yet has not been generally adopted.

Other signs of recovery include movement of limbs, hand grasp, opening the eyes without wrinkling the forehead, speaking or crying, a forceful cough, and lifting the head up off the bed or the operating table. Of these signs most have been found to be unreliable as indicators of ventilatory adequacy. The one exception, perhaps, is elevation of the head.[44] This appears to return only after a patient is breathing actively and moving, and in my experience it has been the most useful clinical sign when actual measuring devices have not been available. A small child, of course, will not attempt to lift his head on command, but one can test him by lifting his shoulders off the bed. If he has the power, he will keep his head on the same level as his body and will not let it fall backward, thus proving the presence of head lifting power.

Rees[45] has a firm conviction that while *d*-tubocurarine is prompely reversed in patients who have been well ventilated gallamine cannot be reversed equally well unless the patient has been hypoventilated and is actually acidotic. This has been studied by Baraka,[45a] whose work supports this concept.

It has been shown by Foldes[41] and by Katz and Papper[46] that the neuromuscular block of *d*-tubocurarine is reduced in an acidotic medium and increased when alkalotic, while gallamine behaves in the opposite manner. This cannot be taken as direct proof concerning reversal, and the point needs clarification. In a small series of cases we have found no significant difference in reversal of the two drugs under clinical conditions of respiratory acidosis and alkalosis (Fig. 14-4).

Rees[45] states that it is extremely rare for complete recovery to require more

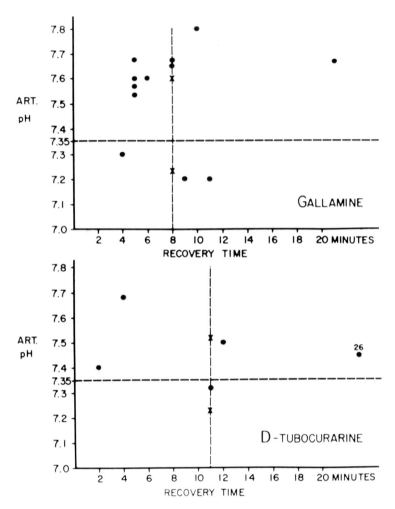

Fig. 14-4. Relationship of reversal time to pH with gallamine and *d*-tubocurarine. Average reversal time with gallamine, 8 minutes; average reversal time with *d*-tubocurarine, 11 minutes, in children with normal arterial pH.

than 10 minutes. My own patients are much less cooperative, and it often takes 10 minutes or more before I feel ready to leave them. Upon testing some of these with a nerve stimulator, it appears that the relaxant has been reversed, but apnea persists due to other causes such as hypocarbia or sedation.

DISADVANTAGES AND DANGERS

From a practical standpoint the use of a relaxant technique for pediatric anesthesia involves both intravenous injection and endotracheal intubation. For major procedures these are inconsequential, but for many relatively simple procedures they seem unjustified. Obviously, the use of relaxants will eliminate respiration and the possibility of using respiratory vigor as a sign of anesthesia.

Complications encountered when using relaxants relate chiefly to various patterns of respiratory depression secondary to neuromuscular block[47] or to cardiac disturbances caused by vagotonic effects of succinylcholine.

Since children show less marked fasciculation and most infants show none at all, muscle pains are no problem.

The respiratory problems noted in children have already been mentioned. Prolonged apnea may be caused by overdosage, by phase II block,[48] by familial deficiency of plasma cholinesterase,[49] and other factors effective in adults.[50-52] The infant is more susceptible to the effect of nondepolarizing drugs[10] and probably more likely to develop phase II block with succinylcholine than is the adult.

Justifiably, much concern has been expressed over the bradycardia associated with succinylcholine, especially upon a second intravenous administration when the patient is under cyclopropane or halothane anesthesia.[53,54] Although fatal outcome has been rare, numerous instances of arrest or near-arrest have been sufficient to make the prophylactic use of atropine mandatory.

Increased intraocular pressure is observed in children with the use of succinylcholine. This is of importance only during the removal of cataracts and in emergency surgery for traumatic rupture of the ocular globe.

Two bizarre complications have been noted with succinylcholine and could be related. Bush,[55] McCaughey,[56] and others have reported deaths in burned children receiving succinylcholine anesthesia 2 to 3 weeks after the burns occurred. Numerous factors were suspected, especially concerning low or inactive plasma cholinesterase. It now appears that trauma and burns cause a delayed rise in serum potassium, which, upon administration of succinylcholine, may reach toxic levels.[57]

An even more perplexing complication has been encountered in the hyperthermic reactions[58,59] recently reported in growing numbers. These hyperthermic reactions frequently start with prolonged generalized myotonic spasm following succinylcholine administration, and they have occurred in patients with preexisting myotonia dystrophica[60] and myotonia congenita.[61] They have occurred more frequently in patients with no known neuromuscular disorder. This complication is included in the discussion on temperature reactions in Chapter 27.

CONTRAINDICATIONS TO USE OF RELAXANTS

Contraindications to the use of relaxants are as follows:
1. *Airway obstruction:* Virtually all anesthetists agree that one should not use relaxants in patients having any significant degree of airway obstruction. To paralyze such patients and then be unable to pass an endotracheal tube or to ventilate them in any way would be an inexcusable and perhaps fatal error. It is preferable either to use an inhalation agent such as halothane or cyclopropane, which will not cause apnea, or to intubate the patient while awake.
2. *Full stomach:* Belief that the relaxants should be contraindicated in a patient who probably has food in his stomach is not held by all, and many anesthetists choose the rapid intravenous injection of thiopental and succinylcholine for this situation and get by with it. I believe that this tech-

nique may cause prompt relaxation of the cardiac esophagus with massive regurgitation of stomach contents and prefer not to use it. (Chapter 24). The use of relaxants when the stomach is actually distended by pressure of contained gas, solid or liquid, is undeniably hazardous and should be accepted by all as being definitely contraindicated.

REFERENCES

1. Beecher, H. K., and Todd, D. B.: A study of the deaths associated with anesthesia and surgery, Ann. Surg. 140:2-34, 1954.
2. Critique of study of deaths associated with anesthesia and surgery, Ann. Surg. 142:138, 1955.
3. Griffith, H. R., and Johnson, E.: The use of curare in general anesthesia, Anesthesiology 3:418-420, 1942.
4. Cullen, S. C.: The use of curare for the improvement of abdominal muscle relaxation during inhalation anesthesia, Surgery 14:261-266, 1943.
5. Smith, S. M., Brown, H., Toman, J., and Goodman, L.: The lack of cerebral effects of d-tubocurarine, Anesthesiology 8:1-13, 1947.
6. Webster, C. F., and Van Bergen, F. H.: Pentothal-curare mixture with endotracheal N_2O and O_2 in infants, Bull. Univ. Minnesota Hosp. & Minnesota Med. Found. 20:525-533, 1949.
7. Anderson, S. M.: Use of depressant and relaxant drugs in infants and children, Lancet 2:965-966, 1951.
8. Stead, A. L.: The response of the newborn infant to muscle relaxants, Brit. J. Anaesth. 27:124-130, 1955.
9. Rees, J. G.: Anaesthesia in the newborn, Brit. Med. J. 2:1419-1422, 1950.
10. Rees, J. G.: The child as a subject for anaesthesia. In Evans, F. T., and Gray, T. C., editors: Modern trends in anaesthesia, New York, 1958, Paul B. Hoeber, Inc., Medical Book Department of Harper & Row, Publishers.
11. Rees, J. G.: Paediatric anaesthesia, Brit. J. Anaesth. 32:132-140, 1960.
12. Telford, J., and Keats, A. S.: Succinylcholine in cardiovascular surgery of infants and children, Anesthesiology 18:841-848, 1957.
13. Churchill-Davidson, H. C., and Wise, R. P.: The response of the newborn infant to muscle relaxants, Canad. Anaesth. Soc. J. 11:1-6, 1963.
14. Churchill-Davidson, H. C., and Wise, R. P.: Neuromuscular transmission in the newborn infant, Anesthesiology 24:271-278, 1963.
15. Bush, G. H., and Stead, A. L.: The use of d-tubocurarine in neonatal anaesthesia, Brit. J. Anaesth. 34:721-728, 1962.
16. Lim, H. S., Davenport, H. T., and Robson, J. G.: The response of infants and children to muscle relaxants, Anesthesiology 25:161-168, 1964.
17. Nightingale, D. A., Glass, A. G., and Bachman, L.: Neuromuscular blockade by succinylcholine in children, Anesthesiology 27:736-741, 1966.
18. Kalow, W.: Relaxants. In Papper, E. M., and Kitz, R. J., editors: Uptake and distribution of anesthetic agents, New York, 1963, McGraw-Hill Book Co.
19. Katz, R. L., and Papper, E. M.: The effect of alkalosis in the action of neuromuscular blocking agents, Anesthesiology 24:18-22, 1963.
20. Zachs, S. I.: The motor endplate, Philadelphia, 1964, W. B. Saunders Co.
21. Hodges, R. J. H.: Suxamethonium tolerance and pseudocholinesterase levels in children, Proceedings of World Congress of Anesthesiologists, Scheveningen, The Netherlands, Sept. 5-10, 1955, pp. 247-251.
22. Kaufman, L., Lehman, H., and Silk, E.: Suxamethonium apnoea in an infant; expression of familial pseudocholinesterase deficiency in three generations, Brit. Med. J. 1:165-167, 1962.
23. Lehman, H., Cook, J., and Ryan, E.: Pseudocholinesterase in early infancy, Proc. Roy. Soc. Med. 50:147-150, 1957.
24. Zsigmond, E. K., and Patterson, R. L.: Plasma cholinesterase activity of neonates and infants. Paper delivered at A.M.A. annual convention, Atlantic City, N. J., June, 1967.

25. Drachman, D. B.: The developing motor-endplate: pharmacological studies in the chick embryo, J. Physiol. **168:**707, 1963.
26. Smith, R. M.: Pediatric patients. In Foldes, F. F., editor: Muscle relaxants, Philadelphia, 1966, F. A. Davis Co., chap. 2; Clin. Anesth. **2:**34-45, 1966.
27. Alver, E. C., and Leek, J. H.: Induced paralysis for endoscopic procedures, Arch. Otolaryng. **62:**399-405, 1955.
28. Farquharson, R. W.: Guide to therapeutics and materia medica, ed. 4, Philadelphia, 1899, Lea Bros. & Co.
29. Lawrence, D. R., Berman, E., and Scragg, J. N.: Clinical trial of chlorpromazine against barbiturates in tetanus, Lancet **1:**987-991, 1958.
30. Christensen, N. A.: A practical approach to the treatment of tetanus, Minnesota Med. **38:**397-400, 1955.
31. Foldes, F. F.: Muscle relaxants in anesthesiology, Springfield, Ill., 1957, Charles C Thomas, Publisher.
32. Smith, S. M.: The use of curare in infants and children, Anesthesiology **8:**176-180, 1947.
33. Foldes, F. F.: Muscle relaxants, Philadelphia, 1966, F. A. Davis Co., chap. 1, The choice and administration of muscle relaxants; Clin. Anesth. **2:**1-33, 1966.
34. Leigh M. D., McCoy, D. D., Belton, M. K., and Lewis, G. B.: Jr.: Bradycardia following intravenous administration of succinylcholine chloride to infants and children, Anesthesiology **18:**698-702, 1957.
35. Love, S. H. S., and Morrow, W. F. K.: Anaesthesia for bronchography in children, Anaesthesia **9:**74-76, 1954.
36. Churchill-Davidson, H. C.: The causes and treatment of prolonged apnea, Anesthesiology **20:**535-541, 1959.
37. Churchill-Davidson, H. C., Christie, T. H., and Wise, R. P.: Dual neuromuscular block in man, Anesthesiology **21:**144-149, 1960.
38. Katz, R. L.: The Block-Aid monitor, Anesthesiology **26:**204, 1965.
39. Gray, T. C.: Personal communication.
40. Gaviotaki, A., and Smith, R. M.: Use of atropine in pediatric anesthesia, Int. Anesth. Clin. **1:**97-113, 1962.
41. Foldes, F. F.: Factors which alter the effects of muscle relaxants, Anesthesiology **20:**464-504, 1959.
42. Salanitre, E., and Rackow, H.: Respiratory complications associated with the use of muscle relaxants in young infants, Anesthesiology **22:**194-198, 1961.
43. Bendixen, H. H., and Bunker, J. P.: Measurement of inspiratory force in anesthetized dogs, Anesthesiology **23:**315-323, 1962.
44. Nielsen, E., and Bennike, K.: The head-lift test after administration of *d*-tubocurarine, Acta anaesth. Scand. **9:**13-20, 1965; abstract in Survey Anesth. **10:**141-142, 1966.
45. Rees, G. J.: Personal communication.
45a. Baraka, A.: Effect of carbon dioxide on gallamine and suxamethonium block in man, Brit. J. Anaesth. **39:**786-788, 1967.
46. Katz, R. L., and Papper, E. M.: The effect of alkalosis in the action of neuromuscular blocking agents, Anesthesiology **24:**18-22, 1963.
47. Katz, R. L., and Katz, G. J.: Complications associated with the use of muscle relaxants. In Foldes, F. F., editor: Muscle relaxants, Philadelphia, 1966, F. A. Davis Co., chap. 7.
48. Churchill-Davidson, H. C.: The causes and treatment of prolonged apnoea. Anesthesiology **20:**535-541, 1959.
49. Kaufman, L., Lehman, H., and Silk, E.: Suxamethoneum apnea in an infant: expression of familial pseudocholinesterase deficiency in three generations, Brit. Med. J. **1:**165, 1960.
50. Corrado, A. P.: Respiratory depression due to antibiotics: calcium in treatment, Anesth. & Analg. **42:**1-5, 1963.
51. Bigland, B., Goetzec, B., Maclagan, J., and Zaimis, E.: The effect of lowered muscle temperature on the action of neuromuscular blocking drugs, J. Physiol. **141:**425-434, 1958.

52. Doremus, W. P.: Respiratory arrest following intraperitoneal use of neomycin, Ann. Surg. **149:**546-548, 1959.
53. Craythorne, N. W. B., Turndorf, H., and Dripps, R. D.: Changes in pulse rate and rhythm associated with the use of succinylcholine in anesthetized children, Anesthesiology **21:**465-470, 1960.
54. Craythorne, N. W. B., Rottenstein, H. S., and Dripps, R. D.: The effect of succinylcholine on intraocular pressure in adults, infants and children during general anesthesia, Anesthesiology **21:**59-63, 1960.
55. Bush, G. H.: The use of muscle relaxants in burnt children, Anaesthesia **19:**231-238, 1964.
56. McCaughey, T. J.: Hazards of anaesthesia for the burned child, Canad. Anaesth. Soc. J. **9:**220-234, 1962.
57. Tolmie, J. D., Joyce, T. H., and Mitchell, G. D.: Succinylcholine danger in the burned patient, Anesthesiology **28:**467-470, 1967.
58. Thut, W., and Davenport, H. T.: Hyperpyrexia associated with succinylcholine-induced muscle rigidity: a case report, Canad. Anaesth. Soc. J. **13:**425-429, 1966.
59. Hogg, S., and Renwick, W.: Hyperpyrexia during anaesthesia, Canad. Anaesth. Soc. J. **13:**429-437, 1966.
60. Kaufman, L.: Anesthesia in dystrophia myotonica, Proc. Roy. Soc. Med. **53:**183-188, 1960.
61. Patterson, I. S.: Generalized myotonia following suxamethonium, Brit. J. Anaesth. **34:**340-342, 1962.

Hypotensive techniques

The intentional lowering of blood pressure to facilitate operative surgery is a dramatic and unphysiologic technique that can be badly missued. In adults, however, there are several rational indications for this "physiologic trespass" and a variety of methods of accomplishing it. In pediatric surgery as well there is a place for the technique, although indications and methods are limited.

INDICATIONS

Situations that justify the use of induced hypotension in children are restricted chiefly to two fields: (1) neurosurgery concerned with highly vascular tumors[1] or dangerous aneurysms and (2) thoracic surgery involving critical hypertension, as in coarctation of the aorta, or technical difficulty in dealing with a greatly enlarged and distended patent ductus arteriosus.[2] Rare situations in which marked hypertension is caused by spinal cord tumor or by pheochromocytoma may also serve as indications for rapid reduction of blood pressure during pediatric surgery.

AVAILABLE TECHNIQUES

Within a period of 5 years four different methods were suggested for the induction of hypotension.

Arteriotomy. In 1946 Gardner,[3] a Cleveland neurosurgeon, introduced the technique of cannulating an artery and allowing blood to run out of the patient into a reservoir until systolic pressure approached shock level. Operative bleeding was so greatly reduced that intracranial operations could be performed much more easily and quickly. After operation the withdrawn blood was transfused back into the patient. Hale,[4] working with Gardner, found this method compatible with anesthetic practice and also reported favorably upon it.

This technique reduces blood volume to a critical level, induces undesirable response associated with shock, and also endangers the blood supply of the hand if arteriotomy is performed upon the radial artery without adequate collateral circulation. This method has been abandoned but served as the forerunner of safer approaches.

Hypotensive spinal anesthesia. In 1948 Gillies[5,6] of Edinburgh introduced the method of reducing systemic pressure by a high level of spinal anesthesia, a technique that has been advocated in America by Greene.[7,8] When used for the purposes it was originally intended, this method has definite advantages in that blood volume remains unchanged, and undesirable shock responses are not elicited. However, the ease with which blood pressure could be lowered led to wide abuse of this technique and caused a high incidence of complications.[9]

The use of the hypotensive spinal technique does not lend itself to pediatric operations because of the greater difficulty of regulating the level of anesthesia and the lability of blood pressure but most of all because of the emotional instability of the children.

Adrenergic blocking agents. In 1951 Laborit and Huguenard[10] introduced their lytic cocktail composed of Phenergan (promethazine), Largactil (chlorpromazine), and Diparcol (diethezine hydrochloride). Chiefly because of the adrenergic blocking effect of chlorpromazine acting at sympathetic end organs, these agents, when used in sufficient quantity, cause release of vasomotor tone and reduction of blood pressure. In addition, body temperature falls and oxygen requirement is lowered. Because of this combination of effects the originators of the technique labeled it "artificial hibernation" and recommended its use in a wide variety of situations, including the treatment of massive blood loss and open heart surgery.

The usefulness of their method has been limited by the difficulty with which it is controlled and its prolonged effect. Hypotension induced by this method may persist 8 to 12 hours and is resistant to standard vasopressor agents. In addition, chlorpromazine has a number of dangerous side effects when used in large amounts.

Although the technique of artificial hibernation as originally devised has not been generally accepted in this country, chlorpromazine has frequently been used in moderate doses in conjunction with hypothermia induced by cooling.[11]

Ganglionic blocking agents. After the successful induction of hypotension by spinal anesthesia, the use of ganglionic blockade by pharmacologic agents naturally followed. The use of pentamethonium by Enderby[12] in 1950 marked the beginning of the clinical application of hypotensive drugs in anesthesia. Of the several agents used for this purpose the most widely accepted have been hexamethonium[13] and the thiophanium derivative trimethaphan camphorsulfonate usually prepared as Arfonad.[14-17] Both agents are given intravenously, the action of hexamethonium being of 15 to 20 minutes' duration and that of Arfonad being so short that administration by constant drip is usually necessary. The ganglionic blocking agents are extremely easy to use, do not interfere with other anesthetics being given, and are rapidly controllable.

Enderby[18] continued to use this approach exclusively, and Eckenhoff[19] has become an enthusiastic disciple of the school.

In 1955 Anderson[20] reported her experience with controlled hypotension in forty-four children, using Arfonad as the agent. She also noted that children required relatively large amounts of the drug and adopted a 0.2% solution for standard use.

It so happens that two of the most important general anesthetic agents are very effective ganglionic blocking agents. Ether and halothane both cause reduction of blood pressure with increasing blood levels. Either drug may be used for this purpose, although halothane will produce this effect more promptly.

USE OF GANGLIONIC BLOCKING AGENTS IN CHILDREN

In the use of ganglionic blocking agents for children two distinctly different situations exist:

1. The patients undergoing neurosurgery have normal blood pressure, which the surgeons wish to be reduced to minimal, safe levels so that unavoidable bleeding will not be excessive. The reduction of blood pressure in patients who are normotensive has brought some difficulty since these patients show marked resistance to the action of hypotensive drugs.

2. In patients undergoing excision of coarctation of the aorta, use of blocking agents is required when extremely high pressures threaten to rupture cerebral vessels. Here the purpose of the blocking agent is not to reduce blood pressure to minimal levels but merely to lower it enough to keep the pressure within its accustomed range.

A patient with a very large, distended ductus arteriosus resembles the neurosurgical patient more than one with coarctation, for here the problem is that of a normotensive patient who may suddenly become exsanguinated if the vessel is torn. Reduction of pressure to minimal levels reduces the danger of rupturing this vessel and also decreases the severity of the ensuing hemorrhage.

Technique for elective hypotension in pediatric neurosurgery. It should be emphasized that there is a distinct difference between the problem of reducing the pressure of a normotensive patient to hypotensive levels and that of bringing a hypertensive patient down into normal range. Our first cautious attempts at the use of both hexamethonium and Arfonad in normotensive children undergoing neurosurgery were quite unsuccessful. At the advice of Nicholson,[21] however, a policy was adopted of using Arfonad in increasing concentration and starting the infusion briskly. Instead of the usual 0.1% mixture obtained by diluting 50 mg. to 500 ml., a 0.4% mixture was used diluting 50 mg. to 125 ml. This solution was used first for a 30-pound, 4-year-old child, who was to be operated upon for an arteriovenous aneurysm of the brain. After induction of anesthesia with tribromoethanol and ether, the child was intubated, and the operation was begun. When the aneurysm was exposed, 40 ml. of the concentrated Arfonad solution was administered rapidly, resulting in a prompt fall of blood pressure to 30 mm. Hg (Fig. 15-1). This marked hypotension was greater than desired and persisted until the administration of 1 mg. of phenylephrine (Neo-Synephrine). The pressure was easily controlled by dosages of Arfonad and phenylephrine for the succeeding 3 hours, and the procedure was successfully terminated. The total dose of Arfonad was 360 mg. This technique has been proved effective in subsequent cases. In most instances suprisingly large quantities of Arfonad have been require to maintain hypotension, and recovery of the preoperative level of pressure has been slow unless hastened by the use of vasopressor agents.

The level at which the blood pressure should be maintained has not been definitely determined. It does not seem prudent to reduce the systolic pressure of the cerebral arteries below 60 or 70 mm. Hg. If the head of the table is to be elevated during operation, it must be remembered that the blood pressure as measured at the brachial artery will be appreciably higher than that in the cerebral vessels. Obviously the hypotensive state should be maintained only while there is indication for it.

During the use of this technique no alteration in the choice of anesthesia is necessary, but the rate of administration can be reduced considerably. When there is no further need for hypotension, the infusion containing Arfonad is discontinued and the apparatus is removed so that additional amounts of Arfonad will not be given by mistake. It is desirable to have the blood pressure return to its normal level before the dura is closed so that all potential bleeding points will be revealed. Phenylephrine may be given in 0.02% drip infusion (5 mg. in 250 ml.), but sudden elevation of blood pressure is to be avoided for fear of initiating hemorrhage. After normal blood pressure has been reestablished, the vasopressor should be reduced as rapidly as possible without allowing recurrence of hypotension.

Use of ether or halothane to control blood pressure in such a case would probably not be successful, for the amount of either drug would be so great that severe myocardial depression might occur. The difficulty in reducing the pressure of normotensive children has been explained by Kilduff[22] on the basis that trimethaphan causes development of tachyphylaxis. Viquera and Terry[23] used pentolinium, which does not have this effect. They described successful application of pentolinium with halothane for removal of a huge facial tumor in a 9-month-old infant.

During hypertensive episodes in neurosurgical procedures. Occasionally in either adult or pediatric neurosurgical procedures, the blood pressure may become markedly elevated because of pressure on the brain or spinal cord.[24,25] If the underlying cause cannot be corrected, a hypotensive agent may be used. In this situation the agent should be used in normal dilution, for the patient will not show the increased tolerance encountered in a normotensive child. It would be reasonable to attempt to control blood pressure with halothane in this case. An electrocardiograph should be used for immediate recognition of any cardiac

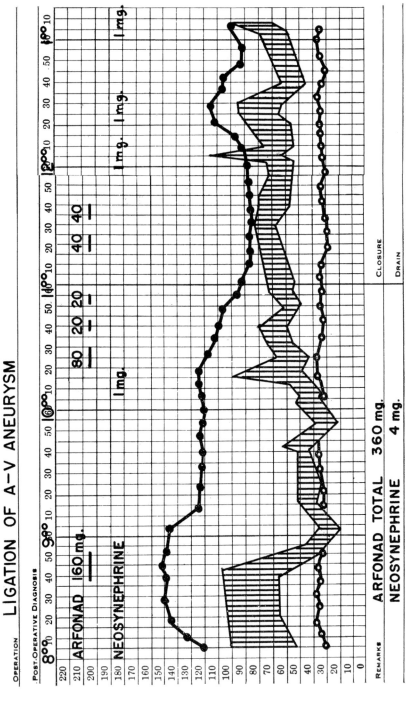

Fig. 15-1. Anesthesia chart illustrating use of hypotensive technique in a 3-year-old child.

disturbance. It would seem reasonable to raise the concentration of halothane as high as 3% or 3.5% if necessary for 3 to 5 minutes, under close observation, to reduce blood pressure.

Ganglionic blocking agents during cardiovascular operations. At present the most frequent indications for controlling blood pressure are encountered in operations on the great vessels.

Coarctation of the aorta. Under usual circumstances the blood pressure of patients with coarctation of the aorta is moderately elevated prior to operation, but after induction of surgical anesthesia with ether or halothane the pressure ordinarily falls to a normal level. Occasionally the pressure remains moderately high until the chest is opened, and then it falls. About one patient in twenty-five will maintain a blood pressure of 170 to 190 mm. Hg until the surgeon is ready to put clamps on the aorta to resect the coarctation. Occlusion of the aorta in the presence of hypertension has been proved dangerous; consequently it seems preferable in such a situation to lower the blood pressure 30 or 40 mm. by the use of blocking agents. Either hexamethonium or Arfonad may be used here with approximately the same degree of success. Our usual choice has been hexamethonium, and a single injection, rarely two, has sufficed. The dosage is calculated on the basis of 25 mg. for a 150-pound patient and is given intravenously about 10 minutes before the aorta is to be clamped. It is our intention to have the systolic blood pressure not over 150 mm. Hg prior to clamping. The hypotensive effect thus achieved lasts 10 to 15 minutes, after which time it may be decided whether more of the agent is needed.

If Arfonad is used in this situation, standard 0.1%, a solution is made by adding 250 mg. to 250 ml. of 5% dextrose and is administered at about 60 drops per minute until two thirds of the desired reduction has occurred. The infusion should then be slowed down to allow for "overshooting" and should be regulated as needed. In order to prevent marked hypotension upon release of the aortic clamps, one must not allow the induced hypotension to be excessive. It is desirable to have a systolic blood pressure not less than 120 mm. Hg prior to release of aortic clamps if shock is to be avoided.

Distended patent ductus arteriosus. To facilitate operations on children who have markedly dilated patent ductus arteriosus, one may use either hexamethonium or Arfonad by intravenous route. Since these patients may show resistance to ganglionic blocking agents and necessitate the use of large amounts of either agent, the greater controllability of Arfonad makes it perferable to hexamethonium. High concentrations of halothane would not be recommended here.

PHEOCHROMOCYTOMA

The methods just described are not effective in managing the hypertensive bouts seen in patients with pheochromocytoma. In these cases specific alpha and beta adrenergic blocking drugs such as phentolamine (Regitine) and propanalol should be employed.[26,27]

REFERENCES

1. Anderson S., and McKissock, W.: Controlled hypotension with Arfonad in neurosurgery with special reference to vascular lesions, Lancet **2:**754-781. 1953.

2. Glenn, W. W. L., Hampton, L. J., and Goodyer, A. V. N.: The use of controlled hypotension in large blood vessel surgery, Arch. Surg. **68:**1-6, 1954.

3. Gardner, W. J.: The control of bleeding during operations by induced hypotension, J.A.M.A. **132:**572-574, 1946.

4. Hale, D. E.: Controlled hypotension, Anesthesiology **16:**1-10, 1955.

5. Griffiths, H. W. C., and Gillies, J.: Thoraco-lumbar splanchnicectomy and sympathectomy; anaesthetic procedure, Anaesthesia **3:**134-146, 1948.

6. Gillies, J.: Anaesthesia for the surgical treatment of hypertension, Proc. Roy. Soc. Med. **42:**295-298, 1949.

7. Greene, N. M.: Hypotensive spinal anesthesia, Surg. Gynec. Obstet. **95:**331-335, 1952.

8. Greene, N. M.: Hypotensive spinal anesthesia, Baltimore, 1958, The Williams & Wilkins Co.

9. Hampton, L. J., and Little, D. M., Jr.: Complications associated with the use of "controlled hypotension" in anesthesia, Arch. Surg. **67:**549-556, 1953.

10. Laborit, H., and Ruguenard, P.: L'hibernation artificielle par moyens pharmacodynamiques et physiques en chirurgie, J. Chir. **67:**631-664, 1951.

11. Dundee, J. W., Mesham, P. R., and Scott, W. E. B.: Chlorpromazine and the production of hypothermia, Anaesthesia **9:**296-302, 1954.

12. Enderby, G. E. H.: Controlled circulation with hypotensive drugs and posture to reduce bleeding in surgery: preliminary results with pentamethonium iodide, Lancet **1:**1145-1147, 1950.

13. Boyan, C. P., and Brunschwig, A.: Hypotensive anesthesia in radical pelvic and abdominal surgery, Surgery **31:**829-838, 1952.

14. Magill, I. W., Scurr, C. F., and Wyman, J. B.: Controlled hypotension by a thiophanium derivative, Lancet **1:**219-220, 1953.

15. Nicholson, M. J., Sarnoff, S. J., and Crehan, J. P.: Intravenous use of a thiophanium derivative (Arfonad RO 2-2222) for production of flexible and rapidly reversible hypotension during surgery, Anesthesiology **14:**215-225, 1953.

16. Sadove, M. S., Wyant, G. M., and Gleave G.: Controlled hypotension. A study on Arfonad (RO 2-222), Anaesthesia **8:**175-181, 1953.

17. McCubbin, J. W., and Page, I. H.: Nature of the hypotensive action of a thiophanium derivative (RO 2-2222) in dogs, J. Pharmacol. Exp. Ther. **105:**437-442, 1952.

18. Enderby, G. E.: A report on mortality and morbidity following 9,107 hypotensive anesthetics, Brit. J. Anaesth. **33:**109-113, 1961.

19. Eckenhoff, J. E., and Rich, J. C.: Clinical experiences with deliberate hypotension, Surgery **59:**286-291, 1966.

20. Anderson, S. M.: Controlled hypotension with Arfonad in paediatric surgery, Brit. Med. J. **2:**103-104, 1955.

21. Nicholson, M. J.: Personal communication.

22. Kilduff, C. J.: The use of Arfonad in controlled hypotension, Lancet **1:**337, 1954.

23. Viguera, M. C., and Terry, R. N.: Induced hypotension for extensive surgery in an infant, Anesthesiology **27:**701-702, 1966.

24. Robertazzi, R. W., Riskin, A. M., and Semeraro, D.: The control and management of hypertensive crises developing during surgical procedures, Anesthesiology **15:**262-271, 1954.

25. Ciliberti, B. J., Goldfein, J., and Rovenstine, E. A.: Hypertension during anesthesia in patients with spinal cord injuries, Anesthesiology **15:**273-279, 1954.

26. Goldfein, A.: Pheochromocytoma: diagnosis and anesthetic and surgical management, Anesthesiology **24:**462-471, 1963.

27. Gebbie, D. M., and Finlayson, D. C.: Use of alpha and beta adrenergic blocking drugs and halothane in the anesthetic management of phaeochromocytoma, Canad, Anaesth. Soc. J. **14:**39-44, 1967.

Induced hypothermia

The use of hypothermia in surgical and nonsurgical patients has passed through many phases. Having played a vital part in the development of cardiac surgery, it now appears to play a role of decreasing importance.

BACKGROUND

The reduction of body temperature is not a new device in medicine. The uses of temperature reduction, though varied, have been based on two bodily responses to cold: anesthesia and lowered metabolic activity.

Ice was used for local anesthesia before the days of ether, and the rapidly vaporizing ethyl chloride spray has been employed for the same purpose. In 1937 Allen[1] again used this principle in his "refrigeration anesthesia," which consisted of covering the arm or leg of a patient with ice and thus inducing anesthesia of the entire limb prior to amputation.

Most of the recent applications of temperature reduction have been based upon lowering metabolic activity and, with it, oxygen demand. In 1940 Fay[2] attempted to arrest tumor growth by cooling several elderly patients to 88° or 90° F. in the hope that the oxygen demands of rapidly growing tumor cells would not be fulfilled and that these tissues would be killed selectively.

It has occurred to many that lowering the temperature of newborn babies might help them to meet their oxygen requirements. Silverman[3] produced evidence that this approach was not only ineffective but actually increased the mortality, and subsequent work has demonstrated that the nonshivering infant, when exposed to cold, has a marked catechol response that causes a large increase in oxygen requirement.[4,5]

The present use of hypothermia as an adjunct to anesthesia is based on its reduction of metabolism rather than upon its anesthetic effect; hence the term "hypothermic anesthesia" should not be used in this connection.

By far the greatest application of hypothermia in relation to pediatric anesthesia has been in the field of cardiac surgery. McQuiston[6,7] deserves credit for the introduction of hypothermic techniques into modern anesthesia. After watching children's temperatures soar to 103° or 104° F. in hot, sunny operating rooms, he devised the water-cooled rubber mattress with which he not only prevented temperature elevation but also reduced the children's temperatures a few degrees (Fig. 16-1). The level of body heat that McQuiston usually hoped to maintain was 95° F. The first patients upon whom this technique was used were children with cyanotic heart disease who were undergoing vascular shunt procedures. The benefit to these critically hypoxic children was great and was instrumental in establishing this field of surgery.

At that time open heart surgery and extracorporeal techniques had not reached the stage of clinical application. Active investigation of hypothermia was being carried on by Bigelow and associates[8,9] in Toronto, Swan an associates[10-12] in Denver, and others[13,14] who hoped to occlude the corporeal circulation completely in order to perform intracardiac operations under direct vision.

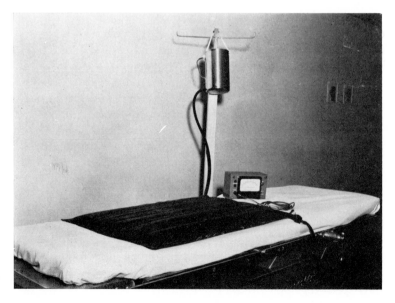

Fig. 16-1. McQuiston water mattress. Water of desired temperature flows from irrigating can into mattress. Electrical thermometer registers esophageal or rectal temperature.

The first successful intracardiac procedure performed with hypothermia was reported by Lewis and Taufic[15] in 1953. This consisted of closure of an atrial septal defect in a 5-year-old girl.

It soon became evident that by cooling patients to 25° to 30° C. it was possible to occlude the circulation for approximately 8 minutes.[16] Shortly thereafter a large number of open heart operations were carried out successfully. These consisted primarily of correction of atrial septal defect, aortic stenosis, and pulmonic stenosis. A classic monograph on the cooling and anesthetic management of these patients was written by Virtue in 1955.[17]

After a period of relative success, the future of hypothermia appeared to be threatened by two great limiting factors: (1) cooling below 25° C. entailed excessive danger of ventricular fibrillation and (2) the allowance of 8 minutes of uninterrupted working time within the heart was sufficient only for correction of simpler defects. With the advent of the pump-oxygenator, which imposed no such limit upon the surgeon, it appeared that hypothermia might be crowded out of cardiac surgery entirely.

Limitations to the value of the pump-oxygenator soon were discovered, however, when repair of complicated ventricular septal defects or aortic regurgitation was attempted. The need for a bloodless, quiet heart led to clinical application of profound hypothermia. This concept, developed by Andjus,[18] Smith,[19] and Gollan, Hamilton, and Menelly,[20,21] was based on the realization that hypothermia approaching 0° C. was compatible with life *provided that adequate perfusion was maintained*. It should be pointed out that in the attainment of successful deep hypothermia, the important change was made from surface cooling methods to cooling by infusion of cold blood, or core cooling, by the "heat exchangers" developed by Sealey, Brown, and Young[22] and Pierce and Polley.[23] Thus, by combining use of the pump-oxygenator with cooling, the barrier of cardiac arrhythmias was overcome and a new field was opened, since by cooling a patient to 15° C., complete arrest of corporeal and extracorporeal circulation could be tolerated for as long as an hour.

This remarkable achievement proved of much value and was used extensively for a variety of procedures. It was found to introduce new problems, especially those of tissue acidosis and increased blood viscosity.

In distinction from cooling by whole body perfusion, local application of cold to the heart has had definite clinical application. By covering the heart with sterile chopped ice, cardiac arrest has been induced for repair of aortic valvular lesions and has been proved to be less traumatic than arrest induced by potassium or anoxic occlusion of coronary circulation. Recently, however, immobilization of the heart has been more easily achieved by induction of ventricular fibrillation by an alternating electrical current.

The early application of hypothermia in neurosurgery was similar but slightly less dramatic.[24,25] After cooling patients to 25° or 30° C., surgeons were able to occlude cerebral vessels for a similar period of 8 minutes[26] in order to excise aneurysms or perform other procedures that under normal circumstances would be prevented by hemorrhage. The use of this technique is now being extended by combining hypotensive methods with hypothermia.[27]

The use of profound hypothermia in neurosurgery at first necessitated establishment of extracorporeal circulation with the full insult of thoracotomy. With development of the external cardiac defibrillator, however, it has been possible to employ deep hypothermia without thoracotomy, the femoral vessels serving as cannulation sites.[28,29] Actually, the use of profound hypothermia in neurosurgery has been relatively limited in adults and is rarely indicated for children.

In relation to pediatric surgery, other applications of decreasing body temperature fall into types that might be termed therapeutic and prophylactic hypothermia.

Therapeutic hypothermia consists of lowering the body temperatures of toxic, critically ill patients before, during, or after operation so that oxygen demands may be more easily fulfilled. Such application has been recommended by Albert and associates[30] for poor-risk patients undergoing major surgery. Albert believes that by reducing body temperature to 32° or 30° C. (89° to 86° F.) cerebral metabolism is lowered appreciably, and he also finds that the postoperative stress response is reduced. Others have used this technique in adults,[31-33] and Lewis, Leigh, and Belton[33] applied the method in a number of pediatric cases with reported success.

The term prophylactic hypothermia applies to the use suggested by Lewis, Leigh, and Belton,[33] Terry,[34] and Kilduff, Wyant, and Hale,[35] who advocate mild cooling of normal patients undergoing routine procedures such as harelip repair or tonsillectomy. This technique has been applied chiefly in pediatric cases and is designed to prevent hyperthermia rather than to invoke any of the physiologic changes seen in marked temperature reduction. Water mattresses are sufficient for this purpose, and temperatures are held at approximately 96° F.

Cooling mattresses or sponging with alcohol to control the temperature of children with high fevers prior to operation is widely used. Since this maneuver is designed to return an elevated temperature toward normal, it is not correctly termed hypothermia. It must be emphasized that surface cooling methods such as sponging with alcohol, application of ice, or use of cold water mattresses can be harmful if applied to a normally responsive patient. Such a patient's reaction will be to vasoconstrict, shiver, and become hyperactive, using 3 or 4 times as much oxygen as would otherwise be necessary. If surface cooling methods are to be employed, such responses must be controlled by anesthesia, relaxants, chlorpromazine, or other methods.[36]

In nonsurgical fields the value of reducing oxygen demands of the central nervous system has been applied to several types of lesions including cerebral anoxia following cardiac arrest, traumatic brain damage, poisoning, and encephalitis.

PHYSIOLOGIC EFFECTS OF HYPOTHERMIA

The literature describing the bodily reactions to hypothermia is now extensive, and numerous reviews and monographs are currently available.[37-39] Briefly, the most important effects of cooling include the following:

1. The unanesthetized patient at first exhibits vasoconstriction, shivering, and increase in pulse rate, blood pressure, and oxygen consumption.

With continued cooling this is succeeded by depression of the organ systems.

2. Under control of general anesthesia or relaxants the early phase of increased activity is not evident, due primarily to the suppression of shivering.
3. As cooling takes place, metabolism is reduced at a slightly diminishing rate. It is calculated that with each temperature reduction of 10° C. the existing metabolic rate is reduced by one half.
4. Carbon dioxide production undergoes a parallel decrease with hypothermia. At 25° C. arterial pCO_2 is about one half the normal value, provided that respiratory tidal volume and rate are constant.
5. Respiration is depressed as cooling progresses.
6. Respiratory acidosis occurs unless ventilation is assisted.
7. The hematocrit falls, denoting a decreased blood volume.
8. Bleeding and clotting time are prolonged.
9. The metabolism and detoxification of drugs are retarded.
10. Adrenal steroid output is reduced.
11. Pain perception is lost at about 31° C. (88° F.), and narcosis supervenes at approximately 28° C. (82° F.).
12. Of most clinical significance are the changes in cardiac automaticity. The heart becomes more irritable with cooling and the action less effective. Auriculoventricular conduction is slowed, and block may occur. Auricular and ventricular fibrillation may occur at temperatures under 28° to 30° C. (83° to 86° F.).

In contrast to earlier views, it is now evident that most essential enzyme systems continue to function until cellular activity is halted by crystallization or denaturization at approximately 0° C.

INDICATIONS FOR HYPOTHERMIA IN CHILDREN

Operations involving occlusion of vessels. As previously outlined, there is ample justification for application of hypothermic techniques during neurosurgical and cardiovascular procedures in which circulation must be curtailed or occluded.

Operations for congenital heart lesions not requiring intracardiac approach. It also appears reasonable to induce mild hypothermia during operation on extremely poor-risk, cyanotic patients such as those with transposition of the great vessels. When vascular occlusion is not required, reducing of temperature to 34° to 35° C. (93° to 95° F.) would seem adequate. It is essential that normal temperature be restored prior to recovery from anesthesia so that patients will not be depressed.

The use of hypothermia for relatively simple procedures such as division of patent ductus would appear to involve unnecessary confusion and delay unless some additional indication exists.

Hyperthermia. The application of cold certainly is justified in children who are toxic and ill, provided that other rational measures are taken to give fluids and antibiotics and to allow time for them to take effect. Reduction of temperature to normal is adequate here without involving subnormal or hypothermic temperatures.

Operations involving extensive blood loss. In resection of the liver for trauma or disease, mortality due to hemorrhage is high and thus far measures to control it have been unsuccessful. By cooling children to 90° F. and administration of chlorpromazine, Welch[40] reports improved survival in hepatic resection. Although our aim has been to prevent heat loss because of danger of cardiac depression, there is justification for the cooling approach in this situation.

Cooling in normal patients undergoing routine procedures. Icing and the use of water mattresses have been advocated for routine procedures simply to prevent temperature elevation. When operating rooms are maintained at a temperature over 70° F., water mattresses are recommended, but these will not be necessary if a cooler environment can be provided by air conditioning.

Cryosurgery. The most recent application of hypothermia has been that of cryosurgery. Using extremely fine control, a liquid nitrogen probe at −180° C. is applied to a local area. The first use was in neurosurgery, but cryotonsillectomy is now reported.* Children must be given general anesthesia to tolerate the procedure.

Nonsurgical application. In nonsurgical situations the induction of moderate hypothermia (90° to 92° F.) may be employed following trauma or anoxia, but there is little definite proof that it is of value. If employed, Rosomoff[41] has found evidence that it must be instituted within 3 hours of the initial trauma to be effective.

If an informed group of physicians were to be faced with the problem of treating a child following cardiac arrest, probably not more than half would choose cooling. My own choice would be to abstain. In the presence of high, uncontrolled fever or continued convulsions, moderate reduction of temperature is indicated. In all applications of cooling it is imperative that shivering is eliminated. McCredie[42] reported considerable success in controlling severe hyperthermic convulsions in children by combining chlorpromazine with cooling to approximately 30° C.

TECHNIQUE

Methods of reducing body temperature consist chiefly of variations of external or surface cooling and direct cooling by perfusion. Surface cooling may be accomplished by sponging with cold fluids, by exposure to cooled air, by the use of the McQuiston type of water mattress or a fluid-circulating mattress,† by covering with chipped ice, or by immersion in an ice water bath. Direct cooling at present usually consists of perfusing cold blood or blood substitute through cannulated vessels, although it may also be produced by pouring ice or saline solution into thoracic or abdominal cavities, by packing chipped ice around the heart, or by irrigating the stomach with chilled solutions.

---

*Medical Tribune, May 17, 1967.

†Therm-O-Rite, Therm-O-Rite Products, Buffalo, N.Y.; Aquamatic-K-Thermia, Gorman-Rupp Industries, Inc., Bellville, Ohio.

Mild hypothermia. Temperature reduction not exceeding 3° to 4° C. may be desired during closed heart operations on cyanotic infants or for nonsurgical patients with neurologic disorders. In such cases the use of the water mattress involves less equipment and bother than the ice bath. The child is prepared for operation in the usual manner and is given adequate sedation. Atropine may be withheld if the temperature is elevated. The water mattress is spread on the operating table and covered with a thin blanket. The child is placed on the blanket, and a thermometer lead is inserted in the esophagus or rectum. If sedation has not been adequate, thiopental may be used to quiet the child. Iced water is run into the mattress, and the child is uncovered and fanned or sponged with alcohol. Shivering will prevent heat loss and should be stopped. This is done most effectively by thiopental induction followed by halothane for maintenance of anesthesia. Once the temperature of the child starts to fall, it may drop well beyond the desired end point unless the cooling process is halted before the goal is reached. Usually the water may be removed from the mattress as soon as two thirds of the desired temperature reduction has occurred. In spite of this measure, it still may be necessary to add warm water (100° F.) to prevent overcooling.

If the temperature is not reduced below 34° C. (93° F.), anesthesia and surgery should progress without the introduction of additional problems. Cardiac arrhythmias are not induced by such mild hypothermia, and the need of monitoring with the electrocardiograph or the electroencephalograph is no greater than during procedures at normal body temperature. Rewarming is accomplished by circulating warm water (105° F.) through the mattress and the addi-

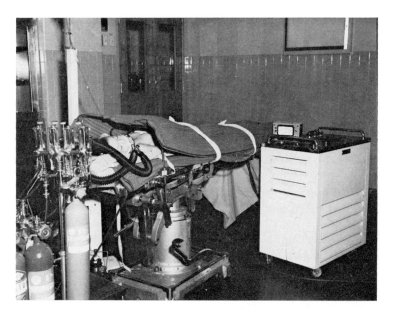

Fig. 16-2. Water-circulating mattress with motor pump and temperature controlling unit.

tion of warm blankets. Shivering on awakening is to be avoided because it increases oxygen needs.

When similar mild degrees of cooling are required in patients who are not under anesthesia, other means may be required to prevent shivering. Chlorpromazine may be administered intravenously in small doses calculated on the basis of 1 mg. per 5 pounds and repeated if necessary at one-hour intervals until shivering is controlled, provided that there is no fall in blood pressure.

Moderate hypothermia for surgical use. The established method of moderate hypothermia for neurosurgical and intracardiac procedures without supplemental pump-oxygenator is achieved either by ice water immersion or water mattress to reach the "safe limit" of 36° C. (86° F.).[43,44] The water mattress has been chosen by many because it is easier to manage and more portable (Fig. 16-2). It is obviously preferable when moderate cooling is used for longer periods in nonsurgical situations.

Prior to operation the child is given mild sedation with atropine, a barbiturate, and a narcotic as indicated by age and bodily condition. The water mattress is placed on the table and is covered by a thin cotton sheet. The child's hands, feet, knees, and elbows are wrapped in sheet wadding for protection. Anesthesia is induced with thiopental or N_2O-halothane. Endotracheal intubation is performed while infusions are being established. Arterial cannulation may be desired for blood pressure reading. The thermometer probe is inserted in rectum or esophagus and electrocardiograph leads are applied. Electroencephalograph leads are also fixed if indicated.

The cotton blanket is then wrapped around the child, after which the water mattress is folded over him. Since this is heavy, it should be supported so that it does not restrict respiration.

Cooling is carried on until the child's temperature falls to 32° C. (90° F.). At this point cooling is discontinued, for the childs' temperature will continue to fall or "drift" several more degrees. The mattress can be used at intervals to maintain the temperature between 30° and 32° C., but this usually will not be required.

The choice of anesthetic in hypothermia is disputed; however, after cooling is established little is necessary. Nitrous oxide supplemented by intermittent administration of succinylcholine has the advantage of being nonexplosive and free from cardiac depression in suitably atropinized patients. Nondepolarizing relaxants would seem to be undesirable since their depressant action should be increased upon rewarming; however, Vandewater and associates[25] have used curare in a large series. Boba[36] favors the use of light ether during hypothermia, in the belief that explosive dangers are easily overcome and of less significance than those with cyclopropane; he believes that the myocardial depression of halothane contraindicates its use. The use of morphine and thiopental in cooled patients has been condemned because these drugs are known to be metabolized slowly in cooled patients. Since this effect is reversed on rewarming, it only means that these drugs will be more effective during the hypothermic period and should be used sparingly rather than cast aside. It appears that many agents are applicable, provided that ventilation is supported, shivering is controlled, and the inherent dangers are recognized. During the process of cooling a moderate decrease in pulse rate and blood pressure should be expected. Blood loss must be replaced as usual, but one should not attempt to maintain the initial heart rate. It has been demonstrated that in cardiac slowing under hypothermia the entire cycle is retarded and that if atropine is employed, the rate is accelerated purely by reducing the resting phase of the heart.[45] One should also remember that blood pressure determined by the standard Riva Rocci method will be markedly reduced by vasoconstriction.

During recovery from moderate hypothermia, excessive shivering again is of potential danger in that it will raise oxygen demands excessively. Rebound hyperthermia is seen frequently, the temperature rising to 102° or 103° F. Here again there is real danger due to increased oxygen demand. This complication can be prevented if rewarming is slowed as the temperature approaches 95° or 96° F. Methods of reversing the warming should be available and should be applied promptly if the temperature exceeds 100° F.

Moderate hypothermia in nonsurgical therapy. The technical aspects of moderate cooling for the treatment of patients not undergoing operation differ somewhat from those just described, in that therapy usually is prolonged to 2 or 3 days or more and patients are not under general anesthesia.

Whether the patient is suffering from the effects of operative cardiac asystole, head injury, or convulsions, it is preferable to organize the treatment in a Special Care Unit or similar area where personnel and equipment are prepared for such situations. The Therm-O-Rite mattress or a similar device is definitely preferable to other methods for continued cooling techniques. Monitoring devices are of more importance, again because of the greater duration of treatment, and should include intra-arterial pressure, electrocardiograph, electroencephalograph, esophageal or rectal temperature, and inlying urinary catheter. Infusion by venous cutdown or catheter, preferably extending into the vena cava, is advisable for certain maintenance of an avenue of administration as well as for use in drawing blood samples and for determination of venous pressure.

In a majority of situations tracheostomy will be indicated, although this is not an invariable rule. Methods of testing mechanical ventilation, such as the Wright spirometer, should be available, as well as apparatus for continued ventilatory support and laboratory facilities for serial determination of blood gases.

Cooling is accomplished with a water mattress as previously described. Shivering will be excessive in most unanesthetized patients, and considerable effort will be required to control it. Although chlorpromazine may be sufficient, it is often more expedient to induce light anesthesia with nitrous oxide or halothane during the early cooling period and depend upon chlorpromazine during maintenance of hypothermia.

For treatment of cerebral edema and hypoxic brain damage, hypothermia is usually continued for 48 to 72 hours or more. During this time provisions are made for fluid and nutritional needs, and ventilation is supported. Vital functions are closely followed and charted. Urinary output is of critical importance and should be measured hourly. In case of failing renal function, mannitol may be indicated.

Several serious complications may occur during prolonged hypothermia. Ventilatory insufficiency and body cooling both lead to acidosis. Measurement of pH, pCO_2, and pO_2 will indicate the source of the imbalance and the therapy required. Sodium bicarbonate or tris (hydroxymethyl)aminomethane (TRIS buffer) may prove invaluable in correction of metabolic acidosis.

Pneumonia is a major problem, especially after 2 or 3 days of cooling. Frequent turning, hyperventilation, and induced coughing are necessary, and the airway must be cleared of all secretions.

Gastric ulcers with severe hemorrhage have caused additional difficulty, perhaps because of stress phenomena. Removal of acid gastric secretions and administration of alkaline solutions (Maalox) are advisable. The termination of this form of therapy will be decided by the clinical course of the patient. Trial warming may be started gradually. If signs of cerebral injury return on warming, cooling is reinstituted; otherwise the temperature is allowed to return to approximately 97° F. and is held there until well stabilized.

Profound hypothermia. The cooling of patients to temperatures below 20° C. is performed only in the anesthetized state, usually for intracardiac or neurosurgical procedures. Cooling is accomplished by direct vascular perfusion by cannulation of major vessels and cooling the blood as it is led through the so-called heat exchanger.[22,46] This may be accomplished gradually, by starting with the blood at normal body temperature, or it may be rapid, by perfusing the body with blood precooled in an extracorporeal oxygenator or special reservoir. With deep cooling the heart arrests at approximately 16° C., and circulation is provided by pump-oxygenator. In rewarming, the heart usually starts automatically as it reaches 16° C. but often fibrillates so that it is necessary to use a defibrillating apparatus.

Probably the greatest additional problem in deeper cooling is rewarming acidosis, which can be sufficiently severe to be fatal. Here monitoring of blood gases and judicial therapy are of extreme importance. Alkaline buffering agents are often indicated. Sodium bicarbonate has been employed using 2 mEq. per pound, and tris (hydroxymethyl)aminomethane or TRIS buffer may be administered, 150 mg. per pound of body weight being the usual initial dose.

APPRAISAL

The value of hypothermia for pediatric use is gradually coming into clearer focus. It has passed through several phases of extreme value, to be replaced by other methods that involved greater safety or efficiency. At present cooling is used only occasionally by some cardiovascular surgeons doing open heart work. Our own principal need for it lies in open repair of tetralogy of Fallot in patients who have previously had a Potts repair. To divide the anastomosis between aorta and pulmonary artery is a hazardous feat. This is greatly facilitated by complete circulatory arrest, which can be accomplished with reduction of body temperature to 75° C. Open correction of aortic valve lesions is also an indication for cooling under most circumstances.

Hypothermic therapy in nonsurgical situations is used following cardiac arrest, head trauma, and similar conditions with a general feeling that it might be beneficial; therefore it should be tried. Those who do not use it under similar conditions can not be criticized.

The future of hypothermic techniques appears less dramatic than formerly believed. With cooling, as with increased oxygen, many early results have been disappointing, and one gradually gains the conviction that animate beings thrive best upon environmental conditions to which they have become accustomed over the millenia.

REFERENCES

1. Allen, F. M.: Local asphyxia and temperature change in relation to gangrene and other surgical problems, Trans. Ass. Amer. Physicians, 52:189-194, 1937.
2. Fay, T.: Observations in prolonged human refrigeration, New York J. Med. 40:1351-1354, 1940.
3. Silverman, W. A.: Respiratory difficulties of newborn infants (Panel discussion: Levine, S. Z., Cook, C. D., Greenwald, P., and Silverman, W. A.), New York J. Med. 58:372-388, 1958.
4. Moore, R. E., and Underwood, M. C.: Possible role of noradrenaline in control of heat production in the newborn animal, Lancet 1:1277-1281, 1960.
5. Stern, L., Lees, M. H., and Leduc, J.: Temperature, oxygen, and catecholamine excretion in newborn infants, Pediatrics 36:367-374, 1965.
6. McQuiston, W. O.: Anesthesia in cardiac surgery, Arch. Surg. 61:892-899, 1950.
7. Bigler, J. A., and McQuiston, W. O.: Body temperatures during anestheisa in infants and children, J.A.M.A. 146:551-556, 1951.
8. Bigelow, W. G., and McBirnie, J. F.: General hypothernia for experimental intracardiac surgery, Ann. Surg. 132:531-539, 1950.
9. Bigelow, W. G., Lindsay, W. K., Harrison, R. C., Gordon, R. A., and Greenwood, W. F.: Oxygen transport and utilization in dogs at low body temperatures, Amer. J. Physiol. 160:125-137, 1950.
10. Swan, H., Zeavin, I., Holmes, J. H., and Montgomery, V.: Cessation of circulation in general hyopthermia. I. Physiological changes and their control, Ann. Surg. 138:360-376, 1953.
11. Zeavin, I., Virtue, R. W., and Swan, H.: Cessation of circulation in general hypothermia. II. Anesthetic management, Anesthesiology 15:113-121, 1954.
12. Swan, H., and Zeavin, I.: Cessation of circulation in general hypothermia. III. Techniques of intracardiac surgery under direct vision, Ann. Surg. 139:385-396, 1954.
13. Cookson, B. A., Neptune, W. B., and Bailey, C. P.: Hypothermia as a means of performing intracardiac surgery under direct vision, Dis. Chest 23:245-260, 1952.
14. Beattie, E. J., Jr., Adovasio, D., Keshishian, J. M., and Blades, B.: Refrigeration in experimental surgery of the aorta, Surg. Gynec. Obstet. 96:711-713, 1953.
15. Lewis, F. J., and Taufic, M.: Closure of atrial septal defects with the aid of hypothermia; experimental accomplishments and report of one successful case, Surgery 33:52-59, 1953.
16. Swan, H., and Blount, S. G., Jr.: Visual intracardiac surgery in a series of one hundred eleven cases, J.A.M.A. 162:941-945, 1956.
17. Virtue, R. W.: Hypothermic anesthesia, Springfield, Ill., 1955, Charles C Thomas, Publisher.
18. Andjus, R. K.: Suspended animation in cooled, supercooled, and frozen rats, J. Physiol. 128:447-556, 1955.
19. Smith, A. U.: Viability of supercooled and frozen mammals, Ann. N. Y. Acad. Sci. 80:291-300, 1959.
20. Gollan, F., Hamilton, W. K., and Menelly, G. R.: Consecutive survival of open-chest hypothermic dogs after prolonged by-pass of heart and lungs by means of pump-oxygenator, Surgery 35:88-97, 1954.
21. Gollan, F.: Physiology of cardiac surgery, Springfield, Ill., 1959, Charles C Thomas, Publisher.
22. Sealy, W. C., Brown, I. W., Jr., and Young, W. G., Jr.: Report on the use of both extracorporeal circulation and hypothermia for open heart surgery, Ann. Surg. 147:603-613, 1958.
23. Pierce, E. C., II, and Polley, V. B.: Differential hypothermia for intracardiac surgery: pre-

liminary report of pump-oxygenator incorporating heat exchanger, Arch. Surg. **67**:521-525, 1953.

24. Botterell, E. H., Lougheed, W. M., Scott, J. W., and Vandewater, S. L.: Hypothermia and interruption of carotid, or carotid and vertebral circulation in the surgical management of intracranial aneurysms, J. Neurosurg. **13**:1-42, 1956.

25. Vandewater, S. L., Lougheed, W. M., Scott, J. W., and Botterell, E. H.: Some observations in the use of hypothermia in neurosurgery, Anesth. Analg. **37**:29-36, 1958.

26. Hebert, C. L., Severinghaus, J. W., and Radigan, L. R.: Management of patients during hypothermia, Anesth. Analg. **36**:24-32, 1957.

27. Dundee, J. W., Mesham, P. R., and Scott, W. E. B.: Chlorpromazine and the production of hypothermia, Anaesthesia **9**:296-302, 1954.

28. Bucknam, C. A., and Galindo, A.: Tolerance of circulatory arrest in deep hypothermia by extracorporeal cooling, J. Neurosurg. **18**:339-347, 1961.

29. Terry, H. R., Daw, E. F., and Michenfelder, J. D.: Hypothermia by extracorporeal circulation for neurosurgery: an anesthetic technic, Anesth. Analg. **41**:241-248, 1962.

30. Albert, S. N., Spencer, W. A., Boling, J. S., and Thistlewaite, J. R.: Hypothermia in the management of the poor-risk patient undergoing major surgery, J.A.M.A. **163**:1435-1438, 1957.

31. Von Luttichau, E. G.: Controlled hypothermia (Laborit) as an aid in the treatment of severe shock, Proc. World Cong. Anesthesiologists, 1955, pp. 117-119; abstract, Survey Anesth. **1**:137-138, 1957.

32. Thierry, N.: Cranial trauma; successful therapy of grave shock and concussion syndrome by artificial hibernation, Anesth. Analg., Paris **10**:454-458, 1953.

33. Lewis, G. B., Leigh, M. D., and Belton, M. K.: Hypothermia in 363 pediatric surgical procedures, Anesth. Analg. **37**:20-28, 1958.

34. Terry, R.: Indications for cooling in pediatric anesthesia, New York J. Med. **57**:105-107, 1957.

35. Kilduff, C. J., Wyant, G. M., and Hale, R. H.: Anaesthesia for repair of cleft lip and palate in infants, using moderate hypothermia, Canad. Anaesth. Soc. J. **3**:102-107, 1956.

36. Boba, A.: Hypothermia for the neurosurgical patient, Springfield, Ill., 1960, Charles C Thomas, Publisher.

37. Hardy, J. D.: Physiology of temperature regulation, Physiol. Rev. **41**:521-606, 1961.

38. Symposium Issue: Hypothermia and effects of cold, Brit. Med. Bull. **17**:1-78, 1961.

39. Smith, R. M., and Stetson, J. B.: Therapeutic hypothermia, New Eng. J. Med. **265**:1097-1103, 1147-1151, 1961.

40. Welch, K. W.: Traumatic lesions of the abdomen. In Benson, C. D., Mustard, W. T., Ravitch, M. M., Snyder, W. H., and Welch, K. W., editors: Pediatric surgery, Chicago, 1962, Year Book Medical Publishers, Inc.

41. Rosomoff, H. L.: Protective effects of hypothermia against pathological processes of the nervous system, Ann. N. Y. Acad. Sci. **80**:475-486, 1959.

42. McCredie, D. A.: The use of hypothermia in pediatric emergencies, J. Pediat **61**:653-659, 1962.

43. Cooper, K., and Ross, D.: Hypothermia in surgical practice, London, 1960, Cassell & Co., Ltd.

44. Crocker, D.: Clinical management of therapeutic hypothermia, Internat. Anesth. Clin. **1**:313-325, 1962.

45. D'Amato, H. E.: Cardiovascular functions in deep hypothermia. In Dripps, R. D., editor: The physiology of induced hypothermia, Washington, D. C., 1956, National Research Council.

46. Conn, A. W., and Mustard, W. T.: Hypothermia for cardiac surgery. In Benson, C. D., and others, editors: Pediatric surgery, Chicago, 1962, Year Book Medical Publishers, Inc.

Chapter 17

Anesthesia for infants under one year of age

Small infants are strikingly different in the problems they present to the anesthetist. As described in Chapter 2, their size, their altered physiologic responses, and the unusual lesions that they bear make them uniquely interesting. Their ability to withstand long procedures, on the one hand, and their high mortality rate, on the other, make the whole situation one of extreme complexity.

It is generally agreed that although other phases of anesthesia may receive more acclaim, the management of the small infant offers greater challenge, calls for more skill, and is much more satisfying when well done.

SURGICAL PROCEDURES

A surprisingly large volume and wide variety of operations are performed upon young infants.[1] These consist mainly of operations for correction of congenital anomalies, with a few additional procedures for such conditions as pyloric stenosis and subdural hematoma.

In order to illustrate the numerous anesthetic and surgical problems encountered in infants, a tabulation was made of 1,000 operations performed at the Children's Medical Center on infants under 1 year of age (Table 17-1). These patients were treated within a period of 13 months.

Obviously each type of case cannot be discussed by itself, but several deserve special consideration because of their difficulty, and others because of the frequency of their occurrence.

Table 17-1. *Distribution of 1,000 operations in infants under 1 year of age*

Thoracic surgery

Tracheoesophageal fistula	23
Diaphragmatic hernia	8
Vascular ring	13
Patent ductus arteriosus	18
Tetralogy, coarctation, and other cardiovascular lesions	6
Esophageal resection or marsupialization	3
Lobectomy	4
Miscellaneous intrathoracic procedures	5
Chest drainage	5
	85

Abdominal surgery

Omphalocele closure	13
Bowel resection, ileostomy, etc. for intestinal obstruction	37
Ileostomy, colostomy closure	10
Gastrostomy	17
Biliary tract exploration	10
Pyloromyotomy	64
Herniorrhaphy, hydrocele repair	193
Abdominoperineal anoplasty	9
Excision of liver or kidney tumor	9
Laparotomy, miscellaneous	29
	391

General and orthopedic surgery

Harelip repair	54
Plastic, to hands or feet	13
Excision of cystic hygroma	6
Esophageal dilatation	40
Cystectomy, cystotomy	9
Perineal anoplasty	23
Excision of sacrococcygeal teratoma	2
Closed hip reduction	23
Miscellaneous (major and minor)	134
	304

Neurosurgery

Craniectomy (for craniosynostosis)	32
Craniotomy (for tumor, hematoma)	30
Ventricular shunt procedures	47
Excision of meningocele, encephalocele	20
Elevation of depressed fracture	5
Ventriculogram, pneumoencephalogram	3
Burr holes and other procedures	11
	148

Otolaryngology

Repair of choanal atresia	2
Tracheostomy	10
Tonsillectomy	1
Mastoidectomy	1
Laryngoscopy	9
Tracheoscopy, tracheogram	17
Bronchoscopy, bronchogram	30
Foreign body removal from esophagus	2
	72

THE INFANT'S RESPONSE TO ANESTHESIA

Much attention has been concentrated upon the infant's reaction to anesthesia and operation, and our management has been altered by experience, better working material, and more information. Small infants require small endotracheal tubes, but the necessity for reducing the size of external apparatus has been questioned. Graff and associates[2] have shown that infants anesthetized with adult circle apparatus do not show evidence of CO_2 retention or increased work. Evidence of this nature has promoted a trend toward development of modified adult equipment for infants and children of all sizes on the theory that such an approach would be more practical. This trend is limited but seems to be growing (Table 17-2). Studies of Podlesch, Dudziak, and Zinganell[3] suggest reasonable concern due to CO_2 increase during halothane anesthesia.

Of rather more importance is information relating to the infant's response to drugs. At present there is considerable uncertainty as to which anesthetic should be used for small infants. Although light ether is occasionally used with nitrous oxide in this country, cyclopropane replaced it as the favored drug some years ago. Now halothane is competing for priority in neonates here, while relaxant techniques are popular in many British centers. Local anesthesia also has considerable value and must not be overlooked.

Small infants are especially resistant to induction by ether, and they will struggle and hold their breath until severely anoxic. Once induced, relaxation is good, but respiration is often irregular and jerking.

Table 17-2. *Agents and techniques for infants*

Agents used in infants 1 year of age*		
	Primary	*Supplementary*
Halothane	537	150
Nitrous curare	65	
Ether	62	
Cyclopropane	10	14
Nitrous oxide		638
Succinylcholine		62
Vinethene		1
Procaine	15	

Anesthetic techniques used in infants under 1 year of age*	
	Primary
T nonrebreathing	638
Infant circle	138
Insufflation	18
Open-drop	12
To-and-fro	8
Adult circle	11
Infiltration	15

*Children's Hospital Medical Center, 1966.

Infants appear to tolerate cyclopropane more easily, and induction may be rapid. However, marked laryngeal obstruction may develop as induction proceeds, and this can be lethal for infants who have cyanotic heart disease or other critical conditions. Cyclopropane has the advantage of promoting conservation of body heat and moisture, of easy control and prompt awakening, and of maintaining both cardiac output and peripheral resistance. Reynolds[4] investigated the metabolic effects of cyclopropane anesthesia in infants and found that in his patients neither respiratory nor metabolic acidosis occurred. This is at variance with the earlier report of Bunker and associates,[5] who found slight metabolic acidosis when cyclopropane was given by to-and-fro technique.

Halothane usually provides the least upsetting induction of all inhalation agents in infants and is greatly preferable for this reason. In addition we know that there has never been any question of halothane toxicity in small children.

Halothane does have disadvantages in its application to neonates. It is a peripheral vasodilating agent, causing decreased peripheral resistance. At the same time it acts directly on the myocardium, reducing cardiac output. The infant normally has relatively active peripheral vasomotor tone, and if any factor reduces this effect, the infant must make up for it by increasing cardiac output. Halothane acts to prevent this reaction, and serious cardiovascular depression may occur. This depression appears to be the chief disadvantage of the drug in infants and is the reason many anesthesiologists continue to favor cyclopropane.

Several clinical impressions of the infant's response to anesthesia have not been satisfactorily explained. Nitrous oxide seems to be much less effective as an induction agent in infants than in older patients. It is so ineffective that I seldom use it in infants under 1 year of age. Infants do not object to halothane and oxygen but appear to enjoy the taste.

The speed of induction and concentration of gases required also deserve explanation. The infant's cardiac output is relatively increased. His alveolar ventilation is said by Avery[6] to be very slightly decreased, but when ether, cyclopropane, or halothane is used, infants appear to require a higher concentration, both for induction and maintenance, than do older patients. Assuming this impression to be true, it could be explained by the higher metabolic activity of the infant. It has been postulated that the highly vascular brown adipose tissue of the neonate might cause this increased uptake.[7]

Blood levels of anesthetics required during infancy have not been extensively documented, but the figures of Reynolds[4] for cyclopropane, varying between 7.1 and 15.2 mg./100 ml., correspond fairly well with those of adults under light anesthesia. Blood levels of halothane in adults approximate those of cyclopropane and should be similar in infants.

The altered responses of infants to muscle relaxants have been discussed in the chapter on that subject, and the use of local infiltration has also been described.

In our hands local infiltration of anesthetics has been extremely useful in abdominal procedures in weak infants, and we prefer to avoid general anesthesia and endotracheal intubation on puny premature infants if possible.

Those who criticize this technique state that such infants become fatigued and need ventilatory assistance. While an infant with respiratory distress syndrome may indeed spend 50% of his total energy output in breathing, infants with normal lungs do not appear to tire, and many have tolerated extensive abdominal procedures under local anesthesia with surprising emotional and physiologic indifference. Definitive measurement of fatigue is difficult. Graff and associates' investigations[7] suggest that increased pCO_2 is probably a sign of the development of respiratory fatigue, and this factor could be employed for clarification of the problem.

THE PREMATURE INFANT

Although prematurity is not an operative lesion, it is one of the greatest threats to survival in both the surgical and nonsurgical infants. The term premature has many definitions, but as used here it means any patient who comes to operation weighing less than 5 pounds, regardless of the gestation period.[9]

The high mortality associated with prematurity is due to a variety of causes. An infant that is premature often has one or more congenital defects, cardiac lesions being very common. The premature infant's lungs are the source of many complications. Respiratory distress syndrome is encountered chiefly in the premature, and the incidence increases in smaller infants. Following operation the reduced respiratory effort of the neonate renders him easy prey to atelectasis, while weakness of protective reflexes often results in regurgitation, aspiration, and either prompt suffocation or subsequent development of pneumonitis. Other characteristic lesions of the premature infant include spontaneous intraventricu-

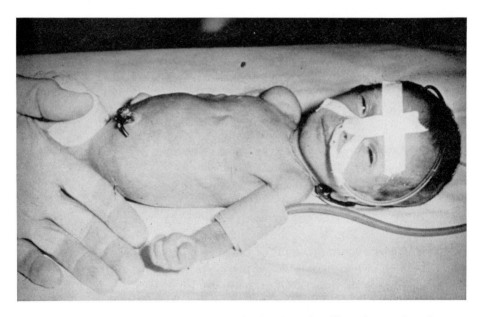

Fig. 17-1. This 2-pound premature infant with duodenal atresia will need warmth and support more than anesthesia. After wrapping the limbs and establishment of an infusion, the operation may be performed under local infiltration.

lar hemorrhage, erythroblastosis, and sclerema.[10,11] Finally, these small patients are especially susceptible to infection, and, in spite of antibiotics, pneumonia is the ultimate cause of a large proportion of the deaths.

The indications for operation on premature infants are limited and consist principally of intestinal obstruction, omphalocele, diaphragmatic hernia, tracheoesophageal fistula, and imperforate anus.

The amount of anesthesia these small patients require is not great, and the anesthetist will have to concentrate more on supporting the infants than on anesthetizing them (Fig. 17-1). Although some babies appear relatively insensitive to pain, they may require relaxation for closure of a distended abdomen or repair of omphalocele, and operations within the chest will require endotracheal anesthesia to maintain ventilation.

In our management of premature infants the choice of anesthesia usually lies between local infiltration of procaine and general anesthesia with cyclopropane. The choice depends largely on the operation, the size of the baby, and his activity. Babies weighing over 4 pounds usually are candidates for general anesthesia. Those over 3 pounds may be given general anesthesia if they appear active, but if they are weak and listless, infants with intestinal obstruction will be good subjects for local anesthesia. Anesthesia for infants under 3 pounds is usually limited to local infiltration for abdominal operations.

It will be better to describe details of anesthetic management with the individual cases.

ANESTHETIC MANAGEMENT OF THE NEWBORN INFANT

If one has dealt previously with a 2-pound premature infant, a strong full-term 7-pound baby will look like a Goliath. He will be active and strong and will resent strenuously an attempt to intubate his trachea without anesthesia. Full-term infants can be sick, however, and those with critical lesions will be nearly as weak as a premature baby.

As previously mentioned, the most lethal surgical conditions of the neonatal period consist of intestinal obstruction of various types, omphalocele, diaphragmatic hernia, and tracheoesophageal fistula with esophageal atresia.

Several preparatory measures are taken with all of these newborn infants. Atropine, 0.1 mg., is given to all unless it is quite certain that the baby will receive only local anesthesia. The anesthetist then prepares full equipment for general anesthesia, for this may be required for support or resuscitation if not for anesthesia. Usual basic equipment for a neonate should include an anesthesia machine, infant circle or T nonrebreathing system, with newborn or premature-sized rubber mask, Magill type (Portex) endotracheal tubes (internal diameter 2.5, 3.0, 3.5, and 4.0 mm.) with adapters, premature and newborn-sized laryngoscopes, polyethylene suction catheters, sized 00 and 0 oral airways, and stethoscope. This equipment is described in Chapter 6.

Upon arrival in the operating room the infant is at once rechecked by the anesthetist, who then assumes responsibility, keeping special watch that the infant's respiration is unobstructed. Unless esophageal atresia is present, the stomach is kept empty by use of a gastric tube.

One of the infant's greatest hazards during the operative period, and one that is badly handled, lies in loss of body temperature.[12,13] Hypothermia may occur rapidly and can result in cardiorespiratory depression, atelectasis, metabolic depression, and sclerema. Physiologic mechanisms involved are described in Chapter 2.

When a neonate is scheduled for operation, one should prepare by warming the operating room to 75° or preferably 80° F. This is unpleasant for personnel but essential until other methods are improved. Emphasis must be placed on prevention of heat loss, rather than allowing loss and relying upon reheating the child on a mattress.

The infant is brought into the operating room in a warmed, covered bassinet and is kept there until surgeons are in the room and ready to operate. Heat loss is most effectively controlled by reducing the exposed surface of the infant. The best method thus far is to wrap the child's limbs in sheet wadding or similar material (Figs. 17-2 and 17-3). Blood pressure cuff and wrapping are applied before removing the infant from the bassinet. (One foot is left free for the infusion.)

A water mattress or heating device is prepared on the operating table and covered with a single layer of blanket (Fig. 17-4). It should be emphasized that the patient's body area that contacts the mattress is relatively small, and buttocks, heels, elbows, back, and occiput are poor heat-conducting areas. Furthermore, when cold or hypotensive, such areas are more easily burned than tissue at normal conditions. Finally, most heating units to date are subject to grossly

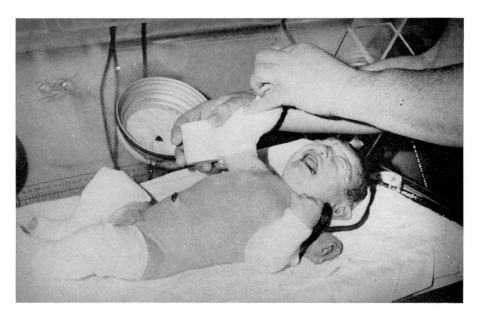

Fig. 17-2. To preserve body heat, infant's limbs should be wrapped in soft sheet wadding before his removal from warmed bassinette.

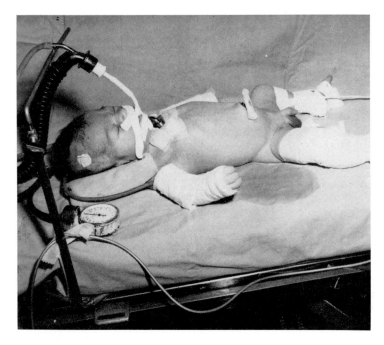

Fig. 17-3. Infant with cutdown intravenous infusion, rectal thermistor, blood pressure cuff, and precordial stethoscope, intubated, wrapped, and ready for laparotomy under halothane anesthesia.

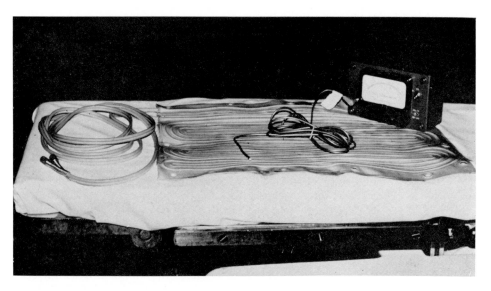

Fig. 17-4. The thermometer is essential in operations upon infants. It must be checked for accuracy before operation. The water mattress is unreliable and potentially dangerous, and it should play a supplemental role in temperature control.

inaccurate calibration and function and have caused serious accidents. *They should be used as supplementary rather than primary methods of temperature control.* No mattress or heating device should ever be warmer than 105° F.

A real effort must be made to keep the infant covered while possible, and to avoid delay. Once covered by drapes, surface heat loss will be diminished. Further losses can occur through wound exposure, nonrebreathing systems, and infusions. Measures to offset these losses include heating of wound area by operating lights, warming and humidification of anesthetic gases, and warming of infusions. Body temperature is monitored by a thermistor, which may be used in the rectum, esophagus, or nose. Thermistors may be stiff and have been known to perforate the esophagus. Nasal temperature is accurate and is to be recommended as the site for monitoring.

The definitive management of neonates will vary considerably depending upon the size and activity of the infant and upon the operation to be undertaken.[14] Our choice of agent usually lies between local infiltration, most often used in premature infants undergoing abdominal procedures, and halothane, which has largely replaced cyclopropane. Cyclopropane is used for some of the weaker infants, if explosive precautions allow it, while nitrous oxide and *d*-tubocurarine are used for poor-risk infants operated upon in the hyperbaric chamber.

Inhalation techniques employed consist chiefly of the Rees modification of the T-piece nonrebreathing method, used with the Bennett heating and humidifying device previously described (Chapter 6) or with the Bloomquist circle apparatus.

Endotracheal intubation is indicated for most operations in the neonatal period, but one must decide whether it will be advisable to intubate the infant without any agent, with a relaxant alone, or under general anesthesia. This is discussed in Chapter 9.

Induction of neonates with halothane is started without nitrous oxide; it progresses by stages to 2.5% until the infant is well relaxed and then is reduced to 1.5% or 1.0%. Cyclopropane is started using a combination of cyclopropane, nitrous oxide, and oxygen, each at a flow rate of 400 ml. per minute.[15] Nitrous oxide appears to decrease the irritant quality of cyclopropane. After the infant is relaxed, nitrous oxide is stopped; the infant is carried on oxygen at 500 ml. per minute, and cyclopropane at 100 to 150 ml. per minute. It is almost always necessary to insert an oral airway shortly after starting anesthesia with either halothane or cyclopropane in neonates. Respiration usually should be assisted or controlled. If respiration is controlled, excessive depth may occur unless concentrations of halothane and cyclopropane are limited to 0.5% and 20%, respectively. Further details are best described with management of individual problems.

An infant blood pressure cuff is fastened in place, but the child is usually so active that it is futile to try to determine the pressure until he is asleep. A stethoscope is not used for blood pressure determination in infants under 2 years of age, systolic pressure being determined by the fluctuation of the pointer on the dial of the manometer.

Blood pressure is a sensitive and important guide to depth of anesthesia and blood volume in infants, and it should be observed closely during any major pro-cedure from birth onward. Suitable equipment is available for all ages (p. 116). Helpful information concerning blood volume is also obtained by observing al-terations in the strength of the pulse; consequently, it is advisable to evaluate a palpable pulse in the radial, axillary, or carotid artery at the beginning of the procedure.

The precordial stethoscope is of greatest importance in the small infant. Here a binaural stethoscope is definitely indicated because best possible hearing of the relatively weak heart and breath sounds is mandatory. Similarly, a full-sized bowl is preferable to any miniature adaptation, since both heart and lungs must be monitored, and for this one wants a moderately large area. When strap-ping the stethoscope to the infant's chest, one should use as little tape as possible, to avoid restriction of rib motion.

Prior to the use of general anesthesia, atropine, 0.1 mg., is repeated if 30 minutes have elapsed since the last dose was given. A cutdown infusion must be established before operation is undertaken. As described in Chapter 26, this should be performed under local anesthesia in most premature infants, and whenever the surgeon is relatively slow, since the procedure may involve from 3 to 45 minutes.

Intestinal obstruction. Many of the smallest infants require surgery for in-testinal obstruction that may be due to atresia of the intestine, meconium ileus, duplication of the intestine, tumors, or other lesion. If the baby is weak and lies limp and uncomplaining, general anesthesia will probably be neither necessary nor justified (Fig. 17-1). A cutdown intravenous infusion can be started under local anesthesia, and then the baby may be prepared for surgery. Arms and legs are gently restrained by wrapping them in sheet wadding and then looping cloth tape around the wrists and ankles. For anesthesia, 0.5% procaine is infiltrated along the site of the incision and where the towel clips are to be placed. A dose of 5 mg./lb. is generally regarded as maximum throughout childhood. A weak baby will show surprisingly little reaction throughout the whole procedure. Oxy-gen should be blown over the face of all premature infants during an operation.

In slightly stronger babies this approach may be satisfactory throughout the major part of the operation, but relaxation may be needed to enable the surgeon to close the peritoneum. Adequate analgesia and relaxation often can be pro-vided by blowing nitrous oxide and oxygen (2 liters of each per minute) over the baby's face. If this is not sufficient, cyclopropane may be required during closure at flows of 500 ml. of oxygen to 150 ml. of cyclopropane.

Infants who are active, cry spontaneously, and resist being handled offer greater difficulty (Fig. 17-5). The use of restraints and local anesthesia constitutes probably the safest course if the operating team has not had previous experience with such undersized patients. If available, however, general endotracheal anes-thesia affords the surgeon much better working conditions.

In the presence of intestinal obstruction or gastric distention, the endotracheal tube is passed while the infant is still awake. Endotracheal intubation is toler-ated easily by newborn infants while awake, and complications are reduced. Im-mediately after intubation the anesthesia apparatus is attached, and the chosen

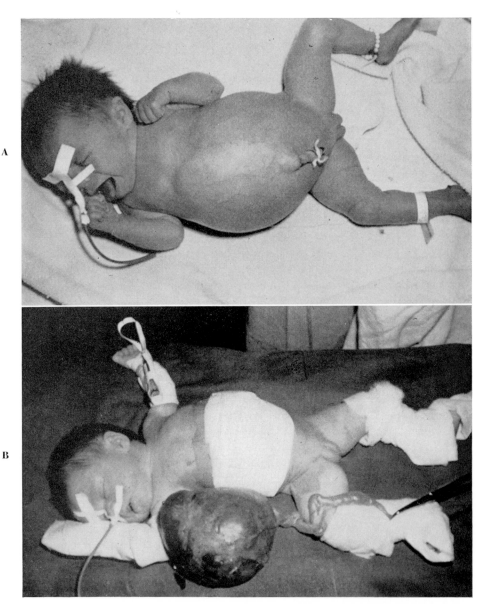

Fig. 17-5. A, Active 3-pound, 10-ounce infant with intestinal obstruction due to large cystic kidney. General anesthesia was necessary for relaxation and respiratory assistance. **B,** Same infant with tumor removed. Note that an arm was used as the site of infusion in case obstruction of the vena cava should retard venous return from the leg.

agents are administered. As previously noted, the choice among general anesthetics lies chiefly between cyclopropane, halothane, and a relaxant–nitrous oxide technique. Let us assume this infant is a 4-pound male neonate with imperforate anus. Cyclopropane would be appropriate, preferably using the revised model of the Bloomquist apparatus, although the infant to-and-fro system and other adaptations are acceptable. If the infant's trachea is already intubated, one can start with flows of 500 ml. per minute of both cyclopropane and oxygen until the child is partially relaxed and breathing quietly. Then cyclopropane is reduced to 150 to 200 ml. per minute and is regulated as necessary.

During the operation the anesthetist relies chiefly upon the stethoscope and blood pressure for monitoring the patient's condition (Fig. 17-6). The rate and volume of the heartbeat tell the adequacy of the cardiovascular system, and breath sounds show the patient's depth of anesthesia as well as the degree of ventilation. The anesthetist gently assists respiration at all times and makes sure that the breathing bag does not become distended enough to cause airway resistance. The strength of the peripheral pulse and the degree of muscle tone are also useful signs to observe.

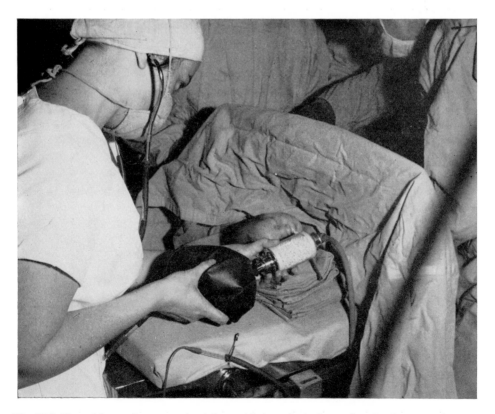

Fig. 17-6. To-and-fro cyclopropane for infant with intestinal obstruction. During operation the anesthetist assists or controls respiration, relying on the stethoscope and on visualization of the field for guidance.

Much of the anesthetist's attention must be directed toward support and protection of the small infant. Special care is taken to keep heavy drapes, instruments, and hands off the baby's chest and abdomen. Blood loss must be replaced, but other fluid therapy usually is not indicated.

A useful supplement to either local infiltration or general anesthesia is the instillation of 4 to 5 ml. of 0.5% procaine in the peritoneal cavity. This measure reduces bowel and peritoneal irritability. Succinylcholine may also be used to facilitate closure of the peritoneum. For this purpose a dosage of 0.5 mg. per pound of body weight is usually adequate and should be given by vein.

At the end of operation the baby is allowed to wake up, move his arms and legs, and open his eyes before the endotracheal tube is removed. If extubation is performed prematurely, apnea may ensue. The infant is covered, given oxygen, and kept in the operating room for 5 or 10 minutes until his condition is stable enough to justify return to his bed.

Omphalocele. It is of utmost importance for anesthetists to understand that the problems formerly encountered in infants with omphalocele now usually can be eliminated by a revised surgical technique using staged closure with plastic mesh, as described in the following paragraphs.

Omphalocele, or exomphalos, is an extension of the abdominal viscera through the unclosed abdominal wall.

Usually a thin-walled sac encloses the omphalocele, but this may become ruptured, allowing uncovered gut to fall unprotected into the bedding (Figs. 17-7 and 17-8).

Therapy is aimed at getting the viscera inside the abdomen and bringing about closure of the belly wall. This can be accomplished by repeatedly painting the intact sac with tincture of benzalkonium chloride, but surgical closure is the usual approach.

Until recently this was such a formidable problem that the outlook for infants born with a large omphalocele was grim. Because the infant's abdominal wall was developed with the viscera outside, there may not be room to allow admission of these organs insides the abdomen without considerable pressure. If the surgeon has to force the organs back into the abdomen, room will be made for them chiefly by pressing the diaphragm upward, often until it is high in the chest and virtually immobilized. The resultant reduction of respiration may be lethal. In the past when there has been danger of severe respiratory embarrassment, the surgeon has not attempted to bring the muscular layers of the abdomen together, but has closed the peritoneum and then brought the skin edges together, expecting to approximate the fascial and muscular layers weeks or months later. Although this skin closure allowed the infant to survive, the ultimate closure often was even more difficult, since the rectus muscle, under no tension, becomes shorter and less yielding. We have had several tragic experiences in which attempts to force liver and other organs under the unyielding rectus muscles have caused compression of the vena cava and death. It has become obvious that if skin closure is used, one should complete the muscular closure during the first month of life, rather than delay it.

The entire problem of closing a large omphalocele has been changed by

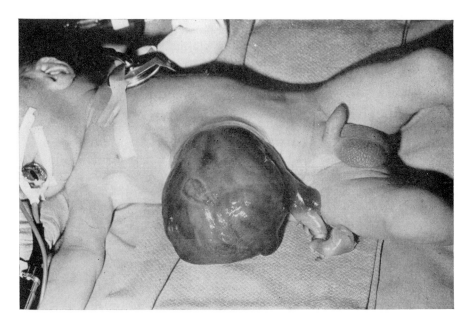

Fig. 17-7. Newborn infant with large omphalocele, sac intact. During operation the chief problem consists of replacing the viscera in the small abdominal cavity.

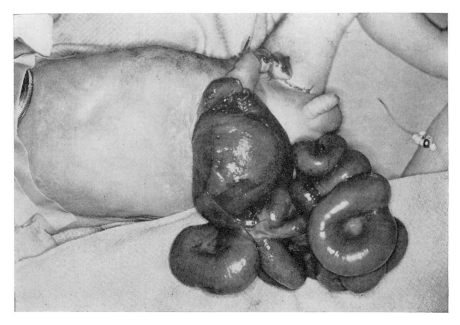

Fig. 17-8. Infant with omphalocele that ruptured in utero.

Schuster's[16] development of the staged closure. The basic principle is the use of plastic material sutured to the rectus muscle on either side of the abdomen. Enough is used to enable the surgeon to cover the viscera and close the abdomen snugly but without pressure. Skin is not approximated. If the sac of the omphalocele is ruptured, an inner lining of smooth plastic is employed to prevent adhesions (Fig. 17-9). The plastic mesh exerts a pull on the rectus muscles, which are stretched evenly and continuously. As the rectus muscle is stretched, it may be pulled gradually toward the midline. Every 3 or 4 days the plastic material may be tightened by resuturing without use of any anesthesia. Final closure of skin and muscle layers can be made within 10 to 14 days, with complete repair of the abdomen.

Under the old system, anesthetic management and support were critical and hazardous. A small omphalocele closed without pressure could be handled without difficulty, but the large ones required endotracheal intubation plus general

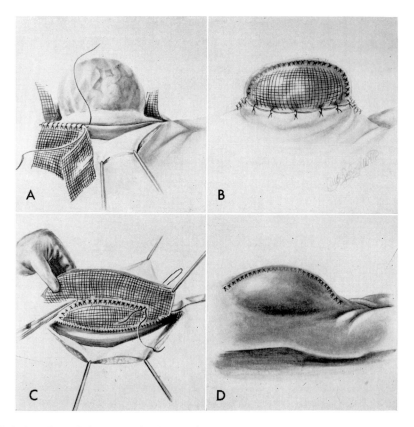

Fig. 17-9. Staged omphalocele repair. **A,** Suturing mesh to rectus muscle. **B,** Mesh closure completed. **C,** Rectus muscle has stretched, allowing reduction of size of mesh. **D,** First skin closure, to be followed by complete removal of mesh with normal abdominal contour. (From Schuster, S.: Surg. Gynec. Obstet. **125**:837, 1967.)

anesthesia. There was difference of opinion as to whether maximal relaxation should be allowed for closure, or whether the child should be allowed to breathe spontaneously at all times. In either case it was often necessary to leave the abdomen so tightly closed that the legs were cyanotic and respiration was definitely impeded, or to use the skin closure.

With Schuster's method, most of the problems have been eliminated. General endotracheal anesthesia may be used, and although spontaneous respiration is favored using halothane or cyclopropane, relaxants are not contraindicated. A minimum of pressure is required for closure, and respiration is not impeded. With subsequent procedures to reduce the size of the sac, anesthesia is needed only at the final closure, when the rectus muscle is actually approximated. Here general anesthesia is indicated, but there will be little or no pressure involved, and the procedure should be uneventful. This surgical approach has been a major achievement in pediatric surgery and has been a boon to the anesthesiologists as well as to the surgeons and the infants.

Diaphragmatic hernia. The anatomic derangement in diaphragmatic hernia arises from a lesion of the diaphragm that allows the stomach, much of the small and large bowel, the spleen, and often part of the liver to reside in the chest (Fig. 17-10). There are several areas in the diaphragm where herniation may occur,[17,18] but herniation at the foramen of Bochdalek is the usual site in neonates.

Respiration is severely impaired by the presence of the viscera in the chest, the affected lung usually being completely unexpanded and exchange often being inadequate in the other lung. The unexpanded lung is underdeveloped and markedly below average weight, and even the lung on the uninvolved side is often slightly hypoplastic.[19]

It is especially important that anesthetists be on the alert to diagnose this condition, for active attempts to ventilate such an infant may cause pneumothorax and hasten his death. Any infant with respiratory distress and increasing cyanosis deserves careful physical and roentgen-ray examination. These will disclose that breath sounds are replaced by bowel sounds on the affected side of the chest, a flat scaphoid abdomen, and x-ray evidence of loops of bowel in the chest. Occasionally these infants will be in such extreme distress shortly after birth that survival will depend upon immediate endotracheal intubation and ventilatory support, to be followed at once by thoracotomy.

Operative approach through the chest wall allows easy access to the diaphragm and may be chosen for this reason. However, many surgeons prefer to use an abdominal incision because malrotation of the bowel is often found in patients with diaphragmatic hernia, and an abdominal approach enables the surgeon to diagnose and correct this malformation at the same time that the hernia is repaired. The pleural cavity will be opened whether the surgeon chooses the thoracic or the abdominal approach; consequently, the anesthetist should have some method of assisting or controlling respiration.

As is the case in omphalocele, the development of the peritoneal cavity has taken place in the absence of part of the usual visceral content; consequently, when the surgeon pulls the viscera from the chest back into the abdomen and

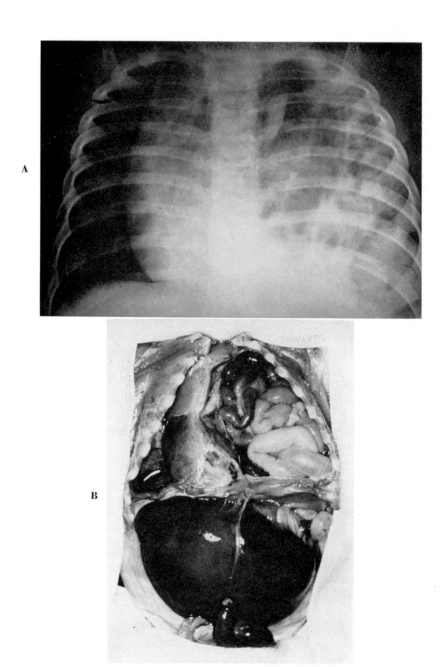

Fig. 17-10. A, Diaphragmatic hernia. Roentgen-ray film showing loops of intestine in the left side of the chest, displacement of the heart to the right, and compression of the right lung. **B,** Diaphragmatic hernia at postmortem examination showing obliteration of the left pleural cavity and severe compression of the heart and the right lung. (Courtesy Dr. A. Colodny, Boston, Mass.)

tries to close the abdominal wall, the diaphragm is pushed up, and respiration is severely limited. Closure under excessive tension may result in failure of respiratory exchange and subsequent death. For this reason operative techniques have been devised for staged repair, closing the skin and leaving the infant with a ventral hernia that is corrected later. This maneuver is less frequently necessary in diaphragmatic hernia than when dealing with omphalocele.

Anesthetic management of infants with diaphragmatic hernia requires full understanding of the situation. Under usual conditions operation is carried out promptly but without undue haste. A nasogastric tube is passed to deflate the stomach. Atropine, 0.1 mg., is administered, and blood is cross matched. After preliminary oxygenation, intubation may be performed when the patient is awake or under anesthesia. One should refrain from assisting ventilation strenuously, limiting pressure to 15 cm. H_2O. I prefer to use intramuscular succinylcholine, intubate, then add halothane or cyclopropane (Fig. 17-11). My choice would be halothane unless marked prematurity or the presence of a congenital cardiac lesion warned me against its use.

During operation motion of the diaphragm must be kept at a minimum. If this cannot be accomplished with gently assisted respiration under halothane, additional intravenous succinylcholine may be employed. The greatest concern of surgeon and anesthetist is prevention of postoperative pneumothorax. Both

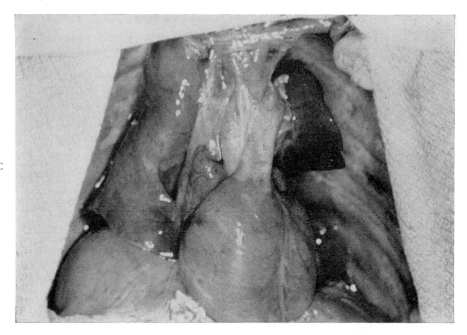

C

Fig. 17-10, cont'd. C, Photograph taken at autopsy showing an infant chest following repair of diaphragmatic hernia; the left lung is dark and unexpanded. Attempts to inflate such lungs during operation have been followed by pneumothorax. Ventilatory pressure should be limited to 15 cm. H_2O pressure.

Dx : DIAPHRAGMATIC HERNIA   Age : 2 DAYS
Operation : REPAIR , ABDOMINAL   Wt. : 2.5 Kg

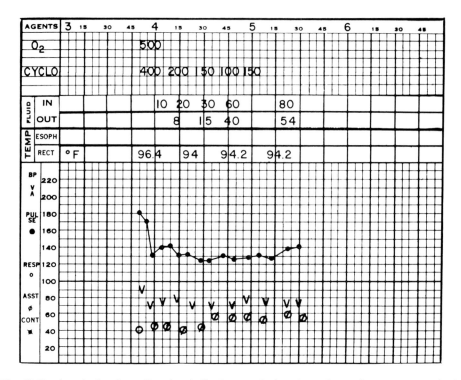

Fig. 17-11. Anesthesia chart. Repair of diaphragmatic hernia under cyclopropane anesthesia using Bloomquist circle system.

lungs are abnormally weak, and even normal ventilatory assistance has been followed by pneumothorax, most frequently on the side of the unexpanded lung, but occasionally on the opposite side as well. As a result of this complication several practices have developed:

1. Anesthetists have refrained from using strong ventilatory pressure (not over 15 cm. H_2O).
2. Anesthetists have refrained from attempting to expand the "collapsed" lung after reduction of the herniated viscera.
3. Surgeons have learned to drain the infant's chest postoperatively.
4. Surgeons have learned to examine the chest roentgenographically daily, or more often if indicated.

The last two steps are most important. Since many of the uninflated lungs are found to be expanded within 24 hours after birth, it seems doubtful if all actually are rudimentary. It seems possible that a gentle attempt to inflate these lungs might hasten their expansion and improve the child's chance of recovery.

During the course of the operation there are two potentially critical periods.

The first comes when the surgeon reduces the herniated viscera and pulls them down out of the chest. This episode may involve considerable reflex irritability, causing apnea and occasionally cardiac irregularity. It usually is short-lived and is easily tolerated if the airway is maintained.

The second critical period is the closure, and this is of considerably greater concern. The problem is for the surgeon to close the abdomen but not to create enough pressure to depress respiration. The anesthetist can either (1) retain spontaneous respiration, thereby rendering closure difficult but ensuring adequate ventilation, or (2) provide complete relaxation to facilitate closure, hoping that respiration will be adequate when the relaxant wears off. This is a matter of individual opinion. If one favors the latter, as I do, one must be very sure that he stays with the patient and supports ventilation until there is no longer any doubt of the adequacy of ventilation. If respiration remains depressed by excessive abdominal pressure, the surgeon must reopen the wound and use a staged repair.

During the last 10 years pediatric surgeons have been reasonably perplexed by a marked increase in the mortality rate in repair of diaphragmatic hernia.[20] After considerable study it became evident that the increased death rate occurred almost entirely in infants operated upon on the first day of life. Until recently few of these very sick infants had lived long enough to be operated upon. More rapid diagnosis and transportation have brought this new group to the surgeon and have thus complicated his problem. By applying lessons of the past on these weaker infants, results are already improving (Table 17-3). The most important factors in this situation probably are the use of chest drainage, daily roentgen-ray examination, and better use of postoperative ventilatory assistance when needed.

Tracheoesophageal fistula with esophageal atresia. One of the greatest challenges in pediatric anesthesia and surgery during the past 20 years has been the infant with tracheoesophageal fistula and esophageal atresia.[21-26] Although there

Table 17-3. *Congenital diaphragmatic hernia (142 cases, 1940 to 1966)**

		Less than 24 hours old	More than 24 hours old	Total
1940–1949	Total cases	6	54	60
	Survival percentage	50%	91%	87%
1950–1959	Total cases	26	27	53
	Survival percentage	46%	100%	73%
1960–1966	Total cases	20	9	29
	Survival percentage	70%	100%	80%
1940–1966	Total cases	52	90	142
	Survival percentage	56%	95%	80%

*From McNamara, J. J., Eraklis, A. J., and Gross, R. E.: Congenital posterolateral diaphragmatic hernia in the newborn, J. Thorac. Cardiov. Surg. **55**:55, 1968.

are several types of esophageal atresia (Fig. 17-12), in those most frequently seen the difficulties are basically the same: the infant cannot swallow food or secretions, and there is an open pathway from the alimentary tract into the trachea. In most cases repeated aspiration of secretions results in the development of pneumonia within 3 or 4 days after birth. Respiration is further impaired by a marked degree of gastric distention caused by passage of air through the fistula into the stomach. In addition, a large number of these infants are either premature or have a variety of complicating congenital anomalies, imperforate anus and congenital cardiac lesions being most frequent. The combination of tracheoesophageal fistula, prematurity, and multiple anomalies is often encountered.

For many years attempts at correction of tracheoesophageal fistula were futile. Successful operations were performed in 1939, however, by Leven of St. Paul and Ladd of Boston, both surgeons using the multiple-stage approach with the construction of an extrathoracic esophagus. In 1941 Haight introduced the primary esophageal anastomosis, which has subsequently been the method of choice. The operative approach to tracheoesophageal fistula and esophageal atresia will vary with the type of patients as well as the institution. Our practice is to perform a gastrostomy as soon as the infant is admitted. This procedure is simple, requires no preliminary preparation, is performed under local anesthesia, and serves an important dual purpose by relieving gastric distention and by draining secretions that might be regurgitated into the lungs.

Division of the tracheoesophageal fistula and anastomosis of the esophagus are performed as soon as the infant can be nursed into satisfactory condition. This may require several days of careful preparation, during which time the proximal esophageal stump must be kept on continuous drainage to prevent aspiration. The anesthetic management of these infants is complicated by respiratory embarrassment due to pneumonia, the open chest, surgical retraction of the lung, and manipulation of the trachea. Endotracheal intubation is clearly indicated. Since the trachea may be injured by operation, it seems wise to employ the least trau-

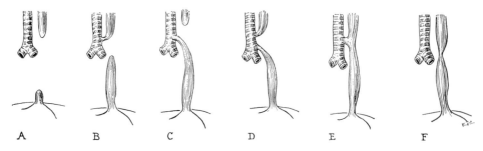

Fig. 17-12. Types of congenital abnormalities of the esophagus. **A,** Esophageal atresia. No esophageal communication with the trachea. **B,** Esophageal atresia, the upper segment communicating with the trachea. **C,** Esophageal atresia, the lower segment communicating with the back of the trachea. Over 90% of all esophageal malformations fall into this group. **D,** Esophageal atresia, both segments communicating with the trachea. **E,** Esophagus has no disruption of its continuity but has a tracheoesophageal fistula. **F,** Esophageal stenosis. (From Gross, R. E.: The surgery of infancy and childhood, Philadelphia, 1953, W. B. Saunders Co.)

matic method of intubation, which is with use of a relaxant, the choice again being succinylcholine administered intramuscularly after preliminary oxygenation. The endotracheal tube should be chosen carefully—a tight fit should be avoided. These infants seem to tolerate halothane or cyclopropane equally well, provided a light plane is employed. Recently relaxants have been used more frequently (Fig. 17-13). A T-piece system is employed when halothane or *d*-tubocurarine is used, while an infant circle is preferable with cyclopropane.

During the course of the operation secretions may block the trachea, and one must be able to use suction effectively at any time. Stethoscopic monitoring is invaluable in detecting such secretions.

Surgical manipulation of the lungs, trachea, and esophagus may also cause complete airway obstruction at frequent intervals. The anesthetist must protect the infant in such situations but occasionally must allow the surgeon intervals of trespass when they are mandatory for the procedure.

The surgical procedure for tracheoesophageal fistula is no longer the problem it once was, and most infants can now be brought safely through long, criti-

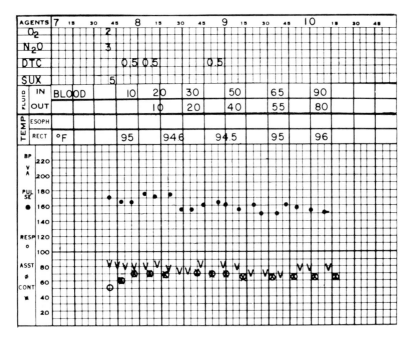

Dx : TRACHEO-ESOPHAGEAL FISTULA
Age: 2 DAYS   Wt. : 2.1 Kg
Operation : DIVISION OF FISTULA, ESOPHAGEAL ANAST.

Fig. 17-13. Anesthesia chart. Repair of tracheoesophageal fistula and esophageal atresia under nitrous oxide relaxant technique using T-nonrebreathing system.

cal operations. Deaths, when they occur, are chiefly in the postoperative period, and it is here that care must be improved.

During correction of tracheoesophageal fistula, blood must be replaced carefully. Blood lost on sponges may be weighed or may be estimated by comparing used sponges to others containing a known amount of blood. Usually 60 to 80 ml. of blood is given to an infant during a 3-hour operation of this nature.

Imperforate anus, meningocele, and other lesions. Infants with *imperforate anus* may require operation soon after birth for relief of intestinal obstruction. If they are extremely distended and ill, colostomy under local anesthesia may be indicated. Usually, however, a corrective perineal or abdominoperineal procedure is performed. These patients present less serious problems than those with tracheoesophageal fistula, but they have the combined disadvantage of being newly born, having distention, and requiring a prolonged operation. The anesthetist should see to it that improper positioning is not added to these problems (Figs. 17-14 and 17-15).

For simple perineal anoplasty, light general anesthesia without endotracheal intubation is usually satisfactory. For the longer abdominoperineal procedure, endotracheal intubation is indicated. If abdominal distention is associated with any of these conditions preoperatively, endotracheal intubation is performed while the infant is awake. Sturdy infants will tolerate general anesthetics or a relaxant technique. Monitoring of blood pressure and temperature is imperative, and supportive therapy must be attended to with great care.

Excision of *sacrococcygeal teratoma* is usually performed in the neonatal period. These tumors are often large (Fig. 17-16), and the operation will involve extensive dissection and considerable loss of blood. Positioning these infants also offers definite problems, and endotracheal intubation is necessary in order to promote adequate respiratory exchange.

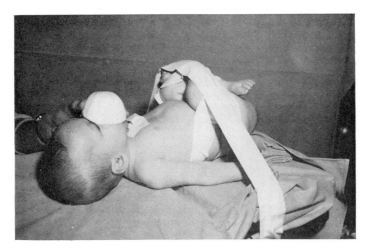

Fig. 17-14. This position offers advantages for the surgeon performing anoplasty, but it impedes the baby's respiration.

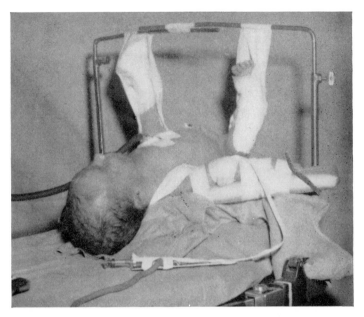

Fig. 17-15. With the legs suspended the operative position is satisfactory and respiration is unobstructed. Obviously the arm should be used for the infusion.

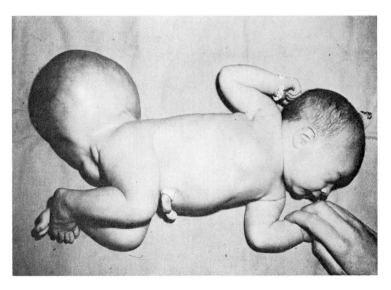

Fig. 17-16. Excision of such a sacrococcygeal teratoma involves marked blood loss as well as difficulties in positioning.

It is especially desirable to avoid circulatory or respiratory depression. Since there is little need for relaxation, very light anesthesia will be sufficient. This can be provided using nonrebreathing or semiclosed methods of administering ether, cyclopropane, or relaxants. When there is danger of marked blood loss, halothane seems less desirable because of its depressant effect on the cardiovascular system.

Infants who have *meningocele* are operated upon as early as possible in order to prevent tearing of the meningocele and subsequent infection. For these patients light halothane or ether anesthesia administered by the T nonrebreathing technique is preferable (Chapter 20).

Various other anomalies requiring operation while infants are in the newborn period may be handled as described in the following paragraphs.

ANESTHESIA FOR INFANTS 1 MONTH TO 1 YEAR OF AGE

Following the neonatal period most operations performed in infants are elective in nature, and time should be allowed for adequate preparation. Infants acquire strength rapidly, and by the time they are a month old they present an entirely different picture from that of the newborn baby.

During this period operation is often indicated for pyloric stenosis, hernia, and harelip, for such tumors as cystic hygroma, for such neurosurgical lesions as hydrocephalus, subdural hematoma, or meningocele, and for intrathoracic pathology, including vascular ring or hamartoma. These operations should be tolerated well by infants, provided reasonable precautions are observed. In general, inhalation agents are employed with open-drop, nonrebreathing, or closed

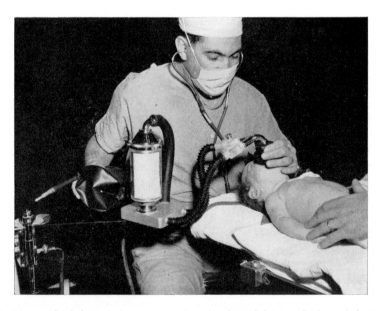

Fig. 17-17. Bloomquist infant circle apparatus is well adapted for use in large infants.

techniques. Infant circle apparatus is useful in many of these older infants (Fig. 17-17), but nonrebreathing systems are usually more practical.

Pyloric stenosis. Pyloric stenosis prevents the normal emptying of the stomach and results in failure to absorb fluid and nourishment. It also causes vomiting and loss of hydrochloric acid. Weight loss, dehydration, and alkalosis result and may be associated with potassium deficiency and anemia.

Correction of these imbalances must be carried out (Chapter 26), and it is often necessary to delay operation for 12 to 24 hours in the process. When prepared adequately, the baby is given atropine, 0.2 mg., and brought to the operating room; the limbs are wrapped in sheet wadding to conserve heat.

The most important step in anesthetic management of these patients is to pass a gastric tube before starting anesthesia (Fig. 17-18). The pyloric stenosis naturally causes retention of stomach contents, and the situation is further complicated by the fact that these infants may be fed sugar water every 2 hours, even in the preoperative stage. If barium has been used for diagnosis, the stomach may have a large amount of this material mixed with the fluid.

The gastric tube should be a 12-Fr. rubber catheter with several holes in the tip; it is passed via the nose into the stomach and strapped in place. As much as 100 ml. of retained fluid and gastric secretions may be removed at this time. If the fluid is relatively clear, one can rinse the stomach a few times with saline and proceed, using general inhalation anesthesia without endotracheal intubation. If curds or barium are found in the stomach wash, it is preferable to use endotracheal intubation. The gastric tube is left in place throughout operation.

Our belief that it is justifiable, under these conditions, to anesthetize infants without endotracheal intubation is based on experienec with 1,139 patients. In them, this practice was carried out without aspiration or other related complication. While endotracheal intubation is justified, it has seemed reasonable to

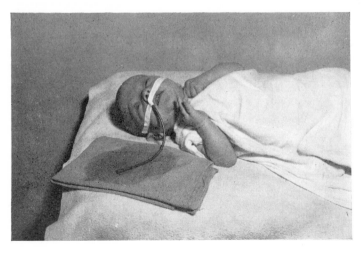

Fig. 17-18. Pyloric stenosis. Before operation the stomach may contain large quantities of fluid. This must be removed before anesthesia is started.

maintain an open policy here, since the potential disadvantages of intubation especially in unskilled hands, may outweigh the advantages. It is to be remembered that pyloromyotomy, like tonsillectomy, is performed in many hospitals where pediatric management is relatively undeveloped.

Anesthesia for pyloromyotomy requires easy, rapid induction and moderate relaxation. Although open-drop ether was used for many of these infants, induction is slow and difficult. Halothane, by nonrebreathing system, is clearly preferable and affords excellent working conditions whether endotracheal intubation is used or not. In this age group, nitrous oxide is not used for induction but may be added later, in 50% mixture with oxygen.

At the end of operation the pharynx is examined; any material is removed, and the stomach tube is aspirated and withdrawn. If the trachea has been intubated, this tube is removed after the infant has reacted and opened his eyes.

Herniorrhaphy. Repair of inguinal hernia is the most common operation of early infancy and is now considered to carry negligible risk in healthy infants. Several types of poor-risk patients may be encountered. These include the child who was born prematurely and continues to be subnormal in development, and

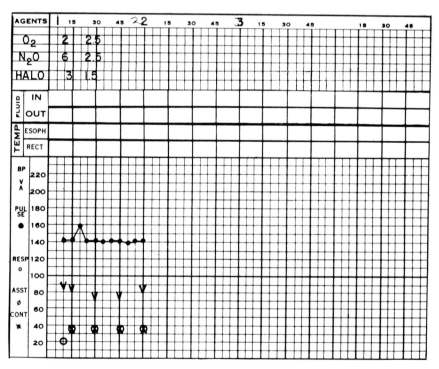

Fig. 17-19. Anesthesia chart. Pyloromyotomy performed on 5-pound infant under halothane and nitrous oxide.

also infants in whom the hernia has become strangulated. Many infants appear with a hematocrit slightly below 10 Gm.%.

Normal healthy infants tolerate a variety of agents, however these infants are often fat and especially prone to develop secretions and airway obstruction if ether or cyclopropane are used. Halothane has been especially advantageous in this age group, and the incidence of respiratory complications has been much reduced. Endotracheal intubation is rarely necessary. These infants make excellent subjects for experience in drop-ether, since they usually awaken promptly and do not appear to be troubled by the aftereffects. For the weaker infants halothane or cyclopropane would be used in preference to ether.

The problem of the child who has low hemoglobin occurs almost every day in a busy pediatric hospital. It is discussed on p. 21.

Harelip and cleft palate. Anesthesia for operations for harelip and cleft palate will be discussed with plastic surgery. Ether or halothane by endotracheal intubation and Y tube is usually preferable.

Tumors about the face and neck. Cystic hygromas and other tumors may occur in the region of the neck and face, and often endanger the airway (Figs. 17-21 and 17-22).

In such situations endotracheal intubation should be attempted prior to induction of anesthesia. Obviously, relaxants should never be used when there is danger of airway obstruction. Older children with airway obstruction may require anesthetic induction prior to intubation. This is performed most effectively using halothane and oxygen without supplementary nitrous oxide. After reaching surgical anesthesia with halothane, it is advisable to add ether to establish

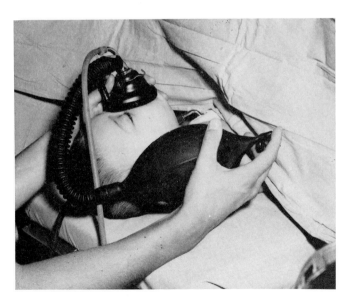

Fig. 17-20. For herniorrhaphy, halothane via nonrebreathing system is excellent. Respiration is most easily assisted by blocking exhale vent with fingertip.

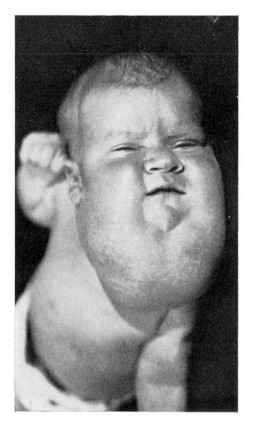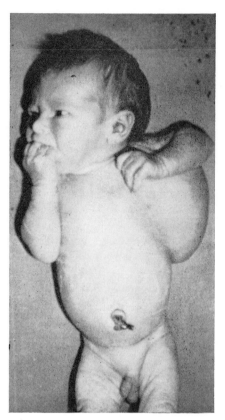

Fig. 17-21   Fig. 17-22

Fig. 17-21. Large cystic hygroma. Tracheostomy is needed but will be hard to perform and difficult to manage after operation.
Fig. 17-22. Removal of a cystic hygroma such as this involves no respiratory problem but may entail considerable blood loss.

maximum safe relaxation that will be of sufficient duration to allow intubation. In massive obstructing tumors it may be necessary to perform tracheostomy at the beginning or conclusion of operation. In either case, an endotracheal tube should be in place prior to performing the tracheostomy.

Maintenance of anesthesia for removal of these large tumors involves several hazards, especially when they occur in the neck. Vagal reflexes are active, and severe cardiac arrhythmias, including three cardiac arrests, have been known to occur. Surgical manipulation may cause dislocation of the endotracheal tube, and all of these tumors may involve severe blood loss from an extensive area. Following operation, tracheostomy may be necessary.[27]

Neurosurgical operations in infants. Many neurosurgical operations are performed on very young infants. Whether the lesion is hydrocephalus, hematoma, or meningocele, patients tolerate endotracheal halothane or ether by the nonrebreathing technique surprisingly well. Even after 3 or 4 hours of anesthesia, these infants maintain easy, rhythmic respiration and wake up and cry as soon as the operation is completed. Maintenance of body warmth is a factor to be watched in air-cooled operating rooms, and fluid replacement always requires a cutdown infusion prior to operation.[15] An attempt should be made to measure blood pressure regardless of the age or size of these infants.

It should be noted that when the T-nonrebreathing technique is used, the proper rate of oxygen flow must be chosen in order to ventilate the patient properly and at the same time to volatilize a suitable quantity of ether or halothane. Investigations by Onchi, Hayashi, and Ueyama,[28] Inkster,[29] and Mapleson[30] have established the correct flow to be two to three times the patient's minute volume when using the Ayre technique as explained in Chapter 7.

Intrathoracic operations in infants. At birth, operation may be necessary for tracheoesophageal fistula or diaphragmatic hernia. During subsequent weeks or months other intrathoracic procedures may include division of vascular ring, lobectomy, or pneumonectomy for cystic lung or hamartoma. These procedures have been performed for several years, and their management has become fairly well understood. Vascular ring is described in the next chapter. Infants with cystic lung require special consideration since attempts to assist ventilation may force additional air into the cystic areas and collapse the remaining lung tissue. All of these procedures may be managed with endotracheal anesthesia using halothane, cyclopropane, or nitrous oxide relaxant techniques.

During recent years there has been a marked increase in the number of operations for correction of congenital cardiac lesions during the first year of life.[31,32] Coarctation of the aorta with cardiac failure, transposition of great vessels, total anomalous pulmonary venous drainage, tetralogy of Fallot, aortic or pulmonary stenosis, anomalous coronary artery, and patent ductus arteriosus now may be definitely diagnosed during early infancy, and the critical condition of the child may leave operation as the only possible solution to an otherwise fatal outcome.[33,34] Correction of these defects may involve use of cardiopulmonary bypass (p. 296), or use of the hyperbaric chamber (p. 306). Anesthetic management must be planned to allow for special cardiac lesions as well as the devices employed in their correction.[35] While cyclopropane has been used successfully for many intrathoracic proceduers in infants, its explosive character prohibits its use with cautery or hyperbaric oxygen. Halothane has been found disadvantageous for patients with intracardiac shunts, and we are left with relaxants as our principal agent for control of muscular activity using light nitrous oxide for sedation.

To date over 250 procedures have been performed under hyperbaric oxygenation for infants with severe congenital cardiac lesions involving either marked hypoxia due to shunting or severe cardiac failure. The series thus far has been remarkably successful.[36,37] Details of management are described in Chapter 18.

Cyclopropane is still used in many infants during less complicated intrathoracic procedures. If inhalation agents are used, two points should be borne in mind: (1) if pulmonary circulation is reduced, as in tetralogy of Fallot, induction will be retarded by the decreased uptake in the lungs; (2) many of these patients are so weak that after induction they will require very little anesthetic, and hyperventilation with oxygen will often prove adequate for considerable periods.

Monitoring of these infants will be especially important. Fluids should be given with great care—while those patients with pulmonary hypertension may easily be overtransfused, those with tetralogy of Fallot may succumb if allowed to become hypotensive.

As noted previously, most of these patients can be brought through operation safely, but the postoperative phase will be the critical period. When there is doubt about a child's condition at completion of operation, the endotracheal tube is left in place, relaxants are not reversed, and the patient is ventilated with a mechanical respirator until greater stability has been established.

POSTOPERATIVE CARE OF INFANTS

At present we are able to keep most small infants alive through the operative procedures, but the first 48 hours following operation gather a great toll. Combinations of fatigue, respiratory depression, and shock appear to cause most of the deaths. To overcome this it is necessary to adopt a more aggressive attitude in caring for these infants, and often there should be continuous physician attendance on these critically ill infants. Positioning the babies so that they have maximal ventilatory exchange is the first requirement, supplemented by intermittent assisted ventilation, if necessary, and meticulous suctioning of upper air passages. Respiratory support with a mechanical ventilator is advised for weak infants who do not breathe well, especially when cardiac failure is a real or potential factor. Cardiac failure, shock, and acidosis must be considered individually and treated definitively.

REFERENCES

1. Gross, R. E.: The surgery of infancy and childhood, Philadelphia, 1953, W. B. Saunders Co.
2. Graff, T. D., Sewall, K., Lim, T. S., Kantt, O., Morris, R. E., and Benson, D. W.: Acid-base balance in infants during halothane anesthesia with use of an adult circle absorption system, Anesth. Analg. 43:583-589, 1964.
3. Podlesch, I., Dudziak, R., and Zinganell, K.: Inspiratory and expiratory carbon dioxide concentrations during halothane anesthesia in infants, Anesthesiology 27:823-828, 1966.
4. Reynolds, R. N.: Acid-base equilibrium during cyclopropane anesthesia and operation in infants, Anesthesiology 27:127-131, 1966.
5. Bunker, J. P., Brewster, W. R., Smith, R. M., and Beecher, H. K.: Metabolic effects of anesthesia in man. III. Acid-base balance in infants and children during anesthesia, J. Applied Physiol. 5:233-241, 1952.
6. Avery, M. E.: The lung and its disorders in the newborn infant, Philadelphia, 1964, W. B. Saunders Co.
7. Rackow, H.: Unpublished data—Lecture at Symposium on the mother, fetus and newborn, Miami Beach, Fla., January, 1966.
8. Graff, T. D., Sewall, K., Lim, T. S., Kantt, O., Morris, R. E., Jr., and Benson, D. W.: The ventilatory reponse of infants to airway resistance, Anesthesiology 27:168-175, 1966.
9. Gross, R. E., and Ferguson, C. C.: Surgery in premature babies, Surg. Gynec. Obstet. 95:631-641, 1952.
10. Collins, H. A., Stahlman, M., and Scott, H. W.: Occurrence of subcutaneous fat necrosis in infant following induced hypothermia used as adjuvant in cardiac surgery, Ann. Surg. 138:880-885, 1953.

11. Bower, B. D., Jones, L. F., and Weeks, M. M.: Cold injury in newborn—study of 70 cases, Brit. Med. J. 1:303-309, 1960.

12. Silverman, W. A., Sinclair, J. C., and Scopes, J. W.: Regulation of body temperature in pediatric surgery, J. Pediat. Surg. 1:321-329, 1966.

13. Roe, C. F., Santulli, T. V, and Blair, C S.: Heat loss in infants during general anesthesia and operations, J. Pediat. Surg. 1:266-275, 1966.

14. Lank, B.: Anesthesia for premature babies, J. Amer. Ass. Nurse Anesth. 21:238-252, 1953.

15. Psaltopoulo-Mehrez, M.: Anesthetic managent of infants, Internat. Anesth. Clin. 1:169-193. 1962.

16. Schuster, S. S.: A new method for the staged repair of large omphaloceles, Surg. Gynec. Obstet. 125:837-850, 1967.

17. Merin, R. G.: Congenital diaphragmatic hernia from the anesthesiologist's viewpoint, Anesth. Analg. 45:44-52, 1966.

18. Creighton, R. E., Whalen, J. S., and Conn, A. W.: The management of congenital diaphragmatic hernia, Canad. Anaesth. Soc. J. 13:124-130, 1966.

19. Roe, B., and Stephens, H. B.: Congenital diaphragmatic hernia and hypoplastic lung, J. Thorac. Surg. 32:279-290, 1956.

20. McNamara, J. J., Eraklis, A. J., and Gross, R. E.: Congenital posterolateral diaphragmatic hernia in the newborn, J. Thorac. Cardiov. Surg. 55:55-59, 1968.

21. Hampton, L. J., White, M. L., and Little, D. L.: Anesthesia for surgical correcton of cardiorespiratory anomalies, Anesth. Analg. 31:105-112, 1952.

22. Wilton, T. N. P.: Anaesthesia for oesophageal surgery in infants and children, Anesth. Analg. 31:267-270, 1952.

23. Zindler, M., and Deming, M. V.: The anesthetic management of infants for the surgical repair of congenital atresia of the esophagus with tracheoesophageal fistula, Anesth. Analg. 32:180-190, 1953.

24. Kennedy, R. L., and Stoelting, V. K.: Anaesthesia for surgical repair of oesophageal atresia and tracheo-oesophageal fistula, Canad. Anaesth. Soc. J. 5:132-136, 1958.

25. Stogsdill, W. W., Miller, J. R., and Stoelting, V. K.: Review of anesthesia for tracheoesophageal anomalies, Anesth. Analg. 46:1-7, 1967.

26. Johnston, A. E., and Conn, A. W.: The anesthetic management of tracheo-oesophageal fistula: a review of five years experience, Canad. Anaesth. Soc. J. 13:28-40, 1966.

27. Macdonald, D. J. F.: Cystic hygroma, An anaesthetic and surgical problem, Anaesthesia 21:66-80, 1967.

28. Onchi, Y., Hayashi, T., and Ueyama, H.: Studies on the Ayre T piece technique, Far East J. Anesth. 1:30-31, 1957; Survey Anesth. 2:352-353, 1958 (Abstract).

29. Inkster, J.: The T-piece technique in anaesthesia; an investigation of the inspired gas concentration, Brit. J. Anaesth. 82:512-518, 1956.

30. Mapleson, W. W.: Ayre T-piece breathing system, Brit. J. Anaesth. 26:323-327, 1954.

31. Cooley, D. A., Berman, S., and Santibaneg-Woolrich, A.: Surgery in the newborn for congenital cardiovascular lesions, J.A.M.A. 182:912-917, 1962.

32. Baffes, G.: Transposition of the great vessels. In Benson, C. D., and others, editors: Pediatric surgery, Chicago, 1962, Year Book Medical Publishers, Inc.

33. Strong, M. J.: Anesthetic management of infants under one year of age with congenital heart disease. In Eckenhoff, J. E., editor: Science and practice in anesthesia, Philadelphia, 1965, J. B. Lippincott Co.

34. Strong, M. J., Keats, A. S., and Cooley, D. A.: Anesthesia for cardiovascular surgery in infancy, Anesthesiology 27:257-265, 1967.

35. Smith, R. M., Crocker, D., and Adams, J. G., Jr.: Anesthetic management of patients during surgery under hyperbaric oxygenation, Anesth. Analg. 43:766-776, 1964.

36. Bernhard, W. F.: Current status of hyperbaric oxygenation in pediatric surgery, Surg. Clin. N. Amer. 44:1583-1594, 1964.

37. Bernhard, W. F., Navarro, R. U., Yagi, H., and Carr, J. G.: The hyperbaric chamber in treatment of cardiac anomalies. In Cassels, D. E., editor: The heart and circulation in the newborn infant, New York, 1966, Grune & Stratton, Inc

Chapter 18

Anesthesia for thoracic surgery

GENERAL PROBLEMS IN ANESTHESIA FOR PEDIATRIC THORACIC SURGERY

All surgical procedures involve certain hazards, but in thoracic surgery the magnitude of the operation plus the initial debility of many of the patients combine to make this a most exacting field for both anesthetist and surgeon.

Preparation. Children undergoing thoracic surgery deserve the best possible preparation, since the outcome can be determined by small details.[1] These patients should be in optimal condition, and time should be taken to allow complete recovery from intercurrent infections and unrelated illness. From the psychologic point of view it is especially important to get the children into a proper frame of mind because emotional outbursts and fatigue can cause severe hypoxia in children with cardiac disease.[2] One must guard aganst the tendency to rush the child about the hospital on the day before operation for roentgen-ray films, electrocardiogram, and laboratory workup. This treatment would completely exhaust and bewilder him and leave him in poor condition on the morning of the operation.

It is especially important for the anesthetist to examine the child thoroughly before operation and to evaluate roentgen-ray films, electrocardiograms, and catheterization data when available. For detailed description of anatomic and physiologic factors one should be familiar with such texts as Nadas,[3] Taussig,[4] and Keith, Rowe, and Vlad,[5] while Keown's[6] monograph offers a useful guide to preoperative evaluation of patients with cardiac disease. An understanding of the operative aspects as described by Gross[7] and in *Pediatric Surgery* by Benson and associates[8] is of fundamental importance to the anesthetist.

Medication prior to operation is indicated in sufficient quantity to bring about vagolytic and antisecretory effects and to have the child in a drowsy, calm state of mind. Atropine, pentobarbital, and morphine are used approximately as suggested in Table 5-1 on p. 88. Although sedation must be carefully suited to each patient, relatively generous atropinization has been our choice for most cases, and morphine has been a reliable and useful agent in many infants and children with severe cardiac lesions.

In order to prevent panic and distress in the early recovery period, it has been helpful to forewarn comprehending children if they are to awaken in an oxygen tent, to reassure them, and to tell them that they will be encouraged to cough and move about.

In this regard it is also advisable to have a physiotherapist make one or two visits to children prior to operation in order to improve breathing mechanics and explain postoperative measures.

Anesthetic requirements. Light, even anesthesia without deep relaxation is desired for thoracic operations. A quiet, unexcited induction is especially important, and it is also essential that gradual, well-controlled establishment of anesthesia be ensured without sudden change of level or cardiovascular load. Either intravenous or inhalation routes may be chosen, depending upon individual factors. Endotracheal intubation is indicated, and the oral route will usually be chosen unless the nasal route is preferred to facilitate postoperative use of a ventilator. Uncuffed tubes are used in children under 8 to 10 years of age, but an airtight fit is essential. Apparatus varies, but at present the nonrebreathing T-piece system is used for most children under 30 pounds, and an adult circle apparatus is used for larger patients (Fig. 18-1). If cyclopropane is used, a Bloomquist infant circle is preferred for children under 30 pounds. The choice of anesthesia usually lies bewteen halothane, cyclopropane, or nitrous

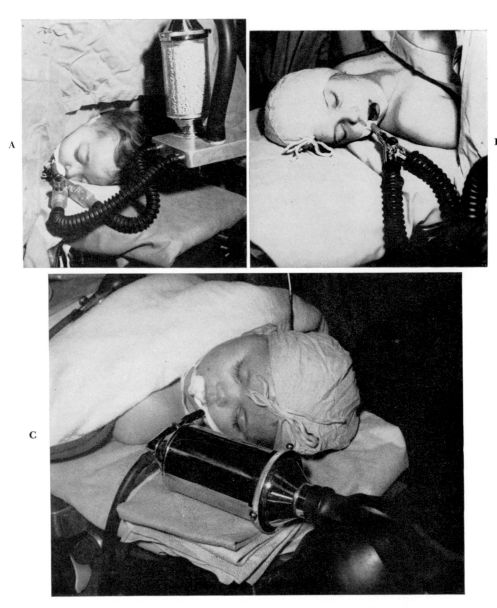

Fig. 18-1. Anesthetic techniques for thoracic operations. **A,** Bloomquist circle apparatus. **B,** Adult circle with Y chimney and straight adapter. **C,** To-and-fro absorption technique.

oxide and relaxants. Assisted respiration is now less popular than controlled ventilation, by manual technique.

Monitoring methods during pediatric thoracic operations are still uncomplicated. The stethoscope is of great value. If the left side of the chest is to be opened, the stethoscope can usually function adequately from the right side of the chest, or an esophageal stethoscope may be used in larger children. While the chest is open, direct visual observation of lung inflation and cardiac action is the most valuable guide available to the anesthetist. Important changes in the force and rhythm of the heart can usually be recognized more promptly by watching the heart than with the use of the electrocardiograph or other instruments; however, the electrocardiograph is used for patients who are suspected of having cardiac irregularity. Central venous pressure determination is indicated when massive transfusion is expected, or when a patient having severe cardiac disease is subjected to an operation that could involve substantial blood loss.

Blood replacement. The great problem common to all thoracic operations is actually not that of ventilation but of blood replacement.[9] The hazard of blood loss and shock is great, but that of overreplacement can be even more perilous. The nature of the problem varies somewhat in each of the different types of operation.

ANESTHESIA FOR OPERATIONS ON LUNGS AND THORAX

Lobectomy and pneumonectomy. If a child has increased bronchopulmonary secretions prior to resection of part or all of his lung, he should be given ample preoperative therapy with antibiotics and postural drainage before admission to the hospital. On the day of operation the patient is given time to clear his pulmonary tree of secretions that have accumulated during the night. Good preoperative care brings the child to operation with a clear airway and makes it unnecessary to perform bronchoscopic suction immediately prior to operation. This procedure is upsetting and irritating and is to be avoided if possible.

Children in reasonably good condition tolerate lobectomy and pneumonectomy without great danger.[10] Halothane or a nitrous oxide relaxant technique would involve less tracheobroncheal irritation than ether or cyclopropane and would now be favored. Adequate provision must be made to suck secretions from the respiratory tract at frequent intervals during the operation. Two points are important here. It will make it much easier if a fairly stiff plastic or polyethylene suction catheter is used, for soft-rubber catheters are difficult to pass down narrow endotracheal tubes. It will also help if one uses a straight metal endotracheal adapter rather than a curved one, for it is next to impossible to insert most catheters through a curved adapter and then down the tube. It is also important to use a suction catheter that does not take up the entire lumen of the endotracheal tube, for this causes rapid removal of alveolar oxygen and bars admission of more oxygen. A plastic tube one third the size of the lumen of the endotracheal tube will usually be effective if good suction is available. One should be reminded that suctioning should not be prolonged but should be interrupted frequently to provide for ventilation.

During pulmonary resection, blood loss is usually appreciable. Measurement may be made of blood lost in sponges and suction bottles, and replacement usually should exceed this by at least 25%.

At the end of the operation extreme care must be taken to clean the nostrils and entire airway of accumulated secretions, as mucopurulent discharges are often copious. Oxygen therapy, humidity, and antibiotics are indicated following pulmonary resection.

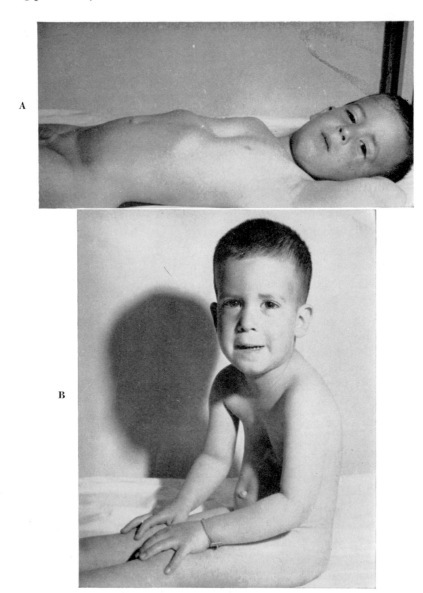

Fig. 18-2. Funnel chest deformity may appear slight when child is supine, **A,** but is greatly exaggerated in usual sitting position, **B.**

Pectus excavatum (funnel chest). This lesion consists of a concave deformity of the sternum, with involvement of ribs and costal cartilages (Fig. 18-2). There are several variations in operations for the correction of pectus excavatum, and although appreciable blood loss and opening of the pleural cavities may occur, the operation often is performed with remarkably little bleeding and with the chest intact.

In addition to these factors one must bear in mind the possible disadvantages associated with the deformity of the chest. It has not been proved that funnel chest interferes markedly with cardiopulmonary function, and some doubt remains as to whether the operation has more than cosmetic value. However, roentgen-ray films may show considerable cardiac displacement, and retraction of the sternum may become so accentuated during operation that some interference with function seems most probable. During anesthesia we have experienced ventilatory disturbances that make us pay particular attention to this factor and monitor both sides of the chest with individual stethoscopes. Possibly due to reduced elimination of carbon dioxide, these patients have shown increased tendency to develop hyperthermia; consequently monitoring of the temperature is of especial importance.

Intrathoracic tumors, tracheoesophageal fistula, and diaphragmatic hernia. Tumors of the lung such as hamartoma, lung cysts, and mediastinal tumors are not uncommon in infants and children. In the presence of lung cysts one must be careful not to use increased airway pressure lest the cyst become overdistended and collapse remaining lung tissue. In intrathoracic tumors general endotracheal anesthesia is required, and the chief problem usually consists of adequate blood replacement and ventilatory assistance.

Tracheoesophageal fistula with esophageal atresia and diaphragmatic hernia were described in the previous chapter.

ANESTHESIA FOR CARDIOVASCULAR PROCEDURES NOT REQUIRING OPEN HEART TECHNIQUES

The problems that arise during operations for congenital heart lesions may include hypoxia, hypercapnia, hypertension, arrhythmias, shock, pulmonary edema, or myocardial depression.[11] In most instances management of the anesthesia is relatively easy, with the airway under control and little relaxation required. The anesthetist will find the origin of most of his troubles to be alterations in hemodynamics; he will be able to function most effectively, first, if he understands the effects of both lesion and operation and, second, if he follows the progress of the operation carefully in order to catch signs of cardiac or pulmonary abnormality at their first appearance. The significant factors in the physiology and management of the major cardiac lesions will be discussed.

Vascular ring (compression of trachea and esophagus by vascular ring). The term vascular ring is used to incude a number of anomalies of the aortic arch and great vessels, all of which act to compress the trachea and/or the esophagus.[12] Those anomalies most frequently seen are (1) double aortic arch, (2) right aortic arch with left ligamentum arteriosum, (3) anomalous right subclavian artery, (4) anomalous innominate artery, and (5) anomalous left common carotid artery.

The double aortic arch is most frequently seen and is the most troublesome because of the marked degree of tracheal and esophageal constriction and also because of the greater difficulty in operative correction (Fig. 18-3). Vascular ring anomalies are not cardiac lesions, and no intracardiac abnormality is involved. The obstruction of trachea and esophagus constitutes the entire clinical problem.

In the symptoms of these anomalies either tracheal or esophageal obstruction may predominate, depending upon which organ is more severely compressed. In mild cases symptoms may be lacking, but in general they appear during infancy in the form of stridor, recurrent respiratory infection, and cough, or in difficulty in eating associated with postprandial vomiting. Infants with marked tracheal compression often lie with their heads arched backward in an opisthotonic position to keep the trachea on the stretch. Diagnosis is made by tracheoscopy and esophagoscopy if a pulsating constriction is seen in either the trachea or the esophagus. Final confirmation is made by roentgen-ray evidence of indentation of the trachea or esophagus by the constricting vessels (Fig. 18-4). Compression of the trachea usually occurs just above the level of the carina.

If the compression is caused by an actual ring of vessels, one sector of the ring must be divided to give relief. In the case of an anomalous innominate ar-

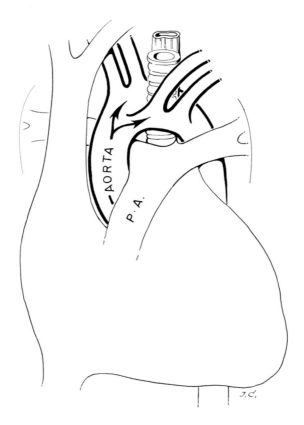

Fig. 18-3. Vascular ring anomaly with double aortic arch encircling trachea and esophagus.

tery or anomalous common carotid artery, the difficulty arises merely from the fact that these vessels lie against the anterior aspect of the trachea and compress it. Relief is gained by removing the thymus and pulling the offending vessel forward, suturing it to the sternum.

In the anesthetic management of these children, the problem of respiratory obstruction is the chief one. If the patient has any difficulty prior to operation, one will hesitate to give preoperative sedation—yet a child who has respiratory obstruction probably gets into greater trouble if excited than if slightly depressed. Consequently, mild sedation is justified, and obviously atropine will be indicated.

Nonrebreathing or closed-system techniques may be used. Induction can be difficult in the presence of tracheal obstruction, and no agent has great preference. Nitrous oxide followed by halothane probably produces the best results. The pleasant, nonirritating induction with cyclopropane may be carried on into an even anesthetic course but can be followed by considerable spasm in patients with airway compression. Succinylcholine may be held in readiness in case its use is indicated to control laryngeal spasm.

Endotracheal intubation is necessary. Several tubes should be prepared because it will be difficult to guess the correct size beforehand. It has been our custom to cut several small holes in the terminal inch of each endotracheal tube for reasons to be stated. It is often necessary to insert the endotracheal tube beyond the point of tracheal compression. If the constriction lies immediately above the carina, there will be a definite possibility that the tube will pass down one main bronchus. By using tubes with additional holes at the tip, the expected obstruction of the other bronchus can be prevented.

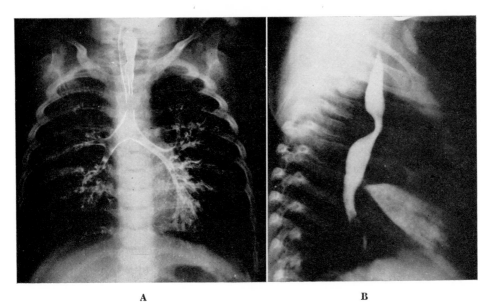

A   B

Fig. 18-4. Roentgen-ray films of patient with vascular ring. **A,** Continuity of tracheal shadow broken above carina. **B,** Marked constriction of esophagus.

Wetchler and McQuiston[13] believe that one should always pass the tube beyond the tracheal compression. Although it is true that this simplifies the anesthetic course greatly, it may increase the postoperative difficulty. It is to be remembered that the trachea does not resume normal shape as soon as the compression is relieved, for the tracheal rings have become deformed and will require time to regain their normal shape. The airway is improved at operation, but obstruction may continue to be critical. If the tracheal mucosa is further irritated by the passage and subsequent friction of the tube, the difficulty may be increased. Since tracheostomy is of little value in these patients, one should observe every precaution.

During the course of the operation the anesthetist must watch the surgical field carefully, for the patient is usually delicate, and the surgeon is working in a dangerous area. Pressure of retractors and instruments may compress the heart, lungs, or trachea, and it is frequently necessary to have the surgeon back away quickly simply in order to keep the infant alive. In the dissection of major vessels there is the ever-present danger of sudden hemorrhage. The anesthetist should be in a position to see this the moment it occurs and also should watch the field in order to estimate the loss from incidental bleeding.

At the end of the operation extubation may be accompanied by serious respiratory obstruction. Extubation should be delayed until full respiratory power has returned but not so long that the child irritates the trachea further by forceful coughing and bucking. After the operation the child is treated with oxygen and humidity to minimize the danger of tracheitis.

Patent ductus arteriosus. The ductus arteriosus, or Botallo's duct, is a normal fetal shunt from the pulmonary artery to the aorta and closes in most infants in the first few weeks of life.[4] Failure of the normal obliterative process allows blood to flow between the systemic and pulmonary circulations (Fig. 18-5). At birth the pressure in the aorta is only slightly greater than the pulmonary artery pressure; the shunting is not significant, nor is it great enough to set up a murmur. In a few months, however, the systemic pressure in the aorta increases and enough blood is forced into the pulmonary artery to set up a murmur, first in systole alone and then both in systole and diastole. This is a characteristic loud, continuous, or "machinery" type murmur.

The hemodynamic effect of the patent ductus is that of a leak from the systemic circulation into the pulmonary artery, a left-to-right shunt.[14,15] During systole a forceful contraction maintains normal arterial pressure, but during diastole peripheral resistance falls sharply because of the free escape of blood through the ductus; hence diastolic pressure is abnormally low. The pulmonary vessels must carry an increased volume of circulating blood, and with large shunts the pulmonary flow may be increased to three or four times normal. The increase vasculature of the lungs is evident by roentgen-ray study, and pulsation of hilar vessels, or "hilar dance," is evident by fluoroscopy.

With a shunt from the aorta to the pulmonary system, blood that has already been oxygenated is ineffectively recirculated through the lungs without going to the tissues. Because the left heart must continue to recirculate this extra load, the left ventricle may show enlargement and failure.

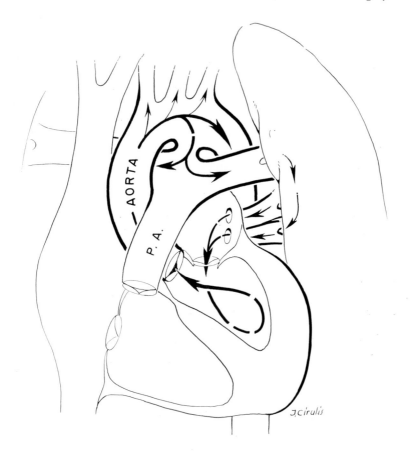

Fig. 18-5. Patent ductus arteriosus.

The clinical effect of a patent ductus is usually slight. With large shunts the child's development may be retarded. Cyanosis is not associated with the lesion unless unusually high pulmonary artery pressure causes reversal of flow through the ductus. Operative ligation or division is indicated to prevent later development of endocardial infection or cardiac failure.[16,17]

The operation and the anesthetic management of ligation or division of the usual patent ductus arteriosus involve little difficulty or danger other than that of hemorrhage from a major vessel.[18,19] In asymptomatic children with small shunts the myocardium is virtually unaffected. In these children operation is performed for prophylactic purposes and may be postponed until the optimum age has been reached. Formerly it was thought best to wait until children were 6 to 8 years old, but improved techniques of anesthesia and surgery have made it possible to operate safely when children are 2 or 3 years old.

Since most of these children are in excellent condition and the increased work of the heart is easily borne, no specific anesthetic agents or techniques are indicated.[20] After sedation with pentobarbital, atropine, and morphine, anesthesia with nitrous oxide and halothane is currently favored, using a T-system for children under 30 pounds and adult circle for larger patients. Cyclopropane, ether, or relaxant techniques are well tolerated by these patients, who represent, in general, the strongest group of children undergoing thoracic surgery. Respiration may be assisted or controlled. For the delicate work of suturing the cut ends of the ductus, the surgeon appreciates a completely quiet field; it is helpful at this time for the anesthetist to control respiration and to be able to stop ventilation each time the surgeon places his suture in the vessel.

Blood replacement deserves special consideration in each type of cardiac lesion.[9] In the presence of a patent ductus arteriosus there is usually an increased blood volume. The transfusion of blood is not obligatory, but because of the danger of sudden hemorrhage from a major vessel, it seems advisable to have blood running during the procedure. The amount given is kept about 10% ahead of the measured loss in sponges and suction bottle.

During operation the child is monitored with stethoscope and blood pressure apparatus, but electrocardiograph offers little advantage. Pulse and blood pressure should remain stable. When the ductus is occluded, there often is an abrupt elevation in the diastolic blood pressure (Fig. 18-6), but this does not always occur. The operation reestablishes normal anatomy, and recovery may be expected to be rapid and uncomplicated. Oxygen therapy usually is unnecessary after the operation. Pain will be moderate after any intrathoracic procedure, and patients usually require morphine or meperidine. The first dosage should be about one half the usual dose (discussion on normal recovery, p. 190). Close

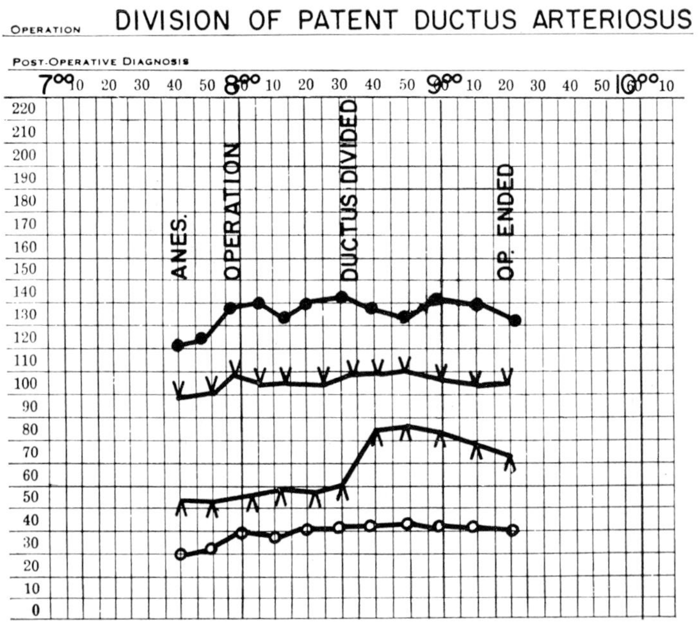

Fig. 18-6. Anesthesia chart of 4-year-old patient during ligation of patent ductus arteriosus. Sharp rise in diastolic pressure is often but not always seen on clamping of ductus shunt.

watch must be kept on all patients following thoracic surgery to make sure that they cough and move about as much as possible.

There is a more serious aspect of patent ductus surgery that involves the abnormally large shunt with pulmonary hypertension and/or increased pulmonary vascular obstruction.[3] An appreciable number of infants and children are now being found who have such high pressure in the pulmonary vessels that reversal of flow occurs in the ductus. The ductus then acts as a safety valve, allowing release of pulmonary pressure by overflow into the aorta. When this occurs, there may be cyanosis of the lower part of the body.

The surgical correction of the large shunts of this nature must be performed in the face of high risk, since death may occur shortly after closure of the ductus. A 50% mortality has been associated with correction of ductus shunts with reversal of flow.[21] In the presence of this problem, the anesthetist's efforts may be concentrated primarily upon preventing factors that might cause further elevation of pulmonary arterial pressure. Consequently, there must be neither struggling nor resistance during induction, nor coughing, bucking, or spasm with intubation. Carbon dioxide excess must be prevented by avoidance of respiratory resistance and deep anesthesia. For sick patients in whom control of anesthesia is of great importance, the use of nitrous oxide and *d*-tubocurarine is of real advantage and has minimal effect on the cardiovascular system.

In patients with large ductus shunts the problem of blood replacement and blood pressure is perhaps the most important, yet the answer is not clear. Because of the danger of vascular overload and heart failure, some believe that blood replacement should be minimal, even though systemic pressure falls to 65 or 70 mm. Hg. Others hold that it is absolutely essential to maintain the systolic pressure well above shock level to ensure passage of blood through the pathologically obstructed pulmonary capillaries. Probably normal blood pressure should be maintained, but, instead of using blood alone, it may be preferable to replace exactly the measured blood loss, relying upon drip infusion of Neo-Synephrine for further support of blood pressure, if this is needed. If a fatality occurs during such an operation, it is most likely to occur about 5 to 10 minutes after closure of the ductus. If the patient survives this period, his chances of ultimate survival are good.

A final and increasingly important aspect of patent ductus arteriosus concerns that encountered in early infancy. Here an excessively large ductus may cause cardiac failure, enlargement, and death unless closure is effected. In such sick young infants, speed is imperative, and simple ligation of the ductus is usually performed rather than division. As described in Chapter 17 a light, even plane of anesthesia with minimal anesthetic concentration is essential.

Tetralogy of Fallot. Tetralogy of Fallot is the most common type of cyanotic heart disease.[4] The syndrome consists of pulmonary valve stenosis, overriding of the aorta, ventricular septal defect, and hypertrophy of the right ventricle. The resultant abnormal circulation is shown in Fig. 18-7, in which returning venous blood enters the right auricle and ventricle, is largely obstructed in its normal course into the pulmonary artery, but deviates through the ventricular sep-

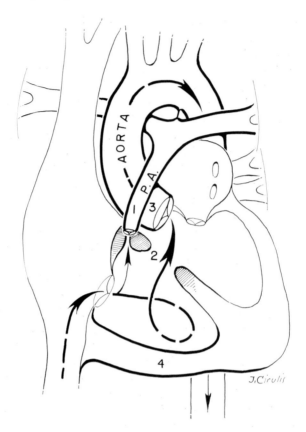

Fig. 18-7. Tetralogy of Fallot. Venous blood is denied entry into obstructed pulmonary artery and passes through septal defect to aorta without oxygenation. Components of tetralogy are the following: **1**, stenosis of pulmonary artery; **2**, ventricular septal defect; **3**, overriding aorta; and **4**, hypertrophy of right ventricle.

tal defect and into the aorta. By this process unoxygenated blood again proceeds to the tissues without passing through the lungs.

Children with this lesion are markedly cyanotic, show clubbing of their fingers and toes, and have greatly decreased exercise tolerance. It is characteristic of young children with tetralogy to squat at intervals when fatigued, and the frequency with which they have to squat is one of the best means of judging the severity of their condition.

Although this lesion is less likely to cause death in the neonatal period than are coarctation of the aorta or transposition of the great vessels, hypoxia increases rapidly in the early months of life, and operation often is indicated in weak infants who already may have experienced hypoxic episodes or cerebral thrombosis.

In the evaluation of the patient one must look for such items in the history and physical examination and then investigate the status of the blood. Hemoconcentration occurs as compensation of hypoxia, but the bone marrow often over-compensates, and the hemoglobin may be 19 or 20 gm.% and the hematocrit as high as 80% or 90%. According to Nadas,[3] elevation of the hematocrit above 75% is of no advantage to the patient. Hemoconcentration involves the risk of thrombus formation. For this reason fluids are encouraged the evening before operation. An added problem is that of excessive bleeding due to the characteristic reduction in circulating platelets.

The operative approach for tetralogy has evolved through several stages. The Blalock end-to-side anastomosis of the subclavian artery to the pulmonary artery,[22] introduced in 1948, was to some extent superseded by the less difficult Potts procedure[23] by which the pulmonary artery is anastomosed to the aorta (side-to-side). Since both of these shunting operations are only compensatory in nature, they were temporarily abandoned when extracorporeal techniques made complete anatomic correction possible. The resultant high mortality in attempted correction of tetralogy influenced many surgeons to revert to a shunting operation as an initial procedure, to be followed, if necessary, by open heart repair after patients develop greater myocardial strength. As a primary operation the Blalock is preferable to the Potts because its shunt is more easily closed at the time of the second procedure. When operation is necessary in young infants, the subclavian artery is difficult to use; consequently anastomosis of ascending aorta to right pulmonary artery (Waterston or Cooley procedure) is often preferable.

For anesthetic management premedication is essential and should be liberal.[20] Morphine is tolerated well, and by quieting the child and reducing his oxygen requirement his color often improves dramatically. If medication has not been adequate, it is better to delay induction than to start with a struggling hypoxic child.

Since the early reports of Harmel and Lamont,[1] McQuiston,[20] and others, cyclopropane has been favored for anesthetic management of children during the Blalock and Potts shunt operations. The value of cyclopropane lies chiefly in its tendency to support cardiovascular action while affording easy, rapid control and maximal oxygenation. The hypotensive effect of halothane has been definitely undesirable. Relaxant techniques are suitable, but they supply less oxygen than when cyclopropane is used.

It will be noted that patients with cyanosis due to decreased pulmonary circulation will at first appear to be remarkably resistant to gaseous induction agents. If a more rapid induction is desired, a relaxant may be given intravenously. Intravenous barbiturates are not well tolerated by severely cyanotic children and must be used with caution. After intubation, cyclopropane is contined using closed or semiclosed technique.

During either the Blalock or the Potts procedure, the anesthetist is faced with two major problems, hypoxia and hypotension.[15] The danger of hypoxia is obvious because of the preexisting cyanosis. With preoperative sedation, cyanosis may decrease, and induction of anesthesia, if quiet and uncomplicated, often results in further improvement. When the child's chest is opened, however, oxygenation may be decreased by partial deflation of one lung. The most critical point of the operation comes when one pulmonary artery is occluded for performance of the anastomosis. If blood flow through the other pulmonary artery is inadequate, the child may not tolerate this procedure. Severe cyanosis and bradycardia will be followed by cardiac standstill. Once committed, the surgeon usually must finish the anastomosis as quickly as possible, while the anesthetist tries to keep the patient alive by ventilating him with unmixed oxygen and adding atropine intravenously to counteract vagotonic reflexes. The use of calcium gluconate may save the day in such a crisis. The dosage has been determined empirically, 300 mg. (3 ml. of 10%) of calcium gluconate being the average intracardiac dose given in critical times of slowing or arrested heart.

Hypotension often is more of a hazard than hypoxia during operation for tetralogy of Fallot. These patients carry a low blood pressure initially, the systolic pressure prior to operation usually being in the neighborhood of 80 to 90 mm. Hg. Induction of anesthesia may lower the pressure appreciably, especially if ether or halothane is employed. Blood loss and myocardial depression also will be mirrored by rapid development of hypotension. Since the children are already hypoxic, hypotension is intolerable. In these patients more than in any others, shock must be avoided.[24,25]

After completion of the anastomosis it becomes important to maintain adequate arterial pressure in order to keep blood flowing through the shunt; otherwise the shunt may thrombose and remain nonfunctioning.

Fluid replacement and support of blood pressure have required special handling in these children. As noted, the tetralogy of Fallot has several unfavorable features including low blood pressure, inability of the heart to increase stroke volume, and chronic hypoxia. The problem is complicated by the fact that plasma is administered instead of blood if the hematocrit is above 55%, and rapid administration of plasma has frequently appeared to cause sudden cardiac depression. This is believed to be due to its low pH and high potassium content.

Calcium gluconate has been most effective in preventing cardiovascular depression. For these operations it has been our custom to use two infusions, one of which is for plasma or blood, the other for an infusion of 5% dextrose and water in which 500 mg. of calcium and 0.5 mg. of Neo-Synephrine are added per 100 ml. of solution. This solution is given at a slow rate throughout the operation and is accelerated to meet special indications. Plasma or blood is administered at a rate that will keep the total infused solution 15% to 20% ahead of the amount of blood loss measured in the suction bottle and sponges. If the blood pressure is under 80 mm. Hg in spite of this replacement, the calcium–Neo-Synephrine solution is speeded sufficiently to return the pressure to normal levels. This mixture is also valuable in the critical situation described previously when bradycardia occurs during the operation and the heart needs more assistance than that afforded by maximal oxygenation.

Although the original belief in the existence of citrate toxicity[26] has been questioned, there is no doubt that calcium has a potent inotropic effect when these cyanotic children become hypotensive.

The usual course of the Blalock or Potts operation is marked by a blood pressure bordering on shock level, moderately rapid pulse, and slightly increased respiratory rate. Respiration is carefully assisted or controlled at all times. The anesthetist follows the color of the patient, the amplitude of his pulse, and the blood pressure with great care. He also monitors the respiratory exchange and cardiac sounds by a stethoscope, but his chief interest is watching the action of the heart. If either the surgeon or the anesthetist notices any change in the character of the heartbeat, he immediately calls it to the attenion of the other so that both can take appropriate steps. If possible, the surgeon interrups his work and allows full oxygenation and relief of constricting forces on the trachea or vasculature. When the normal cardiac activity is reestablished, the operation is resumed.

During the postoperative course the patient is placed in a humidified oxygen tent for 2 or 3 days. Maintenance of blood pressure may continue to be the critical factor for the first day but should stabilize after that. These patients are not normal following such operative shunt procedures but are greatly improved.

In our experience, establishment of palliative vascular shunts in severely cyanotic infants has been more successfully accomplished under hyperbaric oxygenation, described on p. 306, while the anesthetic management of children undergoing open heart procedures for total corrective operation is included in the discussion on extracorporeal circulation.

Pulmonary stenosis with intact ventricular septum. This lesion may appear in early infancy with rapidly developing right ventricular enlargement, a shock-like state, and death. Recently valvotomy has been performed on a number of these infants with success. In its usual form pulmonary stenosis progresses slowly and children bearing the defect show considerably less disability than those with tetralogy of Fallot. The danger is not hypoxia but right ventricular failure.

Repair of pulmonic stenosis has proved to be one of the simplest procedures to do by extracorporeal technique; consequently, this approach is employed for most patients operated upon after infancy.

Coarctation of the aorta. This condition consists of a constriction of the aorta that usually amounts to complete obstruction of flow. Survival depends upon the collateral circulation which may be of two types. In the simple or adult type of coarctation, the type usually encountered, the constriction occurs in the descending thoracic aorta, the ductus arteriosus is obliterated, and collateral circulation passes via the subclavian, internal mammary, and intercostal arteries (Fig. 18-8). In the less frequently encountered variety, the preductal or "infantile" type, the coarctation is situated proximal to the ductus arteriosus, which has remained patent (Fig. 18-9). In these patients the left ventricular output flows via the ascending aorta to the head, arms, and upper body, whereas the lower body and limbs are supplied by the output of the right ventricle, which is carried by the patent ductus arteriosus to the descending aorta. The operative implications of the two lesions are very different.

Simple coarctation usually produces no symptoms during the first 10 years of life. Diagnosis is made during adolescence or early adult life in routine physical examination by the discovery of elevated blood pressure and by the further finding of rib notching and absent femoral artery pulsations. Symptoms, when

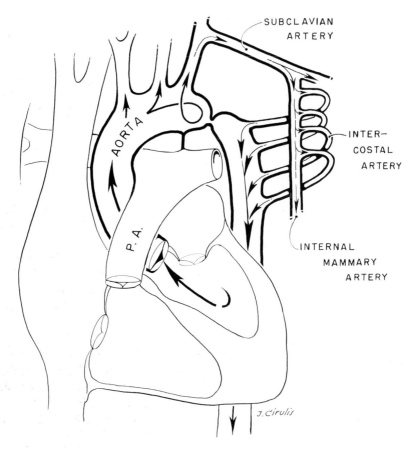

Fig. 18-8. Coarctation of aorta (adult type). Obstruction of descending aorta sends collateral circulation through subclavian, internal mammary, and intercostal arteries to regain distal aortic segment.

present, consist of leg pain on exercise, headache, and fatigue. Although most patients show normal development, some have increased development of the upper torso, arms, neck, and head.

In the preoperative evaluation of patients with coarctation one should determine the patient's blood pressure in both arms and legs and whether or not the patient has any femoral arterial pulsation. It is a better sign if leg pressure and femoral pulsations are poor prior to operation, for this shows that little blood passes the coarctation and sufficient collateral has been established to allow surgical occlusion of the aorta. Adults facing this operation may show left ventricular hypertrophy, bundle branch block, and early cardiac failure, but these are rarely seen in children. One should look for the presence of other complicating anomalies, such as aortic stenosis, in patients who have coarctation.

Operation for coarctation of the aorta[27] involves a very large wound of entry, since it is necessary to expose and free the entire descending thoracic aorta. Be-

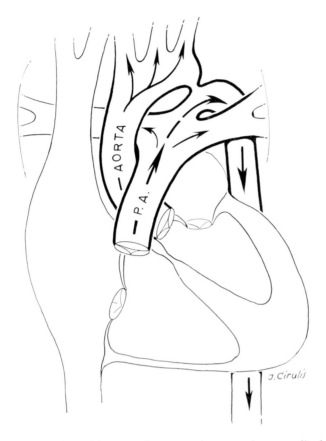

Fig. 18-9. Preductal coarctation, with patent ductus arteriosus entering aorta distal to coarctation.

cause the collateral circulation is carried by the intercostal arteries, these vessels are often extremely large, and the blood loss may be considerable. As the chest is opened and the ribs are divided, blood loss continues, but, after retractors are placed and dissection of the aorta is undertaken, the rate of blood loss is considerably reduced.

Patients requiring operation for coarctation are usually 10 years of age or older and in good physical condition. They tolerate anesthesia and do not offer great problems. The anesthetist should concentrate chiefly on watching the blood pressure and in managing blood replacement. The systolic blood pressure usually is between 150 and 200 mm. Hg prior to operation. Before the aorta is clamped, it is important to have the pressure not above 150 mm. Hg; otherwise occlusion of the aorta may be followed by extreme hypertension and subsequent cerebrovascular accident. Under ether or halothane anesthesia the initially high blood pressure usually falls 30 to 40 mm. during induction and remains in the vicinity of 140 to 150. While the patient is in surgical anesthesia, further reduction of blood pressure is possible by increasing the concentration of the agent. This built-in blood pressure control makes halothane and ether definitely preferable over cyclopropane or a relaxant technique, in which reduction of blood pressure must be accomplished by supplemental use of ganglionic blocking agents.

Although awakening is prompt following halothane, this agent has been reported to increase the rebound hypertension that often follows resection of coarctation.[28,29]

The operation is time-consuming because of the large incision and the careful preparation of the aorta itself. The danger of hypoxia and carbon dioxide retention is appreciable, and the anesthetist must try to prevent this by keeping the left lung partially inflated at all times. At intervals both lungs should be completely expanded.

The two most critical phases of the operation occur with the placing of the clamps on the aorta and later when the clamps are released (Fig. 18-10). In patients who had complete aortic occlusion before operation and had developed good collateral circulation, clamping the aorta produces little change, perhaps a 30-mm. rise in systolic pressure. If the coarctation had not been complete, operative occlusion will bring a greater rise.

In order to perform the aortic anastomosis it is often necessary to clamp the left subclavian artery in addition to the aorta. Because of this added resistance, the systolic pressure may rise as much as 100 mm. Hg. For this reason it is important for the anesthetist to find out prior to aortic occlusion whether the surgeon intends to clamp the subclavian artery as well, in which case additional assurance must be made that adequately low blood pressure exists. In such cases the use of ganglionic blocking agents may be indicated (Chapter 15).

After the aorta is occluded, the maximal blood pressure rise is seen in 5 to 10 minutes, following which the pressure levels off or decreases slightly. Excision of the constricted segment and aortic anastomosis usually requires 20 to 30 minutes to perform.

After completion of the anastomosis, release of the aortic clamps causes a marked reduction in peripheral resistance, and the resultant fall in blood pressure may be severe. If blood replacement has not been maintained, sudden release of the aortic clamps may cause immediate death. Experience has impressed upon us the need for special precautions at this point. Before the clamps are released, one should see to it that blood replacement is satisfactory, that more blood is ready, and that an assistant is standing by to pump it.

The distal clamp may be removed without delay, but the proximal clamp should be released gradually, the anesthetist checking the blood pressure continuously as the instrument is opened. Should the pressure fall below 100 mg. Hg, removal of the clamp is halted, blood is pumped, and the pressure is checked further. Throughout the remainder of the operation the systolic pressure probably should be maintained at not less than 100 mm. Hg.

During the closure of the chest wound an appreciable amount of bleeding may occur. Consequently, the blood pressure must be followed carefully to avoid the unsuspected development of shock. Since much blood is lost in the drapes and gowns in this operation, it is occasionally necessary to give 30% to 40% more blood than that measured in the suction apparatus and sponges.

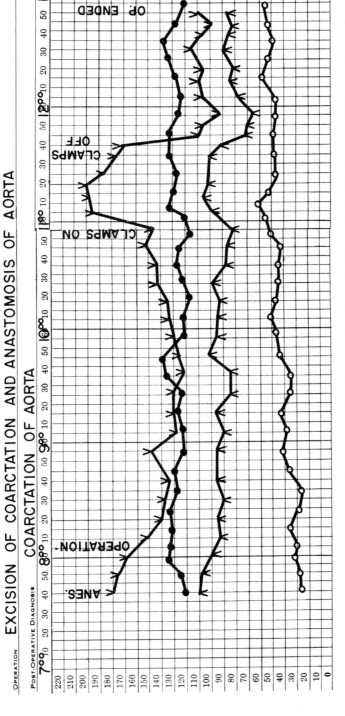

Fig. 18-10. Anesthesia chart during correction of coarctation of aorta, showing typical sharp rise in blood pressure during occlusion of aorta and subclavian artery.

Following the operation continued oozing from the large wound may indicate the use of additional quantities of blood. Oxygen therapy usually is not necessary since aeration should be satisfactory. The wound will be painful and sedation will be required.

There are three variations to the usual picture of aortic coarctation that involve considerably greater operative risk:

1. In infants, coarctation of either the preductal or postductal type may cause marked cardiac enlargement and failure.[30] This type of congenital heart disease is responsible for a large number of infant deaths each year, and operation is often indicated as a lifesaving procedure. Due to the small size of the patient and the cardiac failure, operation under hyperbaric oxygen offers definite advantages (Chapter 17). Hypertension is not a problem at this age, and nitrous oxide–relaxant management is favored.

2. The so-called "infantile" or preductal type of coarctation involving coarctation with a patent ductus arteriosus entering distal to the aortic construction actually may be discovered at any time during life. The absence of collateral circulation has led to an almost prohibitive mortality in attempts at surgical correction of this lesion in older children and adults. The use of the pump-oxygenator may change this situation.

3. The association of aortic stenosis with coarctation also presents problems, since both lesions obstruct left ventricular outflow and increase cardiac strain. Which lesion should be corrected first has led to some dispute. It has been feared that primary repair of aortic stenosis could raise intracranial blood pressure too abruptly, whereas initial repair of the coarctation might render coronary pressure inadequate. In our experience one attempt at initial correction of coarctation resulted in pulmonary edema and cancellation of the operation. Subsequently, however, operations have been successful regardless of which problem was attacked first.

ANESTHESIA FOR OPERATIONS REQUIRING OPEN HEART TECHNIQUES

It is difficult to classify cardiac lesions in relation to the operative procedures, since the approach to each may vary depending upon the severity of the defect, the age of the patient, or the discretion of the surgeon. The most common lesions that are treated under open heart techniques should be familiar to the anesthetist and will be described briefly.

Pulmonic valve stenosis. This lesion offers little difficulty in older children. Correction requires less than 10 minutes of bypass perfusion, and recovery should be prompt. Pulmonic stenosis in small infants can be critical, however, with great cardiac enlargement and failure. Emergency repair under hyperbaric oxygen has been useful for these patients.

Secundum type atrial septal defect. This lesion occurs high in the atrial septum and seldom causes cardiac failure or enlargement (Fig. 18-11). Operation is one of the simplest open heart procedures and one that was formerly accomplished under hypothermia. Anomalous return of right pulmonary veins to the

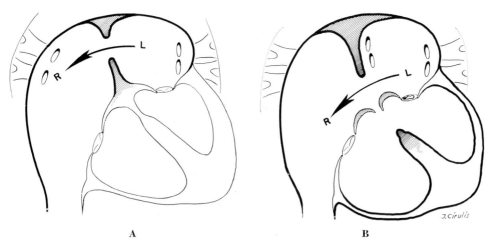

Fig. 18-11. A, Atrial septal defect. Secundum type lesion with defect high in septum, left-to-right shunt, and partial anomalous venous return to right auricle. **B,** Atrial septal defect. Primum type lesion (at base of septum) with left-to-right shunt, left ventricular hypertrophy, and defects of mitral and tricuspid valves.

right auricle occasionally is seen, but correction of this presents little additional difficulty. Mortality should be less than 1%.

Primum type atrial septal defect. This lesion occurs low in the septum and is of much greater concern, since it may involve the conduction system, causing heart block, or may extend into the ventricle or the mitral or tricuspid valve. The resultant left-to-right shunt may be large and involve marked cardiac dilatation and resultant pulmonary artery hypertension.

Ventricular septal defects. Ventricular septal defects (Fig. 18-12), if small, are of little significance and do not require repair if the ratio of pulmonary to systemic shunt is less than 1.7 to 1.[3] In larger shunts open repair is favored in older children, while banding of the pulmonary artery is indicated in infants as a palliative procedure. A mortality for uncomplicated ventricular septal defect of 9% was reported by Kirklin[31] for 1959. Larger ventricular septal defects will involve greater shunting from systemic to pulmonary vessels, with resultant pulmonary artery hypertension.

Pulmonary artery hypertension is a factor of major importance in determining survival.[32] There are two components, that of *quantity of flow,* which may be reduced after operation, and that of *resistance,* which is not significantly affected by operation. High pulmonary artery resistance prior to operation will foretell greater complication and less operative success. Lesions in which operative pulmonary artery hypertension may be encountered are the large patent ductus with preductal coarctation, large atrial septal defect (primum) with mitral regurgitation, large ventricular septal defects, and transposition with ventricular septal defect.

Tetralogy of Fallot. Tetralogy of Fallot has been a major problem. Patients

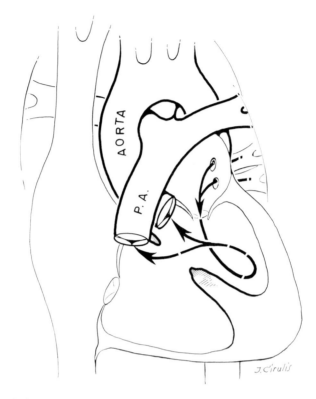

Fig. 18-12. Ventricular septal defect, with pulmonary venous blood circulating through both aorta and pulmonary artery.

with little right-to-left shunting (pink tetralogy) have done well, but those with excessive shunting (blue tetralogy) have had high mortality, especially in younger age groups. Death has usually occurred due to inadequate relief of pulmonary outflow tract and right heart failure. Although Kirklin[33] has had increasing success with total repair, many choose to perform shunts in younger children and withhold total correction until patients are 6 to 8 years old. Total correction of tetralogy always is a formidable procedure requiring prolonged bypass perfusion. It is especially difficult if a previously performed Potts anastomosis must be repaired, since bleeding may be profuse. For this procedure deep hypothermia and total circulatory arrest have been helpful. Following repair, myocardial action often is poor, and hypotension a major problem.

   Transposition of great vessels. Many different procedures have been devised for palliative or corrective repair for this lesion. Although Mustard[34] has succeeded in the total repair of the anomaly, many surgeons prefer palliative measures. There are three forms of transposition of the great vessels[3]: (1) having no ventricular septal defect, (2) with ventricular septal defect and severe pulmonic stenosis, and (3) with ventricular septal defect and no pulmonic stenosis. The palliative procedures for these are (1) creation of an atrial septal defect, (2) cre-

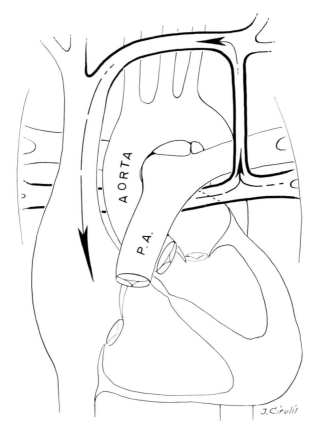

Fig. 18-13. Total anomalous pulmonary venous drainage. One of several variations, this involving union of pulmonary veins, and drainage into right heart via superior vena cava.

ation of shunt (Waterston or Blalock), and (3) banding of pulmonary artery, respectively.

Total anomalous pulmonary venous drainage. Several different varieties of this lesion exist[35] (Fig. 18-13). Cardiopulmonary bypass will not always be required but usually is essential. Postoperative cardiac failure is the greatest problem due to the sudden shift of load to the relatively undeveloped left heart.

Techniques for approaching open heart procedures have included hypothermia, different types of extracorporeal perfusion, and use of the hyperbaric oxygen chamber. Extracorporeal perfusion has widest application but is technically more difficult to apply to infants. Although Cooley's[36] success using perfusion in infants is outstanding, it has been equaled by Bernhard's[37] record using hyperbaric oxygen. Much of Mustard's[34] work in this age group has been accomplished by combining bypass perfusion with hypothermia.

Technical aspects of extracorporeal circulation. The anesthesiologist may play a variable role during extracorporeal procedures, but he should be familiar with technical aspects of the pump-oxygenator as well as the problems of the surgeon.

The development of the pump-oxygenator, like that of the automobile and airplane, was a story of theories, obstacles, and problems through which investigating teams struggled, often with discouraging results. From 1932 to 1950, Gibbon[38] worked almost alone to construct a device that would remove blood from the body, oxygenate it, and pump it back into the circulation. His original combination of screen oxygenator and the De Bakey rotary pump[39] was subsequently used by the Kirklin[40] group at Mayo Clinic with outstanding success. Several oxygenating devices have been developed based on (1) exposing large surfaces of blood to free oxygen, as in screen or disc oxygenators, (2) bubbling oxygen through blood (Lillehei and associates)[41] or (3) the more biologic method of exposing blood to oxygen by means of a semipermeable membrane (Clowes and Neville).[42]

One great problem in development of a pumping device was in the attempt to reproduce the pulsatile flow of the heart. Mechanical valves became stuck, traumatized blood, and were difficult to sterilize. It was some time before it was evident that a continuous nonpulsatile flow[39] would serve the purpose as well or better than the traditional pulsating flow.

Other problems to be met along the way included clotting of blood that contacted glass surfaces, hemolysis due to excessive bubbling or traumatic suction devices, determination of correct rate of perfusion,[43] balancing inflow rate to outflow rate,[41] controlling temperature by perfusion,[44] methods of producing intentional cardiac arrest, accurate anticoagulation methods, and reversal of anticoagulants, combination of moderate hypothermia (85° F.) with bypass methods, and finally use of bypass plus deep hypothermia (65° F.) to prepare for reversible total circulatory arrest.[45] The symposium entitled "Extracorporeal circulation"[46] gives an excellent view of the developing scene in 1958, and Gollan's *Physiology of cardiac surgery*[45] is an unusually informative and enjoyable monograph on the development of extreme hypothermia for cardiac surgery.

The anesthetists and surgeons arriving on the scene today accept the pump-oxygenator as a *fait-accompli,* thereby missing an exciting historical event. However, several problems remain unsolved. Patients who are carried on extracorporeal circulation more than 90 to 120 minutes are subject to several lesions including metabolic acid-base disturbances,[47,48] clotting defects,[49] platelet destruction,[50] cardiorespiratory depression,[46] surfactant washout[51] and renal deficiency.[52,53] Abnormal arteriovenous pulmonary shunting has been especially troublesome[54] and is aggravated in conditions involving pulmonary artery hypertension. Although numerous complications are to be expected due to severe cardiac lesions, these complications are believed to be due in some degree simply to exposure to bypass circulation.

Use of extracorporeal perfusion requires several additional procedures in surgical technique and pharmacologic control. Basic steps in our clinic include the following progression:

1. Establishment of infusions in internal saphenous vein, inferior vena cava, and brachial vein (for anesthetist).
2. Insertion of Foley urethral catheter.
3. Midline sternum splitting incision.

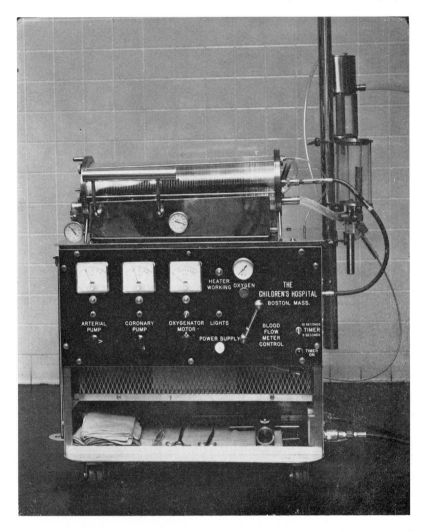

Fig. 18-14. Pump-oxygenator combining disc oxygenator and circular De Bakey pumps. (Courtesy Dr. Robert E. Gross, Boston, Mass.)

4. Construction of arterial inflow line by suturing Teflon plastic sleeve to ascending aorta.

5. Establishment of venous drainage line by passing plastic catheters through right atrium into inferior and superior vena cavae.

6. Administration of heparin anticoagulant, 1 mg./kg.

7. Preparation of pump-oxygenator; De Bakey rotary pump with modified Kay Cross disc oxygenator (Fig. 18-14); adult disc oxygenator contains 114 discs, each bearing in surface; it is primed wtih 3 pints of heparinized whole blood plus 500 ml. Ringer's lactate and 500 ml. 10% dextrose. Infant oxygenator contains 28 discs and is primed with 1½ pints of whole blood.

8. Pump attached to arterial and venous lines; bypass started and regulated to maintain exchange at 100 ml./kg./min. to a maximum of 4,000 ml./min.

9. Suction sumps fixed in atria.

10. If intended operation is to be total repair of tetralogy of Fallot in a patient who previously had Pott's procedure, patient is cooled to 70° F.: otherwise temperature is not altered.

11. If heart is to be intentionally arrested, electric fibrillator is placed under heart, and current applied (110 volts).

12. The corrective repair is performed. Pulmonary artery may be perfused intermittently via Foley catheter, to prevent surfactant destruction.[51]

13. Heart is closed, air removed from ventricles, patient is warmed to 90° F.. and defibrillation is accomplished.

14. If indicated, catheter is inserted into left atrium for sampling and pressure determination, and wires may be implanted in ventricle and chest wall for subsequent use of pacemaker.

15. Caval ligatures are released, pump is stopped exactly as arterial and venous lines are clamped.

16. Calcium gluconate and 50% glucose are administered (adult dose 1 Gm. and 20 ml., respectively).

17. Cannulae are removed; then protamine (1 mg./kg.) is given to reverse heparin, and the dose is repeated in 5 minutes. Dexamethasone (Decadron), 25 mg., adult dose.

18. Epsilonaminocaproic acid given to prevent fibrinolysin formation.[50]

19. Bleeding is controlled, chest tubes are inserted, and the wound is closed.

The steps of such procedures will differ slightly with each team, but the anesthetist should be aware of their significance and should share responsibility for their execution.

Anesthetic management. The anesthetic care of patients undergoing open heart procedures has been well described by several authors.[48,55-60] The reports from the Mayo Clinic by Patrick, Theye, and Moffitt[48] and Theye, Moffitt, and Kirklin[55] are especially to be recommended, as is Conn and Mustard's[60] description of the hypothermic technique used in Toronto.

In the preoperative phase, one takes even more care, if possible, to assess both the emotional and the physical state of the patient. Preparation includes consideration of awakening in the oxygen tent and possible inability to speak (due to endotracheal tube). The degree of risk is evaluated, as in adults, by the child's daily exertion tolerance, the history of failure, digitalis dosage, ascites, arrhythmias, and especially the degree of cardiac enlargement. Cardiac catheterization data should be examined for presence of right-to-left shunting and pulmonary artery hypertension.

Physiotherapists should visit patients before operation to train them to cough and ventilate properly.

Preoperative sedation is ordered, reducing the barbiturate dosage in proportion to the severity of the cardiac lesion. Atropine is used in normal dosage for all patients unless tachycardia is marked.[58] Congenital cardiac lesions are not adversely affected by this agent. Morphine has a desirable effect both on patient and heart; it is especially indicated in children with pulmonic valve stenosis, since it has relaxant effect on the pulmonic infundibulum and often is a specific corrective for severe cyanotic spells seen in children with this lesion or tetralogy of Fallot.[3]

Anesthetic agents and technique. Anesthetic techniques for extracorporeal procedures are usually similar to those in other intrathoracic operations. A humidified T-piece nonrebreathing system is employed if children weigh less than 30 pounds. Adult circle technique is employed in larger patients. A cuffed endotracheal tube is employed in children as young as 7 or 8 years of age, when possible. The choice of anesthetic lies between relaxants and halogenated agents, as described later.

Induction and maintenance. A quiet induction obviously is important. Maximum-risk patients should come to the operating room with a previously established intravenous infusion. After determination of initial heart rate and blood pressure, induction is most quietly accomplished by fractional intravenous doses of morphine (0.5 mg./10 lb.) until the child is relaxed and quiet. Slightly stronger patients tolerate thiopental, but this may cause myocardial depression in weak, cyanotic patients. Children with cardiac lesions of minor severity may be rather fussy but otherwise tolerate standard gentle inhalation induction quite well.

Intubation is accomplished promptly. Usually it is preferable to employ a relaxant rather than deep general anesthesia. Choice between succinylcholine and *d*-tubocurarine is inconsequential. When cardiac function is good, the child may be carried on halothane, but this agent is avoided when cardiac output is limited and when there is marked cyanosis or a large right-to-left shunt. In such cases nitrous oxide and relaxants have proved more reliable in our hands. Although *d*-tubocurarine is more frequently used at present, most of our first three hundred procedures were carried out using intermittent doses of succinylcholine.

The early part of the procedure should be relatively uneventful. When the heart is exposed and manipulated, there may be extrasystoles, but these are usually short-lived. Partial clamping of the aorta to attach the Teflon sleeve is often tolerated better than insertion of caval cannulae, which may cause obstruction of venous return and hypotension. Obstruction of venous return via superior vena cava will result in obvious congestion of the head and face. This should be called to the attention of the surgeon at once.

Unless an anesthetic vaporizer has been incorporated into the pump, intravenous agents must be used for relaxation and sedation during bypass. Our method has been to give *d*-tubocurarine intravenously shortly before bypass in order to establish a relaxed state, and to add enough thiopental into the pump reservoir to provide immediate effect upon establishment of bypass (approximately 1 mg./lb.).

Upon establishment of bypass, one should watch for patient response: (1) movement of legs, (2) diaphragmatic action, (3) opening eyes, or (4) swallowing. Any of these signify inadequate anesthetic control. Most rapid control is achieved by adding thiopental to the pump (the initial dose may be repeated). Mild diaphragmatic action is best treated by a second dose of relaxant, also given via the pump.

Until ligatures are tightened on caval cannulas, the lungs are being perfused, and normal ventilation is required. After ligatures are fastened, preventing the blood from entering the lungs, the gas flows may be reduced (500 ml./min. of both oxygen and nitrous oxide). There is general agreement that the lungs should not be allowed to collapse but should either be held in partial inflation or expanded several times per minute, to prevent atelectasis.

During the course of the perfusion, it is necessary to watch for signs of awakening or movement and to control them, to watch for engorgement of vessels of the head, and to observe signs of blood volume, notably color of skin and conjunctivae, and venous pressure. The nonpulsatile arterial blood pressure will not register on the standard cuff during bypass (Fig. 18-15).

Upon termination of bypass the anesthetist will determine blood pressure immediately and will call for any necessary additional blood, which may be added directly from the pump. Poor myocardial action may be due to hypovolemia, heart block, hypothermia, or myocardial strain, and it should be treated definitively as indicated by signs and monitoring devices.

The next several hours usually are the most eventful for all concerned. Al-

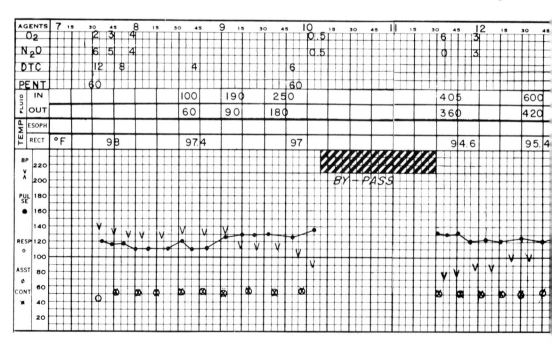

Fig. 18-15. Anesthesia chart. Open repair of atrial septal defect.

though the lesion may have been repaired, the lacerated heart is often unable to bear the altered load and may require a variable period for compensation. Calcium gluconate and 50% glucose stimulate the myocardium and reverse potassium efflux, while isoproterenol has an inotropic effect and also acts to overcome heart block. If these are not successful, wires may be implanted for use with a pacemaker. Digitalization usually is interrupted during the operative period but may be resumed early in the recovery period if indicated.

Arterial blood gases are determined during longer perfusion periods and immediately after termination of bypass. Metabolic acidosis is treated by administration of sodium bicarbonate or tris buffer (4 mEq./kg. of sodium bicarbonate or 150 mg./kg. of tris buffer should elevate pH by 0.1).[61]

The monitoring of patients during bypass operations has been much contested. An esophageal stethoscope, arterial blood pressure cuff, and an esophageal or rectal thermistor are mandatory for all patients.

An electrocardiograph is added when patients have known arrhythmias or are moderately poor risk. Central venous pressure is monitored when patients have shown signs of failure, but this is not mandatory in relatively good-risk patients. Anesthetists should not forget to observe the urinary output, which is one of the best available methods of evaluating adequacy of perfusion during and after operation.

Other useful observations can be made by the surgeon's palpation of the ascending aorta, which can give valuable information on blood volume when instruments fail. The carotid pulse should be followed and carefully evaluated by the anesthetist. It must not only be present but also must be difficult to occlude.

During closure of the chest, nitrous oxide should provide adequate anesthesia. Following less involved procedures such as repair of pulmonic stenosis or secundum atrial defects, the patient should be expected to awaken and recover promptly. Reversal of curarization is carried out, the patient is extubated, and soon after is placed in an oxygen tent in the recovery room, alert, ventilating normally, warm and pink with normal blood pressure.

Following critical procedures involving long periods of perfusion, in patients with damaged or dilated hearts, it is advisable to keep the patient curarized, an oral or preferably nasal endotracheal tube is left in place, and he is taken to the recovery room where respiratory exchange is continued by means of a mechanical ventilator.[62,63] If respiratory assistance appears to be necessary for a period of only 1 or 2 hours and the patient has relatively clear lungs, a pressure-controlled device may be used, but if a longer period is anticipated, or compliance is reduced, a volume-limited ventilator is preferable. Details are described in Chapter 29.

Postoperative care. Critically ill patients should be cared for by an experienced team, preferably in a special care unit near the operating room where suitable equipment and personnel are immediately at hand.

Upon arrival in this area, chest tubes are attached to suction, the ventilator is adjusted, and vital signs are checked. Problems of the recovery phase may be varied, but the most serious complications in our experience have been bleeding, heart block, myocardial failure, and the postperfusion pulmonary syndrome.

Continued bleeding has on several occasions been found to be due to fibrino-lysins, and it has been controlled by use of epsilonaminocaproic acid.[50] At other times thoracotomy has exposed obvious bleeding points, but more often, although no bleeding points were found, removal of clots controlled the hemorrhage. Treatment of tamponade by drainage usually is promptly effective. Heart block may be overcome by use of isoproterenol,[48] but it may require prolonged use of pacemaker control.

The problem of the postperfusion lung syndrome[64,65] has been one of the most perplexing, and still is not satisfactorily explained. Typical signs of this syndrome include cyanosis, dyspnea, fever, and weakness, with widespread rales and rhonchi, diffuse mottling by roentgen-ray examination, and reduced blood gas diffusion. There is widespread atelectasis, congestion, and vascular stasis throughout both lungs, and as the condition progresses the work of respiration becomes greatly increased. Mechanical ventilation will be required; this finally becomes inadequate, leaving the patient to die with virtually solid lungs.

A factor of primary importance in etiology has been found to be obstruction of pulmonary circulation during bypass perfusion. Correction by adequate left atrial drainage has been of great help. It is also believed that failure to expand lungs during perfusion increases atelectasis.

The role of surfactant is still being contested, Mandelbaum and Giammona,[51] having found definite change in pulmonary compliance after bypass perfusion, and others[66] finding no change in compliance. Our own incidence of the perfusion syndrome, once considerable, has been virtually eliminated by (1) adequate drainage of left atrium, (2) ventilation of lung during bypass, (3) intermittent pulmonary artery perfusion, (4) dexamethasone therapy, and (5) postoperative ventilatory therapy in all poor-risk patients, as described in Chapter 29.

ANESTHESIA FOR CARDIAC OPERATIONS IN THE HYPERBARIC OXYGEN CHAMBER

Starting in 1963, a series of corrective or palliative operations under hyperbaric oxygenation has been carried out on critically ill infants with congenital cardiovascular lesions. In 1966 Bernhard and associates[67] reported on 110 infants, and the series has now extended beyond 250. The lesions involve either severe cyanotic disease (transposition of great vessels, pulmonary atresia, tetralogy or tricuspid atresia) or acyanotic disease complicated by severe cardiac failure (pulmonic or aortic stenosis, ventricular septal defect with pulmonary artery hypertension, coarctation of aorta, etc.). All infants were operated upon on an emergency basis and were Class 4 or 5 risk.

Exposure of these infants to 3 atmospheres of oxygen usually effected an increase in oxygen saturation from approximately 20% (initial) to approximately 50% (final).[68] This small elevation appeared sufficient to increase the child's tolerance to operation significantly.

Anesthetic management is governed by the size and debility of the child, the operation, and the environment. As noted previously (Chaper 17), nitrous oxide–oxygen and *d*-tubocurarine have been used in most cases, administered by humidified T-nonrebreathing apparatus.[69]

Dx: AORTIC STENOSIS   Age: 5 Months

Operation: AORTIC VALVOTOMY   Wt. 6 Kg

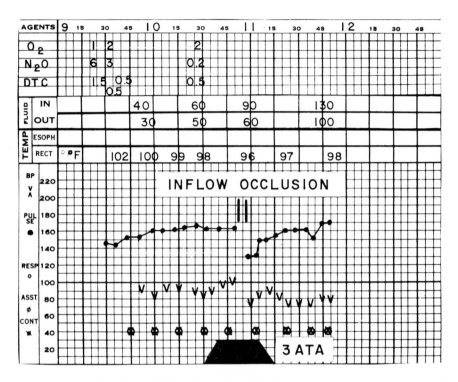

Fig. 18-16. Anesthesia chart of infant 5 months old who underwent aortic valvotomy. Anesthesia consisted of nitrous oxide and *d*-tubocurarine. Hyperbaric oxygenation was used between 10:30 and 11:15, during which time heart was arrested for 2 minutes for valvotomy. Neostigmine was used at end to reverse *d*-tubocurarine.

An infusion is usually established under local anesthesia, the child is intubated with intramuscular succinylcholine and oxygen, the nitrous oxide and *d*-tubocurarine are administered, and the operation is begun. Pressurization is withheld until the chest is open unless the infant's condition demands earlier use (Fig. 18-16).

Pressurization to 3 atmospheres requires 8 to 10 minutes. Agents and drugs are not altered by such pressure, but the partial pressure of a gas such as nitrous oxide will triple if the ambient pressure is tripled; consequently, for the same sedative effect, the concentration of nitrous oxide must be reduced to one third of the starting concentration.[70] In other respects, conduct of the procedures is similar to that of other sick small infants.

Following the definitive part of the operation, which may consist of creating a shunt or an atrial septal defect, the pressure is reduced while the wound is being closed. Total exposure to pressure rarely exceeds one hour. Hyperventilation with oxygen is sufficient for much of the work. If infants have received *d*-tubocurarine, reversal is carried out regularly. Thus far no prolonged apnea has followed the use of *d*-tubocurarine.

The results of this series are impressive in that they surpass previous records at this hospital, as well as that of other hospitals. Although hyperbaric oxygen probably plays a large part, five factors enter the picture: (1) accurate diagnosis, (2) anesthetic experience, (3) detection and correction of acid-base alterations, (4) surgical experience, and (5) improved tissue oxygen availability.

ANESTHESIA FOR CARDIAC CATHETERIZATION, ANGIOCARDIOGRAPHY, AND CARDIOVERSION
Cardiac catheterization

Catheterization studies of the right and left heart involve special problems for the anesthetist. Since the two procedures are distinctly different, they will be discussed individually.

Right-heart catheterization. This procedure is used for the diagnosis of cyanotic heart disease of various types and in lesions involving shunts, the exact nature of which is uncertain. The studies require from one to three hours, and, since measurement of oxygen saturation together with pressure differences constitute the principal goal of the project, it is desirable to avoid the use of oxygen, whether it is mixed with an anesthetic or used purely for supportive therapy. The process of right-heart catheterization usually requires exposure of a vein in the antecubital space and passage of a catheter into this vein and thence into the chambers of the heart. The procedure does not cause excessive pain but is uncomfortable and is something one could hardly expect a small child to tolerate quietly. Sedation is indicated but must be of a type that has a prolonged, even action, without peaking. This has proved to be a difficult problem to solve, and most approaches have fallen short of expectations. Tribromoethanol has been widely used and gives adequate control for a varying period of time. Its disadvantages are that it often is expelled with disturbing results, it has a definite peak in both anesthetic level and depressant effect, and it usually wears off unless repeated doses are given.

Rectal thiopental may be used in single-dose or multiple-dose technique, but it, too, is variable in action and is likely to be depressant when relied upon for the complete effect. Keown and co-workers[71] prefer to use intramuscular thiopental and are satisfied with its use, but in our hands this has been quite unpredictable and certainly does not lend itself to repeated administration. Keats and associates[72] recommend the use of trichlorethylene vaporized by compressed air.

The combination of chlorpromazine, phenothiazine, and meperidine suggested by Smith, Rowe, and Vlad,[73] of Toronto, has been used extensively. The solution is made up as follows:

Phenothiazine	50 mg.	(2 ml.)
Chlorpromazine	50 mg.	(2 ml.)
Meperidine	200 mg.	(4 ml.)
		8 ml. solution

The suggested dose is 1 ml. per 20 pounds of body weight in noncyanotic children and 0.7 ml. per 20 pounds in cyanotic or debilitated children, given intramuscularly 1 hour before intended catheterization.

The prolonged depression caused by chlorpromazine has been disturbing, and for this reason it seems preferable to use a combination of meperidine, 1 mg. per pound, and pentobarbital, 2 mg. per pound, by intramuscular route and supplemented as required by divided intravenous doses during the course of catheterization.

Left-heart catheterization. Formerly general anesthesia was often required for left-heart catheterization that was performed by passing a needle through the chest wall into the heart. A more satisfactory method has now been developed whereby a catheter is passed up the femoral artery and into the left ventricle. This can be done under sedation, as is right-heart catheterization.

Angiocardiography

Whereas formerly the injection of radiopaque solutions into veins and arteries was so irritating and upsetting that anesthesia was required, the development of Renovist* and similar improved media has made the use of anesthesia unnecessary for these studies.

Cardioversion

The electric shock used to revert an irregular heart to normal rhythm is short-lived but most unpleasant and may need to be repeated numerous times in the course of a few weeks. Amnesia with thiopental or methohexital usually is suitable. Precautions must be observed to avoid anesthesia after recent eating or drinking.

---

*E. R. Squibb & Sons.

REFERENCES

1. Harmel, H. H., and Lamont, A.: Anesthesia in the surgical treatment of congenital pulmonary stenosis, Anesthesiology 7:477-498, 1948.
2. McQuiston, W. O.: Anesthetic problems in cardiac surgery in children, Anesthesiology 10:590-600, 1949.
3. Nadas, A. S.: Pediatric cardiology, ed. 2, Philadelphia, 1963, W. B. Saunders Co.
4. Taussig, H. B.: Congenital malformations of the heart, New York, 1947, The Commonwealth Fund.
5. Keith, S. D., Rowe, R. D., and Vlad, P.: Heart disease in infancy and childhood, New York, 1958, The Macmillan Co.
6. Keown, K. K.: Anesthesia for surgery of the heart, ed. 2, Springfield, Ill., 1966, Charles C Thomas, Publisher.
7. Gross, R. E.: Surgery of infants and children, Philadelphia, 1953, W. B. Saunders Co.
8. Benson, C. D., Mustard, W. T., Ravitch, M. D., Snyder, W. H., Jr., and Welch, K. J., editors: Pediatric surgery, Chicago, 1962, Year Book Medical Publishers, Inc.
9. Smith, R. M.: Blood replacement in thoracic surgery for children, J.A.M.A. 161:1124-1128, 1956.
10. Bergner, R. P., and Schafer, G. W.: General anesthesia for pediatric thoracic surgery, Anesth. Analg. 35:194-205, 1956.
11. Strong, M. J.: Anesthetic management of infants under one year of age with congenital heart disease. In Eckenhoff, J. E., editor: Science and practice in anesthesia, Philadelphia, 1965, J. B. Lippincott, Co.
12. Gross, R. E.: Surgical relief for tracheal obstruction from a vascular ring, New Eng. J. Med. 233:586-590, 1945.
13. Wetchler, Z. V., and McQuiston, W. O.: Anesthetic management of infants and children

with double aortic arch, paper presented before American Society of Anesthesiologists, Kansas City, Mo., October, 1956.

14. Burchell, H. B.: Congenital cardiac disease; physiological considerations, Postgrad. Med. 3:321-326, 1948.
15. Smith, R. M.: Circulatory factors affecting anesthesia in surgery for congenital heart disease, Anesthesiology 13:38-61, 1952.
16. Gross, R. E., Emerson, P., and Green, H.: Surgical obliteration of patent ductus arteriosus in 7 year old girl, Amer. J. Dis. Child. 59:554-559, 1940.
17. Gross, R. E.: Complete division for patent ductus arteriosus, J. Thorac. Surg. 16:314-322, 1947.
18. Adelman, M. H.: Anesthesia in surgery of patent ductus arteriosus, Anesthesiology 9:42-47, 1948.
19. Harris, A. J.: Management of anesthesia for congenital heart operations in children, Anesthesiology 11:328-332, 1950.
20. McQuiston, W. O.: Anesthesia in cardiac surgery: observations on 362 cases, Arch. Surg. 61:892-899, 1950.
21. Ellis, F. H., Kirklin, J. W., Callahan, J. A., and Wood, E. H.: Patent ductus arteriosus with pulmonary hypertension. An analysis of cases treated surgically, J. Thorac. Surg. 31:268-285, 1956.
22. Blalock, A., and Taussig, H. B.: Surgical treatment of malformations of the heart in which there is pulmonary stenosis or pulmonary atresia, J.A.M.A. 128:189-202, 1948.
23. Potts, W. J., Smith, S., and Gibson, S.: Anastomosis of aorta to pulmonary artery, J.A.M.A. 132:627-631, 1946.
24. Berger, O. L.: Anesthesia for surgical treatment of cyanotic heart disease, J. Amer. Nurs. Anesth. 16:79-85, 1948.
25. Smith, Code: Anaesthesia for the surgical correction of congenital heart disease, Canad. Anaesth. Soc. J. 2:347-354, 1954.
26. Bunker, J. P.: Citric acid intoxication, J.A.M.A. 157:1361-1367, 1955.
27. Gross, R. E.: Coarctation of aorta; surgical correction of 100 cases, Circulation 1:41-55, 1950.
28. Davis, T. B., Morrow, D. H., Hebert, C. L., and Cooper, T.: An increased incidence of paradoxical hypertension following resection of aortic coarctation under halothane anesthesia, Anesthesiology 22:132-133, 1961.
29. Conn, A. W., and Millar, R. W.: Postocclusion hypertension and plasma catecholamine levels, Canad. Anaesth. Soc. J. 7:443-446, 1960.
30. Bahn, R. C., Edwards, J. E., and DuShane, J. W.: Coarctation of the aorta as a cause of death in early infancy, Pediatrics 8:192-203, 1951.
31. Kirklin, J. W., McGoon, D. C., and DuShane, J. W.: Surgical treatment of ventricular septal defect, J. Thorac. Cardiov. Surg. 40:763-773, 1960.
32. Dammann, J. F., Jr., and Muller, W. H., Jr.: Pulmonary hypertension, In Benson, C. D., Mustard, W. T., Ravitch, M. M., Snyder, W. H., and Welch, K. J., editors: Pediatric Surgery, Chicago, 1962, Year Book Medical Publishers, Inc.
33. Kirklin, J. W.: Tetralogy of Fallot. In Benson, C. D., et al., editors: Pediatric surgery, Chicago, 1962, Year Book Medical Publishers, Inc.
34. Mustard, W. T.: Progress in total correction of complete transposition of the great vessels, Vasc. Dis. 3:177-179, 1966.
35. Cooley, D. A., Hallman, G. L., and Leachman, R. D.: Total anomalous pulmonary venous drainage. Correction with the use of cardiopulmonary bypass in 62 cases, J. Thorac. Cardiov. Surg. 51:88-102, 1966.
36. Cooley, D. A., Berman, S., and Santibaneg-Woolrich, A.: Surgery in the newborn for congenital cardiovascular lesions, J.A.M.A. 182:912-917, 1962.
37. Bernhard, W. F.: Current status of hyperbaric oxygenation in pediatric surgery, Surg. Clin. N. Amer. 44:1583-1594, 1964.
38. Gibbon, J. H.: Artificial maintenance of circulation during experimental occlusion of pulmonary artery, Arch. Surg. 34:1105-1131, 1937.

39. De Bakey, M. E.: Simple continuous-flow blood transfusion instrument, New Orleans M. & S. J. **87**:386-389, 1934.
40. DuShane, J. W., Kirklin, J. W., Patrick, R. T., Donald, D. E., Terry, H. R., Burchell, H. B., and Wood, E. H.: Ventricular septal defects with pulmonary hypertension. Surgical treatment by means of a pump-oxygenator, J.A.M.A. **160**:950-953, 1956.
41. Lillehei, C. W., DeWall, R. A., Read, R. C., Warden, H. E., and Varco, R. L.: Direct vision intracardiac surgery in man using a simple, disposable artificial oxygenator, Dis. Chest **29**:1-8, 1956.
42. Clowes, G. H. A., Jr., and Neville, W. E.: The membrane oxygenator in extracorporeal circulation. In Allen, J. G., editor: Extracorporeal circulation, Springfield, Ill., 1958, Charles C Thomas, Publisher.
43. Gross, R. E.: Discussion on pumps. In Allen, J. G., editor: Extracorporeal circulation, Springfield, Ill., 1958, Charles C Thomas, Publisher.
44. Sealy, W. C., Brown, I. W., Jr., and Young, W. G., Jr.: Report on the use of both extracorporeal circulation and hypothermia for open heart surgery, Ann. Surg. **147**:603-613, 1958.
45. Gollan, F.: Physiology of cardiac surgery, Springfield, Ill., 1959, Charles C Thomas, Publisher.
46. Allen, J. G., editor: Extracorporeal circulation, Springfield, Ill., 1958, Charles C Thomas, Publisher.
47. Patrick, R. T., Theye, R. A., and Moffitt, E. A.: Studies in extracorporeal circulation. V. Anesthesia and supportive care during intracardiac surgery with the Gibbon-type pump-oxygenator, Anesthesiology **18**:673-685, 1957.
48. Carson, S. A., and Morris, L. E.: Controlled acid-base status with cardiopulmonary bypass and hypothermia, Anesthesiology **23**:618-626, 1962.
49. Perkins, H. A., Osborn, J. J., and Gerbode, T.: Problems in coagulation. In Allen, J. G., editor: Extracorporeal circulation, Springfield, Ill., 1958, Charles C Thomas, Publisher.
50. Kevy, S. V., Glickman, R. M., Bernhard, W. F., Diamond, L. K., and Gross, R. E.: The pathogenesis and control of the hemorrhagic defect in open heart surgery, Surg. Gynec. Obstet. **123**:313-318, 1966.
51. Mandelbaum, I., and Giammona, S. T.: Extracorporeal circulation, pulmonary compliance and pulmonary surfactant, J. Thorac. Cardiov. Surg. **48**:881-887, 1964.
52. Mielke, J. E., Maher, F. T., Hunt, J. C., and Kirklin, J. W.: Renal performance during clinical cardiopulmonary bypass with and without hemodilution, J. Thorac. Cardiov. Surg. **51**:229-237, 1966.
53. Lundberg, S.: Renal function during anaesthesia and open-heart surgery in man, Acta Anaesth. Scand. supp. 27, 1967.
54. Hedley-Whyte, J., Corning, H. B., Laver, M. B., Austen, W. G., and Bendixen, H. H.: Ventilation-perfusion relations after heart valve replacement or repair in man, J Clin. Invest. **44**:406-416, 1965.
55. Theye, R. A., Moffitt, E. A., and Kirklin, J. W.: Anesthetic management during open intracardiac surgery, Anesthesiology **23**:823-827, 1962.
56. Smith, R. M., and Engineer, E. H.: Problems related to open-heart operations in children, Anesth. Analg. **39**:104-109, 267-272, 1960.
57. Mendelsohn, D., Jr., Mackrell, T. N., MacLachlan, M. A., Cross, F. S., and Kay, E. B.: Experiences using the pump-oxygenator for open cardiac surgery in man, Anesthesiology **18**:223-235, 1957.
58. Morrow, D. H.: Anesthesia for cardiovascular surgery. In Benson, D. W., editor: Surgical specialties, Philadelphia, 1966, F. A. Davis Co.
59. Cannard, T. H.: Patient response to varying forms of extracorporeal perfusion. In Eckenhoff, J. E., editor: Science & practice in anesthesia, Philadelphia, 1965, J. B. Lippincott Co.
60. Conn, A. W., and Mustard, W. T.: Hypothermia for cardiac surgery, In Benson, C. D., et al.: Pediatric surgery, Chicago, 1962, Year Book Medical Publishers, Inc.
61. Moore, D., and Bernhard, W. F.: Efficacy of 2-amino-2-hydroxy-methyl-1, 3 propanediol (tris Buffer) in management of metabolic lactacidosis accompanying prolonged hypothermic perfusion, Surgery **52**:905-912, 1962.
62. Dammann, J. F., Jr., Thung, N., Christlieb, H., Littlefield, J. B., and Muller, W. H., Jr.:

The management of the severely ill patient after open-heart surgery, J. Thorac. Cardiov. Surg. **45**:80-90, 1963.

63. Brown, K., Johnston, A. E., and Conn, A. W.: Respiratory insufficiency and its treatment following paediatric cardiovascular surgery, Canad. Anaesth. Soc. J. **13**:342-366, 1966.

64. Awad, J. A., Lemieux, J. M., and WuLou: Pulmonary complications following perfusion of the lungs, J. Thorac. Cardiov. Surg. **51**:767-776, 1966.

65. Provan, J. L., Austen, W. G., and Scannell, J. G.: Respiratory complications after open-heart surgery, J. Thorac. Cardiov. Surg. **51**:626-638, 1966.

66. Sullivan, S. F., Patterson, R. W., Malm, J. R., Bowman, F. O., and Papper, E. M.: Effect of heart-lung by-pass on the mechanics of breathing in man, J. Thorac. Cardiov. Surg. **51**:205-212, 1966.

67. Bernhard, W. F., Navarro, R. V., Yagi, H., Carr, J. G., Jr., and Barandarian, H.: Cardiovascular surgery in infants performed under hyperbaric conditions, Vasc. Dis. **3**:33-41, 1966.

68. Bernhard, W. F., Tank, E. S., Frittelli, G., and Gross, R. E.: The feasibility of hypothermic perfusion under hyperbaric conditions in surgical management of infants with cyanotic congenital heart disease, J. Thorac. Surg. **46**:651-664, 1963.

69. Smith, R. M., Crocker, D., and Adams, J. G., Jr.: Anesthetic management of patients during surgery under hyperbaric oxygenation, Anesth. Analg. **43**:766-776, 1964.

70. Special article. Hyperbaric oxygenation: anesthesia and drug effects, Anesthesiology **26**:812-824, 1965.

71. Keown, K. K., Fisher, S. M., Downing, D. D., and Hitchock, P.: Anesthesia for cardiac catheterization in infants and children, Anesthesiology **18**:270-274, 1957.

72. Keats, A. S., Telford, J., Korusu, Y., and Latson, J. R.: Providing a steady state for cardiac catheterization under anesthesia, J.A.M.A. **166**:215-219, 1958.

73. Smith, C., Rowe, R. D., and Vlad, P.: Sedation of children for cardiac catheterization with an ataractic mixture, Canad. Anaesth. Soc. J. **5**:35-40, 1958.

Chapter 19

Anesthesia for general and plastic surgery

ANESTHESIA FOR ABDOMINAL OPERATIONS

General pediatric surgery necessarily encompasses a wide variety of patients among whom are many acutely ill children. Other patients involve increased risk because of tumors, congenital anomalies, or traumatic lesions.

Surgical lesions. Abdominal conditions requiring surgery during the pediatric period may be due to the presence of congenital anomalies, metabolic disorders, and hormonal disturbances and thus may be characteristic of this age group, but they also include the inflammatory lesions, tumors, and traumatic states seen in older patients. The conditions listed in Table 19-1 may be encountered in infants and children.

Anesthetic problems. Some of the anesthetic problems encountered in infants have been mentioned. For the most part the anesthetic requirements for abdominal surgery in children are similar to those in adults. In addition to analgesia,

Table 19-1. *Indications for abdominal surgery in infants and children*

1. Intestinal obstruction	7. Biliary atresia
(a) Atresia	8. Liver cyst
(b) Stenosis	9. Tumor of intestine
(c) Meconium ileus	10. Neuroblastoma
(d) Tumor	11. Wilms' tumor
(e) Volvulus	12. Hirschsprung's disease
(f) Intussusception	13. Portal hypertension
2. Pyloric stenosis	14. Splenomegaly
3. Appendicitis	15. Ruptured viscus
4. Meckel's diverticulum	16. Exstrophy of bladder
5. Hernia	17. Tumors of bladder
6. Undescended testis	18. Adrenogenital syndrome

good relaxation usually is needed, and the use of a potent general anesthetic, muscle relaxant, or regional block will be necessary. In exceptional cases very weak patients may require only analgesic concentrations of anesthetic agents.

For most infants and children halothane affords easy induction and adequate relaxation for abdominal procedures. For procedures such as esophageal resection that require an unusual degree of relaxation, *d*-tubocurarine may be used in supplemental dosage. Cyclopropane may be used for most abdominal procedures, but deep cyclopropane may involve cardiac arrhythmias. Ether is acceptable except for toxic and severely ill patients. Nitrous oxide–relaxant combinations are especially valuable, and methoxyflurane (Penthrane) should be useful here, if anywhere, due to its special relaxant quality. Spinal anesthesia and epidural anesthesia also find their greatest use in abdominal surgery.

Although the first two requirements for abdominal surgery are analgesia and relaxation, a number of other problems confront the anesthetist. The aspiration of regurgitated intestinal contents is always to be feared but is of greatest importance in patients with intestinal obstruction. Gastric suction is always established in such patients prior to anesthesia, and endotracheal intubation will usually be necessary, the tube being left in place until the patient has awakened.

Children facing abdominal surgery may be extremely toxic due to peritonitis, prolonged vomiting, uremia, or cachexia. In fact, of all types of pediatric patients, the sickest may be found among those requiring abdominal operation. Time must be taken for adequate preparation of these children by correction of dehydration, hypovolemia, anemia, and metabolic imbalances.

Blood loss and shock may be the major problems in such long operations as abdominoperineal resection for Hirschsprung's disease, but the danger of shock is especially severe during resection of tumors of the upper abdomen. Excision of tumors of the liver and of retroperitoneal neuroblastomas has proved to be the most shocking of all procedures that we have encountered. In addition to rapid blood loss that might be equaled during thoracic surgery, manipulation of the viscera and of large tumors within the upper abdomen produces tremendous reflex stimulation that intensifies hypotension and the reduction of cardiac output.

Traumatic lesions of the abdomen are most frequently caused by automobile accidents, but bicycles and sleds take an appreciable toll when in season. Ruptured spleen is not uncommon in children, and the resultant hemorrhage may be severe. Trauma to the bladder, kidney, and other organs is less frequently seen.

In addition to the rather general problems just mentioned, other more specific hazards are associated with certain individual lesions or organs. Pheochromocytoma,[1,2] with the extreme variations in blood pressure, carries the same risk as when seen in adults and constitutes a definite contraindication to cyclopropane. The adrenogenital syndrome[3] is occasionally seen in children, and operation is indicated for diagnosis or physiologic alteration. Although the pathology involved in this condition does not suggest any decreased tolerance to anesthesia or surgery, our experience has made us eye these patients with distrust. Sudden depression of respiration and blood pressure has occurred twice in a relatively small series of cases. This was probably due to rapid salt depletion, characteristic of these patients.

Management of typical cases. It seems appropriate to describe the management of a few illustrative conditions in greater detail.

Intestinal obstruction. The anesthetic handling of newborn infants with intestinal obstruction has been described and consists of local infiltration or of awake intubation followed by use of cyclopropane or halothane. The greatest problem with these infants lies in postoperative support.

A variety of lesions many underlie intestinal obstruction, including atresia, stenosis or duplication of the gut, volvulus, malrotation, mesenteric bands, intussusception, meconium ileus, tumors, and imperforate anus. Of this number meconium ileus[4] probably carries the highest mortality. This condition is the infantile manifestation of cystic fibrosis, in which there is a deficiency of proteolytic enzymes throughout the mucus-secreting glands of the body. At birth the infant's abdomen is distended and may feel like moist putty beneath the tight skin. Roentgen-ray films show intestinal stasis and a characteristic ground-glass appearance of the abdominal content. The family history often includes the story of other children who have died during infancy or childhood.

Operation is usually indicated. Following establishment of an infusion, endotracheal intubation, and anesthetic induction, the abdomen is opened to find the gut distended and filled with thick, gummy meconium that cannot be sucked or even squeezed out of the bowel. After the diagnosis is confirmed, attempts may be made to express a little of the material, but ileostomy is usually performed and then the abdomen is closed. Several infants have survived after weeks of ileostomy irrigation with enzyme extracts. The few patient who do survive must be expected to develop the pulmonary manifestations of cystic fibrosis within a short period of time.

Some forms of intestinal obstruction are relatively benign. Intussusception may be serious if it has progressed far, but the condition usually occurs in relatively healthy 1-year-old or 2-year-old babies and generally is diagnosed before the child becomes acutely ill. Gastric suction is established, and anesthesia is induced with nitrous oxide and may be maintained with halothane, ether, or other inhalation agents by nonrebreathing or semiclosed techniques. Endotracheal intubation is preferable but is not mandatory unless distention is present. Fluid therapy may be given by cutdown or percutaneous route.

Incarcerated hernia falls into much the same category as intussusception. These infants are seldom very ill and tolerate most anesthetics well. Occasionally this condition is seen in weak, premature infants, or it may progress sufficiently to cause dehydration and electrolyte disturbance.[5] The choice in such cases probably would be local infiltration, cyclopropane, or halothane. The management of uncomplicated hernia as described on p. 270 consists of simple techniques using nitrous oxide and halothane or ether. Tracheal intubation is performed only if indicated by respiratory obstruction, secretions, or similar complications.

Anesthesia for pyloric stenosis has been described in the discussion on anesthesia for infants.

Appendicitis. Next to tonsillectomy, appendectomy is certainly the operation most frequently performed in children. Appendicitis can occur during infancy but is uncommon in children under 3 or 4 years of age.

If the child has not been ill for more than 24 hours and has not been vomiting or febrile and if physical examination does not suggest peritonitis, operation may be undertaken at once under halothane, cyclopropane, ether relaxant combinations, or spinal anesthesia by those who favor it. Since children seldom feel like eating during the development of appendicitis, it is unusual to find one who has taken any solid food for 8 to 12 hours prior to admission, and the problem of the full stomach rarely exists. Consequently, endotracheal intuabtion will not be required to protect the airway from vomitus but may be used to facilitate control of ventilation and relaxation. Certainly one should always monitor the temperature during operations on the bowel and its appendages.

Gangrenous appendix with peritonitis. The child with perforated appendix presents a more complicated problem that demands a careful approach if mortality is to be avoided.

Formerly, when children were admitted to the hospital with signs of high fever, dehydration, and ketosis, it was believed correct to operate immediately. Convulsions, soaring temperature, dementia, and death occurred with alarming frequency. Some years ago, however, it was shown that these deaths might be prevented if the patients were not taken directly to the operating room but were sent to the ward and given gastric suction, fluid and electrolyte therapy, and antibiotics.

Since the advent of more aggressive use of cooling techniques, many children have been subjected to immediate cooling by sponging or covering with ice and then operated upon with little attention to treatment of underlying electrolyte disturbances.

The rational approach to this problem is to initiate fluid and antibiotic therapy, as outlined on p. 411, and continue until hydration is attested by voiding and until urinary specific gravity and hematocrit are within normal limits. If the temperature has not fallen after 3 or 4 hours of such therapy, it is reasonable to take the child to the operating room, control shivering by induction of general anesthesia with thiopental, cyclopropane, or halothane, and then rapidly cool by bathing or icing the skin. Attempts at cooling that result in shivering will be harmful and relatively ineffective. After insertion of an endotracheal tube, cooling may be effected rapidly by introduction of cold saline solution into the stomach.

The safe time to operate upon such ill patients is difficult to determine, but *as a rule one should not operate until the child has voided, his temperature has fallen below 102° F., and his pulse has fallen below 120.*

Medication is needed for such acutely ill children before operation but should be given with care. Atropine or a similar belladonna-like drug is indicated, but these may cause an iatrogenic elevation of pulse or temperature that could be confused with signs of suddenly increasing toxicity. To prevent such a situation, atropine is not given until the child is in the operating room. In such cases it should be given intravenously.

Pentobarbital and morphine are indicated if the child is alert and apprehensive, but apprehension may be simulated by the rather wild look of an acutely ill patient, who tolerates sedation poorly. In most cases it is better to give very small doses of sedation and to repeat them if necessary.

The anesthesia itself should provide an easy, pleasant induction, high oxygenation, complete analgesia, relaxation, depression of vomiting centers, minimal disturbance of metabolism and fluid control, and rapid recovery. Since patients have been receiving an infusion prior to anesthesia, an intravenous channel is available. Induction is pleasantly accomplished by injection of thiopental, approximately 10 mg. per year of age, after which halothane, cyclopropane, or nitrous oxide and *d*-tubocurarine may be used for maintenance of anesthesia. Endotracheal intubation seems indicated here in order to have the best possible airway in patients who would be unusually intolerant of hypoxia. Although cyclopropane often provides adequate relaxation, arrhythmias occasionally occur even when ventilation appears sufficient. In such instances the concentration of cyclopropane is reduced and relaxation is provided by the use of gallamine or *d*-tubocurarine.

Operations involving the liver. Operations involving the liver bear considerable risk. In some cases this is due to the disturbed function of the liver. In the presence of simple biliary obstruction, as seen in biliary tract atresia, the use of ether appears to be tolerated well. However, in one 6-year-old girl who had inflammatory hepatitis, a liver biopsy performed under ether was followed by rapidly climbing temperature and death. It at once was obvious that ether was the wrong agent to use in this case. Although no drug is actually safe in the presence of hepatitis, relaxants used with nitrous oxide currently appear to be the best choice.

Splenectomy. Splenectomy is indicated for rupture of the organ and also for familial hemolytic jaundice and idiopathic thrombocytopenic purpura. In each of these conditions the red blood cell count may be much decreased. With rupture of the spleen this will be due to loss of whole blood, and the child will be hypovolemic and in danger of developing shock. Naturally, blood transfusion is indicated, and operation should be undertaken as an emergency. If blood is not available, the blood volume may be maintained with plasma, plasma expanders, or 5% albumin (p. 422).

The choice of the best anesthetic agent for children with ruptured spleen is somewhat of a moot point. Cyclopropane is accepted as being preferable for patients who are bordering on shock because it maintains arteriolar tone and sustains blood pressure. However, the fact that it causes splenic engorgement in dogs has led many to question its use for splenectomy in human beings. Ether has the reputation of being undesirable for patients facing shock because of its vasodilating effect, but it causes splenic contraction and from that standpoint would be indicated. Etsten[6] investigated the effect of cyclopropane on the human spleen and found it to be negligible. In any case a reasonable solution is to use both agents so that each will compensate for the weakness of the other. Thiopental, nitrous oxide, and relaxant combinations might be used without appreciably affecting the physiologic picture, but thiopental is considered a poor agent for patients who are recovering from shock.

Splenectomy is generally performed in children through a flank incision, with the patient on his side and with the table arched or broken in the middle. Endotracheal anesthesia and assisted respiration are indicated, and a Levin tube should be inserted to prevent gastric distention.

Children with familial hemolytic jaundice may be markedly anemic. The destruction of the red cells is gradual, however, and the blood volume is not reduced. The use of transfusions to restore the normal red blood cell count may result in bursts of hemolysis, leaving the patient unimproved. For this reason such children are often accepted for operation with depleted red cells. An infusion is started at the beginning of the operation, but blood is not given until the splenic pedicle has been clamped. Endotracheal intubation is advised, and although the ether-cyclopropane combination is sound from a theoretical standpoint, halothane, supplemented if necessary by a relaxant, should be quite satisfactory.

Idiopathic thrombocytopenic purpura involves a different problem. Children with this condition usually receive cortisone prior to operation in order to stimulate platelet formation. Proper steps must be taken to establish and maintain an adequate steroid level before, during, and after operation.

Recently a robust 13-year-old girl with a diagnosis of idiopathic thrombocytopenic purpura entered the hospital for splenectomy. It was known that she had received a course of steroid therapy, and orders were given to maintain adequate cortisone level. The dosage proved inadequate, however—15 minutes after operation the patient developed profound hypotension. The error was immediately recognized, and the patient was revived promptly by the administration of blood and hydrocortisone.

Extensive intra-abdominal procedures. Extensive intra-abdominal procedures (including excision of neuroblastoma, Wilms' tumor, liver tumors, liver cysts, esophageal resection, Swenson or Duhamel pull-through operation, and portocaval or splenorenal shunt) are procedures representing long operations that require much relaxation and moderate to severe blood loss (Fig. 19-1). Although several have individual points of particular vulnerability, the main problems are those

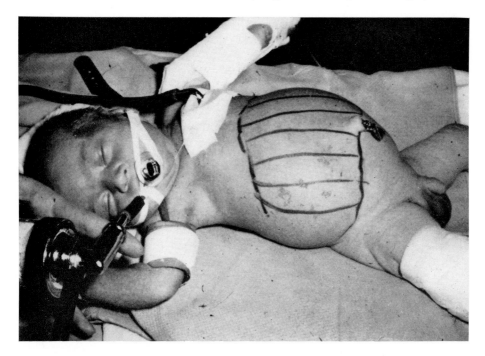

Fig. 19-1. Removal of large abdominal tumors often involves massive blood loss.

of blood replacement and supportive therapy. Preparation of adequate amounts of blood is the first prerequisite. It is reasonable to prepare 1 liter of blood per 20 pounds of body weight beforehand, and to have more available. This blood should be as fresh as possible, and before use should be buffered and warmed to room temperature (details of blood preparation, p. 431).

The room is warmed to 75° F. prior to operation to prevent chilling the patient. An electrocardiograph is prepared, and a defibrillator is made available.

The anesthetic apparatus used will depend primarily on the child's size. For those under 35 pounds, a T-piece apparatus would be suitable if adequately humidified. In larger children a semiclosed apparatus would be used. All patients would require endotracheal intubation. A Levin tube is also used in all except those patients undergoing esophageal resection.

In choosing the anesthetic agent one must consider the need for good relaxation and the effect of the agent in massive blood loss. Cyclopropane conceals blood loss by compensatory vasoconstriction and maintenance of blood pressure, while halothane, in sufficient concentration to give relaxation, causes misleading reduction of blood pressure. Ether, or preferably nitrous oxide and *d*-tubocurarine, would be most suitable for such operations. Both methods afford good relaxation without materially affecting the patient's response to blood loss.

At the start of these operations two reliable infusions are established. In the operations in which the inferior vena cava may be cut or occluded, the arms are used for infusion rather than the legs.

During these procedures patients will usually be in the supine position. For the pull-through procedure the legs will be elevated. A thoracoabdominal approach will be used for esophageal resection and for large Wilms' tumors. This will involve a large initial blood loss that may go unrecognized because the blood may lie unnoticed in the chest and abdomen. It is extremely important that transfusion of blood be started as soon as the skin is incised; otherwise administration of blood may fall seriously behind blood loss. Throughout all of these procedures excessive depth of anesthesia should be avoided. The use of relaxants in either primary or secondary role is of great help.

Particular points are of importance in dealing with these patients. Esophageal varices secondary to portal hypertension bleed copiously, and patients often have cystic fibrosis as the basic pathology. Pulmonary complications and general debility must be expected.

With liver tumors, neuroblastoma, and especially Wilms' tumor, the inferior vena cava may be involved, and surgical dissection may cause laceration or kinking, thereby abruptly interrupting venous return and cardiac action. In all operations involving rapid blood loss, one should keep the amount of transfused blood well ahead of the measured output. One must respect blood pressure readings and keep the pressure above 80 mm. Hg. If pressure falls below 80, the operation must be halted, and either by administration of blood or interruption of manipulative procedures, the pressure must be restored before the surgeon is permitted to proceed.

One should use a stethoscope with the blood pressure apparatus for more accurate observation of blood pressure rather than rely on the fluctuation of the needle of the gauge. Blood loss is estimated as described on p. 424 using weight of sponges, graduated suction bottles, and physical signs as criteria.

After removal of any large tumors extensive bleeding may still occur during closure of the wound, and one should not assume that the danger is over as soon as a large tumor has been disentangled from a patient.

ANESTHESIA FOR OTHER GENERAL SURGICAL PROCEDURES

Operations about the neck, face, and mouth. Surgical lesions that occur in the region of the neck include thyroglossal cyst, branchial cleft sinus, and cystic hygroma. Here, endotracheal anesthesia is indicated to protect the airway from external pressure and to make room for the surgeon. Nonrebreathing techniques are satisfactory (Fig. 19-2), and most of the general anesthetics may be used provided suitable precautions are observed.[7] Cervical masses appear to involve increased danger, since four different cardiac arrests are known to have occurred during relatively simple operations on masses in the cervical region, each arrest seemingly caused by excessive vagal stimulation, surgical manipulation, inadequate atropinization, and use of cardiac-sensitizing anesthetic agents. It seems important to use atropine, at least 0.1 mg. per 10 pounds, avoid excessive manipulation of the head and neck, and especially to avoid pressure at the carotid sinus. Such precautions should make it unnecessary to rule out any desired agent.

At the termination of operations about the neck, the anesthetist should be

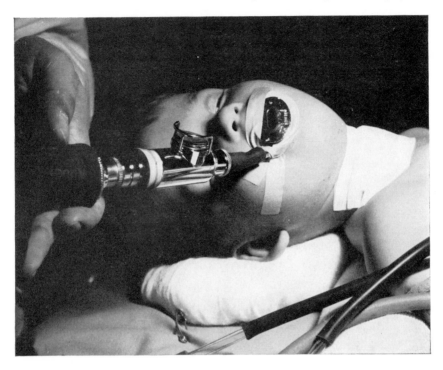

Fig. 19-2. Stephen-Slater nonrebreathing valve used during excision of branchiogenic cyst.

careful to keep the child asleep until the wound is closed and the bandage is applied—"bucking" or coughing may cause renewed bleeding in the tissues adjacent to the trachea.

Other problems may exist when large tumors obstruct the mouth. Hemangiomas and lymphangiomas of the tongue and oral tissues are not uncommon and occasionally reach considerable size (Fig. 19-3). Here, preoperative tracheostomy may be necessary to provide an airway during and after operation. Excessive bleeding may complicate removal of such tumors, and pharyngeal packing will be necessary in addition to endotracheal intubation or tracheostomy.

Esophagoscopy and esophageal dilatation may be included in the sphere of the general surgeon. Patients with congenital, traumatic, or postoperative esophageal stricture may require repeated dilatation. Recently a 16-year-old boy received his one-hundredth general anesthetic for treatment of lye stricture. Although he had refused esophagoplasty for a number of years, this was performed on his one-hundredth admission.

Anesthesia for esophageal dilatation requires relaxation but should afford pleasant induction and rapid recovery. Endotracheal halothane supplemented by succinylcholine for complete relaxation is well suited to this procedure (Fig. 19-4). Here, in an effort to decrease trauma to the glottic region and to give the surgeon maximum working space, we employ a smaller endotracheal tube than usual.

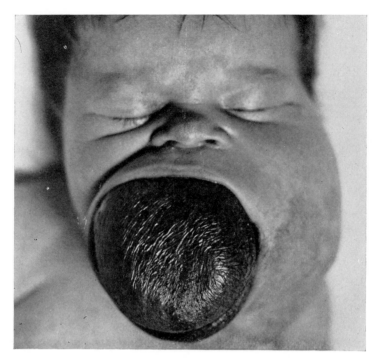

Fig. 19-3. Obstructive lesions about the mouth are not uncommon, but this hemangioma offered exceptional difficulties.

Genitourinary operations. Genitourinary problems represent an extensive branch of pediatric surgery, much of which has thus far been neglected. In dealing with patients in this area, anesthetists have several special considerations to bear in mind. The presence of renal disease may weaken the child as a whole, may create specific electrolyte imbalances, or may make the child less tolerant to certain anesthetic agents. In the presence of decreased renal function, tribromoethanol, divinyl ether, and ether are best avoided.

As with adults, the use of *d*-tubocurarine in the presence of renal disease may result in prolonged effect due to delayed excretion.

Operation upon children who have had low-grade infection of the urinary tract carries danger of sudden dissemination of infection via the bloodstream, resulting in septicemia and/or rapid elevation of body temperature. Either of these complications may be disastrous. As emphasized elsewhere (p. 455), it is extremely important to monitor body temperature in such patients.

The anesthetic management of Wilms' tumor has been discussed in preceding pages. This procedure has carried the highest incidence of severe hemorrhage of any procedure in our experience.

Operations upon the kidney itself usually require having the child in the lateral kidney position, which, if extreme, can impede both respiration and circulation. Endotracheal anesthesia with assisted or controlled respiration will be needed.

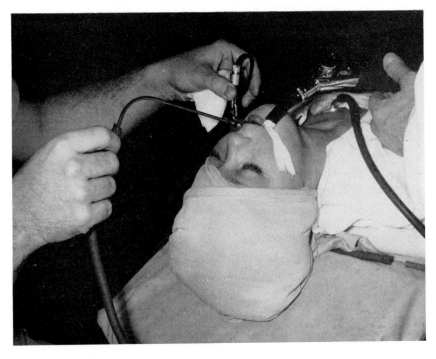

Fig. 19-4. Esophageal stricture may require repeated dilatation. Endotracheal cyclopropane and halothane are both useful and may be supplemented by relaxants if necessary.

As noted by Martin and Feeney[8] anesthesia for cystoscopic procedures deserves consideration due to the combined problem of explosion hazard and a darkened room. In such cases it is usually possible to maintain a shielded light at the patient's head.

Since the introduction of halothane, there has been slight hesitation in choosing this agent for most procedures of this kind. Patients do not require sufficient concentration of the drug to give cardiovascular depression, and the agent is well tolerated by the age groups usually encountered. Intubation is not recommended.

Uncomplicated procedures on the anterior body surface or limbs. When there is no need for endotracheal intubation and relaxants, it does not seem justifiable to use these techniques merely as routine or as labor-saving devices. Consequently, operations on the superficial tissues or limbs of children lying in the supine position may be handled by the least complicated methods. These usually consist of ether or halothane for younger children by various techniques, with additional choice of intravenous combinations for older children.

ANESTHESIA FOR PLASTIC PROCEDURES

Cleft lip repair (cheiloplasty). The management of cleft lip and cleft palate has long been a major problem in pediatric anesthesia. In an effort to provide the surgeon with free access to his field without distortion of the face and in order to overcome the problems of airway obstruction, a multitude of devices and techniques have been introduced.[9-16] Ayre's valuable T-piece nonrebreathing system, which has been so widely adapted in pediatric anesthesia, was originally devised for this procedure.[9,10] The inherent danger of the operation becomes evident when one reviews mortality statistics.

Correction of cleft lip is performed in the neonatal period by many surgeons, whereas others prefer to wait until the child is from 4 to 6 weeks old. In either case general anesthesia provides optimal conditions for the repair, and endotracheal anesthesia is almost always necessary in order to maintain the infant's airway and provide adequate control of anesthetic agents. If an operation is performed during the first days of life, intubation may be performed either awake or under anesthesia.

In infants over 2 weeks old, it is definitely better to intubate under anesthesia. This is most easily accomplished by blowing halothane and oxygen over the child's face with a T-piece system, gradually bringing the mask down on the child's face as he falls asleep.

Induction may be started with divinyl ether and ether, but this is slow and irritating. Cyclopropane is considerably better, but halothane is easily the most effective. Because of the malformation of the lip, which is frequently exaggerated by the presence of a cleft palate, there will be increased obstruction by the tongue and soft tissues, and induction may be prolonged. Intubation is also complicated by the cleft lip, into which the laryngoscope slips. To overcome these difficulties it is helpful to deepen anestheisa by the addition of ether prior to intubation and then to fit a rolled-up sponge into the cleft in the lip, to facilitate use of the laryngoscope. Use of relaxants for intubation is not advised unless one has had considerable experience with this operation.

When the infant is positioned on the table, it is advantageous to extend his head and place a padded roll under his shoulders. This increases respiratory exchange and at the same time makes the face of the child more accessible to the surgeon, who sits at the head of the table. During operation the anesthetic technique must be adapted to fulfill several needs. Apparatus must not involve increased resistance or dead space, and it must not interfere with the surgeon or contaminate the field but should provide means of assisting or controlling the infant's respiration. In spite of many innovations and variations, the Ayre system still appears to answer these demands better than any other. Although there is general agreement concerning this basic technique, there are many different modifications in the type of adapters used and in the method of draping the infant.

In order to minimize resistance and dead space, it is our belief that the vent of the nonrebreathing apparatus should be as close as possible to the infant's mouth and that it should not be covered by surgical drapes (Fig. 19-5). Consequently, the Y piece must remain in the surgical field. In order to maintain the sterility of the area, the Y-tube connections and rubber tubing are sterilized with the surgical instruments. After the endotracheal tube has been inserted, the surgeon cleans it as he prepares the surgical area and attaches the connections. The tube is not strapped in place with adhesive tape but is held in position by a

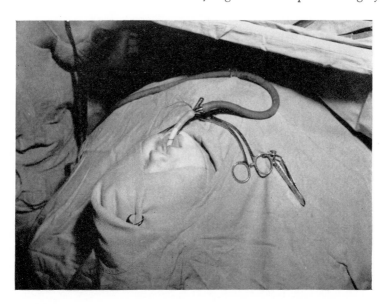

Fig. 19-5. Cleft lip repair. Airway obstruction is minimized when apparatus remains outside of drapes.

pharyngeal pack and subsequently by a tongue suture, which holds the tube to the tongue and at the same time is used to keep traction on the tongue. Since our technique calls for spontaneous respiration, ether is believed to be the best anesthetic agent. It is usually vaporized by a standard copper kettle or Boyle vaporizer. Halothane or cyclopropane may be used for rapid control if the anesthetic level becomes too light.

No method yet devised is completely satisfactory. The disadvantage with this technique is that the exhalation orifice of the Y tube lies in the surgical field and out of the anesthetist's control unless he dons gown and gloves. Actually, since ether and/or nitrous oxide are used, respiration rarely requires assistance. Should this need arise, the surgeon or his assistant may answer it by "thumbing" the open end of the Y tube.

At the completion of the operation extreme care must be taken to remove all blood and secretions from the mouth and hypopharynx. It is mandatory to visualize the hypopharynx to make sure that clots have not formed that might occlude respiration. Since respiratory exchange of these small infants is in extreme danger of obstruction by blood and secretion during recovery, it is especially important that the earliest possible awakening be provided and that the patients be attended continually until they are fully awake. Since it is the tongue that usually causes this obstruction, we have found it of tremendous value to leave a long silk suture in the infant's tongue so that it may be pulled forward and the airway cleared at any moment. The suture is removed after recovery of airway control.

Cleft palate. Repair of cleft palate is usually performed when children are slightly over 1 year of age. Here again the anesthetist is expected to maintain a safe airway without interfering with the surgeon's field. This may be accomplished by using the nasotracheal route, or by using a mouth gag fitted with the Ring modification of the tongue blade, which fits over the endotracheal tube and holds it out of the sight and field of the surgeon (p. 364). Thus far our preference has been for the nasal route largely due to greater experience in its use. This route offers slightly more difficulty, and one should have the child well relaxed before attempting intubation. Choice of the proper tube is extremely important. During operation the tube will be angulated, and there will be danger of kinking. The tube should be the largest that will pass through the naris and should be appreciably longer than would be required for oral intubation. It should be well lubricated before use.

Blind nasal intubation is not recommended in children. The tube is carefully introduced through the naris, and then the glottis is visualized with a laryngoscope and the trachea intubated under direct vision. It may be necessary to use forceps to direct the tip of the tube into the glottis or to have an assistant depress the larynx to meet the oncoming tube. Once in the larynx, the tube should be passed well beyond the cords in order to avoid dislodgement. When the tube is in place, a pharyngeal pack is inserted; otherwise blood may run along the outside surface of the tube and into the trachea.

For palate repair the patient is positioned with the head extended, and the headrest is slightly lowered, as for cleft lip repair. The surgeon prepares the face, cleans the external end of the endotracheal tube, fixes it to the face with sterilized Scotch tape, and then attaches a sterile Y tube and length of rubber tubing to the catheter so that the entire field is relatively uncontaminated (Fig. 19-6). Although the palate that is to be repaired is hardly in a sterile area, introduction of foreign pathogens will increase the risk of wound infection and is definitely to be avoided.

Anesthesia is maintained with halothane or by nitrous oxide supplemented by ether. During operation, special care must be taken to prevent respiratory depression and to watch for obstruction that may be caused by kinking of the endotracheal tube, endobronchial intubation, or blood or secretions that may be present—these causes of obstruction can occur in spite of efforts to prevent them.

Extubation must be accomplished with care. Both the surgeon and the anesthetist should visualize the hypopharynx to see that packing and blood have been removed and that the child leaves the table in the best possible condition. Careful stethoscopic examination of the chest should be performed before and after extubation to check respiratory exchange. Occasionally it will be necessary to use suction in the trachea after operation. During recovery the patient is placed in the prone position and given individual attention until fully awake.

Anomalies associated with cleft palate. Children with cleft palate may have micrognathia or other facial malformations that make intubation extremely difficult. In two instances intubation was impossible, and operation was postponed until the situation was improved by growth of the child.

An association of defects known as micrognathia or the *Pierre Robin syndrome*[17-19] deserves special attention. This consists of a cleft palate, an underde-

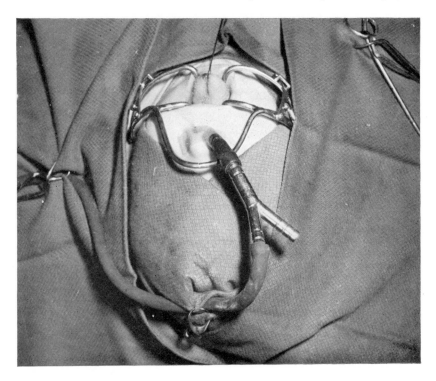

Fig. 19-6. Nasotracheal anesthesia for cleft palate repair.

veloped, receding mandible, and backward displacement of the tongue, a truly dangerous combination. Tracheostomy may be necessary as an emergency measure in early infancy. When these infants are operated upon for palate repair, they present special airway problems before, during, and after operation. Intubation is difficult, and it is usually necessary to use the oral rather than the nasal route. Following operation special nursing care is necessary, and tracheostomy may be indicated at any stage.[20] All of these infants should be kept in the prone position, and a long suture should be left in the tongue for traction.

Although it is possible under some circumstances to anesthetize infants for harelip or cleft palate repair without endotracheal intubation, it is not justifiable to undertake such an operation if the airway is endangered by anomalous conditions that would make intubation difficult in case of emergency.

Because of the problems previously discussed, operations for cleft lip and cleft palate have been associated with an appreciable mortality throughout the country.[21] It has been our good fortune, however, to be associated with an extremely meticulous surgeon whose record consists of 3,636 cleft lip and cleft palate procedures without a death.

Other plastic procedures. In addition to correction of harelip and cleft palate, a variety of plastic procedures may be performed in children, among which are the correction of lop ears, webbed finger repair, skin graft, and others. These provide relatively few problems to the anesthetist in most instances. Lop ear repair is performed in smaller children under endotracheal ether or halothane anesthesia with nonrebreathing technique, whereas intravenous agents may be used in older children if desired. Correction of webbed fingers is usually performed in young children and is a simple but time-consuming procedure. Light general anesthesia is well tolerated, but, due to the duration, one should pay increased attention to maintenance of body temperature, blood pressure, and oxygenation. Endotracheal intubation is rarely necessary. Long duration of anesthesia is not of itself an indication for intubation.

Anesthesia for burned patients. Management of acutely burned patients is described later (p. 388). Burn dressings and subsequent correction of scar contractures may involve additional problems. Children with extensive burns require frequent dressings. The mental anguish of multiple anesthetics may be considerable—these procedures are painful, and attempts to carry them out under heavy sedation or hypnosis have not been highly successful. One important feature in treating these children is to have the same anesthetist put them to sleep each time and pay special attention to them in order to sustain their morale.

Choice of anesthesia has been a serious problem in these critically sick children. Cyclopropane is pleasant and helps to retain body heat, but the explosive hazard is increased because it is necessary to move and turn the child during dressings. Halothane is easy, pleasant, and effective, and its use for numerous anesthetics in the same child has been documented.[22,23] However, although there appears to be slight risk involved, the possibility of sensitivity reaction still exists.[24,25]

The intravenous agent CI-581 is reported by Domino, Chodoff, and Corsson[26] to be well suited to this work, since it affords marked analgesia and very rapid recovery.[27] Because blood loss may be marked,[28] infusions should be established before removal of dressings, and ample provision must be made for blood trans-

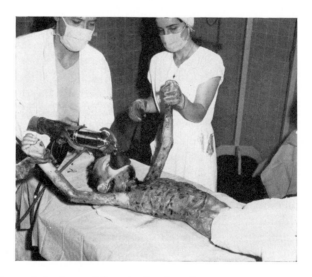

Fig. 19-7. Blood loss and shock may follow the dressing of large burns.

fusion (Fig. 19-7). Exposure of large raw surfaces followed by application of dressings of cold ointment often causes marked heat loss and discomfort on awakening. This may be avoided by warming room, patient, and dressings.

A series of deaths and cardiac arrests has been reported associated with the use of succinylcholine in burned children.[29-31] McCaughey[29] pointed out the odd similarity of these cases. In many of them the children tolerated succinylcholine uneventfully during the first 14 days after being burned. When given succinylcholine during the third week, they promptly suffered arrest, and in many cases it was terminal.

Question has been raised as to whether this period in the recovery from burns renders a child sensitive to succinylcholine due to toxicity, reduced pseudo-cholinesterase, electrolyte imbalance, or other factors. While McCaughey indicts

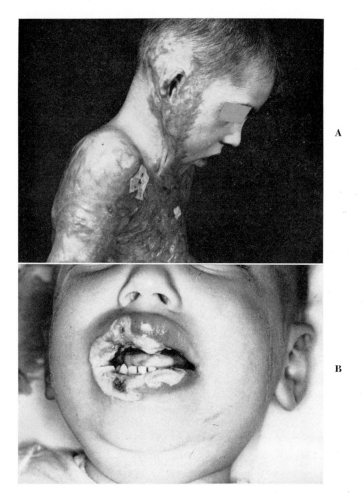

Fig. 19-8. A, Burn contracture of neck. **B,** Electric burn of mouth. (**A,** From Epstein, B. S., Rudman, H. L., Hardy, D. L., and Downes, H.: Anesth. Analg. 45:352, 1966; **B,** Courtesy Dr. A. Colodny, Boston, Mass.

the drug and believes it to be contraindicated during burn therapy, Lowenstein,[32] reviewing a large series of burned children, found only one arrest, obviously due to hypovolemia, and exonerated succinylcholine. Tolmie, Joyce, and Mitchell[33] investigated electrolytes in a burned soldier during four successive procedures showing in each typical cardiac depression or arrest in response to succinylcholine. They found that a significant elevation of serum potassium occurred in each reaction and believe this to be the probable mechanism.

Of the many problems posed by burn contractures, some of the worst are seen in scars around the neck, causing severe retraction of the chin and sometimes making intubation extremely difficult (Fig. 19-8). Awake intubation often frightens small children, and relaxants are ill advised. General anesthesia should be attempted. If additional help is needed, Epstein and associates[34] suggest having the surgeon incise the lateral cords of scar overlying the sternocleidomastoid muscles. This simple maneuver reportedly facilitates intubation greatly.

The repair of epispadias or hypospadias is usually performed when boys are in their early teens and are rather conscious of their deformities. Consequently, adequate preoperative sedation is indicated so that their trip to the operating room will not be unnecessarily embarrassing. For the same reason regional anesthesia, which otherwise might be ideal, is better avoided. General anesthesia with cyclopropane or halothane is chosen because relaxation is desirable, and the unpleasantness of ether should be avoided in patients who must return for a series of operations. Thiopental and nitrous oxide may be used here, but relaxants and endotracheal intubation do not seem justified.

REFERENCES

1. Apgar, V., and Papper, E. M.: Pheochromocytoma, anesthetic management during surgical treatment, Arch. Surg. **62:**634-648, 1951.
2. Thompson, J. E., and Arrowood, J. G.: Pheochromocytoma: surgical and anesthetic management, Anesthesiology, **15:**658-665, 1954.
3. Nelson, W. E., editor: Textbook of pediatrics, ed. 7, Philadelphia, 1958, W. B. Saunders Co.
4. Shwachman, H., Pryles, C. P., and Gross, R. E.: Meconium ileus, a clinical study of twenty surviving patients, Amer. J. Dis. Child. **91:**223-244, 1956.
5. Stephen, C. R.: Anesthesia in infants and young children for major surgical procedures, Arch. Surg. **60:**1035-1044, 1950.
6. Etsten, B.: Personal communication.
7. Macdonald, D. J. F.: Cystic hygroma. An anaesthetic and surgical problem, Anaesthesia **21:**66-80, 1967.
8. Martin, S. J., and Feeney, T. M.: Anesthesia in pediatric urology, J.A.M.A. **148:**180-183, 1952.
9. Ayre, P.: Anaesthesia for hare-lip and cleft palate operations on babies, Brit. J. Surg. **25:**131-132, 1937.
10. Ayre, P.: Endotracheal anesthesia for babies: with special reference to harelip and cleft palate operations, Anesth. Analg. **16:**330-333, 1937.
11. Slocum, H. C., and Allen, C. R.: Orotracheal anesthesia for cheiloplasty, Anesthesiology **6:**355-358, 1945.
12. Leigh, M. D., and Kester, H. A.: Endotracheal anesthesia for operations on cleft lip and cleft palate, Anesthesiology **9:**32-41, 1948.
13. Kilduff, C. J., Wyant, G. M., and Dale, R. H.: Anaesthesia for repair of cleft lip and palate in infants, using moderate hypothermia, Canad. Anaesth. Soc. J. **3:**102-107, 1956.
14. Whalen, J. S., and Conn, A. W.: Improved technics in anesthetic management for repair of cleft lips and palates, Anesth. Analg. **46:**355-363, 1967.

15. Musgrove, R. H., and Bremmer, J. C.: Complications of cleft palate surgery, J. Plast. Reconstr. Surg. **26**:180-189, 1960.
16. Masters, F., Hansen, J., and Robinson, D.: Anesthetic complications in plastic surgery, J. Plast. Reconstr. Surg. **24**:472-480, 1959.
17. Robin, P.: La chute de la base de la langue considéré comme une nouvelle cause de gêne dans la respiration naso-pharyngienne, Bull. Acad. méd., Paris **89**:37-41, 1923.
18. Bougas, T. P., and Smith, R. M.: Pathologic airway obstruction in children, Anesth. Analg. **37**:137-146, 1958.
19. Davenport, H. T., and Rosales, J. K.: Endotracheal intubation of infants and children, Canad. Anaesth. Soc. J. **6**:65-74, 1959.
20. MacCollum, D. W., and Richardson, S. O.: Care of the child with cleft lip and cleft palate, Amer. J. Nurs. **58**:211-216, 1958.
21. Salanitre, E., and Rackow, H.: Changing trends in the anesthetic management of the child with cleft lip palate malformation, Anesthesiology **23**:610-617, 1962.
22. Visser, E. R., and Tarrow, A. B.: Fluothane for multiple burn dressing anesthetics, Anesth. Analg. **38**:301-305, 1959.
23. Bolcic-Wikerhauser, J.: Multiple halothane anesthetics, Brit. J. Anaesth. **38**:228-230, 1966.
24. Popper, H., Rubin, E., Gardiol, D., Schaffner, F., and Paronetto, F.: Drug-induced liver disease. A penalty for progress, Arch. Intern. Med. **115**:128-136, 1965.
25. Davidson, C. S., Babior, B., and Popper, H.: Concerning hepatotoxicity of halothane, New Eng. J. Med. **275**:1497, 1966.
26. Domino, E. F., Chodoff, P., and Corsson, G.: Pharmacologic effects of CI-581, a new dissociative anesthetic in man, Clin. Pharm. Therap. **6**:279-291, 1965.
27. Wilson, R. D., Nichols, R. J., and McCoy, N. R.: Dissociative anesthesia with CI-581 in burned children, Anesth. Analg. **46**:719-724, 1967.
28. Pretorius, J. A.: Blood loss in paediatric surgery, Anaesthesia **15**:424-432, 1960.
29. McCaughey, T. J.: Hazards of anaesthesia for the burned child, Canad. Anaesth. Soc. J. **9**:220-234, 1962.
30. Middleton, H. G., and Wolfson, L. J.: Anaesthesia in burns, Brit. Med. Bull. **14**:42, 1958.
31. Bush, G. H.: The use of muscle relaxants in burnt children, Anaesthesia **19**:231, 1964.
32. Lowenstein, E.: Succinylcholine administration in the burned patient, Anesthesiology **27**:494, 1966.
33. Tolmie, J. D., Joyce, T. W., and Mitchell, G. D.: Succinylcholine danger in the burned patient, Anesthesiology **28**:467-470, 1967.
34. Epstein, B. S., Rudman, H. L., Hardy, D. L., and Downes, H.: Comparison of orotracheal intubation with tracheostomy for anesthesia in patients with face and neck burns, Anesth. Analg. **45**:352-359, 1966.

Chapter 20

Anesthesia for orthopedic surgery

Operations and underlying conditions
Features of orthopedic surgery that concern anesthesia
Anesthetic agents and techniques
    Children under 6 years of age
    Children 6 or more years of age
Anesthetic management of specific problems
    Traumatic lesions
    Spinal fusion
    Operations on patients with cerebral palsy
    Anesthesia for respirator patients
Complications

OPERATIONS AND UNDERLYING CONDITIONS

In a children's hospital that has an active orthopedic service a variety of operations are performed on bones, joints, and tendons. These procedures include open and closed reduction of fractures and dislocations, tendon release or transplant, osteotomy or fusion of long bones or spine, bone graft, amputation, and a number of others. Although such procedures present the anesthetist with a variety of problems, of much greater concern are the many different metabolic and pathologic conditions from which the operative lesions originate. A representative list of orthopedic problems is given in Table 20-1. These and others are described in standard texts of pediatrics[1] and orthopedic surgery.[2]

FEATURES OF ORTHOPEDIC SURGERY THAT CONCERN ANESTHESIA

Each type of surgery has a pattern of its own. In general, orthopedic operations performed on children have the following characteristics:

1. The patients often are chronically ill or have pathologic conditions that affect respiration, structural support, or body metabolism.
2. Many patients must return repeatedly for a series of corrective operations.
3. Operations may be of long duration (3 to 4 hours).

Table 20-1. *Conditions encountered in orthopedic surgery for children*

1. Traumatic conditions	3. Disturbances of growth or metabolism
(a) Fractures, dislocations	(a) Arthrogryposis
(simple, compound, single, or	(b) Idiopathic scoliosis
multiple)	(c) Osteodystrophy
2. Congenital anomalies	(d) Chondrodystrophy
(a) Congenital dislocated	(e) Leg length discrepancy
hip	(f) Streeter's dysplasia
(b) Torticollis	4. Residual poliomyelitis
(c) Congenital clubfoot	5. Bone tumors (benign and malignant)
(d) Sprengel's deformity	6. Cerebral palsy
(e) Absence of tibia, ulna,	7. Osteomyelitis with joint infection
etc.	8. Hemophilia with joint effusion

4. Preoperative skeletal immobilization may complicate preparation and anesthesia.
5. Deep relaxation is seldom necessary.
6. The use of cautery and x-ray may be expected.
7. A tourniquet is often used to control bleeding during operations on the arm or leg.
8. Casts and apparatus may limit postoperative positioning.

The management of anesthesia is determined by adapting the standard pediatric methods to fit the special considerations just mentioned. Usually the demands of the surgeon are not hard to meet. Except for spinal fusion, operations seldom affect vital functions. The main task of the anesthetist often consists of supporting a debilitated child through a procedure of several hours' duration.

The anesthetist's preoperative visit is especially important in orthopedic surgery. The underlying disease may be an unusual disorder, the significance of which will not be recognized. Such conditions as Marfan's syndrome, Morquio's disease, and Streeter's dysplasia are not common, but there are many uncommon diseases, and all combine to make an appreciable number. The anesthetist should learn the nature and the extent of the disease before accepting the child as his responsibility. In such a lesion as Streeter's dysplasia (Fig. 20-1) the deformities of the limbs usually represent the only pathology, but in Marfan's disease organic changes often complicate the problem. Any child who has had poliomyelitis should be investigated thoroughly to determine the extent of residual respiratory impairment. As will be mentioned later, a careful preoperative estimation is imperative before spinal fusion for scoliosis.

The fact that children often must return for several operations makes it necessary to spend extra time with them to keep up their morale and to overcome their apprehension (Fig. 20-2). Preoperative sedation may be a problem if a child is apprehensive but at the same time has poor respiratory function because of muscular weakness. In such cases barbiturates seem to be well tolerated and are ordered in moderate dosage, but narcotics are avoided.

During orthopedic operations the dangers associated with long procedures are especially to be feared. A slight degree of hypoventilation gradually leads to

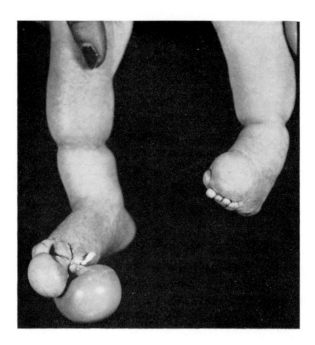

Fig. 20-1. Streeter's dysplasia. Typical circular constriction in legs, with distal deformities.

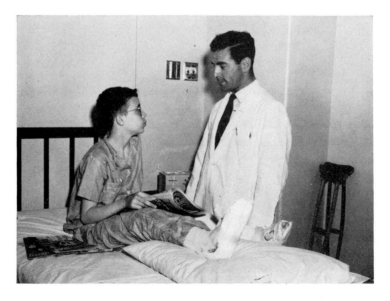

Fig. 20-2. Frequent visits help maintain morale of patients who must return for repeated operations.

serious hypoxia and hypercapnia. Similarly, insidious blood loss during an "uneventful" 4 hours operation may go unnoticed until shock suddenly becomes evident. Since anesthetists often overestimate blood loss and surgeons underestimate it, measurement is definitely advisable in these procedures.

It is especially disadvantageous that many orthopedic patients must return for repeated operations and in addition that each of these operations may be of 3 to 4 hours in duration. This appears to increase the risk of developing sensitivity to halogenated anesthetics. Having encountered this complication twice, it now seems wise to avoid repeated use of these anesthetics if others may be easily substituted.

In some cases surgeons have developed the practice of keeping children in plastic jackets or body casts during anesthesia and surgery.[3] The danger of respiratory embarrassment, the greater difficulty in endotracheal intubation, and the inaccessibility of the chest in case of cardiac arrest are certainly ample arguments upon which to condemn this practice.

The danger of pressure areas and nerve injury makes it imperative to position the patients carefully and to check them frequently. Masks should be removed, and the face should be massaged gently every 10 to 15 minutes to prevent pressure injury or ether burns. Special care must be taken to protect the eyes. When the patient is face down, the head should be repositioned every 15 minutes.

Perhaps the greatest over-all anesthetic problem in such long procedures is derived from the fact that they are not very exciting for the anesthetist and after a few hours may lead to monotony and inattention unless special measures are taken. Such measures, as outlined on p. 180, include the following of a strict routine of check points, frequent visits by instructors or colleagues, and the use of minor changes in anesthetic technique to provide additional interest in the case.

The *use of a tourniquet* occasionally introduces minor complications in orthopedic procedures. A tourniquet applied at the thigh does not produce any generalized signs at first. After a half hour or more it may cause gradual increase in pulse rate and blood pressure and more active respiration. In some cases it may actually be difficult to keep the child anesthetized in spite of using high concentrations of anesthetic agents. The penetration of tourniquet pain in the presence of spinal anesthesia has been reported,[4] and a similar penetration appears to occur during the use of inhalation agents. When the blood pressure and pulse become elevated during such a procedure, one must rule out other possible causes before assuming it to be due to the tourniquet. These include hypoxia, soda-lime exhaustion, hypoventilation, and other forms of sympathetic nervous stimulation.

When the tourniquet is released, the fall in blood pressure usually is prompt and may be marked (Fig. 20-3). When the fall in blood pressure is severe, a peripheral vasopressor agent may be indicated, provided blood replacement has been adequate. If the child had required a strong anesthetic mixture prior to release of the tourniquet, he may suddenly become deeply anesthetized unless the strength of the mixture is reduced.

In the postoperative period casts or traction apparatus may be used that

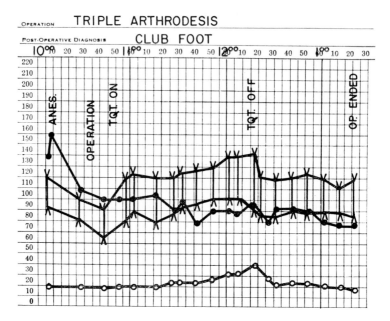

Fig. 20-3. Anesthesia chart of 6-year-old girl showing gradual rise in blood pressure under ether anesthesia while leg is compressed by tourniquet, with distinct fall upon release of tourniquet. Similar changes have been observed with halothane and other anesthetics.

make it necessary for the child to lie flat on his back. If vomiting occurs before the return of gag reflexes, the child may be in serious trouble. Anesthesia for such patients should be chosen to provide rapid return of reflexes. If prompt recovery does not seem likely, an endotracheal tube may be used to protect the airway until the child awakens. In either case the child should remain in the operating room or recovery ward under individual observation until the danger of aspiration has passed.

ANESTHETIC AGENTS AND TECHNIQUES

Children under 6 years of age. Although there is a wide variety in orthopedic procedures at all ages, the management of anesthesia for younger patients may differ basically from that of older children. In small children the operation is less likely to be repetitive. These children are thought to have a high immunity to hepatic toxicity of all types, and they are often less willing candidates for intravenous anesthesia. For these reasons we continue to favor inhalation agents for most smaller children. Ether may be employed, by open, semiopen, or closed techniques, but the explosive hazard now has largely eliminated ether from orthopedic procedures due to the frequent use of cautery or x-ray. One definite advantage of ether is the analgesia provided during early recovery, since these children often awaken in pain unless protected.

Halogenated agents are certainly most widely used in this age group in America, and it is hard to deny the ease of administration and usual freedom from complication. In our experience halothane has been preferable to other halogenated agents for orthopedic work, largely because it has caused considerably less postoperative nausea than related agents. Rapid awakening makes prompt use of analgesia important. Although standard narcotics are quite satisfactory for this, pentazocine has been remarkably effective, using intravenous dosage of 0.4 mg. per kilogram.

As related below, it now seems preferable to avoid repeated use of halogenated agents for orthopedic procedures. After a child has had halothane once, halothane may be used for induction subsequently, if it is discontinued as soon as an infusion has been started. Thereafter intravenous agents, supplemented by nitrous oxide, appear to be safer.

There is often some difficulty in the decision to intubate small children during orthopedic operations. For torticollis correction or procedures on children in prone position intubation obviously is required, but for a 3-hour operation on a child lying supine there are two sides to remember. Although it will be easier to maintain a clear airway in such relatively long operations if the trachea is intubated, it is also true that the longer the operation, the greater is the risk of irritation to trachea and cords. A complication that has occurred several times in patients during prolonged endotracheal anesthesia is occlusion of the endotracheal tube by dried secretions that could not be cleared by suction catheter.

Children 6 or more years of age. The older children who require orthopedic operations more frequently appear to need a series of procedures, often coming at intervals of only 2 or 3 weeks.

It is now our policy to give a halogenated agent only once to these patients, and not use any halogenated agent at a later operation. Although the risk may not be great in proportion to the number of anesthetics administered, it is a risk of death, which for any patient involved is total and permanent. While there may be a warning of developing sensitivity evidenced in postoperative temperature elevation, this can easily pass unnoticed or fail to be noted at the time of the subsequent operation. It seems better to avoid this hazard by not exposing the child to these agents a second time, at least within 6 months.

Fortunately these children usually have easily accessible veins, tolerate venipuncture well, and are candidates for many anesthetic techniques. In general we have replaced halogenated agents by intravenous anesthetics and narcotics, using combinations of thiopental, relaxants, narcotics, and ataractics with nitrous oxide supplementation.[6] Many procedures may be performed with nitrous oxide and thiopental alone, using no more than 20 mg. of thiopental per kilogram of body weight. Relaxant combinations can be used as described in Chapter 14. Recently we have been especially pleased with the combination of morphine and propiomazine (Largon) using approximately 1 mg. of morphine and 2 mg. of propiomazine per 10 kilograms.

Local and regional blocks have been recommended for orthopedic procedures in children. Their use is especially valuable if there has been head injury or recent ingestion of food. If a patient has had poliomyelitis, it is perhaps questionable whether spinal anesthesia would do any further harm, but it would certainly be inadvisable from a legal standpoint, except under the condition that total motor loss were already present. For removal of a kidney stone in a patient with paralysis below the waist, spinal anesthesia might be the best agent to use because it would threaten only that area already damaged beyond repair.

ANESTHETIC MANAGEMENT OF SPECIFIC PROBLEMS

Traumatic lesions. Severe injuries involving a crushed chest or fractures of the skull, vertebrae, pelvis, or long bones may be associated with shock, hemorrhage, or brain injury, all of which demand specific treatment similar to that used for adults. Following blood replacement and adequate stabilization, emergency measures may be accomplished under local or regional block or cyclopropane, if shock is well under control.

More frequently children require treatment for such minor accidents as simple Colles' fractures. Since one can never be sure that such children have not eaten recently, the safest method is to forego general anesthesia and employ a brachial block, preferably by the axillary route (p. 197). If general anesthesia is chosen, one may give sedation with atropine and morphine and then use nitrous oxide–oxygen anesthesa, thus maintaining the gag reflex and protecting the child from the danger of aspiration of vomited food (Chapter 24). If more relaxation is needed, anesthesia is induced with an inhalation agent and the trachea is intubated. The endotracheal tube is then left in place until the child is awake.

Spinal fusion. Children who require fusion of the spine for scoliosis deserve special consideration inasmuch as they often are in poor physical condition before operation, and the operation itself may be a traumatic and shocking procedure.

Scoliosis may be idiopathic in origin, but it often is secondary to poliomyelitis. In either case operation is not usually necessary until the child is 10 or 12 years old.

Prior to operation the patient should be examined carefully as to the cause and extent of the scoliosis (Fig. 20-4). If the deformity is secondary to poliomyelitis, the history of the disease must be investigated to find the degree of respiratory involvement originally present. Further information is then sought concerning the patient's respiratory function, his exercise capacity, and *his exchange when lying in the position he is to assume during the operation.* It is important to know what he has been able to do in the period immediately before operation, whether he has been weakened by immobilization in a cast or has been allowed to walk and exercise. Roentgen-ray films of the spine, thorax, lungs, and heart should be studied by the anesthetist to see the degree of curvature of the spine, the angulation of the ribs, the position of the heart and diaphragm, and the expansion of the lungs (Fig. 20-5). Deformity may be severe enough to cause real limitation of cardiac function that, if not relieved, has been found to lead to cardiorespiratory failure and early death.[8-10] Adequate laboratory studies should be made, and the anesthetist should find out whether the fusion is to involve the thoracic or lumbar area and how many veterbrae are to be exposed.

Preoperative medication usually should be ordered with care to prevent post-

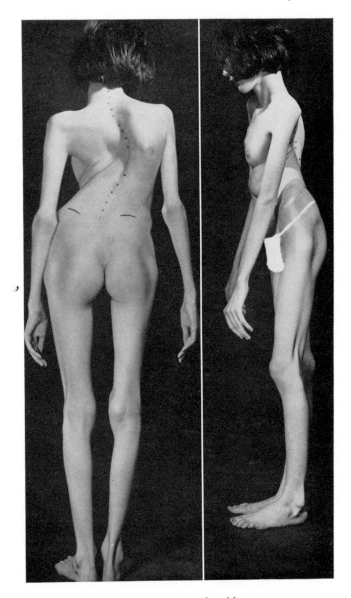

Fig. 20-4. Patients with severe scoliosis are poor operative risks.

operative respiratory depression. Blood should be prepared in generous quantities.

Induction of anesthesia may be accomplished by inhalation or intravenous methods. Thiopental followed by succinylcholine for intubation is often chosen for this age group. Since respiration will be assisted or controlled, a cuffed endotracheal tube is preferable in teen-aged children. A circle absorption system is usually indicated.

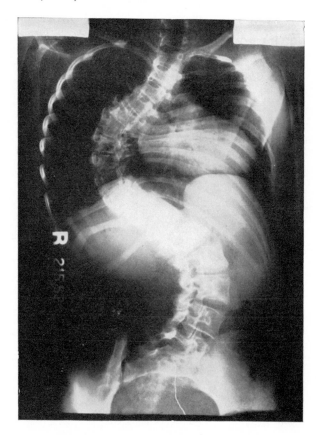

Fig. 20-5. Extreme scoliotic deformity with compression of heart and lung.

For maintenance of anesthesia one has a fairly wide choice. Explosive agents are best avoided, but halogenated inhalation agents, relaxant techniques, or neuroleptanalgesia may be employed provided ventilation is adequately maintained. This operation is one in which use of a ventilating device may be advantageous.

Positioning these patients is extremely important. It is hardly possible to satisfy the surgeon without severely hampering the child's normal respiratory exchange. Consequently, it seems inadvisable to attempt any method relying upon spontaneous exchange, but to assist or control respiration throughout the entire procedure.

Usually supports are placed under the patient to flex the lumbar spine slightly, the arms are extended with elbows flexed, and the knees are slightly flexed. The face is supported in a padded headrest, and one must be sure that the chin is not pressed against the end of the table.

A reliable infusion is mandatory. It is our custom to start infusions in the dorsum of each hand using large-bore needles or catheters.

During spinal fusion the chief dangers consist of hypoventilation, blood loss, and shock. Hypoventilation must be prevented by maintaining a light plane of anesthesia, by assisting respiration, and by stethoscopic monitoring of ventilation throughout the entire procedure. In these patients an esophageal stethoscope usually is more reliable. Blood loss and shock are due to the combined effect of an extensive wound invovling both soft tissue and bone, considerable chiseling and pounding against the thorax, and an additional wound along the lower leg if a tibial graft is taken. When Harrington rods are used for supplementary fixation, considerably more operative trauma and hemorrhage may be expected. Blood pressure should be followed closely, and blood loss should be estimated by weighing sponges and by noting the loss in the suction bottle. The amount of blood administered usually needs to be 100 to 200 ml. more than the measured loss. If signs of shock appear, the surgeons should be asked to halt their work until blood loss is made up and the child's condition becomes stabilized.

At the end of the operation care must be taken not to turn or move the patient too quickly. Children who show any signs of cardiovascular irregularity or shock should be kept face down on the operating table until they are definitely out of danger. As noted by Thomas,[11] it is preferable to keep the endotracheal tube in place until consciousness returns.

Operations on patients with cerebral palsy. Tendon-relaxing operations are often indicated on children with cerebral palsy and other spastic conditions. There are two features of interest here. Although these children often are unable to talk and may appear to be mentally retarded, they may be extremely alert and unusually apprehensive. Consequently, the anesthetist must give them every consideration, explaining the steps to be taken and showing even more patience and gentleness than usual.

The spastic element of the disease may make tendon repair difficult unless additional relaxation is provided. If it is necessary to establish a deeper plane of anesthesia, care must be taken not to expose the patient to overdosage of anesthetic agents or cardiorespiratory depression. Use of relaxants is helpful here, provided a tourniquet has not been applied to the limb on which the operation is performed.

Anesthesia for respirator patients. Patients who are completely paralyzed and depend upon continual support of mechanical respirators occasionally require anesthesia for bronchoscopic suction, tracheostomy, removal of kidney stone, or tendon transplant. Obviously these patients present very definite problems because of their respiratory weakness. In addition, metabolic imbalances will occur whether the patient is in an early acute phase or has suffered prolonged inactivity. Finally, the psychologic problem is a difficult one because these patients become extremely apprehensive if anything threatens the weakened thread upon which their lives depend.

In the anesthetic management of such patients it may be assumed that complete control of respiration must be supplied continuously before, during, and after operation. Although this means that ventilation must be performed meticulously for these sensitive patients, it also becomes evident that there will be little danger involved in the use of sedatives, which ordinarily might act as respiratory depressants. Greater dangers in the use of sedatives and anesthetics lie in the possible stimulation or thickening of bronchial secretions and in depression of the ability to cough and clear the airway after operation. Consequently, drugs that are irritative or drying or that depress the cough reflex are to be avoided.

For bronchoscopy the use of a cuirass respirator[12,13] affords an easy solution to the problem. Anesthesia may be induced with nitrous oxide and relaxant or with cyclopropane. Halothane has very little irritant effect on tracheal mucosa, and the postoperative depression of cough is negligible; hence its choice seems logical.

Similar principles may be applied to anesthesia for respirator patients undergoing such operative procedures as tendon transplant or capsulotomy. Ether is to be avoided, but thiopental, cyclopropane, and relaxants appear to be justified, and, again, halothane is probably the best of all. If bradycardia occurs, enough atropine may be administered to reestablish the original pulse rate. Often tendon transplant is performed on the hand, in which case a cuirass respirator may be used to ventilate the patient throughout operation, and regional block may be employed for anesthesia. At first it seemed best to try to avoid endotracheal intubation. It has been used in a number of cases without subsequent complications, and intubation is now performed with confidence. Whatever agent is used, it is extremely important to clear the airway very thoroughly at the end of the procedure.

Careful supervision must be continued until the respiratory apparatus is replaced and the child is reestablished in his bed on the ward. Frequent postoperative visits are made to check respiratory exchange and to examine the child for evidence of atelectasis or excessive secretions.

COMPLICATIONS

To emphasize the fact that complications can happen during anesthesia for orthopedic surgery, the following experiences are described.

A 10-year-old girl underwent a femoral stapling operation. As a result of faulty positioning she suffered postoperative brachial palsy that persisted for 3 months.

A 12-year-old Negro girl required manipulation of her ankle following poliomyelitis. After a 20-minute ether anesthesia the mask was removed, and the patient's heart stopped completely and permanently. Autopsy showed myocardial involvement of poliomyelitis, but the origin of the arrest was unknown.

A strong 16-year-old boy was operated upon for correction of spondylolisthesis. The surgeon was extremely eager to do the operation with the boy face down, lying in the anterior half of a body cast. With the patient intubated it appeared that this could be done without excessive risk. The procedure progressed for 3 hours under ether, with respiration assisted continuously. There were some secretions, but the patient's condition did not appear critical in any way. As the skin sutures were being placed, the anesthetist hyperventilated the patient with several rather forceful compressions of the breathing bag. The heart action stopped almost instantly. The patient was turned over, his chest was opened, and the heart, which was fibrillating, was defibrillated and resuscitated, but the patient died 8 hours later. The only explanation of this tragedy seemed to be that ventilation had been inadequate, allowing serious accumulation of carbon dioxide. In the manner shown by Young, Sealy, and Harris,[14] the sudden removal of excess carbon dioxide may have mobilized enough free potassium to cause cardiac fibrillation and subsequent death.

All of the preceding complications occurred between 1946 and 1952, and they probably would not occur under present conditions. Of far greater importance are two cases of liver necrosis that occurred during 1967. One child 11 years old received halothane during 3 prolonged procedures, following which she showed rapidly advancing signs of liver failure and died. The second child (9 years old) received halothane for one operation and methoxyflurane for the second, and subsequently showed symptoms of moderately severe hepatotoxicity, but recovered. Thorough examination of each case showed typical course of sensitivity development[15,16] and left little doubt that these incidents were induced by halogenated anesthetics.

REFERENCES

1. Nelson, W. E., editor: Textbook of pediatrics, ed. 7, Philadelphia, 1959, W. B. Saunders Co.
2. Shands, A. R., Jr. and Raney, R. B.: Handbook of orthopaedic surgery, ed. 7, St. Louis, 1967, The C. V. Mosby Co.
3. Denton, M. V. H., and O'Donoghue, D. M.: Anaesthesia and the scoliotic patient, Anaesthesia 10:366-368, 1955.
4. Cole, F.: Tourniquet pain, Anesth. Analg. 31:63-65, 1952.
5. Anderson, S. M.: Use of depressant and relaxant drugs in infants and children, Lancet 2:965-966, 1951.
6. Foldes, F. F., Ceravelo, A. J., and Carpenter, S. L.: The administration of nitrous oxide–oxygen anesthesia in closed systems, Ann. Surg. 136:978-981, 1952.
7. Small, G. A.: Brachial plexus block anesthesia in children, J.A.M.A. 147:1648-1651, 1951.
8. Fischer, J. W., and Dolehide, R. A.: Fatal cardiac failure in persons with thoracic deformities, Arch. Intern. Med. 93:687-697, 1954.
9. Coombs, C. F.: Fatal cardiac failure occurring in persons with angular deformity of the spine, Brit. J. Surg. 18:326-328, 1930.
10. Bergofsky, E. H., Turino, G. M., and Fishman, A. P.: Cadiorespiratory failure in hyphoscoliosis, Medicine 38:263, 1959.
11. Thomas, D. V.: Anesthesia in operations for scoliosis, Anesth. Analg. 36:34-37, 1957.
12. Green, R. A., and Coleman, D. J.: Cuirass respirator for endoscopy, Anaesthesia 10:369-373, 1953.
13. Sleath, G. E., and Graves, H. B.: The use of the cuirass respirator during laryngoscopy and bronchoscopy under general anaesthesia, Canad. Anaesth. Soc. J. 5:330-337, 1958.
14. Young, W. G., Jr., Sealy, W. C., Harris, J. S.: The role of intracellular and extracellular electrolytes in the cardiac arrhythmias produced by prolonged hypercapnia, Surgery 36:636-649, 1954.
15 Popper, H., Rubin, E., Gandiol, D., Schaffner, F., and Paronetto, F.: Drug-induced liver disease. A penalty for progress, Arch. Intern. Med. 115:128-136, 1965.
16. Davidson, C. S., Babior, B., and Popper, H.: Concerning hepatotoxicity of halothane, New Eng. J. Med. 275:1497, 1966.

Chapter 21

Anesthesia for pediatric neurosurgery

DIAGNOSTIC AND THERAPEUTIC PROCEDURES INVOLVED

Neurosurgery in infants and children includes the treatment of trauma to the head, spine, and peripheral nerves, correction of hydrocephalus and various congenital defects, excision of tumors and vascular malformations, treatment of brain abscess and complications of bacterial meningitis, cortical resection for epilepsy, and elective procedures performed for the relief of pain and involuntary movements. In addition, "contrast" diagnostic procedures are frequently performed in the investigation of neurologic disorders.[1] Many of those in infants and children must be carried out under general anesthesia (Table 21-1).

ANESTHETIC PROBLEMS

In planning the management of anesthesia, one must bear in mind several factors characteristic of pediatric neurosurgery:

Table 21-1. *Operative neurosurgical procedures*

---

1. Diagnostic procedures
   (a) Lumbar puncture
   (b) Pneumoencephalography
   (c) Ventricular tap and ventriculography
   (d) Myelography
   (e) Angiography
   (f) Burr holes
2. Therapeutic procedures
   (a) Correction of congenital lesions
       (1) Excision of meningocele, encephalocele
       (2) Shunt procedures for hyrocephalus
       (3) Craniectomy for craniosynostosis
   (b) Treatment for traumatic lesions
       (1) Elevation of depressed skull fracture
       (2) Open reduction of compound skull fracture
       (3) Excision of subdural or extradural hematoma
       (4) Repair of nerve and plexus injury
       (5) Laminectomy and decompression of spinal cord
       (6) Excision of ruptured disc
   (c) Excision of tumors of brain and spinal cord
   (d) Clipping of cerebral aneurysm
   (e) Topectomy, hemispherectomy for degenerative and convulsive disorders
   (f) Relief of postencephalitic conditions
       (1) Excision of subdural membrane
       (2) Decompression of skull
   (g) Drainage of brain abscess

---

1. Although children of all ages are encountered, a great many of the patients are infants *under 1 year of age.*
2. The *preoperative condition* of these children may be poor or critical as a result of severe head injury, advanced malignant tumors, increased intracranial pressure, or destruction of brain tissue.
3. The *positions* required in neurosurgery entail special hazards to the patient. In the prone position respiration is depressed, and there is danger of injuring the face and eyes. The airway can be protected by endotracheal intubation, but the tube may kink, slip out, or become obstructed. In the sitting position there is increased danger of hypotension, air embolism, and postoperative aspiration.
4. *Inaccessibility* of the patient is a real problem. When a small infant is in the prone position and draped to the surgeon's satisfaction, an anesthetist must use considerable ingenuity to remain in contact with the patient. Endotracheal anesthesia is mandatory but solves only part of the difficulty.
5. The *operations usually are prolonged,* making it possible for minor abnormalities to develop into serious complications. The outstanding dangers consist of inadequate ventilation and inaccurate fluid replacement.
6. *Blood loss may be extensive,* either through gradual bleeding over many hours or by rapid, exsanguinating hemorrhage. An added difficulty exists

in the fact that it is practically impossible to measure blood loss. The use of wet sponges and continual irrigation makes the standard gravimetric methods impractical. Fluid replacement has additional risk in neurosurgical patients because of greater danger of cerebral edema.

7. The use of *endothermy* may be expected in all major cases.
8. *Postoperative complications* may be expected to be more common because of the delayed return of consciousness after operations in the vicinity of the brain stem. Tracheostomy will sometimes be indicated to decrease dead space and facilitate removal of secretions.

MANAGEMENT

Diagnostic procedures. Lumbar *puncture* rarely requires anesthesia, but in exceptional cases sedation with pentobarbital or light anesthesia with halothane may be desirable to prevent resistance in patients who are critically ill or highly emotional.

Small infants have tolerated *pneumoencephalography* so poorly that it is seldom performed in patients less than 1 years of age. During the procedure children must be immobilized in the sitting position; they will require enough analgesia to obtund the pain of needle puncture and the subsequent passage of air into the ventricles.

In the past, attempts to perform these procedures under heavy sedation have not been successful, and general anesthesia has been used. Recently, however, newer combinations of sedatives have proved more successful. The mixture of phenothiazine, chlorpromazine, and meperidine has been satisfactory in our hands,* and Corsson and Domino have had excellent results with intramuscular use of a new phencyclidine derivative (Parke-Davis CI-581).

Serious complications may be associated with pneumoencephalography. The most common one is a shocklike state that usually appears when weaker children are moved suddenly following the introduction of air. The blood pressure drops sharply, and the children become pale and ashen. This condition responds to phenylephrine (Neo-Synephrine) given intramuscularly in 2 to 3 mg. doses. If patients are moved with deliberation and care following air injection, this syncopal depression can be avoided.

Deaths have occurred during or shortly after pneumoencephalography. It was formerly believed that these were primarily due to pressure on the brain stem at the foramen magnum, but it has been shown that death may be due to the escape of injected air into the vascular system with resultant cerebral air embolism.[3,4]

Ventricular tap and ventriculography usually are performed with the patients lying on the x-ray table, and positioning creates no problem. This, plus the fact that the procedure often immediately precedes a prolonged craniotomy, influences one to use local infiltration rather than general anesthesia.

Myelography can be a prolonged, difficult procedure. Opaque oil medium is injected into the spinal canal, the child is placed face down on the x-ray table, and the room is darkened. In order to delineate the contours of the spinal canal,

---

*For details, see p. 308.

the roentgenologist repeatedly tilts the table and the patient, first into an abrupt dive and then into a steep head-up position.

Occasionally sedatives alone are sufficient to keep the children quiet, but frequently general anesthesia is necessary. The darkened room, roentgen-ray films, prone position, and continually changing position render any form of anesthesia hazardous. The choice lies chiefly between ether, which supports cardiorespiratory function but entails an appreciable explosive risk, and halothane, which is definitely depressing but is nonflammable. Since only a light plane of anesthesia is required and respiration may be supported, halothane probably is more suitable. The problem of technique then remains, for a highly mobile apparatus is necessary because of the extreme positional changes associated with the tipping of the table. The use of a nonrebreathing apparatus is best suited to this situation.

Study of cerebral vasculature by *angiography* is frequently necessary in children. For most children the use of halothane is advised. Endotracheal intubation is indicated if the vessel is to be dissected out, but it is usually unnecessary if the percutaneous method is used. Blood loss may be appreciable during this procedure, and hematoma may be of even greater concern if it becomes large enough to compress the cervical vessels or the trachea. Patients should be watched carefully for this complication.

Burr holes are often performed as a diagnostic measure to determine the presence of subdural hematoma. The procedure can be performed under local anesthesia, but the child will usually squirm and make it more unpleasant for both the surgeon and himself than it would have been had he received general anesthesia. Since the operation is short and the child lies with his head turned to the side, intubation is not mandatory but usually is preferable. Following sedation as outlined below, anesthesia is induced with nitrous oxide and is maintained with halothane using a nonrebreathing or infant circle system.

Anesthesia for therapeutic procedures. Major neurosurgical operations require light but steady anesthesia, with adequate ventilation and careful maintenance of fluid replacement. If these simple requirements are fulfilled, it is often impressive to see how well even the smallest infants tolerate several hours of surgery.

Because of the similarity of the anesthetic problems involved in most neurosurgical operations, the management of anesthesia usually follows a rather standard formula, which may be modified by the age or condition of the child or by the procedure to be undertaken.

Premedication and induction. Infants under the age of 6 months are given only atropine for premedication, and anesthesia is induced with nitrous oxide and halothane. Since nitrous oxide has relatively little effect on young infants, halothane is used from the outset, starting with a 3:1 mixture of nitrous oxide and oxygen and 1% halothane, then increasing halothane to 3% and cutting the gases back to a 2:2 ratio until time for intubation, after which halothane is reduced to 1%. Children between approximately 6 months and 6 years of age receive atropine and additional sedation is strictly individualized. If children are extremely ill, have increased intracranial pressure, advanced malignancy, or other critical problems, it is often unsafe to use any sedation. However, many children are either normally alert or may be extremely apprehensive due to several previous operations and prolonged hospitalization. It is most important that these children be given the benefit of careful sedation. Pentobarbital, given by rectum (2 to 2.5 mg./lb.) or by mouth (1 to 1.5 mg./lb.) is useful here. Avertin has been used for these children in the past[5,6] and is excellent when ether is the chief anesthetic agent, but if other agents are employed respiration may become excessively depressed. Induction with rectal thiopental or methohexital is also helpful in this age group. A dosage of 10 mg./lb. of either agent is safe but may need supplementation with a second administration of 5 mg./lb. Anesthetic induction in this age group usually is best accomplished by flowing 100% oxygen over the child's face for 2 minutes, then using a 6:1 ratio of nitrous oxide and oxygen for 2 minutes, followed by a 4:1 mixture and addition of halothane.

With older children a similar approach is used, although induction with intravenous agents may be employed, especially in apprehensive children. It should be pointed out that patients with increased intracranial pressure may prove to be remarkably resistant to inhalation anesthetics. Avertin is helpful in such cases since it is absorbed directly and has a slightly depressant effect on cerebrospinal fluid pressure.[6,7] Occasionally it is necessary to perform a ventricular tap, after which anesthetics become effective at once.

It has been noted by Eckenhoff[8] and by Colgan and Keats[9] that the lumen of the airway may be narrower at the cricoid ring than at the glottis and that this may complicate intubation, making it necessary to use endotracheal tubes one or two sizes smaller than would be expected. This has been true in our experience especially when dealing with children who have cranial defects. Outstanding in this group are those who have Apert's syndrome (Fig. 21-1),[10] consisting of gross cranial asymmetry accompanied by fusion of toes and fingers. On several occasions we have found that these children require extremely small endotracheal tubes and have increased danger of postoperative tracheitis. Unfortunately they often require numerous anesthetics for their multiple anomalies.

Intravenous infusion. During the period of induction and intubation, a cutdown infusion is established at the ankle or the antecubital space. For details, see Chapter 26. In larger children a plastic needle may be used rather than the cutdown.

Endotracheal intubation. Endotracheal intubation requires special care in neurosurgical procedures. Precision must be used in choosing a tube of correct size, for a slight error may lead to serious complication in the ensuing hours of operation. A tube that is too large will lead to trauma, whereas one too small will cause resistance.

During operations in the prone and sitting positions the endotracheal tube is in danger of becoming kinked. Furthermore, when the prone position is used, the tube arches back against the posterior aspect of the glottis, increasing the danger of irritation or erosion of the vocal cords. For this reason some prefer to use the latex tubes reinforced with wire (armored tubes). These tubes have other disadvantages, however, and may slip out during anesthesia. We prefer regular Portex tubes and follow the practice suggested by Smith[11] of positioning

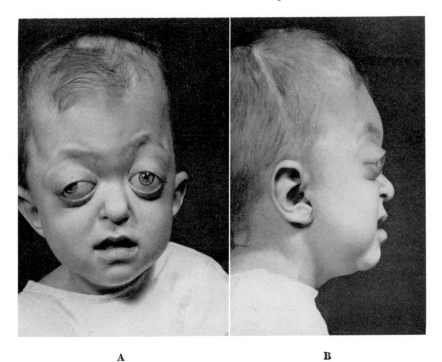

A   **B**

Fig. 21-1. Craniosynostosis has several forms. Apert's syndrome is associated with syndactyly of hands and feet. Cruzon's syndrome, **A** and **B**, shows marked facial deformity and extrusion of eyes due to bony occlusion of orbits. Airway problems are common to all varieties.

the tube in the middle of the mouth, so that its curve can follow the roof of the mouth rather than be held in a horizontal position by the molar teeth and then sharply angulated.

Special care is taken that the tube is not inserted too far and that it is fastened securely. During a long procedure secretions may loosen the tape around the tube and allow the tube to slip out. (If this happens during operations in which the patient is prone, it may be possible to perform blind oral intubation, using the fingers to guide the tube. If the procedure is nearing completion, it may be possible to maintain satisfactory anesthesia by insufflation, if ether is being used.)

Protection of eyes; positioning. Precautions must be taken to protect the eyes from blood and solutions that might run into them and also to guard them against pressure. Isotonic methylcellulose solution may be dropped into the eyes. This is a nonoily liquid plastic that forms a protective coating over the eyes and prevents irritation. In addition it is advisable to tape the eyes shut with nonirritant tape. Before positioning the child on the table the blood pressure equipment and stethoscope are attached, and a temperature-controlling mattress or blanket is placed under the patient. A rectal thermometer is inserted for continuous registration of the child's temperature.

Surgeon and anesthetist share the responsibility of positioning the patient so that the interests of both will be observed. The supine position offers little difficulty, provided that (1) the neck is not too sharply flexed and (2) the endotracheal tube is not allowed to fall forward and kink. Small rolls may be placed under the lumbar area and the knees to prevent hyperextension. In the lateral position a pad is placed under the axilla to prevent pressure on the "down" shoulder, and a thin towel is placed between the knees to prevent chafing.

The prone and sitting positions offer greater problems.[4,12] When an infant is placed in the prone position, he rests chiefly on his abdomen, with little support from his shoulders. Since respiratory exchange in these infants consists, to a large extent, of diaphragmatic breathing, substantial pads must be fixed under the shoulders and upper thighs in order to decrease the pressure on the abdomen (Fig. 21-2). The head is placed gently in a head ring, which is padded to avoid pressure on or near the eyes, and care is taken to see that the chin does not press against the end of the operating table (Fig. 21-3). When the position is satisfactory, the child is fixed to the table by the use of 3-inch adhesive tape passed (1) across the buttocks to either side of the table and (2) from the shoulders, down along the arms, to the sides of the table. The head of the table is then elevated slightly, in position for operation.

Next, the instrument tables are brought up; the patient is prepared, and drapes are applied. This phase is of special concern to the anesthetist, for he must not allow the patient to become hidden beneath the drapes. Tables, screens, and covers must be arranged so that the anesthetist can visualize the child's body and can reach his airway without difficulty in order to check the connection, to assist respiration, or to use suction when indicated. He must be near enough to monitor the child with a stethoscope, feel his pulse, watch his respira-

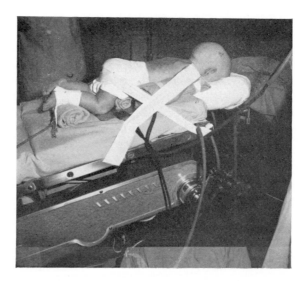

Fig. 21-2. Prone position requires firm support under shoulders and thighs. Adhesive tape prevents infants from slipping during operation. Roll under ankles prevents pressure on feet.

tion, and judge the color of his skin. To provide optimal conditions for the patient and team, an instrument table has been constructed that straddles the operating table and the patient, leaving a foot of free clearance. The anesthetist sits on a low stool beside the patient.

If the patient is to be in the sitting position for posterior fossa operations (Fig. 21-4), endotracheal anesthesia obviously will be necessary. The facepiece of the headrest must be applied with great care to avoid pressure on the eyes. Other parts of the body that may receive pressure are padded generously. The legs are flexed at the hips and knees to reduce muscle tension, and elastic bandages are applied to reduce pooling of blood.[3]

Individual deformities and lesions may lead to further problems in positioning, as in the case of extreme hydrocephalus or large encephaloceles (Fig. 21-5).

Maintenance of anesthesia. Light, stable anesthesia with minimal respiratory depression is definitely preferable in infants and small children.

Ether served well for many years and was especially valuable in providing a stable plane of anesthesia for prolonged periods of time, the child prone or supine, with spontaneous respiration. The risk of explosion due to the use of cautery has never seemed appreciable because of heavy draping and rapid air flow due to air conditioning. The actual reasons for changing to the use of halothane for pediatric neurosurgery were chiefly the anesthetist's greater familiarity with halothane and our failure to dissuade surgeons from using electric hair clippers before the patients were safely protected by drapes.

Halothane has served well for most neurosurgical procedures. The problem of using epinephrine in local infiltrate solution was solved by limiting the surgeons to the use of a 1/200,000 solution using 0.02 ml. per pound of body weight.

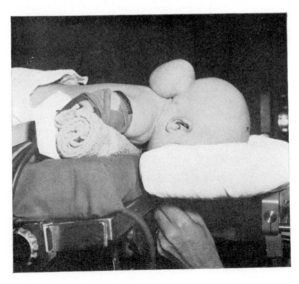

Fig. 21-3. Prone position for removal of encephalocele. Pressure on eyes, face, and chin must be avoided. Suction can easily be applied through the head ring.

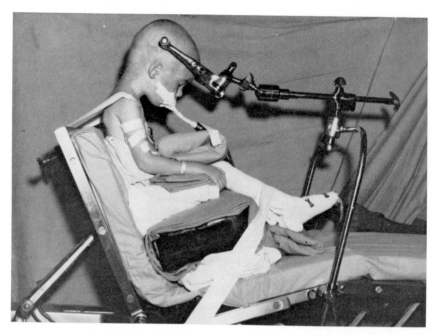

Fig. 21-4. Skull fixation by head tongs ensures stability and prevents pressure on eyes. Elastic bandages prevent venous pooling in legs. Maintenance of airway and blood pressure becomes more difficult when children are in the sitting position. (Courtesy Dr. D. D. Matson, Boston, Mass.)

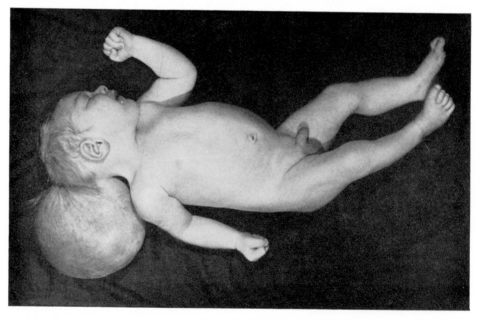

Fig. 21-5. Infant with unusually large encephalocele that creates problems in induction, intubation, and positioning.

Methoxyflurane (Penthrane)[14] has been favored by some for neurosurgical procedures in children. Its high solubility prevents rapid change for anesthetic depth and promises slow, quiet emergence. These features have not proved convincing in our hands as yet.

The use of trichloroethylene and nitrous oxide, once popular in neurosurgery, seems to have little place now that more versatile nonexplosive agents are available. Similarly, nitrous oxide–relaxant techniques are less valuable than previously and are especially undesirable in posterior fossa procedures when it may be important to observe the response of the respiratory center to the operative procedure.

If ether is being used, a simple Ayre T-piece may be employed without any extension on the expiratory piece, since respiration need not be assisted. If halogenated agents are used, the expiratory extension and bag should be added for ventilatory assistance.

Circle absorption systems may be used for neurosurgical anesthesia. The infant Bloomquist is suitable for children under 25 to 30 pounds, the adult system for larger patients. When the child is prone, these systems are somewhat more difficult to manipulate in comparison to nonrebreathing apparatus, but they have the advantage of retaining the patients' heat and moisture. If nonrebreathing apparatus is used, some humidifying device is needed, since the drying effect in a prolonged operation will be considerable. At present the Bennett humidifier appears most effective.

With suitable vaporizing devices, such as the Fluotec or the copper kettle vaporizers, the Ayre technique is effective in children up to 4 or 5 years of age. When using the Ayre system, the flow rate of gases should be sufficient to prevent rebreathing. The standard flow rate should be approximately three times the patient's minute volume to achieve this goal. The vaporizing gas may be oxygen, mixtures of oxygen and air, or oxygen and nitrous oxide.

The relative value of using spontaneous, assisted, or controlled ventilation during pediatric neurosurgery is of practical importance.[15,16] It is essential, in certain operations involving the brain stem, to retain spontaneous ventilation or to be able to produce it on short notice. For most procedures, it is important to be sure the patient is slightly hyperventilated, but the technique is not of critical concern. With ether, most patients will ventilate satisfactorily without assistance, as can many with halogenated agents. In general it is advisable to assist or control patients receiving halothane, although one then is faced with the danger of excessive anesthetic depth. Adequate depth usually is obtained under controlled respiration with the inspired halothane concentration at about 0.5%.

Although mechanical ventilating devices are not widely used in pediatric anesthesia, neurosurgical procedures probably offer reasonable indication for their use since light, even anesthesia is sufficient, is easily maintained, operations are prolonged, and hyperventilation is desirable. Our principal experience has been with the Bird assistor, although Engström and other devices are quite satisfactory.

The management of blood replacement is more difficult during neurosurgical procedures, since the anesthetist cannot visualize the operative field, and the use of continual irrigation makes gravimetric blood loss estimation practically impossible. For these reasons replacement must be guided by judgment of the surgeon, plus the anesthetist's observation of blood pressure and the strength of the child's pulse.

Blood loss is the principal problem in these procedures, but, if the operation involves the brain stem, sudden cardiovascular or respiratory depression may occur. Howland and Papper[17] described a variety of reflex disturbances that may occur during neurosurgical procedures, and Bergman[18] emphasized the dangers associated with repair of meningocele and spina bifida. Correction of lesions such as encephalocele or meningocele, in which the existing capacity for cerebrospinal fluid is reduced or the circulation is altered, may lead to elevation of intracranial pressure with resultant increase in arterial blood pressure and other cardiac and respiratory complications.[19]

Control of body temperature is of major importance during neurosurgical operations. Loss of body heat may occur, and although this may be due to prolonged exposure, the greatest heat loss probably occurs during the early phase while the child is uncovered and is being rinsed repeatedly with chilled antiseptic solutions. Warming mattresses, blankets, and warm operating suites should be employed to maintain the child's temperature at no less than 95° F., and one should try to regain a temperature of 97° F. by the time the child awakens.

Pressure on the brain stem or spinal cord due to tumor, injury, or operative manipulation may also cause sharp elevation in intracranial pressure that will be reflected in increased blood pressure. Management of this problem has been described by Riskin, Semeraro, and Robertazzi[20] and Ciliberti, Goldfein, and Rovenstine.[21] It consists of primary attempts to correct the underlying cause, followed by use of ganglionic blocking agents.

Since relaxation is not required during intracranial procedures, children may be maintained in very light surgical anesthesia. A minor complication seen in such light planes is a marked reduction of pulse rate, which may be associated with cardiac arrhythmia. This appears to be due to vagal stimulation aroused by the endotracheal tube, since it is easily corrected by atropine or deeper anesthesia.

SPECIAL PROBLEMS IN PEDIATRIC NEUROSURGERY

Newborn and critically ill patients. There are several situations in which the use of general anesthesia is unnecessary or unsafe. Local anesthesia may be used for elevation of depressed skull fracture in newborn infants, since the procedure is short and neither relaxation nor airway control is necessary.

For minor procedures on children who are critically ill, local anesthesia may be adequate. However, the necessity for respiratory support will require endotracheal intubation for all major operations, regardless of the child's condition. This may be performed under topical or light general anesthesia.

Elevated intracranial pressure. As previously noted, elevated intracranial pressure may complicate the induction of anesthesia. It may occur during other phases of anesthesia as well, and obviously one must avoid all factors that tend to contribute, such as hypercapnia, airway resistance, and coughing or straining.[22]

Advanced hydrocephalus. Children are seen from time to time whose heads are tremendously enlarged by hydrocephalus. These patients may be mentally retarded and often suffer from motor paralysis or genitourinary dysfunction. Sedation and anesthesia should be administered to these children with caution because they become depressed easily and have poor recuperative powers.

The comatose child. As a result of increased intracranial pressure from hemorrhage or other factors, the child may be comatose prior to operation. Endotracheal intubation is indicated for resuscitation and for protection of the airway. Since relief of pressure may bring return of consciousness during the operation, the anesthetist must be prepared to induce anesthesia at any time. Such awakening is very likely to occur after removal of an extradural hematoma. If the patient shows signs of returning consciousness, the anesthetist can effect induction with the least disturbance by adding thiopental intravenously and supplementing this with nitrous oxide, oxygen and halothane with the nonrebreathing technique. For such induction one may use 25 mg. of thiopental for each year of age (with maximum of 250 mg.) if caution is used to administer the agent very slowly.

Lesions affecting steroid control. Craniopharyngioma stands as an especially complicated neurosurgical problem, since this tumor may involve the hypothalamus, pituitary gland, optic chiasm, circle of Willis, and neighboring neural pathways. The lesion and its removal may cause diabetes insipidus, derangement of sodium metabolism, hypothyroidism, and abnormal reaction to stress unless carefully controlled with cortisone, Pitressin, and thyroid medication.[23]

Measures for the prevention of bleeding during operation. A number of methods have been promoted in order to reduce the vascularity of the brain during neurosurgical operations. These include hypotensive techniques,[24] hypothermia,[25] and more recently hyperventilation with or without the use of a negative pressure phase. Of these approaches hyperventilation probably has greatest safety, yet the possibility of anesthetic overdosage and excessive washout of heat and moisture stand as disadvantages. The sitting position is used to reduce bleeding during operations in the posterior fossa. We have not found it necessary to use any other devices to reduce vascularity. A light stable level of anesthesia and adequate respiratory exchange have provided satisfactory operating conditions.

Anesthesia for electroencephalographic exploration. In operations designed to locate focal areas of irritation in the brain the anesthetist may be requested to anesthetize and intubate a patient for craniotomy and exposure of the cortex and then be able to awaken him at any moment so that his encephalogram may be studied. This task is made more difficult because barbiturates interfere with encephalography and are barred from use. To accomplish the desired effect, the anesthetist may order scopolamine and meperidine for sedation, induce anesthesia with halothane, anesthetize the larynx by topical application, intubate, and then maintain the patient on nitrous oxide supplemented by relaxant and meperidine. The halothane is excreted rapidly, and thereafter the anesthetist can awaken the patient merely by reducing the nitrous oxide.

REFERENCES

1. Matson, D. D.: Neurosurgery of infancy and childhood, ed. 2, Springfield, Ill., 1968, Charles C Thomas, Publisher.
2. Corsson, G., and Domino, E. F.: Dissociative anesthesia: further pharmacologic studies and first clinical experience with the phencyclidine derivative CI-581, Anesth. Analg. 45:29-40, 1966.
3. Jacoby, J., Jones, J. R., Ziegler, J., Claassen, L., and Garvin, J. P.: Pneumonencephalography and air embolism: simulated anesthetic death, Anesthesiology 20:336-340, 1959.
4. Duflot, L. S. M., and Allen, C. R.: Anesthesia for pediatric neurosurgery, South, M. J. 49:1502-1505, 1956.
5. Rossier, J., and VanWagenen, W. P.: Avertin in neurosurgery, Ann. Surg. 103:535-553, 1936.
6. Gardner, W. J., and Lamb, C. A.: Effect of Avertin on cerebrospinal fluid pressure, J.A.M.A. 96:2102-2103, 1931.
7. Stephen, C. R., Woodhall, B., Golden, J. B., Martin, R., and Nowill, W. K.: The influence of anesthetic drugs and techniques on intracranial tension, Anesthesiology 15:365-377, 1954.
8. Eckenhoff, J.: Some anatomic considerations of the infant larynx influencing endotracheal anesthesia, Anesthesiology 12:401-410, 1951.
9. Colgan, F. J., and Keats, A. S.: Subglottic stenosis; a cause of difficult intubation, Anesthesiology 18:265-269, 1957.
10. Apert's syndrome, abstract in Survey Anesth. 10:318-319, 1965.
11. Smith, C.: Lecture at Anesthesia Research Symposium, Bal Harbor, Fla., March, 1964.
12. Slocum, H. C., O'Neal, K. C., and Allen, C. R.: Neurovascular complications from malposition on the operating table, Surg. Gynec. Obstet. 86:729-734, 1948.
13. Eversole, U.: Anesthesia for surgery about the head, J.A.M.A. 117:1760-1764, 1941.
14. Stephen, C. R., and Pasquel, A.: Anesthesia for neurosurgical procedures: analysis of 1000 cases, Anesth. Analg. 28:77-88, 1949.
15. Collins, V. J.: Principles and practice of anesthesiology, Philadelphia, 1952, Lea & Febiger.
16. Teplinsky, L. L., Harris, Z., Cassels, W. H., and Sugar, O.: Anesthesia for neurosurgery, Anesthesiology 10:82-91, 1949.
17. Howland, W. S., and Papper, E. M.: Circulatory changes during anesthesia for neurosurgical operations, Anesthesiology 13:343-353, 1952.
18. Bergman, N. A.: Problems in anesthetic management in patients with spina bifida, Anesth. Analg. 36:60-64, 1957.
19. Schroeder, H. G., and Williams, N. E.: Anesthesia for meningomyocele surgery: some problems associated with immediate surgical closure in the neonate, Anaesthesia 21:57-65, 1966; abstract in Survey Anesth. 10:581, 1966.
20. Riskin, A. M., Semeraro, D., and Robertazzi, R. W.: The control and management of hypertensive crises developing during surgical procedures, Anesthesiology 15:262-271, 1954.
21. Ciliberti, B. J., Goldfein, J., and Rovenstine, E. A.: Hypertension during anesthesia in patients with spinal cord injuries, Anesthesiology 15:273-279, 1954.
22. White, J. C., Verlot, M., Selverstone, B., and Beecher, H. K.: Changes in brain volume during anesthesia: the effects of anoxia and hypercapnia, Arch. Surg. 44:1-21, 1942.
23. Matson, D. D., and Crigler, J. F., Jr.: Radical treatment of craniopharyngioma, Ann. Surg. 152:699-704, 1960.
24. Vanderwater, S. L., Lougheed, W. M., Scott, J. W., and Botterell, E. H.: Some observations in the use of hypothermia in neurosurgery, Anesth. Analg. 37:29-36, 1958.
25. Anderson, S. M.: Controlled hypotension with Arfonad in paediatric surgery, Brit. Med. J. 2:103-104, 1955.

Chapter 22

Anesthesia for eye, ear, nose, and throat operations

GENERAL ASPECTS AND OBJECTIVES

Although this phase of anesthesia may seem less exotic than that for open heart surgery or premature infants, two facts are undeniable:

1. Tonsillectomy has long been one of the most frequently performed of all operations, and therefore it deserves consideration.
2. Emergencies involving the airway, whether from foreign body, post-tonsillectomy "bleeder," or infectious croup, are second to none in excitement and danger.

Most operations about the face and mouth have the following anesthetic requirements in common:

1. Analgesia is needed, but little relaxation is necessary.

2. The child's airway must be protected from obstruction by blood, loose tissues, and the hands and instruments of the operator.

3. The anesthetist must remove himself from the field and leave a minimum of apparatus in the surgeon's way.

The correct preparation of children for these operations includes the preoperative visit, history, physical examination, and laboratory studies. Much of this care is often neglected in patients entering the hospital on a short-term basis, but there is little excuse for such delinquency.

Preoperative medication should be chosen carefully and should include both a belladonna agent and a sedative. A barbiturate is usually indicated, but narcotics may be omitted for the purpose of maintaining gag reflexes and for prevention of vomiting. There are many acceptable forms of sedation for surgery about the face and head, and a phenothiazine derivative might be of special value here for better antiemetic effect.

Local anesthesia was once used widely for many of the operations about the head, but with the advent of reliable general anesthesia the use of local techniques, especially for children, has very largely disappeared. Inhalation anesthesia with endotracheal intubation is indicated for most operative procedures of this class.

OPERATIONS ABOUT THE EYE

Correction of squint (cross-eye) is a common procedure for children 2 or 3 years of age or older. Before anesthesia these patients should be forewarned if they are to wake up with their eyes blindfolded.

Several anesthetic agents and methods can be used for ocular surgery. Induction with nitrous oxide followed by halothane using a T-piece nonrebreathing apparatus is now most frequently employed in children under 6, while a circle apparatus and a semiclosed technique would be chosen for older children. Ether would have some advantage in avoidance of vagal arrhythmias, but proper preoperative atropine medication will provide adequate protection even if halothane is the sole agent.

Some anesthetists prefer not to intubate these patients but to maintain anesthesia by insufflation of ether, using a metal mouth hook. Although this technique can be managed, little is gained by it, and it sets the stage for disturbing situations. Secretions cannot be cleared from the airway easily, and if spasm occurs the whole operation may have to be interrupted for reestablishment of airway control.

The use of intravenous barbiturates, with or without relaxants, may provide more rapid induction and recovery and may be preferred by the experts. If these agents are used, endotracheal intubation seems especially indicated, for depressed or obstructed respiration may be expected.

During operations upon ocular muscles there have been many instances in which traction on rectus muscles, especially medial rectus, has stimulated severe bradycardia and other cardiac disturbances, probably due to an oculocardiac reflex.[1] Local block has been advocated to prevent this complication, but it is time-consuming and unreliable. It should be emphasized that atropine will prevent severe vagotonic disturbances effectively, and its use is definitely indicated in procedures involving traction upon the muscles of the eye.

Glaucoma has long been considered as a contraindication for the use of atropine. It should be noted that this refers to the use of atropine solution in the eye. The use of atropine as a premedicant will have far less action upon the iris and is not contraindicated.

Occasionally an ophthalmologist wants a small child to be quiet just long enough for thorough *eyeground examination,* testing of eyeball tone, or *probing of lacrimal ducts.* The procedure should be scheduled for early morning so that the child will have an empty stomach. No premedication is necessary, but pentobarbital may be used to quiet excitable patients more than 1 year of age. Although we have used divinyl ether or nitrous oxide for many of these procedures and Schwartz[2] in 1957 reported the use of chloroform in 3,200 children for eye examination, both parties now have adopted halothane for the purpose.

Endotracheal intubation would be unnecessary here, and it would be undesirable if patients are to be sent home soon after awakening.

A more complete opthalmologic examination requiring as much as an hour is sometimes necessary. In such cases it certainly is preferable to use endotracheal anesthesia, and it is our preference either to admit the child or to hold him for observation for 2 hours after anesthesia to guard against any postintubation tracheitis.

OPERATIONS ABOUT THE EAR

In some clinics the otolaryngologists perform otoplasty on children with lop ears, but in general this is the work of the plastic surgeon, and the otolaryngologist's efforts consist chiefly of opening bulging eardrums, mastoidectomy, and tympanoplasty.

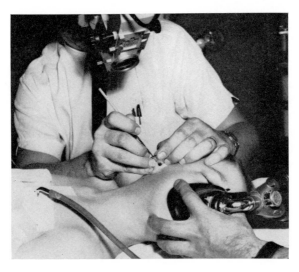

Fig. 22-1. Myringotomy is usually performed as an elective procedure, and patients should be well prepared for general anesthesia.

Incision of the tympanic membrane (myringotomy or paracentesis tympani).
This operation is a short, simple procedure requiring only a momentary period
of analgesia without relaxation. Fortunately it is performed less frequently as
an emergency procedure, and children are brought to the clinic at a preset
time, properly prepared. Under such circumstances a light nitrous oxide and
halothane anesthesia without intubation is quite adequate. The use of premedication often seems to depend upon the child. A quiet, cooperative child who is
not in pain often may be anesthetized without preanesthetic sedation. Neither
the light anesthesia nor the brief myringotomy should invoke troublesome vagal
response, and atropine may be omitted.

The situation is quite different when the child has an acutely inflamed ear,
and the operation is performed as an emergency. These factors may complicate
the picture; such a child will have pain and deserves a preoperative narcotic.

When there is any chance that the child has eaten recently, one should wait
4 to 6 hours if possible. Should one decide to proceed when less than 4 hours
have passed since eating, the anesthetist should try to retain the gag reflex by
using nitrous oxide as the only anesthetic.

At present no topical anesthetic appears to be effective in anesthetizing the
eardrum. Warm Auralgan may have some soothing effect and is advocated by
many otologists. It is possible that dimethylsulfoxide (DMSO) will prove effective in carrying anesthetics through the tympanic membrane.

For children who have a rectal temperature of 102° F. or over it is best to
avoid any general anesthetic until some attempt has been made to reduce the
fever. Divinyl ether is especially contraindicated because of the increased tendency to induce convulsions. Brief anesthesia with nitrous oxide or halothane is
probably justifiable after the temperature has stabilized and the patient is adequately controlled.

What should the busy pediatrician do when, 20 miles from a hospital, he
encounters a child with a bulging eardrum and a temperature of 104° F.?

To move a sick child to the hospital for a 15-second operation seems unwise.
Most pediatricians would open the child's ear using an opiate to reduce the pain.
This would appear a justifiable approach under suitable conditions.

Mastoidectomy. Not long ago mastoidectomy outnumbered most other procedures in children's hospitals. Although it is now indicated much less frequently, the operation is by no means a rarity.

Anesthesia for either simple or radical mastoidectomy need not be complicated. Endotracheal intubation is certainly preferable though not mandatory. Nasal intubation is definitely contraindicated in the presence of any
inflammatory condition about the nose, throat, or ears because of the danger
of spreading inflammation into the eustachian tubes.

Nonrebreathing techniques with halothane as the principal agent are chosen
in children under 8 years old, whereas circle absorpton may be used in older
children, and intravenous agents may be chosen if desired.

Intravenous infusions of dextrose and water usually will speed the patient's
recovery from anesthesia.

Tympanoplasty. Plastic repair of the eardrum is now being performed upon children of all ages. Since a light, even plane of anesthesia must be assured for a relatively long period of time, endotracheal inhalation anesthesia is clearly indicated. Any of the standard agents is applicable, but it will be especially desirable to avoid postoperative nausea and vomiting. Since these operations may last 5 or 6 hours, monitoring of blood pressure, and especially of body temperature, becomes especially important.

OPERATIONS ABOUT THE NOSE

Reduction of fractured nose. The operation requires only light analgesia and scarcely more time than was required for the injury. The chief danger in such cases lies in the possibility that the child may have undigested food in his stomach, plus an unknown quantity of swallowed blood from his fractured nose. Premedication plus light nitrous oxide anesthesia will afford adequate analgesia for reduction in most cases. If a more prolonged procedure is necessary, oral intubation under one of the general anesthetics may be indicated. The pharynx should be packed to prevent passage of more blood into the hypopharynx, and the endotracheal tube should be left in place until the child has awakened in order to prevent postoperative regurgitation and aspiration.

Correction of deviated septum, polypectomy, and other intranasal operations. These operations usually are best performed under oral endotracheal anesthesia, again using nonrebreathing methods in younger children. Nitrous oxide induction, followed by halothane or ether, probably would be best for such procedures. Thiopental may cause objectionable sneezing or coughing if used for operations on the nose and, consequently, seems a poor choice. Packing of the pharynx is indicated in most intranasal operations.

Special consideration should be given to the management of children with cystic fibrosis in whom nasal polyps often occur as a relatively late complication. The polyps are multiple, recur following removal, and frequently are superimposed on considerable local infection. Obviously these children have severe underlying disease, and all anesthetics carry disadvantages. To date our most satisfactory technique has been the use of nitrous oxide and gallamine with endotracheal intubation. This combination allows the surgeon use of epinephrine and electrocautery and precludes the need for atropine, which some believe is undesirable in cystic fibrosis.

Choanal atresia. Occasionally infants are born with bony occlusion of the posterior nares, or choanae.[3] The lesion is suspected if infants are entirely mouth breathers and have a nasal discharge. Diagnosis is confirmed if a catheter cannot be passed through the nose. Choanal atresia is a condition an anesthetist may be the first to discover if he is aware of the possibility.

An infant is badly handicapped by this defect, and operation is undertaken as soon as the mouth is large enough to provide room for surgical approach. The infant tolerates halothane or ether fairly well and may be maintained on the oral endotracheal Ayre technique. The operation consists of laying back a flap of soft palate, chiseling out a passage through the bony obstruction, and replacing the tissue flap.

TONSILLECTOMY AND OTHER OPERATIONS
ON THE PHARYNX, LARYNX, AND ESOPHAGUS

In spite of the large volume and variety of complicated procedures now being performed on children, tonsillectomy still leads the list as the most frequently performed pediatric operation. Although tonsillectomy is usually considered a simple operation, deaths from this procedure contribute heavily to the annual anesthetic mortality.[4-7] Most of these deaths occur in children who were normal and strong before operation, and it is difficult to understand why the toll continues to mount. Probably much of the trouble is simply due to the fact that many people consider this a very minor type of operation and take short cuts.[8,9] Children may receive little or no preoperative care, physical examination and laboratory tests are omitted, and too often children are brought to the hospital on the day of operation to be led directly to the operating room without any premedication. Due to the widespread enthusiasm for removing tonsils, surgeons and anesthetists of varied ability may be called upon. Among them are a great many who are unqualified.[10] In a study of tonsillectomy mortality in Baltimore, Alexander, Graff, and Kelly[11] find the picture much improved during recent years due to use of halothane, better resuscitation techniques, and installation of recovery room care.

Any operation that involves obstruction of the airway by manipulation and bleeding must be considered potentially dangerous, and adequate precautions must be observed.

Precautions necessary for tonsillectomy include those indicated for any elective procedure, i.e., indoctrination by parents, careful history and physical examination with red blood count or hemoglobin, and urinalysis. Medication prior to anesthesia is especially indicated for children with hypertrophied tonsils and adenoids because obstruction and increased secretions make induction more difficult. The benefit of sedation is definitely needed if children are admitted shortly before operation.[12,13]

Many combinations have been suggested. Recently we endeavored to omit all injections while these children are awake. Pentobarbital (Nembutal) or sodium thiopental (Pentothal) is given by rectum to small children, 2.5 mg. per pound 30 minutes before operation, while children over 8 years of age are given pentobarbital orally, 2 mg. per pound. Maximum dose in either case is 150 mg. Shortly after induction has begun, atropine is administered by intramuscular or preferably intravenous route.

Since halothane has become our agent of choice, there has been some excitement upon awakening. For this reason a narcotic has often been added to the medication, either before operation or during the procedure, to take effect as the child emerges from anesthesia.[14]

Induction of anesthesia is accomplished pleasantly with nitrous oxide and halothane. Halothane has been far superior to other inhalation agents for induction in children with large obstructing tonsils, since it neither stimulates secretions nor induces vocal cord irritation.

Whether or not endotracheal intubation is necessary for children undergoing tonsillectomy has been the subject of many bitter debates.[15] When ether was the customary agent, thousands of tonsillectomies were performed both with and without intubation, and complications occurred in both situations.[16-18] The airway is more easily protected under intubation, but if a child is lying head down, in a moderate or Rose position, with pharynx and glottis well exposed, as with Brown-Davis gag, full control of the airway can be maintained without intubation.

Since ether stimulates respiration, adequate ventilation can be maintained using insufflation technique provided the plane of anesthesia does not become too deep.

If any agent other than ether is employed, it seems advisable to use endotracheal intubation, simply because all other agents are respiratory depressants, and adequate ventilation cannot be guaranteed the child by insufflation techniques. It is our preference now to intubate children using nitrous oxide and halothane.

Succinylcholine may be used to facilitate intubation, but actually it is not needed. Two disadvantages will be encountered in using the combination of halothane and succinylcholine for tonsillectomy:

1. If atropine has been inadequate (or forgotten), there may be marked bradycardia.
2. A less easily avoided condition frequently arises when, after the relaxant has worn off often toward the end of operation, the patient remains apneic under very light halothane and then finally awakens abruptly, upsetting the whole procedure. This situation does not occur when halothane is used alone or with nitrous oxide.

The Ring modification* of the Brown-Davis mouth gag has been of great value and has done much to convert surgeons to the use of endotracheal intubation (Fig. 22-2). The notable feature of this gag is the tongue blade, which is made with a groove to fit over an oral endotracheal tube that it presses down into the soft substance of the tongue, and thus out of the surgeon's field.

During tonsillectomy under halothane anesthesia, exchange is carefully monitored by precordial stethoscope. Ventilation should be assisted or controlled during most of the procedure, but the patient should be allowed to breathe spontaneously toward the end of the procedure, so that extubation may be performed safely at completion of the operation. Prior to extubation the anesthetist should inspect the pharynx for the presence of blood and should auscultate both sides of the chest for presence of normal breath sounds and for sounds of blood that could have passed down into the trachea.

Recovery following tonsillectomy must be supervised closely. It is desirable to have children regain their reflexes and consciousness as soon as possible after operation in order to avoid aspiration of blood. Immediately after operation they are placed face down upon the litter or bed, with one arm and one leg flexed and a pillow under the shoulder (T and A position, p. 188). They should be kept in this position until the gag reflex has returned and any evidence of bleeding has disappeared.

---

*Sorenson Co., Salt Lake City, Utah.

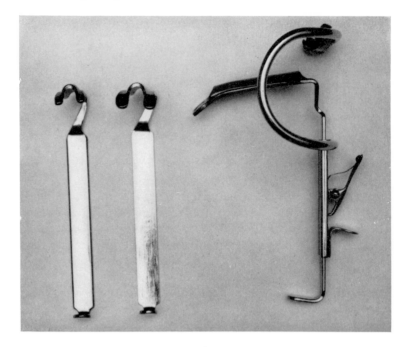

A

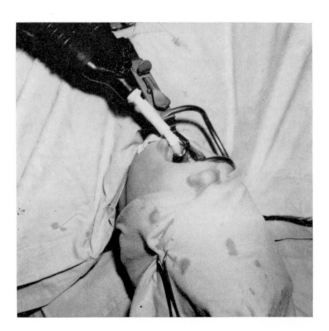

B

Fig. 22-2. **A,** Brown-Davis gag with modified (Ring) tongue blade made with groove to fit over endotracheal tube. **B,** Patient intubated, using modified mouth gag, ready for tonsillectomy.

Postoperative bleeding. Occasionally bleeding will continue after tonsil-lectomy, and it will be necessary to reanesthetize the child in order to remove clots and to pack or suture the bleeding area. This situation involves several hazards and, as noted by Alexander, Graff, and Kelley,[11] failure to initiate prompt action in this situation has been one of the chief sources of tonsillectomy deaths. The child's first medication has worn off and the drying agent will need to be repeated. Repetition of sedation may also be necessary. The child will by this time have been without fluids for several hours and should receive an in-fusion before the second anesthetic is started. The anesthetist must look for evidence of excess bleeding and shock. There may be blood in the bed, but often the child has swallowed most of it, and the loss can be guessed only by pulse, blood pressure, and the color of the skin and mucous membranes. Trans-fusion may be necessary prior to reoperation.[19]

The presence of blood in the patient's stomach introduces the hazard of regurgitation and aspiration, just as if the patient had eaten recently. In this situation it seems definitely advisable to induce the child rapidly with an inhala-tion agent, preferably halothane, intubate the trachea, and leave the tube in place until the child is truly awake, so that there can be no danger of aspirating vomited blood clots. One should attempt to suction the stomach while the pa-tient is still anesthetized. A large tube must be used if clots are to be removed. Davies[20] also emphasized the importance of this complication but reported only 1 death in 546 cases. He, too, stresses danger of using relaxants for this pro-cedure and favors halothane.

Pharyngeal abscess. This condition introduces the danger of sudden release of great quantities of pus that may flood the pharynx and occlude he larynx and trachea. Drainage of the abscess requires little relaxation, and light nitrous oxide anesthesia or halothane may be used without obliteration of protective gag reflexes.[21,22] If deeper anesthesia is desired, endotracheal intubation must be per-formed to prevent pus for entering the larynx. Leigh and Belton's[23] sugges-tion to aspirate pus from the abscess is a good way to reduce the risk.

Ludwig's angina. The problem of how to manage patients with Ludwig's angina has never been answered satisfactorily. In this condition infection, often originating in a tooth, spreads to involve the floor of the mouth in a diffuse cellulitis. The airway may be severely obstructed by the swelling, and the patient may be unable to open his mouth. The inflammatory nature of the process is thought to render the carotid body more sensitive to stimulation.

Anesthesia is required in these cases for deep incision under the ramus of the jaw, but it can be seen that any agent involves serious dangers. Danger of spasm and complete airway obstruction would appear maximum with intrave-nous barbiturates and relaxants. Ether's irritant action would invite airway obstruction and secretions. Halothane and cyclopropane would involve possible vagotonic effects but may be used in mild cases. Local infiltration anesthesia is undesirable in infected areas. A possible expedient might be the use of sub-stantial analgesic medication, followed by nitrous oxide or ethylene with tri-chlorethylene supplementation. Tracheostomy must be considered in all such cases. Bennett[22] and Leigh and Belton[23] suggest the use of topical anesthesia followed by nasotracheal intubation with the patient awake and then the use of nitrous oxide or other agents. Anatomic and emotional difficulties make children poor subjects for this method. Williams and Marcus[24] advise exposure of the trachea under local infiltration and then, with all in readiness for immediate tracheostomy, incision of the inflamed area under thiopental anesthesia. This use of thiopental appears reasonable, and the technique probably is the most suitable for the situation, especially when the lesion is advanced.

Operations on the larynx. Removal of laryngeal papillomas, polyps, or hemangiomas may occasionally be performed, using an endotracheal tube small enough to allow the surgeon to work around it. Then anesthesia offers little difficulty. If the lesion cannot be handled in this manner or if the surgeon wishes to dilate a stenotic larynx, the operation must be performed without an endotracheal tube. In such situations it is usually advisable to establish a relatively deep plane of anesthesia with either ether or methoxyflurane (Penthrane) and supplement this with full topical application of a local anesthetic such as 4% lidocaine. Adequate relaxation and analgesia will be provided with minimal respiratory depression, and inhalation anesthesia may be discontinued, allowing the surgeon 5 to 10 minutes to work unimpeded. If more anesthesia is required, ether can be resumed and the desired plane be reestablished. Apneic techniques rapidly bring hypoxia and are not recommended for this work unless respiration is aided by artificial ventilating devices.[25,26]

Anesthesia for performance of tracheostomy. The indications for tracheostomy and the hazards, complications, and care involved are discussed in Chapter 28. Here we are concerned only with problems of anesthesia for tracheostomy.

In acute severe upper airway obstruction, when the patient is cyanotic and near death, no anesthesia is needed, but an airway must be established at once. Passage of an endotracheal tube with immediate ventilation will usually be the most rapid method available. If a bronchoscope is available immediately, this carries two possible advantages over the endotracheal tube. These advantages are as follows:

1. In case of severe edema of the glottis, as in epiglottitis, the rigid bronchoscope can be introduced more easily than the endotracheal tube.
2. The bronchoscope lying in the trachea makes a better guide for the surgeon as he cuts down into the neck toward the trachea, which is sometimes difficult to locate.

Once ventilation has been reestablished by endotracheal tube or bronchoscope, the tracheostomy can be performed without haste. There is a good chance that the patient might awaken as soon as oxygenation is restored, and that anesthesia would be needed. This can be provided by local infiltration of the wound with 1% lidocaine or procaine, or nitrous oxide and halothane can easily be administered by endotracheal route.

When the surgeon is ready to insert the tracheostomy tube, the endotracheal tube (or bronchoscope) is retracted, but not removed, since several trials may be necessary before a satisfactory fitting is made. After the tracheostomy tube is set in place, the anesthesia inflow tubing is switched from endotracheal tube to tracheostomy tube for further ventilation or anesthesia.

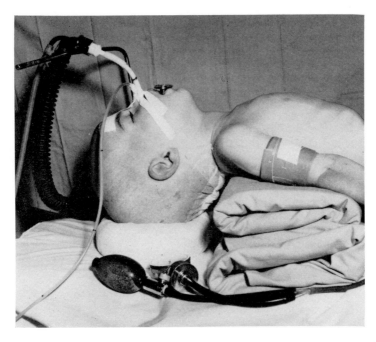

Fig. 22-3. Tracheostomy should be performed only when airway has been established. General anesthesia and careful positioning are advantageous.

Situations may arise in which glottic swelling makes intubation impossible, or it may happen that an emergency arises when there is no bronchoscope or endotracheal tube at hand.[27] For rapid establishment of airway the spear-pointed Shelden tracheotomy[28] has been advocated but can easily cause disastrous injury to vessels and structures of the neck.[29] The insertion of a 15-gauge or 16-gauge needle[27] into the trachea allows one to blow oxygen through it to sustain life while tracheostomy is performed, but this, too, has led to perforation of the esophagus and other complications. If such need should arise for instant relief of obstruction, probably the surest method is to make an incision at the crico-thyroid interspace, where the trachea lies immediately under the skin, and establish an orifice. Then a short hollow tube, like the barrel of a ball point pen, can be inserted into the trachea to ventilate the child.

When children are in only moderate respiratory distress prior to tracheostomy, induction of general anesthesia is advisable. Care must be taken not to increase the respiratory obstruction either by excitement or irritation. Mild sedation is indicated, and induction with nitrous oxide–oxygen and halothane is chosen since this offers minimal stimulation. Once the second plane of surgical anesthesia is reached, a bronchoscope is passed and the tracheostomy is undertaken while the vapor is introduced through the side arm of the bronchoscope.

Tracheostomy may be indicated in patients suffering from Guillain-Barré disease, meningitis, poliomyelitis, or cervical cord injury who are already receiving ventilatory support. If the ventilator being used is one of the current models, it will usually be necessary to detach it and use the anesthesia machine to induce anesthesia. Intravenous thiopental may facilitate this, and maintenance with halothane or halothane-ether is satisfactory.

If the child has been ventilated by a tank ventilator, anesthesia should be induced while the child is still being mechanically ventilated.

In the most severely weakened patients it may be safest to perform the tracheostomy under local infiltration, although this usually is an uncomfortable procedure.

Anesthesia after tracheostomy. When a tracheostomy has been performed in a child, anesthesia is considerably facilitated. Induction is accomplished by removing the tracheostomy tube, inserting a shortened, flexible endotracheal tube into the stoma, and administering gases directly into the trachea. It is also possible to anesthetize the child by dropping divinyl ether and ether on a gauze sponge held over the tracheostomy.

It is preferable, when possible, to use a tracheostomy tube that has a metal collar that may be adapted to standard anesthesia apparatus (Fig. 22-4). With this method the anesthetist can most simply and effectively use gaseous agents, assist respiration, or provide resuscitation (Fig. 22-5).

Foreign bodies in trachea or esophagus. Inhalation or ingestion of foreign bodies is popular with the younger set, especially those in the exploratory years between 2 and 4. Removal of articles from the *esophagus* is not usually a complicated procedure. One first tries to determine what object has lodged in the esophagus and where it is and then inquires as to what food might be in the

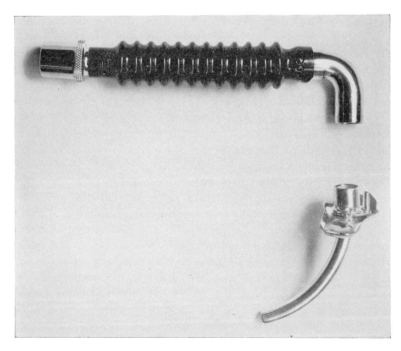

Fig. 22-4. Tracheostomy tube with collar for attachment of anesthetic or resuscitation apparatus.

stomach. Following adequate examination of the child, sedation is given, and subsequently anesthesia is induced with a general inhalation anesthetic. Nitrous oxide and halothane would appear to be the choice here, and endotracheal intubation certainly would be indicated. Following intubation greater relaxation may be achieved by adding succinylcholine, but this should not be necessary.

Unless the anesthetist is reasonably sure that there is no food in the child's stomach, the endotracheal tube is left in place after operation until the child is awake.

When foreign bodies lodge in the *larynx, trachea, or bronchi,* the situation is much more complicated and dangerous, first, because respiration may be seriously obstructed by the presence of the foreign body and, second, because the use of an endotracheal tube will not be possible. Without question, the removal of foreign bodies from the upper respiratory tract is one of the most exciting and exacting procedures known, and success depends greatly on excellent anesthesia.

Obviously oxygenation must be maintained throughout the procedure. This can be done either by using agents that allow spontaneous respiration during relatively deep anesthesia, such as ether or methoxyflurane (Penthrane) or by using agents that depress respiration, then providing oxygenation by some artificial means. Until very recently ether had always appeared to be unquestionably the best agent for such operations, since children do retain satisfactory exchange even when well anesthetized. One should take 10 to 15 minutes to establish a good tissue distribution of the ether and then spray vocal cords, trachea, and carina with 4% lidocaine. Next the mask is replaced, and ether is resumed for 2 or 3 minutes. Finally the patient is hyperventilated with 100% oxygen, the mask is removed, and the surgeon is allowed to begin. After the

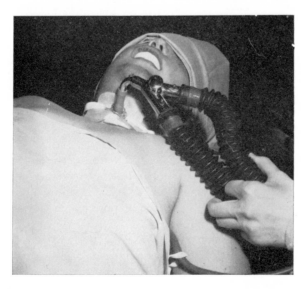

Fig. 22-5. Closed-circle anesthesia by tracheostomy for child with fractured jaw.

bronchoscope has been introduced, nitrous oxide and oxygen in 4:2 ratio may be administered through the side arm of the bronchoscope. Halothane also may be added to maintain anesthesia, if the surgeon does not object. The fumes of ether unquestionably distort one's vision, making instrumentation very difficult, and some believe that halothane has a similar effect.

Should the patient start to cough or awaken during prolonged instrumentation, time may be required to reestablish sufficient depth of anesthesia.

One very important point should be emphasized. Although it may be difficult to locate and grasp the object, the really critical moment comes when the endoscopist finally believes he has it and is ready to deliver it. If at this time the vocal cords have not remained in complete relaxation, it may be impossible to get the foreign body through the cords. It may fall back down into a bronchus, or, worse yet, may remain in the trachea and completely obstruct exchange. This may be fatal, unless the surgeon has the presence of mind to push the object back down into a bronchus.

In order to facilitate the passage of a large foreign body through the vocal cords, one may rely on deep inhalation anesthesia plus topical spray, but in difficult cases probably the best method is to wait until the moment of delivery and then give the patient intravenous succinylcholine (0.5 mg per pound). Complete relaxation should allow rapid removal of the object, and the patient can then be oxygenated by mask or endotracheal tube until awake.[30]

Diagnostic procedures. *Laryngoscopy and tracheoscopy* are frequently indicated for diagnosis of the etiology of stridor and other problems. Laryngoscopy can be performed without anesthesia or with topical anesthesia, but if relaxation is desired, ether anesthesia is preferable since it provides relaxation more quickly than methoxyflurane, and relaxation does not necessitate depression.

Tracheography may be desired for further diagnostic details. In small infants this is most safely done without anesthesia. Aided by a laryngoscope or anterior commissure laryngoscope, a small (18-gauge) plastic catheter is passed through the larynx, 2 or 3 ml. of radiopaque material is injected, the catheter is withdrawn, and the roentgen-ray films are taken.[31]

For older children it is preferable to induce general anesthesia with a nondepressant agent that does not incite laryngeal irritation. Ether and methoxyflurane are most appropriate. After induction, anesthesia is discontinued, allowing several minutes for the instillation of oil and the roentgen-ray exposures. Thorough clearing of the airway is necessary before returning the child to his bed.

For many years *bronchoscopy* in children has been done by the Jackson school[2] without anesthesia of any type, and it is surprising how successful the technique can be in the hands of highly skilled bronchoscopists. However, general anesthesia has become increasingly popular as better anesthesia has been developed.

It may be a hazardous procedure to use the bronchoscope on an infant or child who already has respiratory obstruction or disease, and the agent and technique must be chosen carefully. Preoperatively atropine should be given unless it is specifically desired to obtain tracheal secretions for diagnostic purposes. Pentobarbital without supplemental opiates may be used for preoperative sedation in children over 6 months of age. The use of thiobarbiturates either by vein or by rectum has been recommended for bronchoscopy in children,[32] but in view of the bronchoconstrictor and vagotonic effect, these would seem a poor choice. The worst bout of laryngospasm we have encountered occurred in a small child who was given rectal thiopental and open-drop ether for bronchoscopy. During the procedure the child eliminated the ether and then on withdrawal of the bronchoscope developed such a severe laryngospasm that bradycardia and cyanosis occurred before oxygen could be forced between the closed cords.

The problem of monitoring patients during manipulation of the airway is most important. The stethoscope must be used continuously, as hypoxia may occur rapidly. Lights should be turned on at intervals to inspect the patient and should be under immediate control of the anesthetist.

Usually *bronchography* follows previous bronchosocpy, for which the child has received general anesthesia with ether, methoxyflurane or halothane, plus a topical agent.[33-35] Much of this may have worn off during the procedure, and the child may be moving and coughing when the bronchoscope is finally withdrawn and the anesthetist again takes over. Control of the patient can be regained with halothane and oxygen, and the trachea should be intubated. It will be highly desirable to establish and maintain an airtight system throughout the procedure. If this is accomplished, the bronchography can be done with precision and safety and with free choice of anesthetic agent.

We have used a simple method that has been quite satisfactory. After endotracheal intubation, a **Y** adapter or Rovenstine elbow is attached to the endotracheal tube. One orifice is attached to the anesthesia apparatus, while

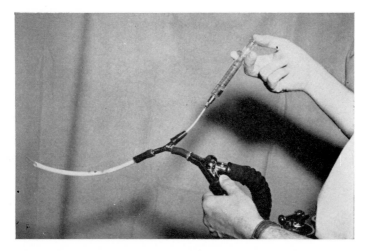

Fig. 22-6. Apparatus for closed-system bronchography. **Y** tube is interposed between endotracheal tube and anesthetic yoke. Plastic catheter for instillation of opaque media is inserted through perforated nipple on **Y** tube and down endotracheal tube.

the other is fitted with a perforated rubber nipple through which a plastic catheter may be passed for introduction of the opaque material. The catheter may be positioned at will, dye injected slowly, and serial films may be taken as each lobe is filled. In larger children and in adults we have passed the plastic catheter into the trachea before intubation and then intubated the patient, thus establishing an undisturbed airtight system. Because control of the catheter is less easily managed, this method is less popular.

If the anesthetist has control of ventilation, halothane and oxygen make a good combination, and succinylcholine may be added if apnea is necessary for the procedure.

If such an airtight system is not maintained, one must revert to ether or methoxyflurane, plus topical spray, and keep the child breathing spontaneously. Control will be poor, and radiologic diagnosis will be less satisfactory.

Under any circumstances, monitoring of these patients is of paramount importance. Here an esophageal stethoscope will be helpful, since a precordial stethoscope would obscure part of the field in the roentgen-rays or would become dislodged during repeated repositioning of the child. Bronchography in children is always a hazardous procedure.

Although the characteristics of ether have made it most valuable for endoscopic work, its flammability influences one to avoid it if possible. Here methoxyflurane (Penthrane) probably has its greatest value. The high solubility of methoxyflurane makes induction slow, but once surgical anesthesia is achieved the patient will maintain relaxation and spontaneous respiration even longer than with ether. In using methoxyflurane, the same procedure should be followed as described with ether: slow, deliberate induction (here requiring 15 to 20 minutes), topical spray, side arm insufflation, and last-moment use of succinylcholine. Halothane is not as useful for such procedures, but it may be used in less critical cases.

Apneic techniques using either long-acting or short-acting muscle relaxants[36] for the entire procedure can be employed, but though more rapid, they entail more hazards. Oxygenation must be maintained by use of an external cuirass,[25] by intermittent interruption of the operation to inflate lungs, use of airtight bronchoscope, or external chest pressure. None of these methods seems as desirable as spontaneous respiration. It is possible, however that in extreme situations, as in removal of an open safety pin, a completely apneic technique will be necessary. The best choice then probably would be to use intermittent intravenous doses of succinylcholine with halothane and oxygen, maintaining respiration by external chest compression plus intermittent lung expansion via the side arm of the bronchoscope.

Respiratory obstruction during injection of the dye is not infrequent, and ventilatory exchange must be observed closely, especially while the room is darkened. This may be accomplished by watching the diaphragmatic excursion under the fluoroscope and by manual assistance of respiration. Cardiac action must also be followed continuously during the procedure, and the lights must be turned on at intervals of not more than 2 or 3 minutes to check the child's condition.

After the procedure the dye is sucked up through the endotracheal tube, and then the tube is removed and suction is administered in the trachea again, since the dye may flow up around the tube and be inaccessible while the tube is in place. The child should be encouraged to cough, and his chest must be clear to stethoscopic inspection before he is returned to his bed. If the endoscopic procedure has been difficult or prolonged, it may be advisable to put the child in a humidified tent or room until any signs of irritation disappear. Close observation is maintained until the child has fully recovered.

REFERENCES

1. Rosen, D. A.: Anaesthesia in ophthalmology, Canad. Anaesth. Soc. J. 9:545-550, 1962.
2. Schwartz, H.: Chloroform anesthesia for ophthalmic examination, Amer. J. Ophthal. 43:27-30, 1957.
3. Jackson, C., and Jackson, C. L.: Diseases of nose, throat, and ear, Philadelphia, 1945, W. B. Saunders Co.
4. Belton, M. K., and Leigh, M. D.: Anesthesia for tonsillectomy and adenoidectomy, Med. Woman's J. 56:15-19, 1949.
5. McKenzie, W.: Risks of tonsillectomy, Lancet 265:958-960, 1963.
6. Cummings, G. O.: Mortalities and morbidities following 20,000 tonsil and adenoidectomies, Laryngoscope 64:647-655, 1954.
7. Tate, N.: Death from tonsillectomy, Lancet 2:1090-1091, 1963.
8. Collins, V. J., and Granatelli, A.: Anesthesia for tonsillectomy in children. Endotracheal technique with cardiovascular observations, J.A.M.A. 161:5-9, 1956.
9. Slater, H. M., and Stephen, C. R.: Anesthesia for tonsillectomy and adenoidectomy, Canad. Med. Ass. J. 64:22-26, 1951.
10. Compton, J., Bader, M. N., Haas, M. V., and Lange, M.: Who is administering anesthesia today? Hosp. Manage. 80:48-52, 1955.
11. Alexander, D. V., Graff, T. W., and Kelley, E.: Factors in tonsillectomy mortality, Arch. Otolaryng. 82:409-411, 1965.
12. Eckenhoff, J. E.: Preanesthetic sedation of children. Analysis of the effects for tonsillectomy and adenoidectomy, Arch. Otolaryng. 57:411-416, 1953.
13. Jackson, K., Winkley, R., Faust, O. A., Cermak, E. G., and Burtt, M. M.: Behavior changes indicating emotional trauma in tonsillectomized children, Pediatrics 12:23-28, 1953.
14. Burnap, T. K.: Anesthesia for operations in ophthalmology and otolaryngology, Internat. Anesth. Clin. 1:195-208, 1962.
15. Granatelli, A., and Collins, V. J.: Advantage of routine endotracheal anesthesia for tonsillectomy in children, New York J. Med. 56:1761-1765, 1956.
16. Bailie, R. W., and Scott, W. E. B.: Massive lung collapse following tonsillectomy and adenoidectomy, J. Laryng. 68:834-841, 1954.
17. Fabian, L. W., Bourgeois-Gavardin, M., and Stephen, C. R.: Anesthesia for tonsillectomy and adenoidectomy, Anesth. Analg. 36:59-62, 1957.
18. Ribeiro, O. V.: Anesthesia for tonsillectomy and adenoidectomy, by dissection, in children. Observations in 8000 cases, Postgrad. Med. 21:22-29, 1957.
19. Holden, H. B., and Maher, J. J.: Some aspects of blood loss and fluid balance in pediatric tonsillectomy, Brit. Med. J. 2:1349-1351, 1965.
20. Davies, D. D.: Reanesthetizing cases of tonsillectomy and adenoidectomy because of persistent postoperative hemorrhage, Brit. J. Anaesth. 36:244-250, 1964.
21. Bougas, T. P., and Smith, R. M.: Pathologic airway obstruction in children, Anesth. Analg. 37:137-146, 1958.
22. Bennett, J. M.: Anesthetic management for drainage of abscess of submandibular space (Ludwig's angina), Anesthesiology 4:25-30, 1943.
23. Leigh, M. D., and Belton, M. K.: Anesthesia for ear, nose, and throat operations in infants and children, Anesth. Analg. 27:41-48, 1948.

24. Williams, A. C., and Marcus, P. S.: Choice of anesthesia in Ludwig's angina, Anesth. Analg. **20:**160-170, 1941.
25. Bayuk, A. J.: Chest respirator for bronchoscopy and laryngoscopy, Anesthesiology **18:**135, 1957.
26. Sleath, G. E., and Graves, H. B.: The use of the cuirass respirator during laryngoscopy and bronchoscopy under general anesthesia, Canad. Anaesth. Soc. J. **5:**330-337, 1958.
27. Reed, J. P., Kemph, J. P., Hamelberg, W., Hitchcock, F. A., and Jacoby, J.: Studies with transtracheal artificial respiration, Anesthesiology **15:**28-41, 1954.
28. Shelden, C. H., and Pudenz, R. H.: Percutaneous tracheostomy, J.A.M.A. **165:**2068-2076, 1957.
29. Smith, V. M.: Perforation of trachea during tracheostomy performed with Shelden tracheo-tome, J.A.M.A. **165:**2074-2076, 1957.
30. Robinson, C. L., and Mushin, W. W.: Inhaled foreign bodies, Brit. Med. J. **2:**324-328, 1956.
31. Flake, C. G., and Ferguson, C. F.: Tracheography and bronchography in infants and children, Pediat. Clin. N. Amer. **2:**279-289, 1955.
32. Helrich, M., Daly, J. F., and Rovenstine, E. A.: Anesthetic management of infants and children during endoscopy, Pediatrics **6:**625-629, 1950.
33. Stephen, C. R.: Elements of pediatric anesthesia, Springfield, Ill., 1954, Charles C Thomas, Publisher.
34. Heerdegen, D. K., and Arrowood, J. G.: Management of anesthesia for otolaryngological procedures, Anesth. Analg. **33:**129-134, 1954.
35. Mushin, W. W., and Lake, R.: Anaesthesia for bronchography in children, Anaesthesia **6:**88-92, 1951.
36. Alver, E. C., and Leek, J. H.: Induced paralysis for endoscopic procedures, Arch. Otolaryng. **62:**399-405, 1955.

Chaper 23

Anesthesia for dentistry in children

The problems involved
Routine pedodontic care
Minor operative cases
Multiple fillings and extractions—dental rehabilitation

THE PROBLEMS INVOLVED

Several problems of slightly different nature arise in connection with anesthesia for dentistry:

1. *Is anesthesia necessary?* Although most human beings are aware of the pain that may be caused by defective teeth, many are critical of the present liberal use of local anesthesia and are seriously opposed to the use of general anesthesia for dentistry, apparently believing that it is safer to endure this type of pain. It is hoped that better anesthesia will gradually eliminate this conviction.

2. *Who gives the anesthetic?* Members of the dental profession have been pioneers in the field of anesthesia and have felt a certain justification in administering both local and general anesthetics themselves.[1] If such men have had adequate training, this may be acceptable, but the use of various agents and especially the intravenous agents has been carried to excess by unskilled persons and has caused a number of deaths. No matter how short the procedure, general anesthesia for dental procedures entails the risk of vomiting, spasm, or apnea, any of which can lead to death. It seems only logical that a qualified person with special training and equipment should be chosen for the work.

3. *Where?* Another practical question concerns whether the patient should be given a general anesthetic in the dental office or should be sent to a hospital.[2] Time and expense are factors here, and many patients will not be treated if hospitalization is required. It seems reasonable to say that if a general anesthetic is to be given in a dentist's office, the patient must be in reasonably good condition, a qualified anesthetist should give the anesthetic, and complete equipment should be available for resuscitation.

4. *What and how?* The actual choice of agents and technique can be discussed in relation to the individual procedures.

ROUTINE PEDODONTIC CARE

The major portion of dentistry for children consists of prophylactic care, the filling of two or three teeth, or the occasional extraction of a deciduous tooth. All this can be accomplished by an understanding dentist without recourse to anesthetics.

If there is to be more than usual discomfort associated with these procedures, the child may be given mild analgesics such as codeine and aspirin half an hour before the appointment.

MINOR OPERATIVE CASES

If the tooth to be removed is firmly fixed, or if two or three teeth require extraction, a local anesthetic may be used for some children, but in most cases a short-acting general anesthetic will be indicated.

This appears to be a very simple type of situation but actually is not the easiest, for it requires the anesthetist to accept an ambulatory child, induce anesthesia quickly and pleasantly, provide analgesia, jaw relaxation, protected airway, and ventilation for 2 or 3 minutes and then have the child wake up promptly, regain normal equilibrium, and be ready to leave within a short period of time.

To fulfill all of these demands requires a well-planned approach that should be started several days prior to the intended procedure. Any child who is to have a general anesthetic should first have a physical examination, which may be performed by the family physician or the pediatrician before admission or by a member of the hospital staff immediately before anesthesia.

Since the child will have little time to become accustomed to the hospital, it will be especially important to build up his morale beforehand by assuring him that no one will hurt him and that he can go home as soon as he awakens.

If the procedure is to be performed in the morning, the child is given no breakfast, but he may be given a mild sedative, such as pentobarbital, before the trip to the hospital. A dosage of approximately 1.5 mg. per pound given by mouth usually helps control apprehension but does not make the child too sleepy to travel. We have used a suspension of chloral hydrate (Chloralixin) with good results. This solution contains 88 mg. of chloral hydrate and 0.1 mg. of atropine per milliliter. The oral dosage has been 1 ml./5 lb., not to exceed 10 ml. If a general anesthetic is to be administered, it is best to have the child lie on an operating table or stretcher rather than sit in a dental chair. Oxygen, suction, oral and endotracheal airways, and a laryngoscope should be at hand for even the shortest procedures. Prior to anesthesia the child should be encouraged to void; his shoes should be removed and his shirt loosened or removed.

A number of agents have been recommended for this type of anesthesia in the past. They include nitrous oxide, divinyl ether,[3] ether, halothane,[4] trichloroethylene,[3,5,6] cyclopropane, and thiopental[7] and have been administered alone or in various combinations. However, ether is too heavy and unpleasant for such use, and thiopental involves a painful venipuncture and some danger of laryngospasm. Nitrous oxide followed by divinyl ether was our choice for years, but the danger of overdosage and convulsion proved to be too great. The combination of nitrous oxide and trichloroethylene is useful and is believed by Slater[8] to be most satisfactory, but in our hands the combination often provided inadequate relaxation and has been followed by considerable nausea. At present increasing familiarity with halothane has enabled us to induce easily and rapidly with nitrous oxide and oxygen, achieve sufficient relaxation for several rapid dental extractions, and allow the child to awaken with minimal disturbance.

Propanidid,[9] a congener of eugenol, is now finding increasing popularity for this type of procedure. Given in 5% solution by intravenous route, the agent acts at once, and it is said to be devoid of respiratory irritation or vocal cord spasm. It is metabolized immediately, allowing the patient to walk out, completely alert, within 5 minutes. This has been used by Ralston[10] in numerous children, but causes some vascular irritation.

Regardless of the agent employed, dental extractions usually involve manipulation of the head and jaw, with definite danger of airway obstruction. During the procedure the anesthetist must keep the jaw firmly supported and warn the dentist if exchange becomes endangered.

Slater[8] overcomes this difficulty by inducing anesthesia with nitrous oxide and inserting a nasoendotracheal tube. Light, controlled anesthesia is then maintained with nitrous oxide and trichloroethylene. Although some may be proficient in this technique, nasal intubation under light anesthesia would be too traumatic for most to attempt.

Following any of these techniques, the child is allowed to awaken completely and then is observed for half an hour before being allowed to leave the hospital.

MULTIPLE FILLINGS AND
EXTRACTIONS—DENTAL REHABILITATION

Because of neglect or oral disease a number of patients come to the dentist with five or six teeth requiring extraction and perhaps ten that need filling. Complete correction of such needs would require appointments over several weeks and would entail excessive hardship on the patient. Another problem is posed by children who, either through mental retardation or simple unmanageability, will not allow a dentist to approach them. A third group is comprised of chronically ill children, such as those with severe congenital heart disease, who do not withstand chair dentistry without danger of excessive excitement and fatigue.

For the past 15 years patients requiring extensive dentistry, those who are entirely unmanageable, and others with severe chronic illnesses have been admitted to the hospital as regular surgical patients and then, under general anesthesia, have undergone complete "dental rehabilitation" in one operation.

Although there was some criticism of this procedure at the outset, it is now regarded as a legitimate form of medicine. As is shown by Karp and Tuescher,[11] Slater and Stephen,[12] and others,[13] the practice is now widely established. Thus far over 2,500 children, many of whom have had severe heart disease, have been treated in our hospital under this regimen. With the exception of one 4-year-old boy who had prolonged cardiovascular depression following glutethimide sedation, none has shown any serious complication during or after operation.

The system of handling such children who enter the hospital for major dental work is as follows: The child is admitted in sufficient time to allow careful preparation and also to allow him to become quieted and accustomed to the hospital. It is believed that these patients deserve the full precautions allowed other surgical patients. Accordingly, before anesthesia the history and physical examination are recorded, and routine blood and urine tests are performed. Special examinations such as electrocardiograms, renal function studies, or chest roentgen-ray films are ordered if indicated. Since, as already stated, the reason for doing such procedures under general anesthesia may be the presence of a neurologic or pathologic abnormality, we believe that anesthesia should not be administered until there has been a real evaluation of the risk involved.

The choice of premedicant and anesthetic may be made from a number of agents, so long as safe principles are applied. Scopolamine or atropine should be given to depress salivation and vagal activity. If tribromoethanol and rectal thiopental are to be used as basal anesthetics, further premedication is best omitted in order to avoid excessive depression. If induction of anesthesia is to be by inhalation or intravenous methods, the patient should have further premedication with barbiturate or opiate, or a combination, in properly chosen dosage.

In our experience children with mental and emotional problems react poorly to pentobarbital premedication and are more easily handled under induction with rectal barbiturate or tribromoethanol followed by nitrous oxide and halothane or ether. Nasal endotracheal intubation is preferable for the dentist and is justified in skilled hands, but it involves greater chance of trauma.

Halothane has the advantages of ease of administration and rapid awakening and is a satisfactory agent; however, since the anesthetist has relatively little access to the head of the patient, signs are more difficult to follow. Consequently, ether seems a better choice until the anesthetist has gained considerable experience both with children and with halothane.

The important factor in administering the general anesthetic is not the agent chosen but the maintenance of a clear airway and prevention of hypoxia. An endotracheal tube is definitely indicated in order to prevent obstruction by packs, soft palate, and tongue, and in order to prevent the aspiration of blood and debris. Packing should be laid in the hypopharynx to prevent blood from running down the outside of the tube and into the trachea.

Throughout the operation the heart and respiration are continuously observed by use of the precordial stethoscope, and the temperature is monitored carefully. An intravenous infusion of dextrose and water is administered during all of these procedures to compensate for the long period of restricted oral intake.

The use of ether in the presence of the dental drill has caused us to evaluate this risk carefully. The possible dangers were thought to lie in the motor, the foot switch, and the drill cord. The motor must be grounded and encased so that vapors may not enter it. The cord is treated by being wiped with liquid graphite to render it conductive. A sparkproof foot switch has been substituted for the standard item. No danger of static or spark has been found in the actual grinding of the drill on the moist tooth, since the drill is grounded by the rotating cord.

The duration of operation is usually 1 or 2 hours. The patients are held in light first plane of anesthesia, just deep enough to tolerate the endotracheal tube without reflex irritation. Throughout the operation the eyes and nose should be covered with moist gauze to prevent the entrance of flying bits of dental debris. The oral packing should be changed during the operation if it becomes soiled with blood or debris, and at the end of the procedure extreme care must be used in cleaning out the mouth and pharynx thoroughly. Bleeding from tooth sockets should also be controlled. Before extubation, suction is used in the trachea and the chest is checked for normal breath sounds. The pharynx is examined with the aid of a laryngoscope, and an oral airway is inserted. It is best to use suction in the tube and then allow the patient to resume normal respiration and finally extubate without suction in order to diminish spasm and the chance of anoxia. After operation the patient is conveyed to his bed and kept in the prone position until conscious.

REFERENCES

1. Seldin, H. M.: The safety of anesthesia in the dental office, J. Oral Surg. 13:199-208, 1955.
2. Foldes, F. F.: Anesthesia consideration in oral surgery and dentistry, Amer. J. Orthodont. 33:379-387, 1947.
3. Stephen, C. R.: Elements of pediatric anesthesia, Springfield, Ill., 1954, Charles C Thomas, Publisher.
4. Harms, B. H.: General anesthesia in 10,500 office tooth extractions, Anesth. Analg. 41:475-477, 1962.
5. Stephen, C. R., and Slater, H. M.: General anaesthesia in the dental office, J. Canad. D. A. 16:183-190, 1950.
6. Bergner, R. P., Herd, R. M., Kline, K., Lawrence, D. R., and Hutton, C. E.: Nitrous oxide, oxygen, and trichloroethylene for office dental anesthesia, Anesthesiology 15:696-699, 1954.
7. Branch, D. R.: Intravenous anesthesia in operative dentistry for ambulatory patients, Anesth. Analg. 33:69-72, 1954.
8. Slater, H. M.: Personal communication.
9. Zindler, M., editor: Intravenous anaesthesia for out-patients, Acta Anaesth. Scand., supp. 17, 1965.
10. Ralston, W. N.: Personal communication.
11. Karp, M., and Teuscher, G. W.: General anesthesia in the difficult pedodontic patient, J. Pediat. 30:317-323, 1947.
12. Slater, H. M., and Stephen, C. R.: Anesthesia in prolonged dental cases, Anesth. Analg. 28:339-345, 1949.
13. Sadove, M. S., and Gans, B. J.: Anesthesia in hospital oral surgery, Anesth. Analg. 29:288-292, 1950.

Chapter 24

Anesthesia for minor and emergency surgery

ELECTIVE OUTPATIENT PROCEDURES

A number of minor procedures may be performed in the outpatient department or in a surgeon's office if adequate precautions are taken and suitable equipment is available.[1] Again it should be stressed that suction, resuscitation apparatus, airways, laryngoscope, and endotracheal tubes should be immediately available if a general anesthetic is to be given. There must also be a suitable area in which a child can be observed during recovery.

Among the procedures frequently scheduled for the outpatient surgeon are excision of skin lesions and superficial tumors, incision of abscesses, circumcision, urethral dilatation, and proctoscopic and similar examinations. Such procedures appear so simple that essential details in treatment may be neglected. Two points are of special significance, however: (1) to impress the parents with the importance of withholding all food and fluid and (2) the use of medication to reduce the child's apprehension and discomfort. Some surgeons believe that if a local anesthetic is to be used, no sedation is necessary. This does not seem logical, for if a child is to remain awake he will be subjected to a number of painful and upsetting experiences and deserves the benefit of medication.

The choice of sedatives for outpatient operations presents a special problem, for here it is desirable that the agent will act quickly and effectively on an alert, apprehensive child, yet be of such duration that the child can get up and walk out soon after the short operation is completed. No sedatives will do exactly this, but the best combination for reasonably cooperative children not less than 1 year of age appears to be morphine and atropine given intramuscularly in standard dosage 20 minutes before operation. Morphine does not induce sleep but provides analgesia and calmness in children. The combination of morphine and atropine does not cause the dizziness, excitement, or disorientation often seen with scopolamine, barbiturates, and meperidine.

For anesthesia in minor elective procedures, one may use local infiltration, regional block, inhalation, or intravenous methods.

If general anesthesia is required to remove a mole from a child's shoulder, the anesthesia obviously is more formidable than the operation. This situation is necessary at times but should be avoided if possible.

Halothane is so well suited to outpatient procedures that one hardly needs to look elsewhere. Ease of induction, adaptability, and rapid recovery are characteristics of halothane that are especially valuable for short procedures. Other agents that have been used are divinyl ether, nitrous oxide either unsupplemented or with trichloroethylene, cyclopropane, and ether. Of these, cyclopropane would be most useful were it not for its explosive qualities.

Intravenous thiopental with nitrous oxide may be used for older children as it is for adults. Prolonged respiratory depression is less likely to occur if patients have not received preoperative sedation with narcotics or hypnotics.

One type of case presents a slight problem. This concerns endotracheal intubation in patients who expect to be discharged immediately after operation. For excision of small lesions about the face, intubation is frequently indicated, but even the remote possibility of postoperative tracheitis is enough to make one hesitate. When intubation is definitely preferable, it may be used with these additional precautions:

1. Patients living within a radius of 10 miles are observed for 2 hours after operation.
2. Patients who live at a distance of more than 10 miles from the hospital are observed for 4 hours or are kept overnight.
3. Parents are told to watch for signs of respiratory obstruction and are instructed concerning steps that should be taken.

EMERGENCY AND UNSCHEDULED OPERATIONS

For many years children were rushed to the hospital for "emergency surgery," which included treatment of lacerations, burns, fractures, appendicitis, peritonitis, intestinal obstruction, abscesses, and a number of other conditions. In the belief that immediate treatment was all-important, and in the surgeon's desire to get the unwelcome interruption out of the way as soon as possible, history and physical examination were omitted, preparation was neglected, and various other shortcuts compounded error upon error and often changed a minor accident into a major catastrophe.

Actually there are very few conditions that demand "emergency" surgery.

Respiratory obstruction, uncontrolled hemorrhage, and acute head injury may deserve immediate treatment, but in most types of acute pathology time must be taken to examine the child thoroughly for other illness or injury, treat shock or fluid imbalance, administer sedatives and antibiotics, and take any other measures indicated to get the child into suitable condition for anesthesia and operation. Thus haste must not lead us into stupid preventable errors. The former attitude of "Emergency Surgery—Hurry" has been replaced by that of "Emergency Surgery—Watch Out."

Problems in minor operations

In the management of children with lacerations, simple fractures, and other minor injuries, the anesthetist meets two major problems, the control of *fear* and the management of *the full stomach*.

Fear. A bloody, begrimed little boy with a gashed head who has been rushed into the hospital by frantic parents is much different from the well-prepared child who is brought into the same department for elective circumcision.

Every effort must be taken to control the child's emotions before any treatment is undertaken. Simply putting the child on a bed in a quiet room and allowing his parents to sit down by his side will help considerably. Further reassurance of the parents and sedation of the child will be repaid by their feeling of relief and grateful confidence.

Although morphine is of some benefit to these children, it will be ineffective in controlling truly excited patients unless excessive doses are given. Other approaches must be considered.

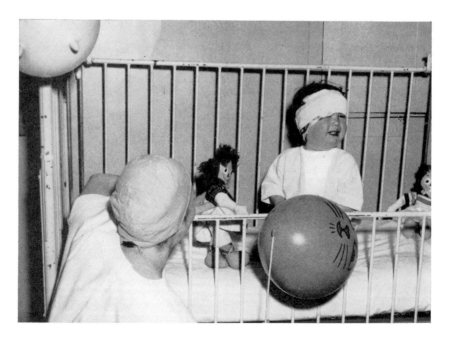

Fig. 24-1. An excited child 1 to 3 years of age is especially difficult to manage.

For the screaming, unmanageable child 1 to 3 years of age (Fig. 24-1) rectal sedation with tribromoethanol or thiopental is undoubtedly the most effective method of sedation for emergency procedures. After receiving a standard dose of tribromoethanol (80 mg./kg.) or thiopental (10 mg./lb.), the child stops crying, becomes drowsy, and quietly goes to sleep within 8 to 10 minutes (Fig. 24-2). This occurs without struggling, resistance, or physiologic disturbance. As the parents watch the child drop quietly off to sleep, they are equally pacified. After such basal induction, the operative procedure may be carried out by supplementation with nitrous oxide–oxygen, local, or volatile anesthetics. If such basal anesthesia is used, the child may sleep 2 or 3 hours after the operation. This is the only real disadvantage of the method and leaves room for improvement.

Recently methohexital (Brevital) given by rectum in doses of 10 mg./lb. has been found to give equally satisfactory induction, with more prompt awakening.

The use of hypnosis is rapidly increasing, and remarkable results can be obtained by this technique in outpatient work. Within a few minutes a child may be induced to tolerate extensive suturing and other procedures that usually are very painful. This method offers the unique combination of rendering sedation unnecessary, avoiding the danger of vomiting and aspiration, and ensuring immediate recovery of consciousness.

Frequently a child comes to the outpatient department and is treated there for his injury but subsequently is admitted to the hospital for further care or observation. In such cases speed of recovery is of less concern. Basal anesthesia

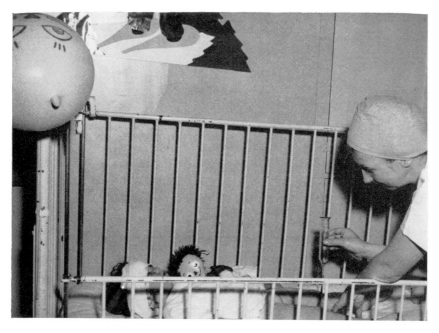

Fig. 24-2. Sedation with tribromoethanol or thiopental by rectum is rapid, pleasant, and effective.

is used on small children, and for older patients the standard combination of atropine, barbiturate, and narcotic has been most satisfactory.

The full stomach. When any child enters the hospital for unscheduled anesthesia, it must be assumed that he has undigested food in his stomach. Care should be taken to find out when and what he was known to eat last, and then allowance should be made for several extra snacks that he probably has picked up in the meantime. It is also important to know how soon after the last meal the accident or injury occurred, for the digestive process often ceases abruptly with excitement, leaving the food in the stomach quite unchanged for many hours.

Although most physicians are aware of the danger of vomiting undigested food, with subsequent aspiration and death, the mortality from this complication continues to be inexcusably high.[2,3]

Several methods of approaching this problem are employed today, each in the belief that it is safe and better than the others. Since this problem is very frequently encountered and is of extreme gravity, each method will be discussed.

Postponement or waiting method. It is believed by some anesthetists that the stomach empties itself in 4 hours, by others that it takes 6 or 8 and that after this time has elapsed anesthesia may be safely conducted under standard "empty-stomach" techniques. Experience has shown that food may remain in the stomach 12 to 24 hours after an injury; consequently, this approach is not justified. A more conservative method is to admit all injured children to the hospital for the night and prepare them for anesthesia next morning. Although this seems safe, it appears to be impractical, especially in a busy area that has many such patients.

Preoperative gastric lavage. It has been an accepted practice to pass a Levin tube into a child's stomach in the belief that gastric contents could be removed in this way. Levin tubes and even large stomach tubes may remove fluid contents, but the dangerous chunks of beef and undigested apple skins will be left in the stomach and the risk will remain the same. Such a tube should be passed *if there is abdominal distention;* however, passage of the tube and irrigation will not give any assurance that it is safe to proceed with standard methods.

Induced vomiting. Another method of trying to empty the stomach is to induce the child to vomit by mechanical irritation of his pharynx, by use of emetic drugs, or by use of open-drop ether just long enough to stimulate vomiting and then make him gag by irritating his pharynx. These methods are very upsetting to the patient emotionally as well as physiologically. Furthermore they are not reliable, for no matter how much the child vomits there usually is more to come.

Gastric balloon. Gastrict tubes with balloons have been constructed to prevent vomiting or regurgitation.[4,5] The tube is passed, and then the balloon is distended and pulled up against the cardiac orifice of the esophagus to block upward passage of stomach contents. Such a tube is not easily passed in children. Furthermore it seems preferable to allow the child to empty his stomach if he can do so safely.

Rapid induction with thiopental and relaxant, followed by intubation. A fifth method is advocated by some but vehemently condemned by many who have used it and experienced serious trouble. This is the use of rapid induction with thiopental and a relaxant, followed by intubation. At first this appears to be a reliable method, but with relaxation the entire gastric content may instantly well up into the pharynx and pour into the paralyzed larynx before anything can be done to control it. A number of deaths have been associated with this technique.

Some have insisted that this so-called "crash" induction is safe if the patient is placed in a steep head-up position. Roe[6] has shown this concept to be false by demonstrating intragastric pressure more than enough to overcome the 19 cm. pressure exerted by gravity.

Each of the five methods just described has some definite disadvantage. There remain three alternatives that have been completely satisfactory in our experience and are recommended for maximum safety and expedience.

Avoidance of general anesthesia. The first and best method is to avoid general anesthesia entirely, if possible. A large proportion of minor lacerations may be handled by combining adequate sedation with local or regional block anesthesia (Chapter 12).

Preservation of gag reflex under nitrous oxide anesthesia. When general anesthesia is indicated, nitrous oxide and oxygen can be used with minimal risk. Although vomiting may occur immediately after operation under nitrous oxide, the gag reflex is retained and usually prevents aspiration. When copious vomiting occurs, one must not rely entirely upon this assumption but should hasten to clear away the obstructing material.

Inhalation anesthesia and prolonged endotracheal intubation. If surgical anesthesia is necessary for relaxation, the most satisfactory method has been not to try to empty the stomach nor wait and hope the stomach will empty itself but to assume the stomach is full and proceed on that basis.[7] A Levin tube is passed only if the stomach is distended, in order to relieve excess pressure. Intravenous anesthetics and relaxants are carefully avoided, but general anesthesia is induced with any of the volatile agents.

Speed is important during induction if one is using a risky technique, but if one is able to control the situation speed is less essential. Since halothane gives the least irritating and most easily controlled induction, this should be the safest agent. One may also use cyclopropane or divinyl ether and ether. The latter agents are irritating and may cause nausea, but during induction the gag reflex will be retained and there is less danger of aspiraton than durng recovery.

There is obviously much difference of opinion as to the safest method of induction. Fortunately there is one basic point upon which all agree. That is that the patient who has eaten presents a major risk, and whatever method is adopted, one must be prepared for trouble and must have a plan of action in readiness. This naturally includes adequate apparatus, as well as special maneuvers with which to meet emergencies. One of the best of these is manual pressure on the cricoid ring, known as Sellick's maneuver.[8] This may be used when a patient starts to vomit; it will close the esophagus effectively and will prevent stomach contents from entering the pharynx. It also should be emphasized that the relaxation of the esophageal sphincter is considerably less under inhalation agents than following administration of succinylcholine.

As soon as anesthesia is induced, a snugly fitting endotracheal tube is passed, and the operation is begun. The stomach may be gavaged during operation, but reliance should not be placed on this gesture. With the use of inhalation agents vomiting is most dangerous during recovery, while the gag reflex is still absent. For this reason *the most important safeguard is to keep the endotracheal tube in place until the child is actually awake.*[9]

The natural tendency will be to remove the tube as soon as the child starts to "buck" and react. This is just the beginning of the danger period, during which the child will vomit copiously for 5 or 10 minutes and be in great danger unless the tube is left in place (Fig. 24-3). Finally, when the child moves his arms and legs, makes facial grimaces, and opens his eyes, it is safe to assume that the gag reflex has returned. After the pharynx, nose, and mouth have been thoroughly cleared of material, the tube may be removed. This procedure has been in effect for the past 20 years and appears to be practically foolproof.

Preparation of equipment. Whalen[10] has correctly emphasized the extreme importance of preparation of equipment prior to anesthesia for children with full stomachs. He lists "an operating table readily adjustable to the Trendelenburg position, proper suction apparatus of a metal pharyngeal type and rubber nasal type, anaesthetic machine with adequately filled tanks, intravenous or

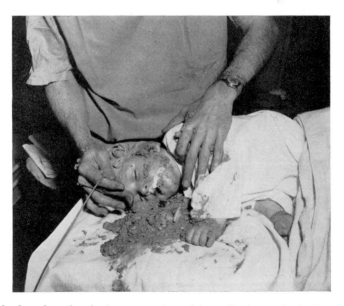

Fig. 24-3. Aspiration of vomitus is the greatest hazard in pediatric anesthesia. It can be avoided by induction with inhalation agents and by endotracheal intubation. The endotracheal tube must be left in place until the child is *actually awake.* (From Smith, R. M.: New York J. Med. **56:**2213, 1956.)

liquid anaesthetic agents and relaxants in complete readiness, airways of proper size, laryngoscope and several endotracheal tubes with connectors attached, adhesive strapping, dental mouth gag, and readily available bronchoscope."*

To this list I should add a stiff suction tube that can be passed easily into the trachea and one or two wide-bore suction tubes fashioned from endotracheal tubes, since standard suction appartus immediately becomes plugged and ineffective when massive vomiting takes place (Fig. 24-4).

Anesthesia for major traumatic conditions

Respiratory emergencies. When children are admitted following severe injuries, the anesthetist first checks ventilation and cardiac activity. Immediate assistance is effected by clearing the airway and providing mouth-to-mouth resuscitation or cardiac massage by external compression of the chest. Respiratory exchange may be endangered by head injury or local injury to the upper airway or chest. The airway can be established by passage of an endotracheal tube or a bronchoscope (Chapter 22). Following initial aeration, a tracheostomy is performed if necessary. Details of anesthesia for this tracheostomy have been

---

*From Whalen, J. S.: Emergency paediatric anaesthesia, Canad. Anaesth. Soc. J. 2:366-373, 1955.

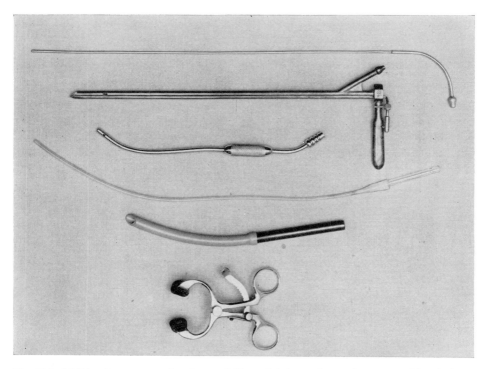

Fig. 24-4. Additional apparatus that is especially useful for patients who are vomiting includes bronchoscope, metal pharyngeal suction tube, stiff plastic suction catheter for trachea, wide-bore suction catheter, and dental bite-block.

described. Subsequent ventilatory assistance must also be supplied if respiration is depressed.

Shock. The treatment of children in shock follows the same rules used for adults. The patient is placed in a horizontal position, and blood volume is restored as rapidly as possible. The best substance to use for blood volume replacement undoubtedly is whole blood. Until this can be procured and cross matched, however, we believe that 5% albumin solution is the most valuable substitute.[11] This material is prepared easily by any standard blood bank and is available commercially. It can be kept prepared in solution, can be stocked for long periods, does not carry hepatitis virus, does not interfere with cross matching as does dextran, and is inexpensive. Lactated Ringer's solution can also be used for rapid replacement of fluid volume.

When active bleeding occurs, it must be controlled; otherwise operative procedures are delayed until the child's blood pressure and pulse are within normal limits and his condition is sufficiently improved to tolerate anesthesia.

Anesthesia must be chosen carefully for patients recovering from shock. Obviously an intravenous infusion must be running prior to induction. Intravenous barbiturates, spinal anesthesia, and ether are best avoided. Cyclopropane or nitrous oxide–oxygen–relaxant combinations are preferable because these agents support vasomotor tone.

Children with *severe burns* rarely require anesthesia during the acute phase of injury. Sedation is allowed, but these patients appear to be shocked into a state of analgesia and do not suffer as much as would be expected.

Acutely ill patients

In children with acute appendicitis and peritonitis, those with intestinal obstruction, large abdominal tumors, brain abscess, and other conditions involving high fever, loss of weight, protracted vomiting, and other debilitating conditions, the problem is not one of speed but of adequate preparation for operation. To rush these patients to the operating room as soon as the diagnosis is made is the surest way to kill them, and although surgeons have known this for years, the mistake is still being made.

Any patient who has a high fever or rapid pulse and who is dehydrated or anemic must be sent not to the operating room but to the ward and treated there until given fluids, antibiotics, and specific therapy sufficient to bring him into a reasonably safe condition for operation (Fig. 24-5). These measures are described in the chapter concerning fluid therapy (Chapter 26).

After such sick children have been brought into optimum condition, premedication and anesthetic must be chosen. Acutely ill children often require little sedation. Certainly each patient must be considered individually, and sedation should be given in reduced quantities. If there has been recent temperature elevation, atropine is not given at the usual time 45 minutes before operation but is withheld until the child reaches the operating room and then is given intravenously. This precaution is taken to avoid an iatrogenic pulse elevation that could not be distinguished from one arising from a sudden exacerbation of the underlying disease.

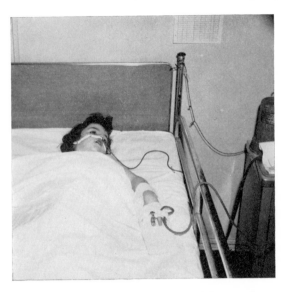

Fig. 24-5. Emergency treatment of a child with an acute abdomen often consists of hydration and antibiotics to be *followed by operation.* (From Smith, R. M.: New York J. Med. **56:**2213, 1956.)

Anesthesia for small infants that are critically ill may well consist of local infiltration. If relaxation is needed, cyclopropane combines controllability with rapid recovery and is well tolerated. In very sick children it is better to use very light cyclopropane and to supplement it with a relaxant than to attempt a greater depth of cyclopropane alone.

Sick children 3 or more years of age who come to the operating room following special preparatory treatment usually have an infusion running. Induction is most humanely accomplished by adding thiopental (approximately 1 mg. per pound) via the infusion. After the child has fallen asleep, anesthesia may be continued, using halothane, cyclopropane, or nitrous oxide–relaxant combinations. Ether is tolerated satisfactorily if the patient has been well hydrated and adequately prepared. Spinal anesthesia and epidural anesthesia have been recommended for appendectomy and other abdominal operations in sick children. If the patient is adequately hydrated and prepared, these methods may be used, but an ill, poorly prepared child is no better candidate for spinal anesthesia than for general anesthesia.

The problem of high fever in the patient requiring emergency surgery is familiar to all.[12] It is generally recognized that it is extremely dangerous to operate upon children with elevated temperature, yet few have arrived at a reasonable solution. Our approach is to administer fluids, antibiotics, and rectal aspirin until normal hematocrit and urinary flow give evidence of adequate hydration (hematocrit, 30 to 35%; urine specific gravity, 1.005 to 1.035).

If the temperature remains elevated, the child is taken to the operating room, anesthetized, and then cooled by application of ice and alcohol sponges

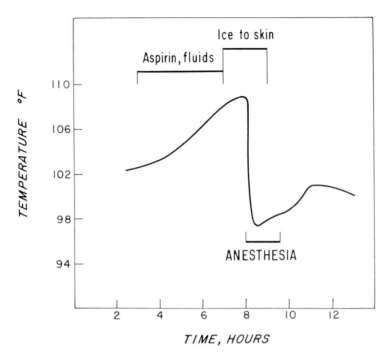

Fig. 24-6. Temperature curve of 9-year-old boy with peritonitis. Treatment with rectal aspirin and intravenous fluids failed to control temperature. Surface cooling caused shivering and further elevation of temperature, until general anesthesia was induced. When shivering was controlled, temperature dropped, and operation was undertaken.

(Fig. 24-6). Temperature is observed closely throughout the operative and post-operative phase. The anesthetic agent for patients who have had a high temperature is less important than the supplementary methods of temperature control. Most agents are safe if the temperature remains below 102, but few if any are safe if the temperature rises above that. Since halothane promotes dissipation of body heat, this is recommended.

Unscheduled operations on newborn infants

The baby who is born with a cystic lung, a diaphragmatic hernia, or with intestinal obstruction sends no warning in advance; therefore these situations fall into the class of emergency or unscheduled surgery. Operations for these conditions actually comprise a large part of the unscheduled procedures in most pediatric surgical services and present the anesthetist with many problems. Although the anesthetic management of the newborn infant has already been discussed (Chapter 17), it may be repeated that any anesthetist who deals with infants and children must be prepared to care for critically ill, newborn infants. When preparation is made for such cases, two factors are of great importance: (1) to have a complete stock of equipment on hand for infant anesthesia and (2) to have a clear understanding of the special pathologic problems involved.

REFERENCES

1. Editorial: Anaethesia in outpatient departments, Brit. Med. J. **1**:505-506, 1954.
2. Merrill, R. B., and Hingson, R. A.: A study of incidence of maternal mortality from aspiration of vomitus during anesthesia occuring in major obstetric hospitals in the United States, Anesth. Analg. **30**:121-135, 1951.
3. Morton, H. J. V., and Wylie, W. D.: Anaesthetic deaths due to regurgitation or vomiting, Anaesthesiology **6**:190-201, 1951.
4. Guiffrida, J. G., and Bizzari, D.: Intubation of the esophagus—its role in the prevention of aspiration pneumonia and asphyxial death, Amer. J. Surg. **86**:329-334, 1957.
5. Gilman, S., and Abrams, A. L.: Prevention of aspiration of gastric contents during general anesthesia, New Eng. J. Med. **255**:508-509, 1956.
6. Roe, R. B.: The effect of suxamethonium on intragastric pressure, Anaesthesia **17**:179-181, 1962.
7. Smith, R. M.: Anesthesia for emergency surgery in pediatrics, Clin. Anesth. **2**:99-119, 1963.
8. Sellick, B. A.: Cricoid pressure, Lancet **2**:404, 1961.
9. Smith, R. M.: Some reasons for the high mortality in pediatric anesthesia, New York J. Med. **56**:2212-2216, 1956.
10. Whalen, J. S.: Emergency paediatric anaesthesia, Canad. Anaesth. Soc. J. **2**:366-373, 1955.
11. Kevy, S. V.: Transfusion therapy, Internat. Anesth. Clin. **1**:287-298, 1962.
12. Brayton, D., and Lewis, G. B.: The use of hypothermia in general pediatric surgery. A preliminary report, Ann. Surg. **145**:304-310, 1957.

Chapter 25

Special problems in pediatric anesthesia

Toxic and critically ill patients
Presence of acute or chronic respiratory disease
Mumps, measles, and whooping cough
Children with cardiac disease undergoing noncardiac operations
Anesthesia in the presence of liver and kidney disease
Blood dyscrasias and leukemia
Metabolic disorders
    Diabetes
    Gargoylism (Hurler's disease)
    Neimann-Pick disease and Gaucher's disease
Mongolism, mental retardation, and epilepsy
Myasthenia gravis and amyotonia congenita
Familial dysautonomia (Riley-Day syndrome)
Hereditary angioneurotic edema
Separation of conjoined (Siamese) twins
Adrenogenital syndrome

Patients who are critically ill, those who have infections, metabolic disorders, organic lesions, or other complicating problems, may require individualized preparation and anesthetic management. Certain general principles apply to most of these patients. They include the reduction of preoperative sedation, the use of light planes of anesthesia, and a special effort to avoid hypoventilation, spasm, and metabolic disturbance and to produce rapid recovery.

TOXIC AND CRITICALLY ILL PATIENTS

Although a child with acute appendicitis and peritonitis may be nursed into fair condition by preoperative hydration and antibiotics prior to operation, one who has advanced malignancy (Fig. 25-1) or recurrent intestinal obstruction may not respond to any form of preoperative therapy and may require operation while in extremely poor condition. Local anesthesia is indicated if it will permit the surgeon to do his work satisfactorily. In all poor-risk patients an

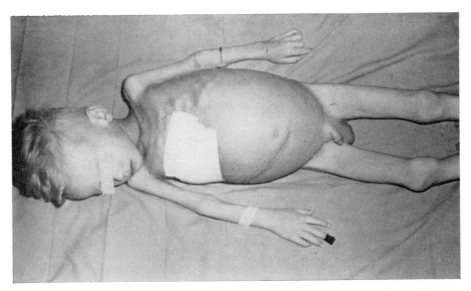

Fig. 25-1. Children with advanced malignancy require minimal amounts of anesthetic agents.

infusion should be started before the operation, both for supportive therapy and for administration of minimal amounts of short-acting sedatives or relaxants should they prove necessary. Oxygen is administered throughout all such procedures.

When general anesthesia is needed for sick children, light cyclopropane anesthesia supplemented by succinylcholine can be used, although it is surprising how much can be accomplished simply with 50% nitrous oxide and oxygen. Recently we encountered a 12-year-old girl whose appendix had ruptured 2 weeks previously and who was admitted in virtually moribund condition with azotemia, draining abdominal sinuses, and peritoneal abscesses. She was in delirium and also had toxic myocarditis with heart block. After allowing time for hydration and reduction of fever, the surgeons performed a thorough abdominal exploration and wide drainage. Nitrous oxide and oxygen not only provided analgesia but also produced adequate abdominal relaxation.

PRESENCE OF ACUTE OR CHRONIC RESPIRATORY DISEASE

Although it is hardly a serious problem, a troublesome and extremely common situation arises when a child who is scheduled for operation appears to have a cough or a runny nose. If there is fever, pharyngeal inflammation, or any sign of pulmonary infection, operation is cancelled. Evidence of upper respiratory infection is also taken as a strong contraindication to the use of endotracheal intubation for fear of postoperative otitis or tracheitis. However, if the child seems to be recovering from a mild upper respiratory infection and the operation is one that should not wait, it may seem permissible to go ahead. In this case halothane, because of lack of irritating and secretory effects, is probably the best agent.

Bronchial asthma is seen relatively frequently in children and will vary in degree from an insignificant finding to an incapacitating affliction. Although all agents have been administered to such patients, is seems advisable to omit thiobarbiturates and cyclopropane. In mild states of the disease children tolerate premedication with standard agents. If there is appreciable respiratory obstruction prior to operation, induction with tribromoethanol (Avertin) is especially useful.[1,2] Maintenance with halothane or ether is advised. If bronchospasm develops during anesthesia, epinephrine may be administered during ether, and aminophylline may be given (3 mg./lb.) during either halothane or ether anesthesia.[3] Following use of either of these agents a child's asthma may be remarkably improved.[3a]

Pancreatic fibrosis (cystic fibrosis of the pancreas, mucoviscidosis)[4,4a] is actually a generalized disease involving the mucus-secreting glands of the entire body and also is characterized by absence of intestinal trypsin. The earliest form of this disease is meconium ileus, seen in the neonatal period (p. 253). An infant who survives this will next be easy prey to several other phases of the illness. As the disease progresses the child appears malnourished and develops an emphysematous chest and a protruding abdomen.

Although lack of intestinal enzymes can be treated successfully, chronic infection of the lungs is more difficult to overcome. Masses of staphylococci plug the bronchioles, causing recurrent bouts of pneumonia, abscess formation, bronchiectasis, emphysema, cor pulmonale, and ultimately death. Prolapse of the rectum is common among younger children having cystic fibrosis, and nasal

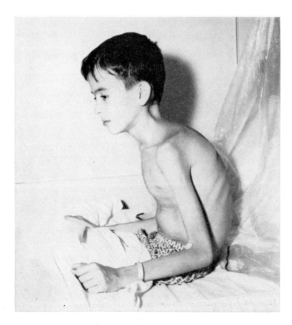

Fig. 25-2. The advanced stages of cystic fibrosis bring wasting, bronchiectasis, emphysema, and cor pulmonale.

polyps occur in older children—the nasal polyps often become necrotic and destroy the turbines and sinuses. Numerous therapeutic and diagnostic procedures may be required in these children, including colostomy, bronchoscopy, lobectomy, pneumonectomy,[5] tracheostomy, repair of prolapse, and excision of nasal polyps.

Sick, coughing thick heavy sputum, apprehensive, and often febrile, these children present a pathetic picture and a real anesthetic problem (Fig. 25-2). Premedication should be light. Pediatricians have feared that use of atropine would cause increased airway obstruction, but our experience[6] and that of Salanitre[7] do not bear this out. Any operation should be preceded by postural drainage, antibiotics, and maximum pulmonary preparation. In patients with copious purulent secretions the prone position may be indicated. Halothane will be the most useful agent in general, but for excision of nasal polyps a relaxant–nitrous oxide technique is chosen so that epinephrine may be used.

Tracheobronchial lavage has been tried in patients with cystic fibrosis, using repeated instillations of n-acetyl cysteine,[8,8a] saline, or other fluids. This has proved to be a relatively dangerous procedure, and enthusiasm for it seems to be waning.

MUMPS, MEASLES, AND WHOOPING COUGH

It is not unusual for a child to develop a surgical lesion during the active stage of an acute communicable disease.[9] The management of these cases will vary with the disease involved, but some factors are common to all.

If fever is present, hydration and temperature-controlling devices may be indicated to reduce the temperature to safe level (below 102° F.) before operation.

Since respiratory irritation is associated with most diseases of this nature, secretions and spasm will be more troublesome. For this reason bronchodilating and nonirritant agents are preferred. Preoperative sedation may be used in reduced quantities. Tribromoethanol probably is superior in children with pertussis for induction and halothane for maintenance. Thiopental is to be avoided in such cases because of its bronchoconstricting qualities. Relaxants are undesirable under such conditions since attendant intubation in the presence of infection about the mouth increases the hazard of spreading organisms. Local anesthesia may be used for conditions other than pertussis, but coughing is best controlled by a general anesthetic during operation. During and after operation the usual precautions must be taken to prevent dissemination of communicable diseases.

CHILDREN WITH CARDIAC DISEASE
UNDERGOING NONCARDIAC OPERATIONS

Children who have heart disease occasionally require elective or emergency surgery as do normal children.

If the patient is asymptomatic and leads a normal life in spite of his cardiac lesion, anesthesia may be chosen as for a normal child, although it may be expected that shock and hypoxia will be tolerated poorly; hence, anesthesia must be conducted with increased care.

When children have symptomatic heart lesions with easy fatigability, dyspnea, cyanosis, cardiac hypertrophy, or pulmonary hypertension, further precautions should be observed. The necessity for operation should be indicated clearly, and any procedure that is not definitely essential for the health of the child should be deferred. If general anesthesia is to be used, no matter how simple the intended procedure, it is wise to hospitalize the child the night before operation for complete preparation and for maximal psychologic conditioning.

Moderate sedation is allowable and will improve the oxygenation of cyanotic children. General anesthesia with cyclopropane is well tolerated, and there is no contraindication to small amounts of thiopental or relaxants. Very light ether anesthesia is tolerated well but may prolong recovery and disturb the fluid balance. In our experience halothane has been tolerated poorly in children with cyanotic heart disease, but it is useful in noncyanotic cardiac patients. Although spinal anesthesia has merits in patients with cardiac failure, such anesthesia used in children with heart disease may lead to undesirable apprehension and straining, with resultant increase in oxygen demand.

When patients with rheumatic fever require anesthesia, a similar approach is indicated. In addition, one must be sure to find out whether cortisone or other steroids have been used and must take the proper precautionary steps (p. 77).

During anesthesia for all cardiac patients, supplemental oxygen must be used, blood pressure should be followed closely, and cardiorespiratory activity should be monitored by stethoscope. During operations on children with serious cardiac lesions or preoperative conduction defects, the use of an electrocardiograph will be indicated.

Fluid management will also require special consideration. Hypotension must be prevented by the use of intravenous fluids, blood, or vasopressors, as indicated. In cyanotic children with hemoconcentration the restriction of preoperative fluid intake may lead to thrombosis of cerebral or peripheral vessels. Consequently, infusions are indicated preoperatively to counterbalance the restriction of oral intake.

ANESTHESIA IN THE PRESENCE OF LIVER AND KIDNEY DISEASE

Since the presence of severe liver or kidney disease is considered a contraindication to most anesthetic agents, children with these lesions present further problems. Infants with biliary atresia often show marked jaundice. However, since this is an obstructive form of jaundice, the liver is still functionally effective, and such infants tolerate most agents relatively well. Hepatitis, on the other hand, usually involves serious functional impairment, and all agents involve some danger. Minimal amounts of cyclopropane, local anesthesia, or nitrous oxide and curare may be used guardedly.

Use of halothane in the presence of hepatic disease is decidedly questionable. Popper[9a] states that halothane gives increased liver perfusion and is the anesthetic of choice in hepatic pathology not caused by drugs, but that any drug toxicity should be considered a contraindication to halogenated anesthetics.

Children having phenylpyruvic oligophrenia (phenylketonuria) have a complex type of pathology involving brain, liver, and endocrine glands. Those under dietary treatment are in danger of severe hypoglycemic episodes because of glycogen depletion of the liver. One death has occurred in our vicinity following strabismus correction under ether anesthesia.

The presence of nephritis occasionally complicates operative problems. Preoperative sedation with chloral hydrate is usually preferred, and anesthesia with nitrous oxide, oxygen, and succinylcholine has definite advantages. Patients with nephrosis may be managed similarly. It has been found that when medications are given to these children by subcutaneous or intramuscular route, it may take several hours for them to be absorbed. This should be borne in mind if sedatives or narcotics are employed.

BLOOD DYSCRASIAS AND LEUKEMIA

Sickle cell disease, being restricted to the Negro race, is seen frequently in the southern states and occasionally in the north. The disease is characterized by the presence of elliptic red blood corpuscles of increased fragility, which have a tendency to produce a sludging effect in the blood with thrombus formation throughout the body.[10] As emphasized by Shapiro and Poe,[11] this disease presents several problems to the anesthetist, among which anemia and sickling crises are especially important. Extremely low hemoglobin levels are common and should be corrected prior to anesthesia, since shock carries exaggerated danger in these patients. Bouts of increased sickling are induced by a number of causes, including hypoxia, electrolyte imbalance, and low blood pressure. Consequently, increased care must be taken to prepare patients thoroughly, to avoid depressant sedatives and anesthetics, and to provide full oxygenation during anesthesia. Shapiro and Poe also mention the danger of localized stasis, which may follow the use of spinal anesthesia, faulty positioning, or hypothermia.

Children who are scheduled for splenectomy deserve special attention. Elective splenectomy usually is performed to correct either familial hemolytic anemia or idiopathic thrombocytopenic purpura, and both of these conditions involve pitfalls for the anesthetist.

In familial hemolytic anemia the low hemoglobin level would ordinarily be an indication for transfusion. However, administration of blood may precipitate renewed hemolytic episodes and be of no benefit to the patient. Consequently, it may be preferable to wait until the spleen has been removed before starting transfusion.

Children with idiopathic thrombocytopenic purpura often receive cortisone preparations in order to stimulate platelet formation. Suitable therapy must be undertaken to control this hazard (p. 77).

Leukemia in an early or advanced stage may be an indication for diagnostic sternal biopsy or may be present as a complicating factor in patients with other operative conditions. Cortisone is almost always part of the complicated therapy employed here. For sternal biopsy, nitrous oxide, oxygen, and halothane give adequate analgesia and minimal disturbance. Since these children have a short life expectancy, it seems unnecessary to add to their troubles by transfusion or additional cortisone therapy to prepare them for diagnostic procedures.

METABOLIC DISORDERS

Diabetes. The preoperative and anesthetic management of diabetic children is similar to that of adults.[12] Ordinarily one attempts to establish the patient on NPH insulin prior to operation and aims to have the patient continue to show a slight trace of sugar in the urine. It is advisable to give the patient half of his daily dose of NPH insulin prior to operation, administer 5% glucose during the procedure (approximately 5 ml. per pound in 2 to 3 hours), to be followed by the second half of the insulin dosage after operation. The urine should be tested at intervals throughout the day and the results used as a guide to further therapy. It is preferable to have the child awaken as soon as possible so that he may take fluids by mouth.

Gargoylism (Hurler's disease). Gargoylism is an osteochondrodystrophy in which there are lesions of the bones of the hands, the vertebrae, and the long bones.[13,14] The facies of these children is characterized by heavy eyebrows, snub nose, protruding eyes, and large tongue (Fig. 25-3). In addition there are hepatosplenomegaly and accumulation of firm masses of lymphoid tissue in the mouth and neck. Operation may be indicated for splenectomy, liver biopsy, or lesions unrelated to the underlying disease.

When these patients are anesthetized, the lymphoid tissue in the mouth and neck may cause severe respiratory obstruction. On two occasions we have encountered great difficulty in establishing an airway. The airway in one child

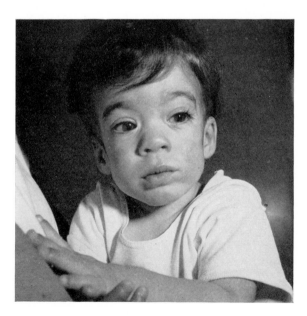

Fig. 25-3. Children with Hurler's syndrome (gargoylism) develop increasing respiratory obstruction from lymphoid hyperplasia.

became completely obstructed, and it was impossible to visualize the glottis. Immediate tracheostomy barely saved his life. Another case of this nature has been described in which the child died.

Because of these experiences, children with gargoylism are approached with great respect, and if there is evidence of lymphoid hyperplasia, preparations for tracheostomy are made. The use of intravenous barbiturates and relaxants is definitely contraindicated in such types of airway obstruction. Light sedation and generous atropinization, followed by nitrous oxide, oxygen, and halothane should give the most reliable anesthesia.

Niemann-Pick disease and Gaucher's disease. Niemann-Pick disease[15] and Gaucher's disease[9] are disorders of lipid storage, in which marked lymphoid hyperplasia may occur about the mouth and pharynx, as well as in the spleen. Niemann-Pick disease is characterized by apathy, pancytopenia, hepatosplenomegaly, emaciation, and death in early childhood. Gaucher's disease represents a slightly less severe disorder, which has both acute and chronic forms. Pancytopenia is absent, but a pseudobulbar syndrome is typical. Muscle hypertonia, laryngeal spasm, and trismus also are present. Both diseases present problems to the anesthetist that are due to severe malnourishment and chronic liver dysfunction. The greatest problem is associated with lymphoid hyperplasia about the pharynx, causing marked respiratory obstruction and rendering intubation extremely difficult.

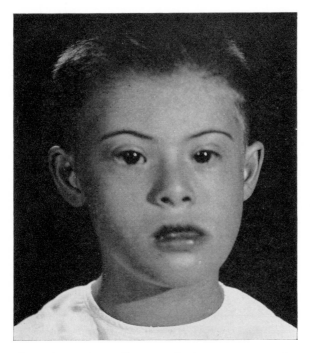

Fig. 25-4. In Down's syndrome (mongolism) anesthesia may cause marked cardiorespiratory depression.

MONGOLISM, MENTAL RETARDATION, AND EPILEPSY

Children with mongolism (Down's syndrome) exhibit recognizable traits of slanting eyes, epicanthal folds, large tongue, and mental retardation[16,17,17a] (Fig. 25-4). In addition they have increased susceptibility to infection, and many of them have congenital cardiac lesions. In relation to anesthesia it has been stated that they do not tolerate atropine well. However, this appears to refer chiefly to pupillary responses rather than to any generalized reaction.[18] We have found that they behave very much like patients with hypothyroid disease. On two occasions mongoloid children have shown marked cardiorespiratory depression following anesthesia and have taken several hours to recover. The first child had received ether, the second *d*-tubocurarine and nitrous oxide. It appears that sedation for mongoloid children should be reduced and that minimal amounts of anesthetic agents should be used.

Incidentally, there has been a noticeable increase in the number of these patients during recent years. Many infants with tracheoesophageal fistula or intestinal obstruction and numerous older children with cardiac anomalies have tolerated cyclopropane, halothane, or relaxant techniques without complication.

Children who are physically normal but mentally retarded respond poorly to attempts at preoperative conditioning. If they are not antagonistic, mild sedation may be successful and should be followed by carefully controlled, light anesthesia. When such children appear antagonistic, they may become excited and unmanageable after barbiturate medication. A better approach has been to put them to sleep in their own beds with tribromoethanol or rectal thiopental.

Quite frequently a physician calls in the warning that a child he is admitting for operation is subject to epileptic seizures, implying that he is more likely to convulse with anesthesia. This, of course, is not true, for an epileptic patient is benefited by sedation and general anesthesia and presents no problem to the anesthetist from this standpoint. If he is mentally retarded, treatment should be altered accordingly.

MYASTHENIA GRAVIS AND AMYOTONIA CONGENITA

The pathologic physiology of myasthenia gravis is localized in the myoneural junction, where depression of end-plate potential results in generalized muscular weakness. As is well known, patients with this disease show markedly exaggerated response to relaxants and ether, and these agents are best avoided.

When children are to undergo thymectomy or other procedures, belladonna agents are especially important to control excess secretions stimulated by therapeutic anticholinesterases.[19] Opiates and sedatives must be given in reduced dosage to prevent respiratory depression and postoperative depression of cough reflex. Adriani[9] notes that subclinical forms of myasthenia are more common than is suspected and are more frequently seen in children. For induction and maintenance of anesthesia, cyclopropane or halothane offers advantages of easy controllability and rapid recovery, with little effect upon the underlying disease. It is advisable to reduce the dose of neostigmine prior to operation in order to avoid postoperative overreaction. Decreased neostigmine requirement should be expected after thymectomy, and administration should be delayed until definitely indicated. Supervision must be maintained until adequate respiratory exchange has been reestablished through active function or by use of a mechanical ventilating device. During the recovery period, depression of respiration and cough and excessive secretions will be the principal hazards, whereas neostigmine overdosage may be a complicating factor. Articles by Chang, Harland, and Graves[19] and Mathews and Derrick[20] and the review by Foldes and McNall[21] may be consulted for details of management.

Amyotonia congenita is also characterized by extreme muscle weakness. In this disease the primary pathologic changes occur in the central nervous system and include defective anterior horn cells, deficient myelinization of peripheral nerves, and decreased Betz cells. In addition the muscles are pale and small, and muscle cells are diminished in number.

Patients with amyotonia exhibit an unforgettable picture of limp, flabby tissue. Children often are unable to sit up, and infants usually cannot even hold up their heads. Such patients not infrequently are scheduled for muscle biopsy, for diagnostic laryngoscopy because of airway obstruction, for muscle transplant, or for treatment of lesions not related to the underlying disease.

As in the case of myasthenia gravis, the inability to cough and expel secretions postoperatively poses the greatest anesthetic problem. When possible, local anesthesia is chosen, but unfortunately this is often unsuitable for the particular operation. Cyclopropane, with careful supervision of airway and exchange, has been used with most satisfactory results; however, halothane, which has remarkably little irritant effect, might be an even better choice.

Although patients with myotonia congenita rarely require muscle relaxants, these children, as well as those with myotonia dystrophica, are known to show generalized muscle spasm in response to succinylcholine.[22]

FAMILIAL DYSAUTONOMIA (RILEY-DAY SYNDROME)

Children with familial dysautonomia (Riley-Day syndrome),[23] a disorder of the autonomic nervous system, present special problems during anesthesia because of hypertension, postural hypotension, swallowing difficulty, excessive sweating, vomiting, and recurrent bronchopneumonia. Administration of catecholamines may give rise to exaggerated response. McCaughey[24] described his experience in anesthetizing one child several times. He found that although most anesthetics caused marked blood pressure reduction, methoxyflurane was successful if maintained on an inspired concentration not exceeding 0.5%. It probably was the greatly reduced concentration rather than the specific drug that deserved the credit here.

HEREDITARY ANGIONEUROTIC EDEMA

Children who have hereditary angioneurotic edema, a rare biochemical defect, may be exposed to high risk when anesthetized. Slight trauma, as of the passage of an endotracheal tube, is sufficient to precipitate a catastrophic bout of laryngeal edema. Reasonable safety from this complication can be obtained by preoperative transfusion with fresh human plasma.[25]

SEPARATION OF CONJOINED (SIAMESE) TWINS

Now that open heart surgery is commonplace, the most spectacular operation in pediatric circles probably is the separation of conjoined twins. Because of the rarity of this condition, few can give firsthand advice on the subject, but several cases have been reported accurately by Hall, Merzig, and Norris,[26] Aird,[27] Allen, Metcalf, and Giering,[28] and others.[29,30]

When the union is superficial and positioning offers no problem, the situation is easily managed. One anesthetist cares for each infant and treats him as an individual.

Major difficulties arise, however, when unions involve airway problems, as in the brow-to-brow position (Fig. 25-5), or when vital organs are shared. Here the unusual conditions make it important to organize plans for anesthetic, supportive, and operative management before the time of operation.

In the preoperative care of conjoined twins the usual laboratory studies are made and the infants are nursed into optimal condition before operation is undertaken. An important point made by Aird[27] and stressed by Allen, Metcalf, and Giering[28] is the possibility that the adrenal development of one twin may be defective, and death may occur after separation unless provision is made for this by adequate cortisone administration before, during, and after operation.

At the time of operation cutdown infusions are started in both infants, and one anesthetist is assigned the position of infusionist. In addition, each infant is cared for by an individual anesthetist. The surgical team is planned so that after separation, operation on both infants may be completed simultaneously.

Endotracheal intubation of the infants will be indicated in all but the simplest types of union. In small infants awake intubation is preferable. In

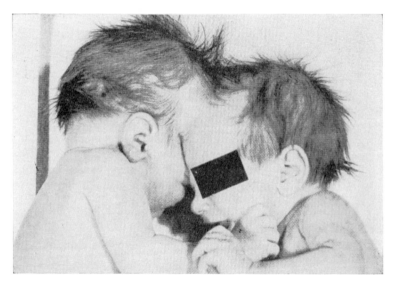

Fig. 25-5. Craniopagus conjoined twins introduce unusual problems. (From Hall, K. D., Merzig, J., and Norris, F. H., Jr.: Anesthesiology **18:**908, 1957.)

strong, resistant infants anesthesia may be necessary, but the use of relaxants should be avoided if intubation promises any difficulty, for the child may become apneic, leaving the anesthetist unable to intubate or ventilate him. Time should be taken for inhalation induction and for the establishment of a satisfactory plane of anesthesia before intubation is attempted in such infants.

When there is circulatory communication between the two twins, there will be increased danger due to the possibility of one infant "bleeding out" into the other. This complication was encountered by Bachman[30] during operation and occurred during the preoperative phase in Allen, Metcalf, and Giering's case.[28] One child was held over the other to facilitate intubation. The uppermost infant immediately showed cardiovascular collapse, and death was narrowly averted by lowering him immediately.

ADRENOGENITAL SYNDROME

It has been our experience that children with adrenogenital syndrome present markedly increased anesthetic risk. Sudden cardiovascular collapse has occurred during anesthesia in three instances in such children, without any obvious precipitating cause. Gross obesity may play a large role, as well as abnormal

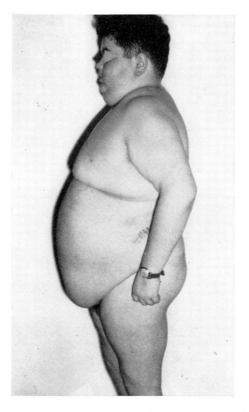

Fig. 25-6. Adrenogenital syndrome may cause obesity, acute salt deficiency, and abnormal catechol response.

catechol response (Fig. 25-6). Many of these children, like those with craniopharyngioma, excrete large quantities of salt, and if replacement is neglected during operation, acute salt depletion can cause acute myocardial depression. Children with adrenogenital syndrome may require operation for excision of tumor or clitoridectomy.

REFERENCES

1. Converse, J. G., and Smotrilla, M. M.: Anesthesia and the asthmatic, Anesth. Analg. **40:**336-342, 1961.
2. Schnider, S. M., and Papper, E. M.: Anesthesia for the asthmatic patient, Anesthesiology **22:**886-892, 1961.
3. Gold, M. I.: Pulmonary mechanics and blood gas tensions during anesthesia in asthmatics, Anesthesiology **27:**216-217, 1966.
3a. Gold, M. I., and Helrich, M.: A study of the complications related to anesthesia in asthmatic patients, Anesth. Analg. **42:**283-293, 1963.
4. Shwachman, H.: Therapy of cystic fibrosis of the pancreas, Pediatrics **25:**155-163, 1960.
4a. di Sant'Agnese, P. A., and Talamo, R. C.: Pathogenesis and pathophysiology of cystic fibrosis of the pancreas, New Eng. J. Med. **277:**1287-1294, 1344-1353, 1359-1408, 1967.
5. Schuster, S. R., and Shwachman, H.: Pulmonary surgery in cystic fibrosis, J. Thorac. Cardiov. Surg. **48:**750-760, 1966.
6. Smith, R. M.: Anesthetic management of patients with cystic fibrosis, Anesth. Analg. **44:**143-146, 1965.
7. Salanitre, E., Klonymus, D., and Rackow, H.: Anesthetic experience in children with cystic fibrosis of the pancreas, Anesthesiology **25:**801-807, 1964.
8. Doershuk, C. F., and Matthews, L. W.: Cystic fibrosis: comprehensive therapy, Postgrad. Med. **40:**550-553, 1966.
8a. Hacket, P. R., and Reas, H. W.: A radical approach to therapy for the pulmonary complications of cystic fibrosis, Anesthesiology **26:**248, 1965.
9. Adriani, J.: Anesthesia for patients with uncommon and unusual diseases, Anesth. Analg. **37:**1-7, 1958.
9a. Popper, H.: Lecture at Twenty-first Postgraduate Assembly in Anesthesiology, New York State Society of Anesthesiologists, Dec. 12, 1967.
10. Murphy, R. C., and Shapiro, S.: Pathology of sickle cell anemia, Ann. Intern. Med. **23:**376-397, 1946.
11. Shapiro, N. D., and Poe, M. F.: Sickle-cell disease: an anesthesiological problem, Anesthesiology **16:**771-780, 1955.
12. Goodman, J. I.: Management of diabetes mellitus during ketoacidosis, acute infection, and surgery, J.A.M.A. **159:**831-835, 1955.
13. Gilbert, E. F., and Guin, G. H.: Gargoylism, Amer. J. Dis. Child. **95:**69-80, 1958.
14. Leroy, J. G., and Crocker, A. C.: Clinical definition of the Hunter-Hurler phenotype, Amer. J. Dis. Child. **112:**518-531, 1966.
15. Crocker, A. C., and Farber, S.: Niemann-Pick disease. A review of 18 patients, Medicine **37:**1-95, 1958.
16. Krivit, W., and Good, R. A.: Leukemia and mongolism, Amer. J. Dis. Child. **91:**218-222, 1956.
17. Benda, C. E.: Mongolism and cretinism, New York, 1949, Grune & Stratton, Inc.
17a. Lejeune, J.: Autosomal disorders, Pediatrics **32:**326-337, 1963.
18. Priest, J. H.: Atropine response of the eyes in mongolism, Amer. J. Dis. Child. **100:**869-872, 1960.
19. Chang, J., Harland, J. H., and Graves, H. B.: Anesthetic aspect of thymectomy for myasthenia gravis, Canad. Anaesth. Soc. J. **4:**13-21, 1957.
20. Mathews, W. A., and Derrick, W. S.: Anesthesia in the patient with myasthenia gravis, Anesthesiology **18:**443-453, 1957.
21. Foldes, F. F., and McNall, P. G.: Myasthenia gravis; a guide for anesthesiologists, Anesthesiology **23:**837-873, 1962.

22. Patterson, I. S.: Generalized myotonia following suxamethonium, Brit. J. Anaesth. 34:340-343, 1962.
23. Riley, C. M., Day, R. L., Greeley, D. M., and Langford, W. S.: Central autonomic dysfunction with defective lacrimation, Pediatrics 3:468-478, 1949.
24. McCaughey, T. J.: Familial dysautonomia as an anaesthetic hazard, Canad. Anaesth. Soc. J. 12:558-568, 1965.
25. Freedman, S. O., and Dolovich, J.: McGill University Medical Clinic of the Montreal General Hospital, Montreal, Canada.
26. Hall, K. D., Merzig, J., and Norris, F. H., Jr.: Case report: Separation of craniopagus, Anesthesiology 18:908-910, 1957.
27. Aird, I.: The conjoined twins of Kano, Brit. Med. J. 1:831-837, 1954.
28. Allen, H. L., Metcalf, D. W., and Giering, C.: Anesthetic management for the separation of conjoined twins, Anesth. Analg. 38:109-112, 1959.
29. Grossman, H. J., Sugar, O., Greeley, P. W., and Sadove, M. S.: Surgical separation in craniopagus, J.A.M.A. 153:201-207, 1953.
30. Bachman, L.: Personal communication.

Chapter 26

Fluid therapy and blood replacement

The ability of children to survive long surgical procedures depends largely on two factors, pulmonary ventilation and fluid balance. The essential features of ventilation are generally recognized, but fluid therapy in children undergoing surgery is difficult to put into practical terms and is poorly understood. The approach adopted here is designed to eliminate unnecessary detail and to divide the subject in such a way that additional reading may be more intelligible. An effort will also be made to point out the most common errors in fluid therapy, many of which are avoidable.

Much confusion can be cleared at the start by dividing the subject into several practical aspects and considering each one separately.

BASIC CHARACTERISTICS CONTROLLING FLUID BALANCE IN CHILDREN

The problems that arise in fluid replacement in children can be dealt with more logically if it is understood how the child differs from the adult in control of body fluid.

Total body water. At birth the body fluids of the infant constitute a larger proportion of body weight than in later life. Approximately 80% of the total body weight of the newborn infant consists of fluid; this figure drops to 75% in the young child and to 55% to 60% in the adult[1] (Fig. 26-1).

Since clinical measurements are commonly in terms of extracellular volume (plasma plus interstitial fluid), it is important to note that extracellular volume of the infant is also relatively increased and constitutes about 40% of the body weight at birth in comparison to 25% in adult life.

Blood volume. The term total body water, signifying intracellular, extracellular, and intravascular fluid, is not to be confused with blood volume. Blood

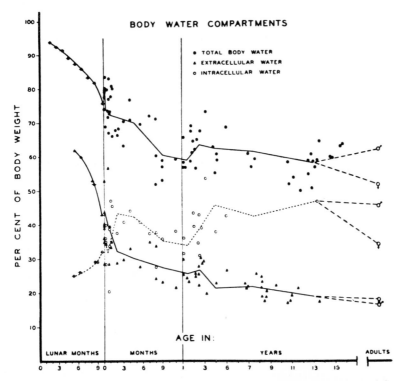

Fig. 26-1. Changes in total, extracellular, and intracellular water during fetal life and from birth to 16 years of age, and extended to corresponding normal values in the adult female and male subject. (From Friis-Hansen, B.: Acta paediat., supp. 110, 1957.)

volume is believed to be relatively greater in infants also, however, and represents about 10% of the total fluid volume throughout life. The blood volume in infants is approximately 80 ml. per kilogram of body weight, that in adult males 65 to 70 ml., and that in females 55 to 65 ml. per kilogram, varying inversely with the amount of body fat present.[2]

Body fluid compartments. The distribution of fluid within the body compartments in the infant differs from that in the adult, as shown in Figs. 26-1 and 26-2. In the adult 50% of the body weight is intracellular fluid, whereas in

Table 26-1. *Extracellular chemical values of adults and newborn infants**

	Adults	*Infants*
Sodium (mEq./L.)	140	140
Potassium (mEq./L.)	3.8–6.0	3.8–6.0
Chloride (mEq./L.)	103	110
Bicarbonate (mEq./L.)	27	20
Phosphate (mg./100 ml.)	2.5–4.5	5.0–8.0
Protein (Gm./100 ml.)	7	5
Osmotic pressure (m. osmol/L.)	310	310

*From Bland, J. H.: The clinical use of fluid and electrolyte, Philadelphia, 1952, W. B. Saunders Co.

ADULTS

INFANTS

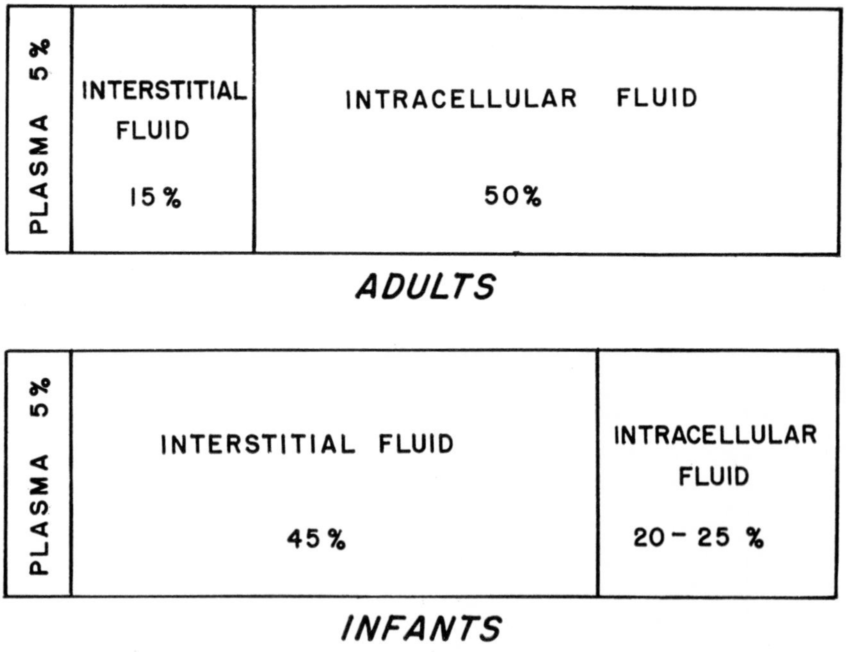

Fig. 26-2. Comparison of fluid compartments in adults and newborn infants. Observe that the interstitial fluid compartment of the infant is much larger than that of the adult and the intracellular compartment much smaller by comparison. (From Bland, J. H.: The clinical use of fluid and electrolyte, Philadelphia, 1952, W. B. Saunders Co.)

infants intracellular fluid comprises only 20% to 25% of the body weight, the interstitial compartment being considerably greater.[3]

Blood chemistry. The chemical elements in the blood show small but important differences at birth (Table 26-1).[3,4] The plasma chloride in infants is 110 mEq. per liter while 100 mEq. per liter is normal for the adult. This leads to a hyperchloremic acidosis with a lowered plasma pH.[5] A partial compensatory respiratory alkalosis with a decreased plasma bicarbonate is also normal for the infant. The ability of an infant to buffer added amounts of acid or base is limited and should be considered when parenteral replacement therapy is ordered. Lowered plasma protein is also typical of the newborn infant.

Renal control. Although the infant kidney has been considered to be functionally less adequate when measured by adult standards,[6,7] it is remarkably well adjusted to excrete a dilute urine (specific gravity, 1,010-1,020). This ability is important in view of the large extracellular fluid compartment and the normally dilute diet of infancy. However, the ability of an infant to excrete a concentrated urine above 800 m.osmols/L. is limited (1,600 m.osmols for the adult). Therefore, the ability to conserve water is small, and dehydration may develop rapidly. Limited renal function also restricts the excretion of sedative and anesthetic drugs. Fluid replacement should be given on a continuous 24-hour-a-day basis to avoid dilution of extracellular electrolytes and effective water balance.

Water metabolism. The rate of water metabolism in infants and children is an especially important factor. During the first 3 or 4 days of life, water metabolism is chiefly negative, there being loss via skin, lungs, and excretions with little intake. As soon as the baby begins to take feedings, however, fluid metabolism accelerates rapidly. When the infant is about 2 years old, water metabolism reaches its peak, with a daily turnover of 15% of the total body water content compared to that of 9% in the adult.[8-10] This reflects a higher metabolic rate in proportion to weight and results in higher insensible (skin and lungs) and renal water losses. For clinical guidance a 5%, 10%, or 15% loss or gain of body weight will result in mild, moderate, or severe dehydration or overhydration. For a 2.5-kg. infant a deficit of 250 ml. of fluid in a 24-hour period may exceed the limits of safety.

In brief, the infant and small child have excess body water content, rapid fluid turnover, limited renal function, low plasma protein, and high chlorides—all of these factors cause increased danger of fluid overload and edema formation. Decreased bicarbonate and buffer activity set the stage for the second threat, that of acidosis.

INDICATIONS FOR FLUID THERAPY IN SURGERY

Many preventable errors occur in failure to correct fluid imbalance existing prior to operation, the toxic child with peritonitis being the outstanding example. Another costly mistake lies in the failure to appreciate the need for fluid replacement until operation is well under way. To start an infusion in the collapsed vein of an infant covered by voluminous drapes is difficult and time-consuming, and the delay may be fatal.

Usually the indications for fluid therapy are clear-cut and predictable. They fall into three categories, preoperative, operative, and postoperative.

Preoperative indications. The degree and direction of fluid, electrolyte, and acid-base abnormalities seen in the infant will vary with the type of pathology and duration of illness. The changes resulting from infection and fever will differ from those relating to intestinal obstruction and require a different replacement fluid. Although many of the deficits may be predicted, hematocrit, electrolyte determinations, parameters of acid-base status, and urinalysis are essential for a rational program designed to correct the metabolic abnormalities. The most frequently encountered indications for preoperative administration of fluid are dehydration, alkalosis, ketosis, anemia, and low blood volume.[11] These conditions may exist alone or in combinations. The degree and direction of fluid, electrolyte, and acid-base abnormalities seen in the infant will vary with the type of pathology and the duration of the illness. Mild dehydration may be due to fever or poor fluid intake, and it can be corrected by administration of 5% dextrose and water. Fluid should be given until there is return of tissue turgor, reduction of fever below 102° F., and voiding.[12]

If dehydration is severe, it usually will be accompanied by electrolyte imbalance. A common form of electrolyte and fluid disorder in the preoperative period is that seen in infants with *pyloric stenosis.* Failure to correct the hypochloremic and hypokalemic alkalosis and dehydration prior to surgery accounts for the major mortality in this disease today.[13]

A typical case is described for illustration:

M. E., a 6-week-old white male infant weighing 8 pounds, was admitted with a 2-week history of postprandial vomiting, projectile and not containing bile. Diapers were dry for 12 hours. A pyloric tumor was felt in the right upper quadrant.

The child was listless, skin turgor was absent, mucous membranes were dry, and eyes were recessed. The hematocrit was 48%; electrolytes: Na 122 mEq./L., K 2.8 mEq./L., Cl 89 mEq./L., and CO_2 42 mEq./L.

An intravenous route was established, and fluid therapy was started. Hydration and electrolyte balance were achieved within 24 hours. Following the pyloromyotomy feedings were begun, and an adequate oral intake was given by the end of the first postoperative day.

Comment: Although the diagnosis was evident on admission, a full day was devoted to repairing the severe fluid, electrolyte, and acid-base imbalances prior to operation. An immediate general anesthesia and surgical procedure with the added fluid loss and acid-base changes might have exceeded the limited reserves of this infant.

The volume and content of the replacement fluid must be precise. A deficit of electrolyte content in the fluid given will further dilute the abnormally low extracellular fluid concentrations of sodium, chloride, and potassium.

Suggested replacement program (pyloric stenosis):

1. Total fluids 25 ml./lb. body weight in 8 hours
    15 ml. 5% dextrose in saline
    10 ml. 5% dextrose in water

2. Potassium: 1 mEq./kg. body weight in 8 hours added to the preceding
   solution

This 8-pound infant was given 200 ml. of fluid and 4 mEq. of potassium within the first 8 hours. At that time he had not voided and was still dehydrated. He was given two more "sets" of fluid for a total of 600 ml. within the 24 hours prior to surgery. Generally a child with pyloric stenosis will require only one or two "sets" of fluid to achieve adequate hydration.

The empiric formula presented will offer electrolytes and fluids at a rate slow enough to allow adjustments between the intracellular and extracellular compartments. Alkalosis is more easily corrected than acidosis, and the addition of acidifying solutions such as NH_4Cl is not commonly required.

The effects of *dehydration, hypovolemia, acid-base, and electrolyte disturbances* following a severe infection in a child are graphically illustrated by the following case report.

E. F., a 2-year-old child who had a history of vomiting and abdominal pain of 5 days' duration, was admitted to the surgical service with a presumptive diagnosis of *perforated appendicitis and generalized peritonitis.* The child appeared listless and pale. The respiratory rate was 50, pulse, 150-160 per minute, temperature, 104° F. rectally, and weight, 32 pounds.

The hematocrit was 48%; W.B.C., 3,200 with a marked shift to the left. The urine obtained by catheter showed a specific gravity of 1,039 and 3+ acetone. The serum electrolytes were Na 125 mEq./L., Cl 92 mEq./L., K 3.3 mEq./L., and CO_2 18 mEq./L.

Comment: Here the need for early surgical drainage of the peritoneum is obvious. However, a general anesthetic and surgical procedure on admission in this acute and chronically ill child would incur an unnecessary risk.

Physiology of generalized peritonitis with appendicitis follows:

1. Water loss—decrease in total body water
   a. Insensible water loss (lung and skin) increased with high metabolic rate and fever
   b. Intraperitoneal inflammation—fluid drawn into the peritoneal cavity
   c. Vomiting
   d. Water lost in the bowel lumen with ileus

Except for the insensible water loss by lungs and skin, the remainder of the fluids lost contain electrolytes in varying concentrations and proportions. The direction and degree of the sum can be estimated by determination of the serum electrolytes. The amount of water loss is estimated as a percentage of body weight by the degree of hemoconcentration (HCT), volume, and specific gravity of urine and the subjective signs of skin turgor, hydration, of mucous membrane, and filling of neck veins.

2. Blood volume—decreased plasma volume, hemoconcentration, increased viscosity of blood

The intraperitoneal inflammatory process damages the capillary bed and plasma is lost. This volume of plasma loss is related to the extent of infection. In a generalized peritonitis with a broad surface involved, a large volume loss follows in a short period. The hypovolemia is compounded by the decrease in total body water and shrinkage of the extracellular space.

3. Acidosis—partially compensated metabolic acidosis with a lowered pCO_2, HCO_2, and lowered pH
   a. Starvation—no oral caloric intake in the face of an increased caloric demand outstrips the reserves of glucose and glycogen; the metabolism of fat reserves increases the serum ketone levels.
   b. Increased blood viscosity with decreased rate of blood flow through capillary bed leads to a relative tissue anoxia and a high level of acid metabolic products.
   c. Elevated diaphragms due to distention and irritation by the inflammatory process decrease the capacity for a compensatory respiratory alkalosis.

The metabolic rate, caloric requirements, and cardiac output are maximum in a child with the stress of a generalized infection and hyperthermia. Correction of the metabolic defects and volume rate and cardiac output by control of body temperature and adequate antibiotic therapy are necessary prior to surgery.

A large intravenous cannula was placed in the saphenous vein, and a nasogastric tube was passed and placed on suction. A Foley catheter was left in the bladder.

In a 4-hour period a total of 300 ml. of plasma, 400 ml. of 0.3 N dextrose in saline solution with 15 mEq. of potassium chloride was given. One million units of aqueous penicillin were added to the intravenous fluid, and 150 mg. of streptomycin were given intramuscularly. Aspirin, 0.6 Gm., was given by rectum. At the end of this time the urine output increased from 3 to 5 ml. to 20 ml, per hour, and the temperature dropped to 101.5° F. The heart rate was 100 to 110 per minute.

The appendectomy was completed without incident.

Preoperative management and replacement program in a child with sepsis follows:

1. Delay surgery to allow adequate preparation and decrease the risk of anesthesia and surgery.
2. Nasogastric tube to empty the stomach and avoid bowel distention.
3. An adequate venous cannula or needle for fluid administration.
4. Fluids and antibiotics started immediately:
   a. 5% dextrose in saline—10 ml. per pound may be given safely within a 4-hour period.
      5% dextrose in water—may follow at a slower rate depending on the degree of dehydration; urine output is observed closely; a Foley catheter may be indicated.
   b. Plasma at a rate of 10 ml./lb. may also be needed if hemoconcentration and the degree of hypovolemia warrant.
   c. Penicillin (aqueous) is given intravenously in large doses—up to 10 million units a day for a 50-lb. child.
      Streptomycin—10 mg./lb. intramuscularly and repeated twice daily.

d. Hyperthermia is treated by intravenous fluids, rectal aspirin, and exposure of the skin.

The body temperature should be monitored closely.

The operation is delayed until an adequate response to the preceding treatment is noted. The temperature is checked—it should fall below 102° F. rectally, and the pulse should fall below 120 per minute before the start of a general anesthetic. The 3-hour to 4-hour period in so preparing a child may avoid an intraoperative crisis.

Anemia existing prior to operation should be corrected. If an operation is elective in nature, it may be wiser to give the child oral therapy until the deficit is made up. When an operation is imperative, small transfusions of blood or packed cells are indicated in order to have normal conditions established before anesthesia is started.

Low blood volume, frequently seen in adults suffering from malignancy or chronic illness,[14,15] is not unknown in children. Several very bitter experiences have convinced us that children with large abdominal tumors have remarkably poor tolerance for blood loss (Fig. 26-3). Merely with the vasodilatation of anesthesia these children may develop profound shock. It is essential that such pa-

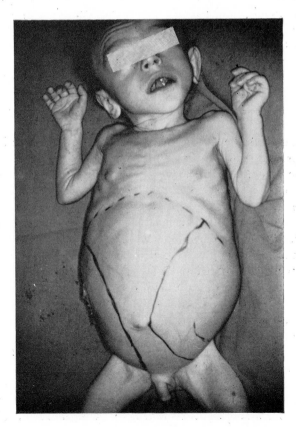

Fig. 26-3. Children with large abdominal tumors have been extremely poor operative risks.

tients be prepared most carefully before surgery is begun and that transfusion is not delayed until after the operation is started.

Indications for fluid therapy at start of operation. Assuming that all deficits are corrected when the child comes to surgery, certain types of operation may be taken as definite indications that infusions be established at the start of operation for administration of fluid or blood. Among these are the following:
1. Intracranial operations
2. Intrathoracic operations
3. Major abdominal operations
4. Open bone surgery
5. Major plastic procedures
6. Miscellaneous (anoplasty, hygroma, etc.)

The first two classifications do not require any explanation "Major abdominal" may be taken to mean any upper abdominal procedures, as well as bowel resections, but not to include uncomplicated herniorrhaphy or appendectomy. "Open bone surgery" includes spinal fusions and other procedures in which bone is actually laid open as in triple arthrodesis and in osteotomy. Plastic procedures, although often involving only superficial wounds, may cause severe blood loss. The dressing of large burns is an outstanding example. The amount of blood lost in harelip and palate repair varies considerably with the surgeon, and blood should be given if the loss is more than minimal. Among other procedures that usually involve considerable blood loss are excision of cystic hygroma, anoplasty, and excision of sacral teratoma.

Closure of a colostomy in an infant can be misleading. Although a relatively small operation, Davenport[16] noted more blood lost than during an average patent ductus ligation. Closure of colostomy is considered a real indication for cutdown and blood transfusion.

It is our practice to use cutdown or catheter infusions in all intracranial and intrathoracic procedures regardless of the patient's size or age. Rapid administration of large amounts of blood may be necessary, and for this purpose the cutdown infusion is definitely more reliable than the percutaneous needle. Cutdown infusions are also preferable in all small infants undergoing major surgery, since percutaneous infusions are far more difficult to maintain in small veins.

Two additional factors that should be taken as indications for starting infusion of water and saline or glucose before operation begins are the duration of operation and the time at which operation starts.

Duration of operation. If the procedure is expected to last more than $1\frac{1}{2}$ hours, it seems wise not to wait until dehydration or shock becomes evident but to use fluids from the outset.

Time of operation. When surgery is not scheduled until late morning or afternoon, the child may not resume oral intake until late afternoon or the next day, and for this reason he deserves parenteral therapy. Hot weather or overheated operating rooms will also cause increased loss of body fluids and will be a reasonable indication for early administration of intravenous fluid.

Indications for starting infusions during an operation. If infusions are started at the beginning of operation for the indications just noted, one will not often be troubled by the need to set up an infusion during operation. However, occasional unpredicted events occur that alter the situation. Unexpected blood loss due either to sudden or to prolonged bleeding may occur in any type of surgery, and treatment by immediate transfusion is the only remedy. Unexpectedly prolonged operations may result from any number of factors. We have set up an empiric rule whereby any child under anesthesia for more than 1½ hours is to receive intravenous fluid. Unexpected losses of body fluid, such as by marked sweating, may also provide indication for parenteral fluid.

In the unusual event of convulsion during anesthesia, dehydration must immediately be suspected. An infusion should be instituted at once, both for fluid therapy and for administration of specific anticonvulsive agents.

As previously noted, if a child continues to have vascular oozing after tonsil-

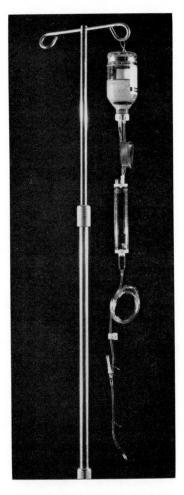

Fig. 26-4. Intravenous fluid equipment composed of plastic tubing with reservoir, visible adjustable drip, and side arm for addition of other agents or for pumping fluid.

lectomy and requires a second anesthetic on the same day, an infusion is indicated to maintain fluid intake, and occasionally blood replacement will be required.

APPARATUS AND TECHNIQUE

Many avoidable errors are due to the use of inadequate apparatus and to failure in the mechanics of establishment and maintenance of the infusion. Suitable sets for pediatric infusion have been difficult to obtain but are now available.

The important features of a set for pediatric fluid therapy are a finely calibrated scale to determine the amount of fluid administered, a reservoir or method for preventing accidental administration of excessive amounts, a fine visible drip, and a method whereby the fluid can be pumped into the patient rapidly. Several manufacturers now produce acceptable apparatus (Fig. 26-4).

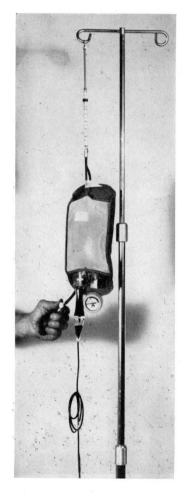

Fig. 26-5. Blood transfusion equipment. Blood is stored in plastic bag, shown here suspended by measuring scale, and held in pneumatic sleeve that can be compressed to accelerate flow.

For storage of blood, plastic containers offer many advantages. When administering blood, pressure may be applied to the system by use of an external pneumatic cuff. The amount of blood infused is measured by a spring scale (Fig. 26-5).

A very simple and accurate method that is valuable during operations on small infants is merely to attach a 10-ml. or 20-ml. syringe and plastic extension tube to the cutdown catheter (Fig. 26-6). The syringe is placed beside the infant's head, and the anesthetist administers the fluid in desired quantities as needed. This method offers the greatest insurance against inadvertent use of excess fluid, although errors in judgment still may occur. When pumping blood, plastic syringes are far superior to glass, since they do not stick.

It is helpful to have several types of needle available. For short-term use an 18-gauge or 20-gauge steel needle may suffice in larger patients. Often the 19-gauge hubless scalp vein is preferable, being more comfortable and easier to keep in place (Fig. 26-7). Several plastic needles and catheters are available for long-term use, and often these render a cutdown infusion unnecessary. For most small infants, however, and for critical procedures in which extensive blood loss may occur, we prefer a standard cutdown infusion with a polyethylene catheter that is fitted over the end of a blunt steel needle.

It has now become a routine matter to warm blood when it is to be given to small infants or when it may be required rapidly in large quantities.[17] This may be accomplished by immersing the blood in a pan of water at body temperature prior to transfusion or by passing a coil of the infusion tubing through a pan of water during the administration of the blood.

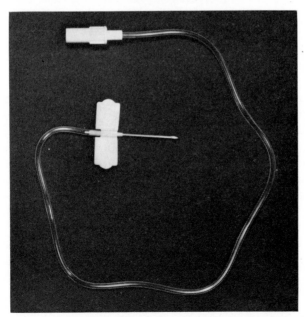

Fig. 26-6. Scalp vein set consisting of hubless needle and 8-inch length of plastic tubing.

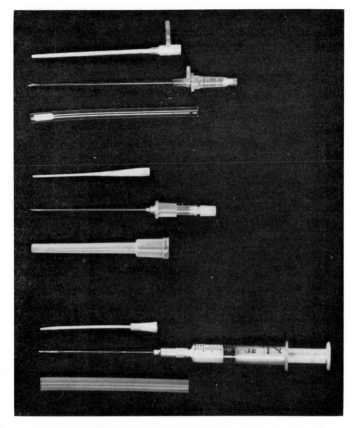

Fig. 26-7. Plastic needles for intravenous infusion.

To establish a dependable infusion in a 4-pound or 5-pound infant is no easy task, and to have a surgeon or anesthetist who can do this quickly and consistently makes a great different to all concerned.

If the person starting the infusion is reasonably experienced and the patient is in good condition, it is preferable to induce anesthesia and then to perform the cutdown. If the patient is a premature infant or in critical condition, or if the infusionist is inexperienced, it is better to perform the cutdown under local anesthesia some time before operation and not to take the chance of prolonging the anesthesia an extra half hour or more.

The best site for the cutdown infusion is usually the internal saphenous vein at the ankle. The vein is extremely consistent in its position as it passes anterior to the internal malleolus and then swings backward toward the calf and dives into the deeper structures. A horizontal incision immediately anterior and superior to the malleolus is made, the wound is separated, and a stiff probe or hook is drawn firmly along the surface of the tibia to locate the vein. The vein will usually be unmistakable when it is delivered and in general will appear larger and stronger than expected. Two silk sutures are passed around it, the distal one tied and used for traction (Fig. 26-8).

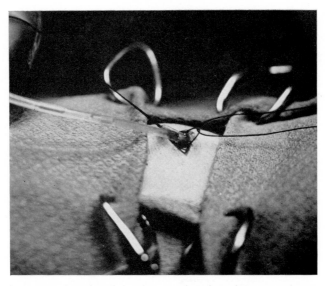

Fig. 26-8. Sutures are passed around the vein, and a plastic catheter is inserted. (From Gross, R. E.: The surgery of infancy and childhood, Philadelphia, 1953, W. B. Saunders Co.)

The infusion set is prepared, and a good point is trimmed on the plastic catheter. With scissors or a fine scalpel blade the vein is then incised deeply enough to expose the lumen, and the catheter is threaded up into the vein. It is desirable to use the largest catheter possible, and a 20-gauge tubing can ordinarily be inserted into the saphenous vein of a 3-pound or 4-pound baby. The catheter may be larger than the collapsed vein, but the vein stretches readily. The catheter is advanced about one third of the way up the lower leg and is secured by tying the proximal suture.

Next, one should test the infusion by drawing blood back into the tubing and by seeing that fluid runs in readily and does not leak from a pierced vein to reappear in the wound. Then the wound is closed and the catheter is anchored firmly in place with adhesive tape (Fig. 26-9). At this time one should be sure that the infusion is not allowed to run into the patient unchecked.

Occasionally the leg will not serve as the site of infusion. If the child has been operated upon several times already, both ankles may have been used previously. In certain cases the ankle should be avoided by choice. If the infant is to be in the lithotomy position for anoplasty, or if operation for a large abdominal tumor or omphalocele threatens to obstruct blood flow through the inferior vena cava, it is better to start the infusion in the arm. Here the antecubital veins usually offer the best selection. These veins are small, superficial, and much less constant in their position than is the saphenous vein, the arm is more difficult to position, and the procedure is definitely more exacting. If an incision is made one-half inch distal to the antecubital crease (Fig. 26-10) and if the wound is separated carefully, two or three fragile veins may be found lying in a superficial plane. One must not expect to find anything but the meanest strands to work with in the arms of infants.

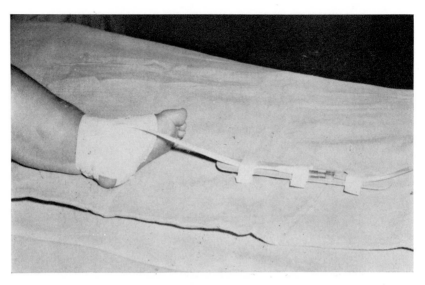

Fig. 26-9. Internal saphenous cutdown infusion completed. Plastic catheter must be taped securely so that it will not be pulled out of vein and will not become kinked.

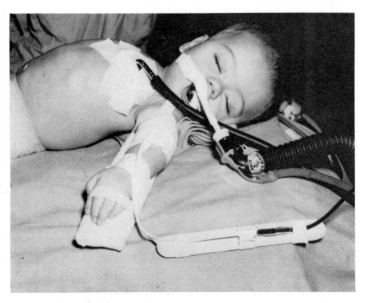

Fig. 26-10. Antecubital space is site for infusion when venous return from inferior vena cava is jeopardized.

In older children undergoing relatively minor operations, percutaneous vein puncture may be used. In this case the antecubital space should be avoided carefully, for, regardless of the restraint, almost any child can squirm enough to dislodge the needle and drive it into his arm. The dorsum of the hand can be immobilized effectively and usually provides the best veins. No smaller than a

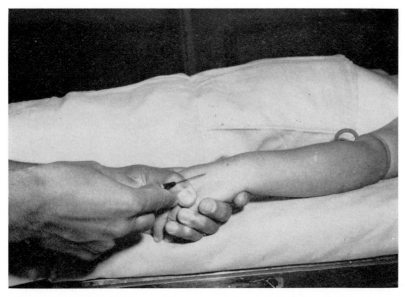

Fig. 26-11. For percutaneous infusions, the dorsum of the hand should be chosen.

21-gauge needle should be used if blood is to be administered by gravity flow (Fig. 26-11).

Occasionally the internal saphenous vein or vessels on the dorsum of the foot or the external jugular vein may be used for percutaneous venipuncture.

TYPES OF FLUID

Much confusion arises from the array of combined electrolyte mixtures suggested by biochemists and acid-base experts. During the operative period it is best to use simple mixtures. The following fulfill most purposes: (1) 5% dextrose in water, (2) 10% dextrose in water, (3) 5% dextrose in saline, (4) 5% dextrose in half strength (0.45%) saline, (5) 5% dextrose in one-third strength (0.3%) saline, (6) lactated Ringer's solution, (7) potassium chloride prepared from 20-ml. (40 mEq.) ampules, (8) normal (0.9%) saline, (9) whole citrated blood (ACD or CPD), fresh or bank blood, (10) packed red blood cells, and (11) albumin in 5% solution.

For the majority of needs No. 1 through No. 3 solutions will suffice. Ideally the requirements of each patient are evaluated and a proper mixture of 5% dextrose in water and 5% dextrose in saline is prescribed.[18] In order to avoid the mixing of fluids by the bedside and risking possible contamination, a group of premixed fluids is now available (No. 4 to No. 6). The maintenance fluid for a routine postoperative patient on intravenous replacement without serious extrarenal losses is 5% dextrose in 0.3% saline.

All infusions are started with 5% or 10% dextrose solution rather than with saline solution because there is always a chance that excess fluid will be allowed to run in by mistake, and dextrose would involve considerably less danger. To provide water and calories, dextrose solutions are satisfactory. Invert sugar has theoretical advantages of additional carbohydrate utilization, but this is not of critical importance.

The 10% dextrose in water solution is of some advantage in the neonate with a small glycogen and glucose reserve. The high caloric content defers the need for metabolism of fat and proteins.

In a patient with desalting loss such as intestinal obstruction, more Na and Cl are provided in 5% dextrose in 0.45% saline.

The intraoperative use of lactated Ringer's solution has recently achieved much popularity due to the work of Shires, who, with Williams and Brown,[19] reported marked loss of extracellular fluid during operation. This fluid may be used when a single unit of blood would otherwise be administered.

Shires, with Jenkins and Gieseke,[20] also suggests that 10 ml. of lactated Ringer's solution be administered per pound of body weight per hour, to overcome the extracellular fluid loss. This concept may have value during prolonged bowel operations in children, such as for correction of Hirschsprung's disease, but addition of excess Na or fluid would involve increased risk in neurosurgical and cardiac procedures, and in most small infants. Although supported by Viguera,[21] this concept has been applied to pediatric surgery to a very limited degree. The resultant improved urinary output does not appear to be of sufficient advantage to warrant the attendant use of an inlying urinary catheter.

Whole citrated blood is used for replacement under ordinary circumstances. A solution containing citrate, phosphate, and dextrose (CPD),[22] which is less acid than the standard ACD mixture, has been used as a whole blood preservative for several years.

For emergency use as blood volume sustainer we store 5% albumin in ready-mixed 250-ml. vials. Albumin in a physiologic suspension is an excellent plasma expander and source for calories and protein for the neonate on a long-term postoperative replacement program.

Potassium chloride is employed occasionally to restore the losses that occur in prolonged vomiting associated with pyloric stenosis. It should be noted that dehydration must be treated before potassium is administered, otherwise the heart may be dangerously depressed.[23]

AMOUNT AND RATE OF INFUSION

Thus far an attempt has been made to correct several sources of confusion and preventable errors. This leaves the main problem, the amount to be administered, in clearer detail.

The amount of fluid needed depends upon three factors: the *preexisting deficit,* the rate of *operative loss,* and the *daily requirements.* The relaitve importance of these factors depends upon whether the infusion is to be given before, during, or after the operation.

Preoperative fluid replacement. The amount of infusion to be given before operation will be determined largely by the preoperative deficits, which may include body water, electrolytes, and blood constituents. Dehydration can be evaluated by clinical signs of failure to void, dry skin, and sunken fontanels. Laboratory evaluation of the hydrogen ion concentration carbon dioxide, sodium, chloride, and potassium may help to assess critically ill infants but usually is not necessary.

Pure dehydration ordinarily is mild. Correction is accomplished by giving 5% dextrose in distilled water, the dextrose being added to give water osmotic power and incidentally to supply calories. This solution is administered in amounts to provide 10 ml. per pound of body weight and then is repeated if necessary until the clinical signs of dehydration have been corrected. When dehydration is severe, it is almost invariably associated with acidosis or alkalosis. The management of such cases from clinical evaluation has been outlined.

A more accurate estimation of needed repair solutions for sick children can be made by finding the infant's weight loss and measuring his electrolyte concentrations, serum pH, and serum CO_2[24,25]; e.g., a 4-kg. infant with pyloric stenosis is found to have a chloride ion concentration of 90 mEq./L.; therefore, his chloride deficit is $103 - 90 = 13$ mEq./L. If 75% of his body weight is fluid, his body fluid $= 75/100 \times 4$ kg. $= 3$ kg. or 3 liters. His deficit then equals $3 \times 13 = 39$ mEq. of chloride. Normal saline solution has 150 mEq. of chloride per liter. The infant needs 39/150 liter, or $39/150 \times 1,000$ ml. $= 260$ ml. NaCl. Other electrolyte needs are calculated in similar fashion.

When the hemoglobin is low, the amount of blood needed to raise the hemoglobin 1 gram per 100 ml. is estimated as approximately 10 ml. per pound of body weight or preferably half this volume of packed red cells.

Amount of replacement needed during operation. The amount (and type) of fluid replacement during operation should depend chiefly upon current losses since preoperative deficits should be replenished prior to operation. Losses during operation may be of two types, body fluids exclusive of blood and blood loss.

Fluid replacement. During all surgical procedures, body fluids are lost at variable rates in respiration, sweating, and evaporation from the wound. During short operations on healthy patients, this loss is usually small and is made up soon after operation. In longer operations (over one and one-half hours) in which blood loss is not appreciable, an infusion of 5% dextrose in 0.45 N saline is allowed to drip at such a rate that the patient receives 2 ml. per hour per pound. This may be increased if there is marked sweating, but children do not often perspire actively in reasonably cool operating rooms. Infants during the first three days of life receive no fluids unless blood loss is appreciable, in which case the blood is replaced.

Replacement of blood loss. This is the greatest problem in the operating room. Since there is no way to predict how much blood will be needed, estimation of blood requirement must be based on several guides. The most useful guides are the "10 ml. per pound" rule, the measurement of blood loss, and clinical signs.

PREDETERMINED RULES. There is one rule of thumb that has a basic but limited value. This provides that for infants weighing less than 20 pounds an infusion of 10 ml. of blood per pound will be of appreciable value to an average patient without involving danger of overloading him. Many patients will require more than 10 ml. per pound, but this establishes a "safe limit." Until this figure is exceeded, one feels a certain assurance that at least he is not doing the patient any harm. For a number of operations in which blood loss is not excessive, as in most bowel surgery, this rule will prove rather an adequate guide.

On the basis of a careful survey Davenport[16] suggested an excellent rule whereby blood loss under 10% of the child's blood volume does not justify transfusion, loss of 10% to 14% justifies replacement, and loss of more than 14% demands transfusion.

MEASUREMENT OF LOSS. In all major pediatric operations a real effort should be made to measure blood loss. This can be approached by several methods:

1. *Measurement of suctioned blood:* This is always possible, simply by use of a calibrated suction bottle. The use of an antifoaming agent in the suction bottle will help considerably.

2. *Gravimetric system:* During operations in which dry sponges may be used, the blood lost in sponges may be accurately determined by using sponges of known weight and reweighing them after use. This gravimetric method was introduced by Wangensteen in 1942 and has served as our principal guide for several years, with the use of the adapted dietary scale described by Gross[26] (Fig. 26-12). This technique is simple and is as accurate as many of the newer methods. Furthermore, it can be repeated at short intervals throughout the operation.

(a) A nurse keeps a running account of blood loss in the suction bottle and sponges, as well as the fluid and blood administered. This "in and out" balance is recorded in a chart posted on the wall or on a blackboard that the whole team can refer to at will. In estimating replacement this actual measured loss is considered the baseline, to which

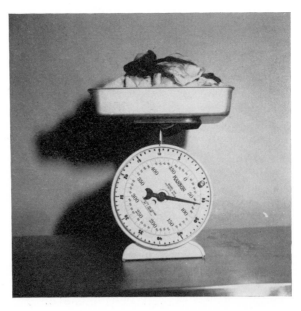

Fig. 26-12. Adapted dietary scale for measurement of blood lost in sponges.

an additional 10% or 20% must be added for unmeasured loss in gowns and drapes.

(b) Recording the blood administered and lost serves as an excellent guide in all thoracic operations.

(c) Continuous recording is especially valuable in specific situations. When there is extensive or rapid blood loss, frantic efforts to replace blood may lead to confusion and bad mistakes unless a reliable check is available.

(d) In long operations blood loss often occurs at very different rates at various phases of the procedure. Fig. 26-13 illustrates how closely the changing needs may be followed through at 6-hour procedure.

(e) Finally, when patients are in critical condition and can tolerate neither deficit nor excess, continuous measurement offers the nearest approach to accuracy.

3. *Visual estimation of blood on sponges:* When dry sponges cannot be used, as in abdominal procedures, the blood loss on sponges should be calculated by visually checking them against sponges stained by known amounts of blood (Fig. 26-14).

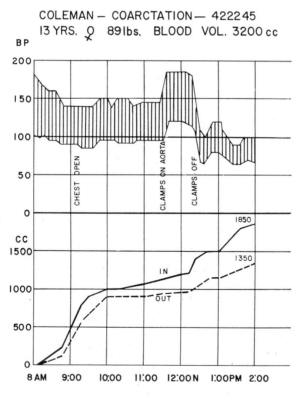

Fig. 26-13. Changing rate of blood loss during the repair of coarctation of the aorta in a 13-year-old child. (From Smith, R. M.: J.A.M.A. **161**:1124, 1956.)

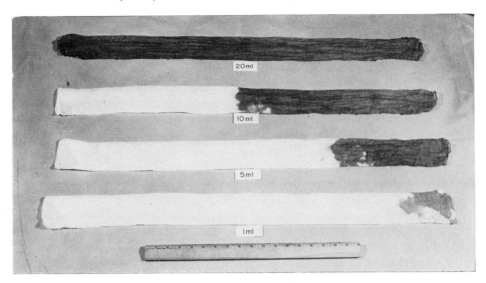

Fig. 26-14. Sponges containing 1, 5, 10, and 20 ml. of blood may be used as standards for visual estimation of blood loss.

CLINICAL SIGNS OF BLOOD LOSS. It is of utmost importance to watch closely for clinical signs of blood loss and to regard them with respect. There are several that are valuable:

1. Blood pressure is always an important guide, and even in newborn infants it gives valuable information. Cuffs may be fitted to all sizes. When arms are not available, the thighs may be used. The blood pressure stethoscope is not always effective on small arms; however, systolic pressure can be determined by watching the fluctuation of the needle or feeling the pulse. The "flush method" may be employed, whereby the return of color is noted with release of the tourniquet, and this denotes the "mean" arterial pressure. The systolic blood pressure should be above 80 mm. Hg in all patients, and anything under this or failure to determine blood pressure should be regarded as a sign of shock, except in neonates in whom the pressure was low initially. Occasionally a newborn infant will show pressures between 65 and 80 mm. Hg without other evidence of shock. Here it is essential to rely on maintaining the infant's initial pressure.

2. The pulse rate is not a reliable sign concerning blood loss in children because it is often rapid prior to hemorrhage and may show no further change in the presence of shock until severe hypoxia causes terminal bradycardia. On the other hand, should the pulse show a significant increase, one must consider blood loss a probable cause.

3. The pulse volume, however, is definitely helpful in estimating blood loss and should be followed carefully. Even small newborn infants usually have a palpable radial pulse. This should be evaluated at the start of operation and checked at short intervals. Weakening or absence of the pulse is a reliable indication of decreased blood volume.

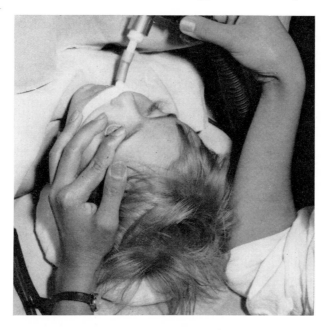

Fig. 26-15. Conjunctival circulation is one of the most valuable indications of blood volume.

4. Color of the skin should be followed closely but will blanch with cold and with relaxants. The color of the lips is more reliable than that of the skin. The most useful visual sign of blood volume is undoubtedly found in the conjunctivae (Fig. 26-15). Normal capillary circulation will completely disappear with appreciable blood loss, and the conjunctivae will appear bloodless. Blood replacement will immediately be evidenced by capillary engorgement. With infants less than 1 year old, repeated manipulation of the eyelids may cause edema and should be avoided; however, in older children this is an invaluable guide.

5. Another sign of special value in infants is the *volume of the heart sounds*[27,28] as heard by means of the precordial stethoscope. In severe blood loss the cardiac contraction is so weak that the heart sounds become faint and then entirely inaudible. This is a sign of marked but not irreversible shock and is a signal for immediate administration of blood.

6. If patients who have been maintained with a fixed concentration of anesthetic suddenly appear more deeply anesthetized and show increasing flaccidity or dilated pupils, these signs may denote inadequate blood volume.

7. The central venous pressure is believed by many to be of great value as a guide to blood replacement during operation, especially in distinguishing between inadequate blood replacement and cardiac failure. It must be emphasized, however, that many intraoperative factors such as endotracheal intubation, prone position, and assisted ventilation, will alter venous pressure greatly. In the postoperative period,

when these forces are not present, venous pressures will give more reliable guidance.[29]

8. Urinary output, as determined by an inlying urinary catheter, will also give basic evidence of the adequacy of blood flow. Normal urinary output for an adult is considered to be 50 ml./hr.

A word of warning should be given here. At the end of operation we have been faced several times with the problem of a child who had neither blood pressure nor palpable pulse, yet because considerably more blood had already been given than the measured loss, we were hesitant to add more. Almost invariably we have found that there had been continued hemorrhage into the chest or abdomen and that the signs of shock were not misleading. These mistakes have convinced us that, although measurement is extremely helpful, when doubt arises, greater reliance should be placed upon the clinical signs.

Postoperative requirements. It is certainly desirable for children to resume oral feeding as quickly as possible after operation, and many children will not require any parenteral fluids during this period. Following most major operative procedures, however, orders will be needed concerning continuation of intravenous therapy, and the anesthetist should be able to assume part of this responsibility.

The first consideration may concern the amount of blood that will be required to complete the replacement of operative loss and to allow for expected postoperative bleeding. This must be judged by individual situations and will depend upon the size and type of the wound, the final control of bleeding, clinical signs, and other factors.

One must next consider the future fluid needs, and here the determining factor is the *daily fluid requirement,* to which must be added replacement of fluid and electrolytes lost by vomiting, drainage tubes, or ileostomy.

The daily fluid requirement in relation to body weight varies markedly since metabolism is a function of body surface area rather than of body weight. Actually, the basal fluid requirement of the body when related to surface area is constant, remaining 1,500 ml. of fluid per square meter per day.[30] For practical purposes, however, it is easier to follow a table such as Table 26-2, which is based on both age and weight.

For children who will resume oral fluid intake on the day of operation, the problem is relatively simple. Orders for fluids may consist merely of adding enough blood to replace the expected additional loss, plus enough glucose and water to replace half of the daily fluid need. Thus, for a 40-pound child who received adequate blood replacement during operation and not more than 10 ml. of supportive fluid per pound, a reasonable postoperative allowance would be $40 \times 30/2 = 600$ ml. of 10% glucose in water.

For sustained parenteral support a more comprehensive regimen must be followed, and in addition to fluid and caloric needs one must consider electrolyte, protein, and vitamin requirements, which will vary with individual patients. Such children usually will be on either nasogastic or bowel drainage and will thus be losing extra fluid and electrolytes. The losses must be measured and replaced. Children who are on simple gastric suction may be given their basic daily fluid

Table 26-2. *Daily requirements of infants and children during the operative period**

Age or weight	Daily (ml. per pound) fluid requirement
Newborn	No fluid for 36 to 48 hours
Premature infants	20 to 30
3 to 4 days old	20 to 30
10 to 20 pounds	45
20 to 30 pounds	40
30 to 40 pounds	35
40 to 50 pounds	30
50 pounds and over	25

*From Wrenn, E.: Fluid therapy for infants and children. Symposium on infant anesthesia, Ninth Postgraduate Assembly, New York, December, 1956.

Table 26-3. *Postoperative electrolyte maintenance for infants and children**

First 24 hours	No electrolytes
After 24 hours	1. NaCl, 0.5 gram per 10 pounds
	2. KCl, 1 to 1.5 mEq. per pound
	3. $CaCl_2$ or Ca gluconate, 20 mg. per pound

*From Wrenn, E.: Fluid therapy for infants and children. Symposium on infant anesthesia, Ninth Postgraduate Assembly, New York, December, 1956.

allowance plus replacement of suctioned fluid, planned in such a manner that two thirds consist of 10% glucose in water and one third of 0.5% saline solution in water. A guide to postoperative electrolyte maintenance is shown in Table 26-3.

Proteins in the form of blood, plasma, or concentrated albumin will be needed in small amounts each second or third day during parenteral supportive therapy. A guide to dosage of these factors is provided in Table 26-4.

Finally, it must be remembered that vitamins should be administered in adequate quantities during the operative period. This applies to preoperative use of vitamin K in the newborn infant, as well as postoperative administration of vitamins B and C. The use of these vitamins is outlined as follows*:

1. Vitamin K: Given to newborn and jaundiced babies before operation; normal newborn infants receive 2.5 mg. per day; jaundiced infants receive 1 mg. per day.
2. Vitamin C: 100 mg. per 10 pounds to be given throughout period of parenteral support.
3. Vitamin B complex: 1 ml. per day during parenteral therapy.

COMPLICATIONS IN FLUID AND BLOOD REPLACEMENT

The foregoing details concerning fluid therapy were considered indicated because complications are frequent, they occur rapidly, and they may be extremely

*From Wrenn, E.: Fluid therapy in infants and children. Symposium on infant anesthesia, Ninth Postgraduate Assembly, New York, December, 1956.

Table 26-4. *Guide to postoperative protein administration in infants and children**

Blood	10 ml. per pound
Plasma	10 ml. per pound
Albumin	1 to 2 ml. per pound
Protein hydrolysate	5% hydrolysate in 10% glucose with 5% alcohol

*From Wrenn, E.: Fluid therapy in infants and children. Symposium on infant anesthesia, Ninth Postgraduate Assembly, New York, December, 1956.

serious. Such complications are caused by inadequate or excessive administration of fluid or various components or by reactions to specific substances.

Inadequate replacement. Most anesthetists have learned that insufficient fluid replacement can lead to dehydration, shock, and death. In addition, deficits of electrolytes may result in alkalosis, acidosis, or specific imbalances.

Excessive replacement. In dealing with children the hazard of overinfusion is more marked in the postoperative period, but it is also present during operation. Signs of overinfusion are a slowing heart, engorged veins, generalized plethora, and a full pulse. The copious, watery, or bloody pulmonary secretions are a late sign of fluid excess. Premonitory signs may consist of increased resistance of the lungs to inflation and of rales heard by stethoscope.

The treatment of overinfusion consists, first, of discontinuing the infusion and then instituting symptomatic therapy, which may include elevation of the head, application of tourniquets, venesection, and the use of oxygen, morphine, vasopressors, diuretics, and digitalis, depending upon the circumstances. The use of ganglionic blocking agents also seems rational in treatment of pulmonary edema resulting from fluid excess. If overtransfusion occurs during intrathoracic surgery, the best expedient may be for the surgeon to withdraw 50 to 200 ml. of blood directly from the heart. This has appeared to be a lifesaving maneuver in two instances in our experience.

Following operation the danger of overinfusing small patients is a great hazard, and extreme precautions must be observed. Not more than half of the day's requirement should be ordered at one time, and the rate of infusion should be specified in drops per minute when dealing with infants. Intravenous sets for fluids are now constructed with reservoirs in which limited amounts of fluid may be held in order to prevent accidental overinfusion.

Electrolyte imbalance may be associated with overhydration. Harned and Cooke[31] reported four children who developed hyponatremia following infusion of large quantities of water. Convulsions typical of water intoxication followed, and, although three patients responded to therapy with 3% saline solution, the fourth, a 2-day-old infant with tracheoesophageal fistula, died. These authors reported two other children who developed hyponatremia associated with hyperpotassemia. The patients had undergone correction of cardiac lesions and then had developed cardiac failure. Hyperpotassemia was evident by electrocardiograph, as well as by bradycardia and generalized weakness. Both children were treated with 3% saline solution, but here again one infant died in spite of therapy.

Reactions to specific substances. Transfusion reactions may occur in infants and children of any age and will follow the same patterns see in adults.[32]

Problems of massive rapid transfusion. The complications associated with rapid infusion of large amounts of blood have been particularly evident in pediatric surgery. We have seen children who had exsanguinating hemorrhage and who continued to live through the period of maximum reduction of blood volume, only to die after the blood was replaced.

We have considered several different explanations and now believe that a number of factors probably act together; consequently, they all should be combated.

The possibility of citrate intoxication has been disputed but not resolved.[33-35] However, it has been obvious many times in our experience that during transfusion failing heart action has been abruptly stimulated immediately after administration of calcium chloride or gluconate. Consequently, during any case in which blood is given rapidly in large amounts (one third or more of the patient's blood volume), 10% calcium gluconate is given. The dosage of calcium is not well established, but 100 mg. per 200 ml. of blood has been taken as a maximum. A reasonable amount would be approximately 100 mg. per 20 lb. body weight.

Administration of calcium actually is best determined by electrocardiographic evidence of low calcium concentration, signified by peaked T waves, QRS slurring, or prolonged Q-T interval.[36]

In children with high hematocrit levels, as in tetralogy of Fallot, plasma is often used for blood volume replacement. On numerous occasions we have observed sudden cardiac depression during rapid infusion of plasma. This has been most effectively treated by administration of 10% calcium gluconate as noted previously, or preferably as a prophylactic measure. During Blalock or Potts procedures for tetralogy it has been advantageous to have one infusion for plasma or blood and a second in which a solution of 500 mg. of calcium gluconate, 5 mg. of Neo-Synephrine, and 150 ml. of 5% glucose is administered throughout the operation.

It is highly probable that acidity[18,37] and temperature[38] of bank blood is of much greater danger than the citrate content. The pH of ACD bank blood when fresh may be 7.0 to 7.2, and then it falls daily (Fig. 26-16), whereas CPD blood is only slightly less acid. Obviously a large transfusion of blood with pH of 6.8 or less can by itself be fatal. To counteract this danger it is advisable to buffer blood prior to infusion.[39] This may be done by testing pH and adding tris(hydroxymethyl)aminomethane (THAM), 150 mg. of which should raise the pH of 1 kg. of blood 0.1. In an emergency, it is expedient to add 1,200 mg. of THAM to each unit of bank blood without titrating it. If THAM is not available, it is advisable to administer sodium bicarbonate to the patient. One ampule containing 44 mEq. of sodium bicarbonate may be used as an effective dose for an adult.

Having seen cold blood used to stop the heart intentionally for open-heart procedures, it is easy to realize that we probably have done exactly the same thing

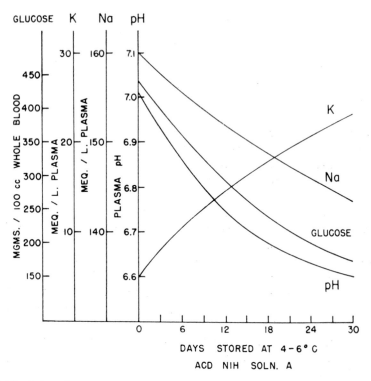

Fig. 26-16. The lesion of storage. Changes in the plasma of blood that is stored in ACD reflect (1) the effect of accumulation of metabolites on the pH of the plasma (because of continuing gly- colysis) and (2) the effect of the disturbance in the transport of cation on the levels of sodium and potassium. (From Gibson, J. G., II, Murphy, W. P., Jr., Scheitlin, W. A., and Rees, S. B.: Amer. J. Clin. Path. 26:855, 1956.)

when we have transfused small children with cold bank blood and had cardiac arrest. The heart stops at 16° C., and bank blood is stored at 4° C.

This realization has led us to adopt several countermeasures:

1. Blood that is to be given to small infants or that is to be given rapidly is prewarmed to near body heat. Blood may be warmed prior to administra- tion by immersing the container in a water bath, or by passing it through a warming device during administration. Blood warmers are available commercially,[40] or may be home constructed, using a small bucket, a thermometer, and an additional 10-foot coil of intravenous tubing. Over- heating the blood will cause hemolysis, and the bath temperature should be about 100° F.

2. Special effort is made to maintain the child's temperature; otherwise the heart will be dangerously near the critical temperature prior to transfusion.

3. If asystole occurs that might have been caused by infusion of cold blood, warm saline solution is poured over the heart as it is massaged.

Stetson made the interesting observation that dogs survive cold blood trans- fusions given by intraarterial route better than those given by intravenous route, since blood given via the arteries is warmed by passage through tissue capillaries prior to reaching the heart.[41]

REFERENCES

1. Friis-Hansen, B.: Changes in body water compartments during growth, Acta paediat., supp. 110, 1957.
2. Moore, F. D., McMurray, J. D., Parker, H. V., Magnus, I. C.: Body composition: total body water and electrolytes: intravascular and extravascular phase volumes, Metabolism 5:447-467, 1956.
3. Bland, J. H.: The clinical use of fluid and electrolyte, Philadelphia, 1952, W. B. Saunders Co.
4. James, L. S., Weisbrot, I. M., Prince, C. F., Holaday, D. A., and Apgar, V.: The acid-base status of human infants in relation to birth asphyxia and the onset of respiration, J. Pediat. 33:379-394, 1958.
5. Smith, C. A.: Physiology of the newborn infant, ed. 2, Springfield, Ill., 1951, Charles C Thomas, Publisher.
6. McCance, R. A.: Renal physiology in infancy, Amer. J. Med. 9:229-241, 1950.
7. Strauss, J., and James, L. S.: Renal function in the first hours of extrauterine life, Amer. J. Dis. Child. 102:486-488, 1961.
8. Gamble, J. L.: Early history of replacement therapy, Pediatrics 11:554-567, 1953.
9. Gamble, J. L.: Chemical anatomy, physiology and pathology of extracellular fluid, ed. 5, Cambridge, 1947, Harvard University Press.
10. Gamble, J. L.: Companionship of water and electrolytes in the organization of body fluids, Lane Medical Lectures, Stanford, Calif., 1951, Stanford University Press.
11. Percheson, P. B., and Carroll, J. J.: Difficulties in paediatric anaesthesia, Canad. Anaesth. Soc. J. 5:115-132, 1958.
12. Gross, R. E.: The surgery of infancy and childhood, Philadelphia, 1953, W. B. Saunders Co.
13. Hill, F. S.: Practical fluid therapy in pediatrics, Philadelphia, 1954, W. B. Saunders Co.
14. Nicholson, M. J., and Jensen, F. G.: Importance of blood volume studies in management of surgical patients, Anesth. Analg. 31:27-34, 1952.
15. Clark, J. H., Nelson, W., Lyons, C., Mayerson, H. S., and DeCamp, P.: Chronic shock: the problem of reduced blood volume in the chronically ill patient, Ann. Surg. 125:618-646, 1947.
16. Davenport, H. T., and Barr, M. N.: Blood loss during pediatric operations, Canad. Med. Ass. J. 89:1309-1313, 1963.
17. Boyan, C. P., and Howland, W. S.: Cardiac arrest and temperature of bank blood, J.A.M.A. 183:58-61, 1963.
18. Terry, R. N., and Trudnowsky, R. J.: Intraoperative fluid therapy, New York J. Med. 64:2648-2651, 1964.
19. Shires, T., Williams, J., and Brown, F.: Acute change in extracellular fluids associated with major surgical procedures, Ann. Surg. 154:803-810, 1961.
20. Jenkins, M. T., Gieseke, A. H., Jr., and Shires, G. T.: Electrolyte therapy in shock: management during anesthesia, Clin. Anesth. 2:39-59, 1965.
21. Viguera, M. G.: Fluid therapy during paediatric surgery, Canad. Anaesth. Soc. J. 13:290-300, 1966.
22. Gibson, J. G., Gregory, C. B., and Button, L.: Citrate-phosphate dextrose solution for preservation of human blood, Transfusion 1:280-287, 1961.
23. Darrow, D. C.: Body-fluid physiology: the role of potassium in clinical disorders of body water and electrolyte, New Eng. J. Med. 242:978-983, 1014-1018, 1950.
24. Frank, H. A., Hastings, T. N., and Brophy, T. W.: Fluid and electrolyte management in pediatric surgery, Western J. Surg. 60:25-31, 1952.
25. Hand, A. M., and Leininger, C. R.: Parenteral fluid therapy in children, Med. Clin. N. Amer. 34:53-70, 1950.
26. Gross, R. E.: Scale for measurement of blood which is lost in surgical sponges, J. Thorac. Surg. 18:543-545, 1949.
27. Smith, R. M.: Blood replacement in thoracic surgery for children, J.A.M.A. 161:1124-1128, 1956.

28. Bosomworth, P. P., Dietsch, J. D., and Hamelberg, W.: The effect of controlled hemorrhage on heart sounds, Anesth. Analg. **42**:131-140, 1963.
29. Talbert, J. L., and Haller, J. A., Jr.: Recent advances in postoperative management of infants, J. Surg. Res. **6**:502-509, 1966.
30. Harris, J. S.: Special pediatric problems in fluid and electrolyte therapy in surgery, Ann. New York Acad. Sci. **66**:966-975, 1957.
31. Harned, H. S., Jr., and Cooke, R. E.: Symptomatic hyponatremia in infants and children undergoing surgery, Surg. Gynec. Obstet. **104**:543-550, 1957.
32. Seldon, T. H.: Reactions to transfusions during operation, Surg. Clin. N. Amer. **29**-1129-1135, 1949.
33. Bunker, J. P.: Citric acid intoxication, J.A.M.A. **157**:1361-1367, 1955.
34. Marshall, M.: Potassium intoxication from blood and plasma transfusions, Anaesthesia **17**:145-148, 1962.
35. Corbascio, A. N., and Smith, N. T.: Hemodynamic effects of experimental hypercitremia, Anesthesiology **28**:510-516, 1967.
36. Marshall, M.: Potassium intoxication from blood and plasma transfusions, Anaesthesia **17**:145-148, 1962.
37. Howland, W. E., and Schweizer, O.: Acid-base lesion of bank blood, Anesthesiology **25**:102-108, 1964.
38. Boyan, C. P., and Howland, W. S.: Blood temperature a critical factor in massive transfusion, Anesthesiology **22**:559-563, 1961.
39. Moore, D., Bernhard, W. F., and Kevy, S. V.: Method for control of hydrogen ion concentration in stored heparinized blood prior to use in cardiac surgery, Ann. Surg. **159**:1000-1006, 1963.
40. Howland, W. S., and Schweizer, O.: Blood warming and hemolysis, Anesthesiology **26**:223-224, 1965.
41. Smith, R. M., and Stetson, J. B.: Therapeutic hypothermia, New Eng. J. Med. **265**:1147-1151, 1961.

Chapter 27

Anesthetic complications

Respiratory complications
    Respiratory depression
        Preoperative respiratory depression
        Respiratory depression during operation
        Continued respiratory depression following anesthesia
    Airway obstruction
        Nonpathologic airway obstruction
            Obstruction by tongue
            Excessive secretions
            Crowing and reflex spasm of vocal cords
            Airway obstruction during endotracheal anesthesia
        Aspiration of intestinal contents
        Pathologic airway obstruction
    Inadequate source of oxygen
        Abnormal respiratory rate and rhythms
        Extubation spasm
        Acute postoperative cardiorespiratory collapse
        Postoperative tracheitis
        Cyanosis following operation
Cardiovascular complications
    Tachycardia
    Bradycardia and arrhythmias
    Unexplained cardiac arrest
        Anesthetist's role in the treatment of cardiac arrest
    Heart failure during anesthesia
    Blood pressure variation
        Hypertension
        Hypotension and shock
    Illustrative treatment of shock
Complications of the central nervous system
    Convulsions and other motor disturbances
        Classic ether convulsions
        Convulsions due to local anesthetic agents
        The ether shrug
        Divinyl ether convulsions
        Shivering and muscle tremors
        Postoperative convulsions
    Hyperthermia in anesthetized patients
        Malignant hyperthermia
        Prophylaxis and therapy

Gastrointestinal complications
 Distention of the stomach
 Silent regurgitation
 Vomiting
  The well-prepared child
   Induction
   Vomiting during anesthesia
   Postoperative vomiting
  Vomiting in the presence of full stomach
Hepatorenal complications

RESPIRATORY COMPLICATIONS

Of the many problems that may upset the course of anesthesia and recovery, respiratory complications are by far the most common.[1] These may occur at any stage of the procedure, and although some may be insignificant, others may lead to immediate death. The origin and pattern of complications may appear varied, but actually most of them fall into three categories: respiratory depression, airway obstruction, or inadequate oxygen supply. Regardless of the nature of the complication, therapy will usually be most effective if it is directed toward the three essential steps of *clearing the airway, promoting ventilation,* and *increasing the oxygen supply.* Correction of any one or two of these factors may not be adequate if the third is neglected.

Individual complications should be approached with this underlying plan in mind and with the realization that any complication should be corrected at once; otherwise minor problems will rapidly assume major proportions.

Respiratory depression

Preoperative respiratory depression. A child's ventilation may be reduced before operation because of illness or preoperative sedation, either as a result of gross overdosage or apparently increased sensitivity to medication. In the event of mild hypoventilation, anesthesia by the open-drop technique would be inadvisable, but if a technique is used that allows ventilatory assistance, and if there is no cardiovascular depression, it seems reasonable to go ahead with the procedure rather than to postpone it.

Respiratory depression during operation. Inadequate ventilation is not easily recognized, and it is difficult to tell what comprises sufficient exchange. Clinical signs and the respiratory rate are no measure of alveolar ventilation or tissue oxygenation. Consequently, the best plan is to provide slight hyperventilation at all times by use of light ether anesthesia or by use of assisted or controlled respiratory technique. At present the use of a stethoscope is the most practical method by which to monitor ventilatory exchange and prevent hypoventilation.

Continued respiratory depression following anesthesia. If a child's exchange is decreased at the end of operation because anesthetic agents have not been eliminated, ventilation certainly must be assisted until the child regains his full exchange and his normal respiratory pattern. If relatively deep inhalation anesthesia has been used and respiration is controlled, it may take 5 or 10 minutes for return of adequate spontaneous respiration. Such depression is unusual and is not a sign of good anesthetic technique.

If depression continues, one should look for other causes. If narcotics have been used for preoperative sedation, overdosage may be treated with an antagonist such as nalorphine (Nalline) or levallorphan (Lorfan). For adults narcotic overdosage is treated by intravenous administration of 5 to 10 mg. of nalorphine or 1 to 2 mg. of levallorphan. If incomplete response is obtained, one half of the original dose may be repeated in 10 minutes. The dosage for children should be modified in relation to the size of the child. The usual dose for newborn infants suspected of narcotic depression is nalorphine, 0.2 to 0.4 mg., and levallorphan, 0.05 to 0.1 mg.

If relaxants have been employed, apnea or hypoventilation may be even more prolonged. Nondepolarizing agents such as *d*-tubocurarine and gallamine should be reversed with prostigmine. Apnea following succinylcholine is more difficult to overcome and usually requires ventilatory assistance and investigation as described in Chapter 14.

If there is apnea or complete absence of spontaneous respiration, the anesthetist usually will provide adequate support for the patient. There is actually greater danger for the patient after he has begun to breathe for himself, for the anesthetist, seeing signs of spontaneous exchange, often makes the mistake of assuming that respiration is adequate and will allow the patient to continue by himself. Such a patient may become severely hypoxic. One must expect to continue respiratory assistance long after the first reappearance of the patient's efforts.

Following neurosurgical operations lesions of the brain may cause lasting respiratory depression. In such cases tracheotomy and use of ventilatory machines may be needed.

Airway obstruction

The causes of airway obstruction are many and varied. They may be divided into nonpathologic and pathologic types.

Nonpathologic airway obstruction. Ventilation is often impaired by anatomic relaxation, spasm, secretions, and other factors.

Obstruction by tongue. Unless the trachea is intubated the tongue may fall back into the hypopharynx and interfere with respiratory exchange. The angle of the chin must be supported to bring the mandible forward if this is to be prevented. During induction the patient may be rolled on his side until anesthesia is sufficient to allow the use of an oral airway.

Excessive secretions. Although respiratory exchange may be obstructed at any time because of excessive secretions, this is most likely to occur during induction of anesthesia. Suction apparatus must always be available, but, if the secretions appear early in the course of induction, the use of suction will stimulate the child and cause him to waken. It may be preferable to turn the child on his side and lower the head until he has passed the excitement stage. As soon as possible the airway should be cleared completely.

After suction has been used on the pharynx there may still be sounds of moist airway obstruction. Usually, if a laryngoscope is used to expose the larynx, a few drops of secretions will be seen in the glottis and may easily be removed. Occasionally it is necessary to pass the catheter down into the trachea to clear secretions from the trachea and bronchi.

If secretions continue to be troublesome, atropine or scopolamine may be repeated in slightly reduced dosage by intravenous route. It was once believed that such drying agents should not be given if secretions were already present for fear of reducing the fluid to tenacious sticky plugs. This has not occurred in our experience.

Crowing and reflex spasm of vocal cords. Stridor or spasm may be encountered with any agent and during any operation, but it is most frequently seen with ether anesthesia during orchidopexy or other operations that involve reflex stimulation. Often the crowing may be relieved by adjusting the patient's head or the position of the airway. It is even more helpful to maintain continuous positive pressure in the patient's airway for 30 to 40 seconds, trying to deepen the plane of anesthesia. It seems likely that Fink[2] is correct in his statement that inspiratory stridor denotes too light a plane of anesthesia.

When severe spasm occurs, one's first tendency is to try to force oxygen through the constricted cords. However, this often increases the irritation, and one usually does better to wait 20 to 30 seconds to see if the child will breathe for himself. During this time one prepares succinylcholine in case intubation becomes necessary. If spasm does not break, one can attempt to force oxygen through the cords, but it is best to avoid excessive pressure (not over 50 cm. H_2O) and to watch for gastric distention. If such methods are ineffective, succinylcholine should be administered, and then the trachea may be intubated. Succinylcholine is best administered by vein, but if a small infant does not have easily accessible veins it may be best to employ intramuscular injection that will be effective in 60 to 90 seconds.

Airway obstruction during endotracheal anesthesia. The presence of an endotracheal tube does not exclude the possibility of airway obstruction. The tube may become kinked, filled with secretions or blood, or have been obstructed before introduction. One should always check the lumen of the tube prior to use, for tubes have been used that had no lumen or that were occluded by marbles, beans, or pipe cleaners.

Either bronchus may be occluded if the tube is passed beyond the carina, or the tube itself may be obstructed by an overinflated cuff.

If the anesthetist is unable to inflate the patient's chest and the endotracheal tube appears to be patent and properly placed, bronchiolar spasm may be present. In this case the anesthetist should continue to attempt to ventilate the patient until the spasm is conrolled. Foldes[3] recommends the use of isoproterenol (adult dose, 0.1 to 0.3 mg.) or aminophylline (3 mg./kg.)

Aspiration of intestinal contents

Aspiration of intestinal contents is one of the most serious causes of airway obstruction. Should it occur, the airway must be cleared immediately by exposing the glottis with a laryngoscope and sucking away all obstructing material. Bronchoscopy or tracheotomy may be necessary if large chunks of food have been aspirated. Prevention of this complication was discussed in detail in Chapter 24.

Although definite evidence is difficult to obtain, there is general agreement that steroids such as dexamethasone (Decadron) will help prevent postaspiration pneumonitis. A dosage of 0.3 mg./kg. every 4 hours seems reasonable.

Pathologic airway obstruction. Respiratory exchange may be impeded by congenital anomalies such as choanal atresia and laryngeal stenosis, by tumors, inflammation, foreign bodies, or the familiar tonsils and adenoids.[4,5] When such lesions are present, obstruction may be evident before operation and show the path that must be taken, or the danger may not become apparent until the procedure is under way and then may cause sudden and complete airway occlusion. For relief of upper airway obstruction, nasal or oral airways, endotracheal tube, or bronchoscope may suffice. Occasionally tracheostomy may be indicated, but an endotracheal tube or bronchoscope should be passed before this is undertaken. In an emergency one may pierce the trachea with a hollow needle and administer oxygen through it.[6] It must be remembered that tracheostomy will not help when obstruction occurs in the lower trachea or bronchi. Endobronchial intubation with catheter or bronchoscope may be required in such a case.

Inadequate source of oxygen

When open-drop anesthesia or nitrous oxide is employed, one may easily administer less than 20% oxygen to the patient. If slightly hypoxic mixtures are delivered for prolonged periods, damage to the central nervous system may result. This hazard must be averted by adding oxygen when using open-drop techniques and by observing safe standards in the administration of nitrous oxide.

In addition to the respiratory complications caused by depression, obstruction, and inadequate oxygen supply, others may be caused by increased apparatus dead space, irregular respiratory rhythm, and postoperative collapse.

Abnormal respiratory rate and rhythms. Infants and children are subject to great variation in respiratory pattern. A rapid rate is not especially harmful unless it is so fast that it reduces the tidal exchange. An infant's respiratory rate preferably should remain under 100 per minute, but it is the alveolar ventilation that determines adequate exchange. If ventilation appears inadequate, it may be supplemented by manual assistance. Slow respiration rarely is a problem unless the child has been severely depressed. In such a case intubation and artificial ventilation may be indicated.

Irregular respiration may take the form of apneustic gasping, Cheyne-Stokes breathing, tracheal tug, or many other variations. The first two complications do not appear to have a definite etiology but may occur in premature babies, in ill children, or in normal infants following a difficult induction marked by screaming or excitement. If a light, even plane of anesthesia is maintained, respiration is assisted, and supplemental oxygen is administered, one can make up for the irregular pulmonary exchange.

The presence of a tracheal tug[7] during anesthesia is almost always the sign of inadequate ventilation due to obstruction, deep anesthesia, or carbon dioxide excess. All possible steps should be taken to eliminate this truly important sign. These include decreasing the anesthetic concentration, hyperventilating the patient, checking the carbon dioxide absorbent, clearing the airway, and checking the entire chest by stethoscope. The use of a relaxant is to be avoided here, for it will merely obliterate an important signal of danger without correcting the cause.

Hiccough occasionally is seen during induction with inhalation agents or following administration of thiopental or methohexital (Brevital). It is usually eliminated when surgical anesthesia is established. Under any circumstances respiration should be assisted or controlled until the hiccough stops, for ventilation may be seriously embarrassed. In attempting to find the source of the hiccough one first considers gastric distention or some irritation of the diaphragm or phrenic nerve. In most situations the condition lasts only a few minutes, but should it persist a relaxant is used, followed by intubation and the use of controlled respiration. If hiccough persists and does not appear to be due to an organic cause, Steinhaus[8] advises slow intravenous administration of 1% lidocaine (Xylocaine) in dosage of 1 ml. per 50 pounds of body weight.

The application of a suction catheter to the nose has also been described as a remarkably effective measure to control hiccough during anesthesia.[9]

Extubation spasm. Extubation spasm is described on p. 187.

Acute postoperative cardiorespiratory collapse. A small infant may tolerate herniorrhaphy, pyloromyotomy, or harelip repair uneventfully under general anesthesia, wake up and respond, and then 10 minutes later suddenly become limp, apneic, and pulseless. Usually active resuscitation by mouth-to-mouth ventilation, bag-and-mask technique, or intubation will result in prompt recovery, but several deaths have been reported and many more barely averted under such circumstances. This very serious complication is characteristic of small infants but has not been satisfactorily explained. It seems probable that it is caused by hyperventilation during anesthesia with resultant removal of carbon dioxide and consequent loss of respiratory stimulus. The possibility of such an unexpected complication makes strict observation of greatest importance during the early recovery period.

Postoperative tracheitis. Irritation and edema of trachea and vocal cords may occur following endotracheal anesthesia, causing hoarseness, stridor, and retraction in varying degree in children. Although its incidence and severity can be greatly influenced by scrupulous precautions, it has been difficult to avoid entirely. There are several factors that affect it. As Bachman and Freeman[10] reported, this complication occurs most frequently in children 1 to 3 years of age, as does infectious croup. It also is seen more frequently during winter months. Certainly it occurs more frequently following operations around the neck, and in the prone position.

Although one can not alter the preceding factors, other causative factors are more controllable. Tubes must be clean and nonirritant. Much emphasis has justly been placed on cleaning tubes and keeping them clean, but it seems probable that ethylene-oxide and other sterilizing techniques may introduce an irritant action unless great care is used to rinse or air tubes sufficiently. Following sterilization with ethylene oxide, equipment should be aired 18 to 20 hours.

Size of the tube and motion of the tube are two important controllable factors. The tube should be small enough to pass the cords and cricoid without any resistance. It should be inserted gently without trauma. It also must not rub back and forth during anesthesia. Finally, any preexisting irritation of the glottis definitely will increase the incidence of postoperative edema.

Following bronchoscopy patients are routinely placed in humidified tents. Other patients are placed in tents upon appearance of hoarseness or stridor, and, if it appears marked, dexamethasone (Decadron), approximately 0.3 mg./kg., is administered as recommended by Deming and Oech.[11]

Should respiratory obstruction become severe, one must choose between reinsertion of an endotracheal tube and tracheostomy. At present insertion of a nasotracheal tube for a period of 12 to 24 hours is favored.

Cyanosis following operation. If at the end of operation a child's color is dusky or cyanotic, immediate and systematic steps should be taken to determine the cause. The first step is to check with a stethoscope the cardiac and respiratory sounds throughout the chest. Pulse and blood pressure are observed in order to rule out inadequate circulation. Suction is used in the nares, the pharynx is exposed with a laryngoscope, and the pharynx and the trachea are cleared of any offending material. The lungs are hyperventilated with oxygen. The temperature is taken, for the patient may be extremely cold.

If the answer still has not been found, a roentgen-ray film of the chest may be ordered to rule out atelectasis. If the operation had involved opening the chest, drainage tubes should be checked and irrigated in case there might be hemothorax or pneumothorax. The patient should be encouraged to cough. In case there is any sign of aspiration of foreign material or a mucus plug, thorough suction of the trachea should be performed or bronchoscopy should be employed.

CARDIOVASCULAR COMPLICATIONS

Abnormal variations in the heart rate or rhythm or in the blood pressure occur with less frequency than do respiratory irregularities, but they may give good reason for alarm. Circulatory failure or cardiac arrest may follow.

Tachycardia

It is difficult to fix the limits of normal heart rate during anesthesia, for there may be wide variation. In general, the pulse will accelerate 10 to 20 beats per minute under thiopental or cyclopropane and about 40 beats under ether anesthesia. Should these limits be exceeded, tachycardia may be said to exist, and the cause should be sought. One first checks blood loss and fluid replacement and then turns to dead space, soda lime exhaustion, depth of anesthesia, reflex stimulation, or prolonged use of a tourniquet. If no fault is found, it may be advisable to use the electrocardiograph to rule out paroxysmal tachcardia, in which case vagal stimulation may be an effective therapeutic measure.

In several patients who had repeated or persistent tachycardia of undetermined origin, the use of edrophonium (Tensilon) in doses of 0.1 mg. per 20 pounds was effective.

Bradycardia and arrhythmias

Slowing of the heart during anesthesia may be due to hypoxia, vagal stimulation, or direct myocardial depression.

With increasing depth of halothane anesthesia the reduction of heart rate is a useful sign. This slowing is due both to vagal stimulation and to direct myocardial depression.

More severe bradycardia may occur when succinylcholine is administered intravenously[12,13] (Fig. 27-1). This has been discussed (p. 162), as has that which may occur during operations on the eye. In both instances the bradycardia is due to vagal stimulation and may be prevented or corrected by atropine.[14,15]

Moderate slowing of the heart during ether anesthesia occurs if the plane of anesthesia becomes light. This is often seen during neurosurgery or similar procedures requiring endotracheal intubation but slight relaxation. The anesthetic plane of the patient may become light enough to evoke vagal laryngeal reflexes and sinus arrhythmia or bradycardia. Use of atropine or deeper anesthesia corrects the situation quickly.

During cardiac surgery bradycardia may signify heart block. Diagnosis may

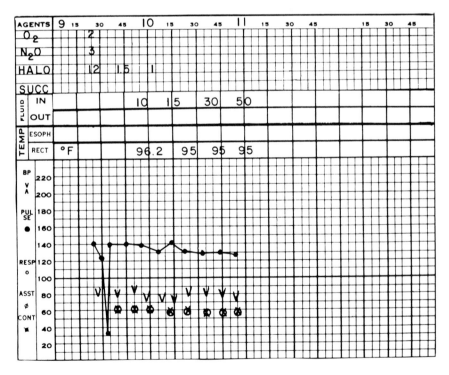

Fig. 27-1. Severe bradycardia resulting from combination of halothane and intravenous succinylcholine.

be confirmed by electrocardiograph, and treatment with isoproterenol (Isuprel) or ephedrine will probably be indicated. Other cardiac arrhythmias may be noted rather frequently if the patient is monitored by electrocardiograph. A number of transient irregularities are encountered that have little significance. Those more commonly seen include atrioventricular nodal rhythms, occasional ventricular premature contractions, ST deviation, wandering pacemaker, and bigeminy.[16]

Most inhalation anesthetics may be complicated by the appearance of cardiac arrhythmias, but with cyclopropane and halothane arrhythmias are commonly seen, usually in the form of coupled beats, bigeminy, and premature ventricular beats. Deep anesthesia or hypoventilation may play a part in causing this, as may surgical manipulation of the viscera. Steps to correct these factors are first taken, and atropine may be useful. One then may choose between discontinuing or supplementing the agent or using a drug to decrease the sensitivity of the heart. Propranolol, a beta adrenergic blocking drug, has been used for this purpose. Since halothane has adrenergic blocking properties, the addition of a beta blocking agent could be markedly depressing, on theoretical grounds. Craythorne and Huffington[17] report that propranolol reduces cardiac output significantly when used with cyclopropane but merely decreases cardiac rate in dogs anesthetized with halothane. As yet, use of these agents in human beings is not well documented and requires restraint.

Irregular rhythms are known to occur with trichloroethylene.[18] Their appearance should be taken as an indication for more oxygen and less anesthetic.

Although ether less often causes cardiac irregularities, we have had two in-

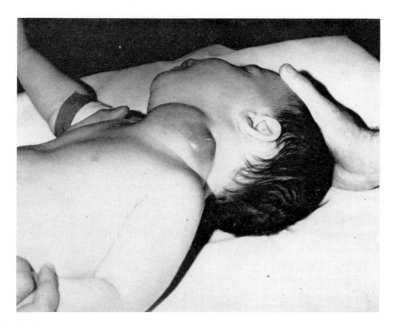

Fig. 27-2. Cardiac arrest has been reported during several operations on cervical masses.

stances of severe paroxysmal tachycardia under this agent, and another patient showed a peculiar auriculoventricular dissociation upon several different occasions when anesthetized with ether.[19]

Unexplained cardiac arrest

Although many excellent articles have been written on the subject,[20,21] the term cardiac arrest has been widely used and often with rather loose meaning. Some writers apply the term to any type of sudden death; others appear to read into it some inescapable and unassailable quality, as though it were an act of God, calling for neither explanation nor blame.[22]

Any death must have a specific cause or chain of events leading to it. When recognizable, it should be named. At present the term cardiac arrest is acceptable only because there are deaths the causes of which are not evident. It will be used here to denote sudden unexpected cardiac standstill or fibrillation in situations that gave neither warning nor obvious explanation of the calamity. Obviously hemorrhage is not one of these situations. If all patients were watched with meticulous care and each heartbeat and respiration monitored, it seems probable that most of these so-called cardiac arrests would be averted, for without doubt many of them are due to preventable but unrecognized insults such as hypoxia, carbon dioxide excess, or blood loss. Sudden cardiovascular collapse has been known to occur in three children during operations on cervical masses (Fig. 27-2). Such catastrophes have convinced us that one can never be sure of the safety of the patient.

Statistics have indicated that cardiac arrest is more common in pediatric anesthesia. This will be discussed in Chapter 30.

Anesthetist's role in the treatment of cardiac arrest. The excitement that immediately follows recognition of cardiac arrest may cause utter confusion unless surgeon and anesthetist act according to an organized, predetermined plan.

On failure to obtain the pulse or heartbeat, the anesthetist can make several important moves *within a very few seconds.* He notes the time, washes out the anesthetic, notifies the surgeon, calls for additional operating room personnel and surgical assistance, ventilates the patient, again checks the heart by carotid pulse and auscultation, and calls for a check of blood measurements and for rapid infusion if indicated. In the meantime he must look for possible causes of the arrest and take steps to correct them. The most probable causes are hypoxia, exsanguination, anesthetic overdosage, and overinfusion.

If an endotracheal tube is in place when the arrest occurs, the patient is immediately ventilated with 100% oxygen. If the patient is not intubated, it is preferable to oxygenate the patient by mask several times and then intubate, thus avoiding additional seconds of hypoxia required for intubation.

Ventilation should be adequate, but not excessive. Overzealous bag squeezing in such an emergency will prevent venous return and nullify other restorative measures.

The surgeon immediately feels for pulsation of abdominal aorta or heartbeat if working in the abdomen or chest. Fortunately, he no longer must make the great decision to open the chest. Without a moment's hesitation, he can begin external cardiac massage.[23,24] In small infants pressure is applied at mid-sternum, rather than at the lower third, as in adults. If the infant is on a firm bed or table, adequate effect may be obtained by pressing on the sternum with three fingers, but this will be unsatisfactory if the child is not supported. It is more effective to grasp the child's chest in the hands, with thumbs at midster-num, and squeeze the heart rhythmically (Fig. 27-3, *A*).

Several deaths have occurred due to compression and rupture of the liver and stomach during cardiac massage. This danger may be averted by reversing

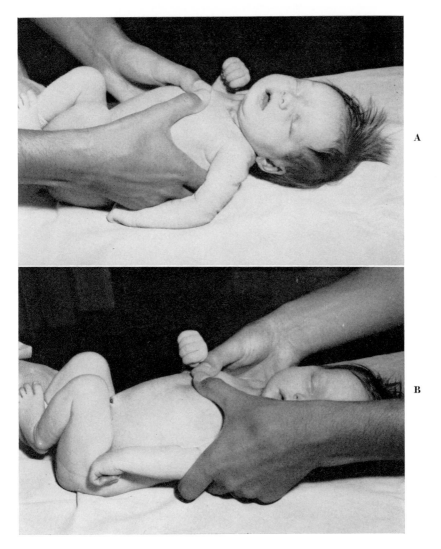

Fig. 27-3. A, Closed cardiac massage. Thumbs properly placed at midsternum, but hands may compress and rupture descending liver and stomach. **B,** Preferred method producing same cardiac compression but allowing free descent of abdominal viscera.

one's position so that the hands encircle the chest rather than the abdomen (Fig. 27-3, *B*). In order to increase venous return it is advisable to elevate the child's legs on a pillow or rolled-up sheets. If cardiac action does not return at once, further diagnostic and therapeutic action is indicated. Cardiac stimulants and buffering agents are important adjuncts, and an electrocardiograph should be put into prompt use. Intracardiac injections are best made by substernal approach, thereby avoiding the lungs (Fig. 27-4).

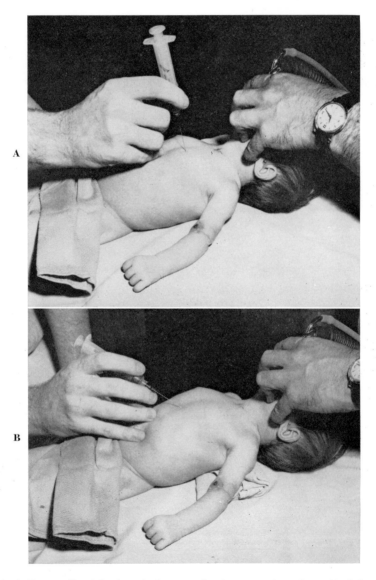

Fig. 27-4. A, Intracardiac injection via intercostal space may pierce lung. **B,** Substernal route provides greater safety.

Dosages for drugs are suggested in Table 27-1. These have never been accurately evaluated, but they have proved clinically effective. Epinephrine is tolerated well by children, and tolerance is increased in hypoxic states.[25,26] The 1/1,000 concentration is now believed to be acceptable and practical. Calcium, epinephrine, and glucose all may be given directly into the heart by intercostal, or preferably substernal, injection. Concentrated glucose is effective as an inotropic agent and has been shown to reverse the potassium efflux that may occur during hypoxic states.[27]

Buffering agents, sodium bicarbonate or tris buffer, tris (hydroxymethyl) aminomethane, should be administered within 5 minutes after arrest, or sooner if hypoxia was present prior to arrest. Either of these agents is satisfactory. Tris buffer acts more rapidly and has immediate intracellular effect; however, this drug causes hypoglycemia and respiratory depression. It should never be used unless effective ventilatory assistance is available. Hypoglycemia may be averted by mixing the agent in glucose solution. A 1.5 molar solution is prepared by dissolving 36 Gm. of tris in 180 ml. of 5% dextrose; then each milliliter contains 200 mg. An initial dose of 150 mg. per kilogram is expected to raise the pH by 0.1.[28]

Sodium bicarbonate may be used in the same manner. One ampule containing 3.75 Gm. is considered a standard initial dose for an adult. Either tris or sodium bicarbonate may be repeated several times without danger if indications exist.

The effectiveness of cardiac massage must be noted by palpation of peripheral pulses, by continued normal color of skin and mucous membranes, and especially by maintenance of contracted pupils. Adequacy of ventilation is attested by stethoscopic ausculation or direct observation of the lungs. Open cardiac massage can be avoided in most situations, but it may prove more effective when other methods fail. If arrest has occurred in a basically sound child in the operating room, it seems advisable to open the chest after 10 minutes of unsuccessful closed massage.

If the heart has been chilled by cold blood, direct warming may be indicated.

Table 27-1. *Drugs used for reversal of cardiac arrest*

		Dose	
Agent	*Concentration*	*Under 10 lb.*	*Over 10 lb.*
Epinephrine	1/1,000 (0.1%)	0.2 ml.	0.25 ml./25 lb.
Calcium gluconate	100 mg./ml. (10%)	1 ml.	1 ml./15 lb.
Glucose	500 mg./ml. (50%)	1 ml.	1 ml./15 lb.
Sodium bicarbonate	3.75 Gm./50 ml. (44.6 mEq./50 ml.)	3–4 ml.	1 ml./ 3 lb.
Tris (hydroxymethyl) aminomethane (THAM)	200 mg./ml. (1.5 M.)	3–4 ml.	1 ml./ 3 lb.
Isoproterenol (Isuprel)	1/5,000	0.2 ml.	0.1 ml./15 lb.

If there is intrathoracic hemorrhage or if the arrest follows cardiac surgery, thoractomy may be advisable.

Further considerations in the treatment of arrest have been described exhaustively.[29,30]

The final duty of the anesthetist during this catastrophe is that of official recorder. For this he will need an assistant, who should be told to do nothing but stand by and record each step that is taken. When all is completed, the anesthetist should immediately write out his own detailed report of the entire event.

Heart failure during anesthesia

Normal children rarely develop heart failure during operation, but this may occur in children with heart disease. Signs of a failing heart during anesthesia are distended veins, slow capillary refill time, weak, irregular pulse with tachycardia or bradycardia, irregular respiration, faint heart sounds, failing blood pressure with narrow pulse pressure, electrocardiographic signs of myocardial failure (T-wave changes, widened QRS, etc.), enlarged liver, and pulmonary edema. If this occurs during intrathoracic surgery, the heart can be seen to enlarge and its force become weaker.

Treatment will include placing the patient with head slightly elevated, restriction of fluid, the use of intermittent positive pressure oxygenation, vasopressors to sustain the blood pressure, and rapid digitalization, accomplished by the use of digitoxin, initial dosage approximately 0.02 mg. per pound.[31]

Blood pressure variation

Hypertension. Elevation of blood pressure may occur during anesthesia as a result of carbon dioxide retention, the use of a tourniquet to control operative bleeding, increased pressure on the spinal cord or brain, or the presence of coarctation or pheochromocytoma. Treatment is directed at correction of the cause. Rapid temporary reduction of blood pressure may be effected by use of ganglionic blocking agents such as trimethylene thiophanium (Arfonad) or hexamethonium[32,33] (Chapter 15).

Hypotension and shock. Problems associated with hypotension in pediatric anesthesia are more frequent and more severe than those seen in adults because they occur with greater speed and the signs are less obvious.

The treatment of hypotension is very often approached in an extremely unintelligent manner. In the attempt to restore the pressure to its previous level, one often resorts to pumping blood or to the use of vasopressor agents without considering the mechanisms involved. Gradual or abrupt fall in blood pressure may be due to many different factors, and definitive treatment should be employed.

Most of the causes of hypotension during operation fall into one of three classes: myocardial failure, decreased peripheral vascular resistance, or decreased blood volume.

Myocardial failure may result from disease, hemodynamic overload during congenital heart surgery, overinfusion, or excessive depth of anesthesia. Specific therapy will be indicated for each, and transfusion is rarely helpful.

Decreased peripheral resistance may occur as a result of reflex vascular vasodilatation, spinal anesthesia, adrenocortical insufficiency, operative brain trauma, transfusion reaction, sepsis, or sudden carbon dioxide washout.[34,35] Definitive treatment is also indicated in these cases. Here vasopressors will occasionally be indicated, but transfusion will play a small part.

When a vasopressor is needed, 0.5 ml. of 1% phenylephrine (Neo-Synephrine) may be added to 100 ml. of 5% dextrose solution and infused as required. This relatively concentrated mixture is advised in order to avoid excess fluid administration.

Decreased blood volume has been our commonest cause of hypotension during operation and is a definite indication for blood replacement. Guides to blood replacement have already been described (Chapter 26).

The response of the body to prolonged or acute blood loss[36-38] entails a chain of reactions that should also be considered if intelligent therapy is to be undertaken. Local vascular constriction occurs first; then general compensatory mechanisms are set off by decreased venous return and falling blood pressure. Tachycardia, adrenal response, ganglionic stimulation, outpouring of epinephrine, hyperglycemia, selective vasoconstriction, elevation of plasma potassium, shift of body fluid, and lactate and pyruvate build-up follow in sequence[39,40] and terminate in generalized vasomotor paralysis, organ hypoxia, and death. If one can estimate how far this process has advanced, treatment can be shaped accordingly. It may happen, however, that, instead of helping, treatment will actually strike the fatal blow by way of transfusion reaction, sepsis, or overdigitalization.

Illustrative treatment of shock

In spite of many theoretical considerations, prompt, coordinated action is necessary in treatment of shock. Three specific situations are presented with appropriate corrective measures:

1. *Sudden hemorrhage during great vessel operation in a 4-year-old child, with heart slowing and blood pressure unobtainable:* Treatment (primarily directed toward correct replacement of blood):
    (a) Shut off anesthetic and rinse apparatus with oxygen; then ventilate the patient at moderate rate and pressure.
    (b) Pump blood and measure the lost and administered blood continually.
    (c) Have surgeon massage heart if its action lags.
    (d) Give 10% calcium chloride, 1 ml. per 200 ml. of blood pumped.
    (e) Replace blood until the infused amount is at least 10% to 15% in excess of loss and the blood pressure is above shock level.
    (f) Repeat atropine intravenously if bradycardia persists.
2. *Hypotension during excision of abdominal mass in a 2-year-old child:* Treatment (to control blood loss and reflex vasodilatation):
    (a) Stop anesthesia and give oxygen.

  (b) Stop operation.
  (c) Have surgeon remove packs and retractors and relieve abnormal position of patient.
  (d) Replace blood loss with moderate excess and add 10% calcium chloride, 1 ml. per 200 ml. of blood.
  (e) Administer phenylephrine (Neo-Synephrine) by drip method, or 1 mg. intravenously, for rapid correction of reflex vasodilatation.

3. *Postoperative hypotension. Blood pressure of 10-year-old child gradually falls to 60/40 one hour after lobectomy:* Treatment (management demands continued effort at correct diagnosis):
  (a) Check catheters for chest drainage.
  (b) Auscultate chest for hemothorax and atelectasis.
  (c) Check blood measurements.
  (d) Give oxygen and check airway.
  (e) Add 100 ml. of blood and watch response.
  (f) Examine chest roentgenographically.
  (g) Test vasoconstrictor response with 1 mg. of phenylephrine (Neo-Synephrine).
  (h) If response is good, add blood; if response is poor, give 100 mg. hydrocortisone intravenously.
  (i) Consider blood dyscrasia, afibrinogenemia, etc.
  (j) Take electrocardiogram.

The use of ganglioplegic drugs for treatment of hypotension and shock[41] may have real justification. As yet this technique has not been evaluated in pediatric patients.

COMPLICATIONS OF THE CENTRAL NERVOUS SYSTEM

Minor complications involving the central nervous system consist of postoperative dizziness, headache, vertigo, excitement, and transient psychic disturbances. Excitement following cyclopropane and halogenated agents is seen occasionally and may be controlled by intravenous administration of a sedative or narcotic.

Nerve palsies may occur as the result of faulty positioning during operation.[42,43] Care must be taken to pad arm boards and braces and to avoid traction or unnatural positioning under anesthesia. A new danger was brought to light when two children developed transient ulnar nerve palsies apparently due to pressure from the strap of the blood pressure stethoscope.

Serious complications involving the central nervous system may appear during anesthesia or in the postoperative period. Most of them are caused by hypoxia,[44,45] resulting either from inadequate ventilation or deficient cerebral circulation. The extent of the damage will vary with the degree and duration of physiologic trauma.

Delayed awakening may follow minor degrees of hypoxia, whereas more serious insult may cause spasticity, blindness, or decerebration. These complications may be either transitory or permanent in nature. Postoperative convulsions also are seen as a result of severe hypoxia during anesthesia, but other causes such as water intoxication[46] or operative brain damage should be considered.

Children show remarkable powers of recuperation. Following severe complications progress may be slow, but hope may be sustained as long as any improvement is seen. Two children have been encountered, one in our experience and one in a neighboring hospital, in which cardiac arrest was followed by coma and decerebration from which the children did not arouse for 1 and 4 weeks, respectively. When consciousness returned, both children were found to be blind. Sight slowly returned to these children throughout subsequent weeks, and now both are believed to be completely normal.

Cerebrovascular accidents are not to be expected in normal children but have occurred in two patients during operation for coarctation of the aorta. Hemorrhage in these cases probably was the result of the preexisting vascular lesions plus the additional strain imposed by occlusion of the aorta.

Convulsions and other motor disturbances

The incidence of anesthetic convulsions has always been high in children, and it is generally accepted that youth, dehydration, and fever, plus ether, are the most common factors in this complication.

The problem is actually a most complex and confusing one about which much has been written but very little is known. Originally, our difficulty was chiefly concerned with convulsions that occurred with ether. The subject has become even more complicated since other anesthetic agents have entered the picture.

As Bergner[47] pointed out, almost every anesthetic may be associated with some sort of motor spasm. However, there appears to be considerable difference in the significance of these phenomena, and the term convulsion should not be extended loosely to include them all. The term convulsion or seizure should be used only to describe a motor spasm having a central manifestation in the cortex demonstrable by an electroencephalogram. Several of the abnormal motions seen during or after anesthesia do not fit this definition.

The different motor phenomena seen during anesthesia may be divided into five groups: (1) classical ether convulsions, (2) those seen with local anesthetics, (3) the ether shrug, (4) divinyl ether convulsion, and (5) nonspecific shivering.

Classic ether convulsions. These are seen almost exclusively in patients who are toxic, dehydrated, or overheated.[48] The convulsion is Jacksonian in type, starting with twitching about the mouth or eyes or occasionally the fingers, and then it may develop into a typical grand mal type of seizure with the hands and arms held in flexion. This suggests a cortical focus and certainly deserves the term convulsion.

True ether convulsions have become an extreme rarity in hospitals in which operating rooms are reasonably cool (below 70° F.) and in which children are well prepared for operation.

The mortality associated with ether convulsions has been estimated as being 25% to 50%; consequently, they should be regarded as an extremely dangerous complication.

The treatment of an ether convulsion must be started immediately and should be specific as well as symptomatic. The anesthetic is discontinued and the child is ventilated with oxygen. In order to terminate the seizure as quickly as possible, thiopental or a relaxant may be used intravenously. Succinylcholine may be given by vein, or if a promising vein is not evident, it may be injected intramuscularly, 1 mg. per pound of body weight (up to 60 mg.). The effect will usually appear in less than a minute.

General measures consist of oxygenating the patient and of starting fluid therapy. If the patient appears hot, ice is applied to the face, axillae, and other exposed surfaces, and cold saline solution may be used to irrigate the stomach.

In addition to youth, illness, and fever, a long list of factors has been given as the basic cause of ether convulsions.[49] These include hypoxia,[50,51] hypercapnia,[52] hypoglycemia,[53] ketosis, hypocalcemia,[54] ether impurities, and many other contradictory and unconfirmed ideas.

Hauser[55] listed three basic causes of convulsions: hypoxia, hypoglycemia, and increased neuronal excitability, all of which lead to a defect in binding acetylcholine, metabolic loss of glutamic acid, failure of cellular Na and K exchange, and finally interference with adenosine triphosphate (ATP) metabolism.

A renewal of interest in this problem is seen in the work by Owens, Dawson, and Scott,[56] who showed that temperature is probably the most critical factor in anesthetic convulsions. Pittinger and his group[57] confirmed this concept and further showed halothane to have the least tendency to arouse convulsive activity, divinyl ether being the most dangerous in this respect.

Convulsions due to local anesthetic agents. The actual seizure caused by toxicity of local anesthetics appears identical with an ether convulsion. As an underlying factor, however, preexisting illness of the patient plays a small part, the primary cause usually being overdosage or rapid absorption.[58] This type of convulsion may be followed rapidly by myocardial depression and death unless treatment is prompt and specific. Intravenous barbiturates are known to help in controlling the seizure but should be used with caution because they may aggravate the myocardial depression. The patient must be oxygenated, and cardiac massage may be necessary.

The ether shrug. There is a second type of muscular contraction that is seen rather frequently with ether but that apparently has been overlooked. This consists of a rhythmic shrugging of the shoulders associated with pronation of the hands and extension of the arms. It occurs almost exclusively during induction with ether, more frequently when the open drop method is used, and usually appears as anesthesia is being induced rapidly. It is seen in normal, well-prepared children.

The character of this motion is unmistakable. There is no facial grimace and no spastic twitching, but at regular intervals, usually with every third inspiration, the hands pronate slightly, and then as induction is continued this motion becomes more pronounced and the arms and shoulders also take part. Normal respiration continues without interruption. The fact that there is pronation and extension and not flexion suggests a mesencephalic focus or temporary decerebrate rigidity.[59]

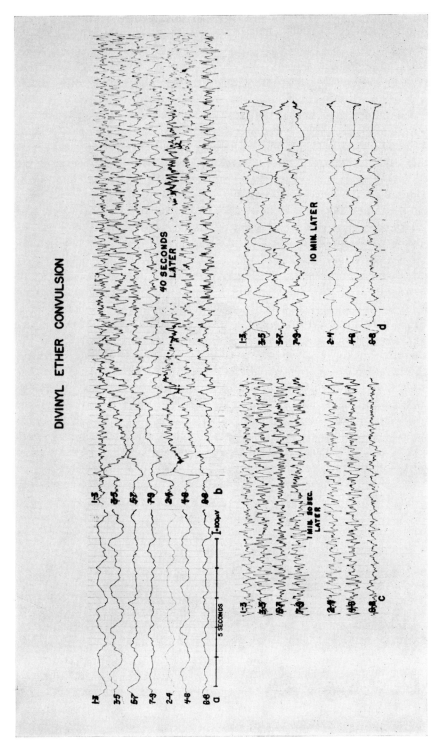

Fig. 27-5. Electroencephalogram of 1-year-old child during divinyl ether anesthesia. **a**, Normal initial pattern under light anesthesia. **b**, Overt convulsive seizure with irregular high-voltage tracing. **c** and **d**, Seizure patterns persisting after disappearance of momentary convulsion.

Divinyl ether convulsions. The muscular spasms seen with divinyl ether are well known.[57,60,61] These, too, have a characteristic pattern. During rapid induction or relatively deep anesthesia with this agent, patients usually hyperventilate, open their eyes in a fixed stare, and then extend their arms and legs, arch their backs, and next, holding themselves in this position, become apneic and then cyanotic until the seizure ends.

If the premonitory signs are recognized, this reaction may be aborted by interrupting the anesthetic. After a minor episode of this nature, one may resume the use of the anesthetic. This convulsion appears to be a specific reaction to divinyl ether and may happen with normal children, but illness increases the incidence.

Investigation of the seizure pattern by electroencephalogram has demonstrated that the convulsion is generalized and Jacksonian in nature. We were especially alarmed by one patient who showed clinical seizure manifestation for only 30 seconds but who continued to show seizure patterns by electroencephalogram for the next half hour (Fig. 27-5).

Shivering and muscle tremors. During recovery from anesthesia a variety of tremors may occur that may be mistaken for convulsions. As infants awaken after ether anesthesia, their arms and legs may shake with a jerky, clonic movement, but evidence of central disturbance is lacking. This appears to be either a form of shivering or the irregular return of muscle control.

Following thiopental, many patients show a generalized shaking tremor. This has been studied and found to have no central electroencephalographic manifestation.[62] Its increased incidence in cool operating rooms and its prompt response to warming give strong evidence that it is true thermal shivering. This shivering probably is seen more frequently after thiopental because of barbiturate depression of adrenal activity. Other than the fact that shivering increases oxygen demand, this tremor is harmless. A similar type of activity is seen during awakening from halothane.

Postoperative convulsions. Shivering and other tremors that occur during awakening are usually limited to the immediate postoperative period. Convulsions that occur several hours after operation are probably the result of hypoxia, brain damage, or water intoxication.[46] These complications have already been described.

Hyperthermia in anesthetized patients

Temperature elevation associated with anesthesia is far less common than the hypothermia noted in infants, but it carries much more danger.[63-65] There appear to be two varieties of situations in which hyperpyrexia occurs, although the entire picture still remains poorly defined. The first consists of patients who develop gradual temperature elevation, usually with demonstrable environmental or pathologic cause, while the second is an alarming reaction that has but recently been recognized, usually appears to be associated with succinylcholine and/or halothane and the appearance of sustained muscular spasm, and is followed by a high incidence of deaths.

The *gradual elevation of temperature* during operation is to be expected whenever heat production exceeds heat loss. Although this rarely occurs in infants, there is an increased incidence in young children who have high metabolic rate and easily develop febrile reactions to mild infections.

One should always look for intraoperative temperature changes; however, special precautions should be taken under the following conditions:

1. Recent history of fever, especially the recently controlled fever of peritonitis
2. Any underlying infection, especially of the genitourinary tract
3. Unexplained rectal temperature above 99° F. immediately before operation
4. Prolonged operations
5. Operations starting late in the day, after prolonged fluid restriction
6. Unfavorable environment: room temperature above 70° F. for children over 1 year old, poor air circulation, humidity over 50%
7. Blood transfusion

Under any of the preceding circumstances the patient's temperature must be monitored.

Temperature elevation usually occurs gradually at first but after reaching 101° or 102° F., the rate of increase often accelerates suddenly; thus it is of great importance to recognize the problem and correct it promptly. If not recognized until the temperature reaches 105° to 106° F., the situation is likely to be beyond control.

Therapy in hyperthermia follows logical steps and should be aimed at sev-

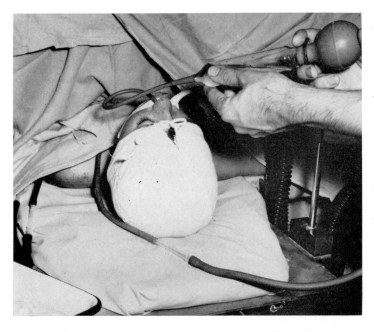

Fig. 27-6. Internal cooling by iced-saline gavage is much more effective than surface methods.

eral underlying factors including hypoxia, acidosis, CO_2 retention, and dehydration.

For temperature of 100° F.:
1. Cool and ventilate room.
2. Expose skin as possible, loosen drapes.
3. Hyperventilate.
4. Use semiclosed or nonrebreathing technique.
5. Check hydration of patient and administer fluids as needed.

If temperature exceeds 102° F.:
1. Follow preceding steps, plus.
2. Apply ice water to head, neck, all possible exposed areas, especially hands, feet, axillae, groins.
3. Use iced saline gastric lavage, (Fig. 27-6).
4. Give sodium bicarbonate (I.V., 4 mEq./kg.)

If temperature exceeds 104° F., add following steps:
1. Turn off strong lights.
2. Pour cold solutions into operative wounds, especially chest and abdomen, if open.
3. Inject chlorpromazine (I.V., 1.0 mg./kg.)
4. Give calcium gluconate, 100 mg./5 kg., to counteract possible potassium excess.
5. Use electrocardiographic monitor.
6. If patient shows any bodily activity, use relaxant to control it, and minimize oxygen demand.

In high temperature elevation, use *rapid internal cooling methods.* Do not rely on mattress, sponging, or other surface cooling devices. The anesthetic agent is probably of minor importance, Halothane favors vasodilatation and heat loss, but *nonrebreathing hyperventilation* with high oxygen supply is essential to accommodate increase of oxygen demand and high carbon dioxide production. *Treatment of rapidly developing acidosis is also essential.* When 103° F. is exceeded, convulsive activity may occur and will accelerate all unphysiologic mechanisms. This should immediately be controlled, preferably with *d*-tubocurarine.

Malignant hyperthermia. During the last 5 years at least 35[63,71] cases have been reported in which patients developed marked hyperthermia, with a strikingly similar combination of features, notably fever of 103° to 109° F., which appeared in previously afebrile patients but usually following administration of succinylcholine or halothane and the appearance of prolonged, severe generalized muscular spasm. Age does not seem an important factor, since many have been adults. Underlying infection has not been noted, but several patients did have neuromuscular disorders.[64,70] Some patients had the same response on more than one occasion; it has also occurred in siblings. It has been fatal in more than half of the cases[64-75] (Table 27-2).

In analyzing the nature of this response, several phases deserve consideration. There appears to be an underlying sensitivity that is touched off by succinylcholine or halothane and causes prolonged muscular spasm. This has not

Table 27-2. *Malignant hyperthermia—summary of cases*

Disease	Age	Sex	Operation	Agent	Spasm	Temperature	Remarks	Result*	Author
Hernia	47	M.	Herniorrhaphy	Succinylcholine, N₂O, halothane		108.5° F.		S	Saidman and Eger[64]
Hypertrophied adenoids Myotonia congenita	12	F.	Adenoidectomy	N₂O, halothane	3+	108° F.		D	Saidman and Eger[64]
Hypertrophied tonsils	5	M.	Tonsillectomy and adenoidectomy	Succinylcholine and methoxyflurane	4+	104.2° F.	Serum K, 19.0 mg.	D	Thut and Davenport[66]
Equinovarus	22	M.	Correction	Thiopental and halothane	4+	110° F.		D	Hogg[68]
Arthrogryposis	3	F.	Heel cord lengthening	Succinylcholine and halothane	4+	107.4° F.		D	Relton[69]
Strabismus (two operations)	5 mo.		Postponed	Succinylcholine and halothane	+	101.6° F.		S	
	5 mo.		Correction	Halothane, N₂O	+	106.7° F.		S	Relton[69]
Scoliosis	10	F.	Spine fusion	Thiopental, succinylcholine, methoxyflurane	+	108.5° F.		S	Relton[69]
Mesenteric adenitis	8	M.	Appendectomy	Succinylcholine and cyclopropane	0	107° F.		S	Cullen[71]
Carcinoma of uterus	32	F.	Hysterectomy	Succinylcholine and halothane	0	109.5° F.		D	Cullen[71]
Gallbladder disease	24	F.	Cholecystectomy	Succinylcholine and halothane	3+	108° F.	K 4.5	D	Davies[73]
Breast tumor	44	F.	Mastectomy	Thiopental, succinylcholine, halothane	3+	108° F.	K 7.8	D	Purkis et al.[74]
Scoliosis	12	F.	Spine fusion (postponed)	Succinylcholine, d-tubocurarine, N₂O	3+	37.8° C.		S	Relton et al.[75]

*S, survived; D, died.

been explained adequately, although patients with myotonia are known to show spasm after injection of succinylcholine.[72] It seems probable that the subsequent hyperpyrexia may be a reasonable result of the spasm, with the attendant increased O_2 demand, CO_2 production, and, most important, perhaps, rapid and excessive rise of serum potassium.

Dripps[76] noted that muscle contraction promotes rapid elevation of plasma potassium. When prolonged muscle spasm occurs in the hyperthermic syndrome, potassium rise should be expected. In one case reported the serum potassium was 19 mg.%.[66]

The role of catecholamines in heat regulation has recently been explored by Feldberg,[77] who finds that epinephrine and norepinephrine release acts to prevent shivering and favor temperature reduction, while 5-hydroxytryptamine has the reverse effect. A possible relationship of catechol response to hyperthermia may exist in the fact that while ether and cyclopropane cause catechol response and rarely evoke shivering, halothane and thiopental cause little or no catechol stimulation, and often these agents evoke strenuous shivering.

Fifteen cases of hyperthermia were described by Wilson and associates,[67] twelve of them having received a halogenated agent. These authors point to an enzyme failure as a possible cause, and they show that in dogs oxidative phosphorylation of 2-4 dinitrophenol will be blocked by halothane with fatal results.

Prophylaxis and therapy. Major points should be stressed in regard to handling the so-called malignant hyperthermia. They are as follows:

1. Persistent generalized myotonia occurring during anesthesia should stimulate alarm and action.
2. Steps should be taken to monitor temperature and provide for all therapeutic measures described in the previous section on hyperthermia, especially central cooling and hyperventilation.
3. In addition muscle spasm should be controlled if possible with *d*-tubocurarine, repeated doses of Demerol, or even spinal anesthesia.

Other phenomena may cause hyperpyrexia. Modell[78] reported 6 patients whose postoperative fever was proved to be due to pyrogens. We have had only one patient with severe hyperpyrexia in 100,000 anesthetics. This proved to be due to myoglobinemia. The 18-year-old patient's temperature climbed to 108° F. during arthrotomy of his right hip. With gastric lavage of ice and external cooling, his temperature was controlled, and after 2 days of semicoma he recovered completely.

GASTROINTESTINAL COMPLICATIONS

Gastrointestinal complications are limited chiefly to gastric distention, silent regurgitation, and vomiting.

Distention of the stomach

Distention of the stomach[79] may occur in any patient, but it is more likely to be found under particular circumstances. Obviously patients with preexisting intestinal obstruction, abdominal trauma, or head injury may be expected to have distention prior to operation.

In pediatric anesthesia irregular gasping respiration is the commonest cause of distention. An infant who cries and struggles during induction may gulp down so much air that the inflated stomach will actually interfere with respiration. In such instances a tube should be passed to deflate the stomach as soon as possible.

Marked distention may occur without apparent cause. In one child a tremendously dilated stomach was noticed by fluoroscopy during bronchography.

Inflation of the stomach is to be expected when there is deep total relaxation. This may occur with the use of curarizing agents but is almost certain to occur if ventilation of a moribund patient is attempted without endotracheal intubation. As previously suggested, it seems best to ventilate the moribund patient briefly by whatever method is available regardless of distention, but, after initial aeration, it is definitely preferable to intubate the patient.

Two iatrogenic complications may cause gastric distention: (1) the passage of an endotracheal tube into the esophagus and subsequent inflation of the stomach and (2) distention of the stomach by nasal oxygen.

Silent regurgitation

Children, like adults, may regurgitate gastric contents during anesthesia without any outward signs of vomiting or choking. Tracheal irritation due to acid stomach contents has been emphasized in the literature but has been less annoying than mechanical obstruction. Late effects of regurgitation have not been evident in our patients.

The use of an endotracheal tube will prevent aspiration of large quantities of fluid, but some gastric fluid may flow around the tube and into the trachea. This can be averted by use of a tightly fitting tube, a cuffed tube, or a pharyngeal pack, but in small children these precautions seem more dangerous than the complication itself.

Aspiration of regurgitated fluid can be recognized most easily by stethoscopic monitoring of respiration. Sounds of moisture in the airway will be sufficient indication for removal of the material by suction. During any operation the anesthetic mask should be removed at intervals to look for visible evidence of regurgitation.

Vomiting

Infants less than 6 months old rarely vomit during anesthesia or in the recovery period. As they grow older, however, children's reactions become similar to those of adults, and active vomiting may seriously upset induction or maintenance of anesthesia as well as the recovery period. If children are prepared adequately and their stomachs contain neither food nor intestinal contents, the consequence may not be severe. However, if the stomach contains large amounts of material, vomiting may lead to aspiration and fatal respiratory obstruction.

The well-prepared child. The management of problems associated with vomiting depends to some extent upon the time at which this complication occurs.

Induction. Sudden vomiting may occur early in induction under inhalation agents. If this happens, the mask must be removed, and time must be taken to clean up the patient and area for a fresh start. During suction of the mouth and pharynx of such a child, anesthetists often jab stiff catheters against the posterior pharynx with hard rapid strokes, much as a woodpecker attacks a tree, and with similar damaging results. The suction catheter must be used gently and with intelligence.

When a child's gag reflex is present, it is often better not to push the catheter beyond the base of his tongue. If his head is turned to one side, he will bring the material up into his mouth, and the anesthetist can remove this without jabbing at his pharyx or making him gag.

When ready for the second attempt to start induction, it is often better to change to cyclopropane for an easier and more rapid induction.

If, during induction, the well-prepared child merely begins to swallow and retch slightly, it is often better to watch him very carefully but to proceed with induction, trying to carry him through this period as quickly as possible.

Vomiting during anesthesia. To allow a patient to vomit during anesthesia is usually a serious and inexcusable mistake. There are a number of signs that should warn the anesthetist in ample time before vomiting actually takes place. These include irregular respiratory rhythm, active eye motion, and muscular movement, as well as moderate reduction in pulse rate. In addition, the anesthetist has specific evidence of the impending complication if he rests one finger over the child's larynx. Before vomiting, patients almost always make a series of swallowing motions that are easily felt as the larynx moves up and down. Should vomiting appear imminent, pressure on the cricoid ring (Sellick's maneuver)[80] may be used to compress the esophagus and block passage of gastric contents into the pharynx.

If vomiting occurs, steps must be taken at once to clear the pharynx and trachea in order to prevent aspiration and asphyxia.[81] It may be extremely inconvenient for the surgeon to have the patient cough and retch at this time, but he should be notified of the accident and should allow the anesthetist to rectify it as soon as possible. Exposure of the glottis with a laryngoscope and initial clearing of the airway should be followed by intubation. The patient can be controlled quickly with addition of cyclopropane, following which further steps may be taken to complete the cleansing of the respiratory tree.

When the child has vomited and starts to waken during anesthesia, one might think of using a relaxant to control the situation, but this would relax the cardiac sphincter of the stomach and cause immediate regurgitation of all the remaining stomach contents.

If an appreciable amount of material has been aspirated, the usual soft rubber catheter may be less effective than a stiff plastic tube or metal suction tube. A metal mouth gag may be valuable in keeping the jaws open during such treatment. Bronchoscopy should be considered if other methods are not successful.[82]

If there are signs of retained material or inadequate ventilation following anesthesia, repeated tracheal aspiration, bronchoscopy, roentgen-ray, examination, and steroids may be indicated. Dexamethasone (Decadron) is probably the steroid of choice, administered intravenously, 3 mg. for infants under 1 year of age and 8 mg. for older children, to be repeated in 6 and 12 hours.

Postoperative vomiting. Some vomiting during recovery from anesthesia is to be expected. Following nitrous oxide–oxygen anesthesia, a child usually retches and vomits a small amount of fluid secretions immediately after the operation but subsequently is bothered no more. Following other anesthetic agents the incidence of vomiting appears to be greatest with ether and methoxyflurane, whereas that following nitrous oxide, thiopental, and relaxants is only slightly less. The incidence of nausea and vomiting following cyclopropane and halothane has been significantly less than that with the other agents mentioned.

In general, children do not appear to be greatly troubled by the act of vomiting, and they recover quickly. Prolonged nausea occasionally occurs, however, and should be given attention. Usually it is wise to stop the use of morphine, temporarily avoid oral feeding, and try the use of chlorpromazine (Thorazine), using 0.3 mg. per pound of body weight by intramuscular injection three times a day.

Several other agents, such as perphenazine (Trilafon), have been suggested as being superior as antiemetics. Since all carry some side effects, as yet not established, there is some advantage in using chlorpromazine, which is reasonably predictable.

Vomiting in the presence of full stomach. When a child is not prepared for operation but is given anesthetics with undigested food in his stomach, the possibility of vomiting becomes a major problem. This is discussed in Chapter 24.

HEPATORENAL COMPLICATIONS

Postoperative disturbances of the liver and kidneys are rare in pediatric anesthesia. Several years ago, however, one child with hepatitis was inadvisedly given ether anesthesia for performance of a liver biopsy. Her postoperative course consisted of a rapid temperature elevation and death, presumably due to liver failure. It is to be noted, however, that many infants with biliary atresia (an obstructive lesion) have received ether without any adverse effect.

Although hepatotoxicity following halogenated anesthetics had not been known to occur in children, two very severe reactions occurred in our hospital during 1967. In the first, a healthy 11-year-old girl had three orthopedic operations at 2-week intervals, receiving halothane each time. The procedures were long, but entirely uneventful, except that after the first operation the child had a temperature elevation to 103° F. without obvious cause (Fig. 27-7). After the third procedure classic signs of acute liver necrosis progressed until death. No cause other than halothane could be suspected under the circumstances.

The second child was a 5-year-old girl who had two 5-hour orthopedic procedures, the first under halothane, the second under methoxyflurane. Here also there was a temperature elevation after the first procedure. Several days after the second operation the patient was listless and had a tender, enlarged liver, but

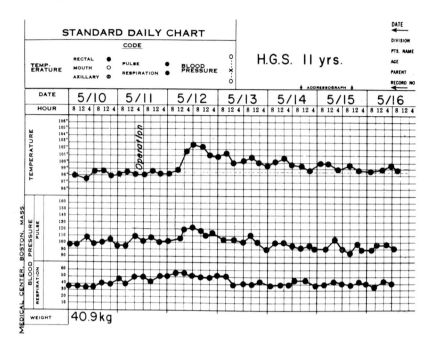

Fig. 27-7. This postoperative temperature elevation was the single warning sign of developing halothane sensitivity. Subsequent exposure was followed by acute liver necrosis and death.

gradually recovered. She had not received blood, and the anesthetic agents appeared to be the most reasonable cause of the complication. This experience leads us to believe that although halogenated agents cannot be shown to have direct toxic effect on the liver,[83-85] a sensitivity phenomenon can occur that may have fatal results. As noted by Popper,[86,87] the best warning that such a response has occurred is an unexplained temperature elevation following anesthesia, with or without jaundice. Such a complication should be taken as an absolute contraindication for subsequent halogenated anesthesia of any kind for at least 3 months.

Urinary retention is an extremely rare complication, but catheterization may be indicated on occasion. Inlying urethral catheters are used routinely following intracardiac operations in order to estimate the efficiency of kidney function.

REFERENCES

1. Smith, R. M.: Complications of anesthesia in pediatrics, Anesth. Analg. 27:227-231, 1948.
2. Fink, B. R.: The etiology and treatment of laryngeal spasm, Anesthesiology 17:569-577, 1956.
3. Foldes, F. F., editor: Muscle relaxants, Philadelphia, 1966, F. A. Davis Co.; chap. 1, The choice and mode of administration of relaxants.
4. Bougas, T. P., and Smith, R. M.: Pathologic airway obstruction in children, Anesth. Analg. 37:137-146, 1958.
5. Robinson, C. L., and Mushin, W. W.: Inhaled foreign bodies, Brit. Med. J. 2:324-328, 1956.
6. Jacoby, J. J., Reed, J. P., Hamelberg, W., Gillespie, B., and Hitchcock, F. A.: Simple method of artificial respiration, Amer. J. Physiol. 167:798-799, 1951.

7. Harris, T. A. B.: The mode of action of anaesthetics, Edinburg, 1951, E. & S. Livingstone, Ltd. (Printed in the United States by The Williams & Wilkins Co.)
8. Steinhaus, J.: Unpublished findings.
9. Salem, M. R.: An effective method for the treatment of hiccups during anesthesia, Anesthesiology **28**:463-464, 1967.
10. Bachman, L.: Personal communication.
11. Deming, M. V., and Oech, S. R.: Steroid and antihistaminic therapy for post intubation subglottic edema in infants and children, Anesthesiology **22**:933-936, 1961.
12. Leigh, M. D., McCoy, D. D., Belton, K. M., and Lewis, G. B.: Bradycardia following intravenous administration of succinylcholine to infants and children, Anesthesiology **18**:698-702, 1957.
13. Williams, C. H., Deutsch, S., Linde, H. W., Bullough, J. W., and Dripps, R. D.: Effects of intravenously administered succinyldicholine on cardiac rate, rhythm, and arterial blood pressure in anesthetized man, Anesthesiology **22**:947-954, 1961.
14. Jones, R. E., Turndorf, H., and Deutsch, S.: Effects of atropine in cardiac rhythm in conscious and anesthetized man, Anesthesiology **22**:67-73, 1961.
15. Gaviotaki, A., and Smith, R. M.: Use of atropine in pediatric anesthesia, Internat. Anesth. Clin. **1**:97-113, 1962.
16. Smith, R. M., and Wiley, H. P.: Evaluation of electrocardiography during congenital heart surgery, Anesthesiology **18**:398-412, 1957.
17. Craythorne, N. W. B., and Huffington, P. E.: Effects of propranolol on the cardiovascular response to cyclopropane and halothane, Anesthesiology **27**:580-583, 1966.
18. Norris, W., and Stuart, P.: Cardia arrest during trichloroethylene anaesthesia, Brit. Med. J. **1**:860-863, 1957.
19. Gold, S. M., and Smith, R. M.: Repeated cardiac arrhythmia during ether anesthesia, Amer. Heart J. **54**:448-451, 1957.
20. Turk, L. N., and Glenn, W. W. L.: Cardiac arrest. Results of attempted cardiac resuscitation in 42 cases, New Eng. J. Med. **251**:796-803, 1954.
21. Lam, P. T. C., Wrzesinski, J. T., and Walske, B. R.: Cardiac arrest, Amer. J. Surg. **89**:593-599, 1955.
22. McQuiston, W. O.: Editorial, Survey Anesth. **1**:510, 1957.
23. Kouwenhoven, W. B., Jude, J. R., and Knickerbocker, G. G.: Closed-chest cardiac massage, J.A.M.A. **173**:1064-1067, 1960.
24. Safar, P.: Closed chest cardiac massage, Anesth. Analg. **40**:609-613, 1961.
25. Darby, T. D., Aldinger, E. E., Gadsden, R. H., and Thrower, W. B.: Effects of metabolic acidosis on ventricular isometric systolic tension and the response to epinephrine and levarterenol, Circ. Res. **8**:1242-1253, 1960.
26. Jones, R. S.: The acid base changes due to cardiac bypass. In Evans, F. T., and Gray, T. C., editors: Modern trends in anaesthesia, vol. 2, London, 1962, Butterworth & Co.
27. Feldman, S. A.: Effect of changes in electrolytes, hydration, and pH upon the reactions to muscle relaxants, Brit. J. Anaesth. **135**:546-550, 1963.
28. Moore, A. A. D., and Bernhard, W. F.: The efficacy of 2-amino-2 hydroxy methyl-l, 3-propanediol in the management of metabolic lactacidosis, Surgery **52**:905-912, 1962.
29. Martin, S. J.: Management of sudden cardiac collapse, Anesthesiology **27**:738-750, 1961.
30. Benson, D. W., Williams, G. R., Spencer, F. C., and Yates, A. J.: The use of hypothermia after cardiac arrest, Anesth. Analg. **38**:423-428, 1959.
31. Nadas, A. S.: Pediatric cardiology, ed. 2, Philadelphia, 1963, W. B. Saunders Co.
32. Robertazzi, R. W., Riskin, A. M., and Semeraro, D.: The control and management of hypertensive crises developing during surgical procedures, Anesthesiology **15**:262-271, 1954.
33. Ciliberti, B. J., Goldfein, J., and Rovenstine, E. A.: Hypertension during anesthesia in patients with spinal cord injuries, Anesthesiology **15**:273-279, 1954.
34. Dripps, R. D.: The immediate decrease in blood pressure seen at the conclusion of cyclopropane anesthesia: "cyclopropane shock," Anesthesiology **8**:15-35, 1947.
35. Young, W. G., Jr., Sealy, W. C., and Harris, J. S.: The role of intracellular and extracellular electrolytes in the cardiac arrhythmias produced by prolonged hypercapnia, Surgery **36**:636-649, 1954.

36. Brannon, E. S., Stead, E. A., Warren, J. W., and Merrill, A. J.: Hemodynamics of acute hemorrhage in man, Amer. Heart J. 31:407-412, 1946.

37. Phemister, D. B.: Mechanism and management of surgical shock, J.A.M.A. 127:1109-1112, 1945.

38. Wiggers, C. J.: Physiology of shock, New York, 1950, The Commonwealth Fund.

39. Huckabee, W. E.: Relationships of pyruvate and lactate during anerobic metabolism. I. Effects of infusion of pyruvate or glucose and hyperventilation; II. Exercise and formation of O_2 debt; III. Effect of breathing low-oxygen gases, J. Clin. Invest. 37:244-248, 1958.

40. Greene, N. M.: Lactate, pyruvate and excess lactate production in anesthetized man, Anesthesiology 22:404-412, 1961.

41. Boba, A., and Converse, G. C.: Ganglionic blockade and its protective action in hemorrhage: a review, Anesthesiology 18:559-572, 1957.

42. Slocum, H. C., O'Neal, K. C., and Allen, C. R.: Neurovascular complications from malposition on operating table, Surg. Gynec. Obstet. 86:729-734, 1948.

43. Nicholson, M. J., and Eversole, U. H.: Nerve injuries incident to anesthesia and operation, Anesth. Analg. 36:19-33, 1957.

44. Gebauer, P. W., and Coleman, F. P.: Postanesthetic encephalopathy following cyclopropane, Ann. Surg. 107:481-485, 1938.

45. Courville, C. B.: Ether anesthesia and cerebral anoxia, Anesthesiology 2:44-58, 1941.

46. Harned, H. S., Jr., and Cooke, R. E.: Symptomatic hyponatremia in infants and children undergoing surgery, Surg. Gynec. Obstet. 104:543-550, 1957.

47. Bergner, R. P.: Convulsions during anesthesia, J. Kentucky Med. Ass. 55:519-521, 1957.

48. Cassels, W. H., Becker, T. J., and Seevers, M. H.: Convulsions during anesthesia, Anesthesiology 1:56-68, 1940.

49. Ray, B. S., and Marshall, V. F.: Convulsions during general anesthesia, Ann. Surg. 118:130-148, 1943.

50. Belinkoff, S.: Convulsions under anesthesia in children, Anesth. Analg. 28:40-48, 1949.

51. Seevers, M. H., Cassels, W. H., and Becker, T. J.: Role of hypercapnia and pyrexia in production of "ether convulsions," J. Pharmacol. Exp. Ther. 63:33-34, 1938.

52. Williams, D., and Sweet, W. H.: The constitutional factor in anesthetic convulsions, Lancet 2:430, 1944.

53. Lundy, J. S.: Convulsions associated with general anesthesia, Surgery 1:666-687, 1937.

54. Raab, A.: Hyperventilation and alkalosis, Anesth. Analg. 15:295-297, 1936.

55. Hauser, H. M.: Convulsive disorders in medical disease, Dis. Nerv. Syst. 17:5-16, 1956.

56. Owens, G., Dawson, R. E., and Scott, H. W.: Experimental production of "ether convulsions," Anesthesiology 18:583-593, 1957.

57. Pittinger, C., Mitchell, C., Aleu, F., and Page, W.: Convulsive phenomena in hypothermic dogs during anesthesia, Anesthesiology 22:893-896, 1961.

58. Moore, D. C., and Tolan, J. F.: Anesthesia for surgery of the nose, pharynx, larynx, and trachea, Arch. Otolaryng. 63:275-288, 1956.

59. Best, C. H., and Taylor, N. B.: The physiological basis of medical practice, ed. 5, Baltimore, 1950, The Williams & Wilkins Co.

60. Dawkins, C. M. J.: Convulsions occurring under vinesthene anaesthesia, Brit. Med. J. 1:163-164, 1940.

61. Di Giovanni, A. J., and Dripps, R. D.: Abnormal motor movements during divinyl anesthesia, Anesthesiology 17:353-357, 1956.

62. Smith, R. M., Bougas, T. P., and Bachman, L.: Shivering following thiopental sodium and other anesthetic agents, Anesthesiology 16:655-664, 1955.

63. Stephen, C. R., Dent, S. J., Hall, K. D., Knox, P. R., and North, W. C.: Body temperature regulation during anesthesia in infants and children, J.A.M.A. 174:1579-1585, 1960.

64. Saidman, L. J., Harvard, E. S., and Eger, E. I., II: Hyperthermia during anesthesia, J.A.M.A. 190:1029-1032, 1964.

65. Denborough, M. A., Forster, J. E., Lovell, R. R. H., Mapleston, P. A., and Villiers, J. D.: Anaesthetic deaths in a family, Brit. J. Anaesth. 34:395-399, 1962.

66. Thut, W., and Davenport, H. T.: Hyperpyrexia associated with succinylcholine-induced muscle rigidity: a case report, Canad. Anaesth. Soc. J. 13:425-429, 1966.

67. Wilson, R. D., Nichols, R. J., Dent, T. E., and Allen, C. R.: Disturbances of oxidative phosphorylation mechanism as a possible etiological factor in sudden unexplained hyperthermia occurring during anesthesia, Anesthesiology 27:231-233, 1966.

68. Hogg, S., and Renwick, W.: Hyperpyrexia during anesthesia, Canad. Anaesth. Soc. J. 13:429-437, 1966.

69. Relton, J. E. S., Creighton, R. E., Johnston, A. E., Pelton, D. A., and Conn, A. W.: Hyperpyrexia in association with general anaesthesia in children, Canad. Anaesth. Soc. J. 13:419-425, 1966.

70. Editorial, Canad. Anaesth. Soc. J. 13:415-416, 1966.

71. Cullen, W. G.: Malignant hyperpyrexia during general anaesthesia: a report of two cases, Canad. Anaesth. Soc. J. 13:437-444, 1966.

72. Patterson, I. S.: Generalized myotonia following suxamethonium: a case report, Brit. J. Anaesth. 34:340, 1962.

73. Davies, L. E., and Graves, H. B.: Hyperpyrexia and death associated with general anesthesia, Canad. Anaesth, Soc. J. 13:447-448, 1966.

74. Purkis. I. E., Horrelt, O., de Young, C. G., Fleming, R. A. P., and Langley, G. R.: Hyperpyrexia during anesthesia in a second member of a family, with associated coagulation defect due to increased intravascular coagulation, Canad. Anaesth. Soc. J. 14:183-192, 1967.

75. Relton, J. E. S., Creighton, R. E., Conn, A. W., and Nabeta, S.: Generalized musclar hypertonicity associated with general anesthesia: a suggested anaesthetic management, Canad. Anaesth. Soc. J. 14:22-25, 1967.

76. Williams, C. H., Deutsch, S., Linde, H. W., Bullough, J. W., and Dripps, R. D.: Effects of intravenously administered succinylcholine on cardiac rate, rhythm and arterial blood pressure in anesthetized man, Anesthesiology 22:947-954, 1961.

77. Feldberg, W., and Myers, R. D.: Effect on temperature of amines injected into the cerebral ventricles. A new concept of temperature regulation, J. Physiol. 173:226-237, 1964.

78. Modell, J. H.: Septicemia as a cause of postoperative hyperthermia, Anesthesiology 27:329-330, 1966.

79. Leigh, M. D., and Belton, M. K.: Pediatric anesthesia, ed. 2, New York, 1959, The Macmillian Co.

80. Sellick, B. A.: Cricoid pressure, Lancet 2:404, 1961.

81. Onchi, Y., and Fujita, M.: Pediatric anesthesia, Tokyo, 1958, Nankodo & Co., Ltd.

82. Marshall, B. M., and Gordon, R. A.: Vomiting, regurgitation, and aspiration in anaesthesia, Canad. Anaesth. Soc. J. 5:274-282, 1958.

83. Bunker, J. P., and Blumenfeld, C. M.: Liver necrosis after halothane anesthesia: cause or coincidence? New Eng. J. Med. 268:531-534, 1963.

84. Subcommittee on the National Halothane Study. Possible relation between halothane anesthesia and post-operative hepatic necrosis, J.A.M.A. 197:121-136, 1966.

85. DeBacker, L. J., and Longnecker, D. S.: Prospective and retrospective searches for liver necrosis following halothane anesthesia, J.A.M.A. 195:157-160, 1966.

86. Collins, W. L., and Fabian, L. W.: Transaminase studies following anesthesia, Southern Med. J. 57:555-559, 1964.

87. Popper, H., Rubin, E., Gardiol, D., Schaffner, F., and Paronetto, F.: Drug-induced liver disease, Arch. Intern. Med. 115:128-133, 1965.

88. Davidson, C. S., Babior, B., and Popper, H.: Concerning hepatotoxicity of halothane, New Eng. J. Med. 275:1497, 1966.

89. Babior, B. M., and Davidson, C. S.: Post-operative massive liver necrosis, New Eng. J. Med. 276:645-653, 1967.

90. Lindenbaum, J. and Leifer, E.: Hepatic necrosis associated with halothane anesthesia, New Eng. J. Med. 268:525-530, 1963.

91. Editorial. Hepatitis: drug or viral? Amer. J. Med. 41:491-496, 1966.

92. Dykes, M. H. M., Walzer, S. G., Slater, E. M., Gibson, J. M., and Ellis, D. S.: Acute parenchymatous hepatic disease following general anesthesia, J.A.M.A. 193:339-344, 1965.

Chapter 28

Diagnosis and treatment in respiratory emergencies

Respiratory resuscitation has been taught as a first aid procedure, and learned by thousands of lay and professional people as a *routine* to be applied to anyone who has stopped breathing. Anesthetists often take this mechanical approach. Treatment, no matter how simple, should be governed by intelligent on-the-spot thinking. *Diagnosis and treatment* are both essential in the management of respiratory emergencies.

466

Deaths due to respiratory depression or airway obstruction occur in the home, on the street, and on the medical wards, as well as in the delivery and operating rooms. A great many of them could be prevented by prompt application of a few simple mechanical procedures. These procedures may be modified in many details, but even under the most elaborate conditions they include only three basic steps:

1. Clearing the airway (aspirate!)
2. Establishing ventilation (ventilate!)
3. The addition of oxygen (oxygenate!)

Although reference has already been made to several types of respiratory complication and treatment has been discussed, it seems important to present a concise approach that can be of immediate practical use.

CLEARING THE AIRWAY

The last act of an expiring infant often consists of the regurgitation of all its stomach contents into the mouth and hypopharynx. If a hasty attempt is made to ventilate this moribund child, the regurgitated material may be blown into his lungs, thereby ending his life.

Upon finding an infant in cardiorespiratory collapse, probably the best thing to do is perform external cardiac massage actively, about 15 times in approximately 5 seconds. This will stimulate the heart, circulate blood, and by this forced expiration, push any regurgitated material out of the trachea and phar-

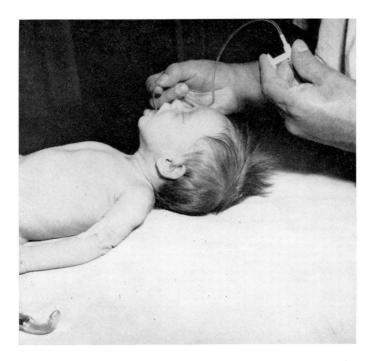

Fig. 28-1. Suction: mouth and airway must be cleared before air is blown into the lung.

ynx, allowing air to enter the lungs each time the chest expands. Time can then be taken to remove the obstructing material. This is performed most effectively by use of a laryngoscope and suction apparatus or by an aspirating bulb, which should be at hand in operating or delivery rooms (Fig. 28-1). Under other circumstances airway clearance should be attempted by holding the child's head downward to allow secretions to drain from the trachea and pharynx and then by sweeping other material from the mouth with the finger.

If the airway is obstructed by thick or solid material, bronchoscopy may be required.[1] Removal of foreign bodies is discussed on p. 369. If the passage of air is such that the patient is rapidly becoming asphyxiated, and if intubation is not possible, an emergency tracheostomy may be necessary. In such cases it is performed by making an incision at the interspace between thyroid and cricoid cartilages. When this situation arises outside a hospital, two widely available objects that may then be used as tracheostomy tubes are the emptied barrel of a ball-point pen and the central shaft of a coffee percolator. Tracheostomy and nasotracheal intubation for less acute situations are discussed on p. 476.

VENTILATION

Mouth-to-mouth technique. Establishment of a free airway may enable the patient to breathe for himself; otherwise one must immediately provide exchange for him. Although many mechanical devices may be used, none is essential since mouth-to-mouth resuscitation remains one of the most effective techniques.[2] Unless other apparatus is within reach, this method should be applied at once.

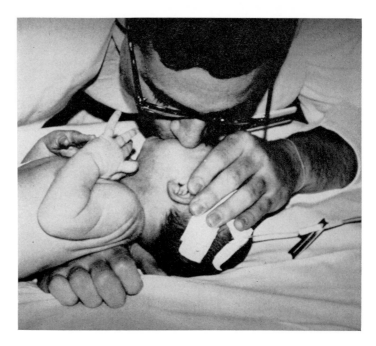

Fig. 28-2. Mouth-to-mouth resuscitation. Chest is elevated, head extended.

When performing mouth-to-mouth resuscitation upon an infant, the thorax should be elevated to promote exchange; the head should be extended and the chin supported firmly, so that the tongue will be held forward (Fig. 28-2). Because of the small size of the baby's face, it is usually necessary for the anesthetist to place his mouth over both nose and mouth of the infant. One hand is placed on the child's stomach to prevent it from becoming distended. Then the anesthetist blows into the patient's airway. He should be able to see the chest rise with each inflation. When resuscitating neonates, one must avoid using excessive volume or pressure. This can be accomplished by blowing mouthfuls of air into the child, rather than by using one's rib cage for the driving force. The rate of induced respiration should vary from about 40 per minute in an infant to about 16 per minute in an adult.

To facilitate mouth-to-mouth resuscitation one may insert an oral airway to support the infant's tongue. Another modification of the mouth-to-mouth method consists of holding an anesthesia mask against the patient's face and blowing against the hole in the back of the mask.

Bag-and-mask method. For emergency use the self-inflating (Ambu type) bag (Fig. 28-3) is valuable and may be placed at critical areas throughout the hospital together with additional resuscitation apparatus (Figs. 28-4 and 28-5). The mask must be applied snugly and the bag compressed briskly in order to have an air-tight fit and activate the valve (Fig. 28-6). The chest should rise with inflation.

When the bag-and-mask technique is used on completely relaxed patients, the stomach may become distended as it does during application of the mouth-to-mouth approach. In such cases the stomach should be compressed and aspirated and endotracheal intubation employed as soon as possible.

Endotracheal intubation. For infants and children who are apneic or severely depressed, endotracheal intubation and subsequent passive ventilation offer the

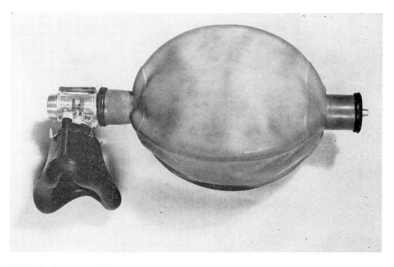

Fig. 28-3. Self-inflating bag with mask.

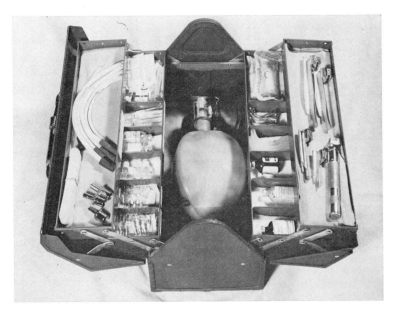

Fig. 28-4. Resuscitation kit with bag and mask, endotracheal apparatus, airways, and medications.

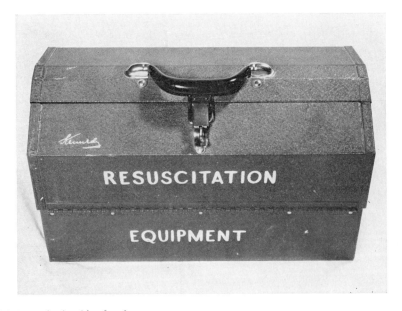

Fig. 28-5. Resuscitation kit, closed.

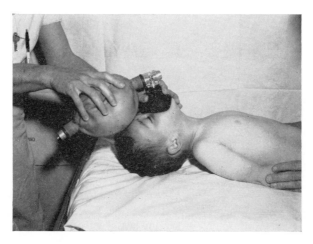

Fig. 28-6. Ventilatory resuscitation with bag and mask.

surest method of obtaining effective ventilatory exchange and airway control. Although there has been great hesitancy in the intubation of newborn infants, such a conservative attitude does not seem justified. Intubation is easily performed on relaxed, anoxic patients, and the hazard of trauma is far less than that of prolonged anoxia. Instruments and techniques for intubation are described in previous chapters.

When the endotracheal tube has been inserted, the anesthetist can ventilate the child by attaching the Ambu bag to the endotracheal tube (Fig. 28-7) or by blowing gently into the tube until the patient's chest begins to rise. At this time a stethoscope should be applied to the patient's chest to test the adequacy of exchange and to confirm the correct position of the endotracheal tube. If wet or absent breath sounds are noted, a fine plastic catheter should be used for suction of the trachea prior to further ventilation. Once a clear exchange has been established, the patient's lungs are inflated rapidly but gently, with continued stethoscopic auscultation.

OXYGENATION

As soon as initial ventilatory exchange has been accomplished, greater oxygen concentration than that in expired or room air should be provided. If special equipment is not at hand, the anesthetist can improvise by allowing oxygen to run into his mouth as he blows on the endotracheal tube, or oxygen tubing may be connected to the tail of the self-inflating bag.

Best results will be obtained if 100% oxygen is used in resuscitation; consequently an endotracheal tube and an undiluted supply of oxygen are necessary. Self-inflating bags, even with supplemental oxygen, are not adequate for prolonged use here, since oxygen is always diluted with room air and rarely exceeds 40%.

Throughout the process of resuscitation the rate and quality of the heartbeat should be observed. This is accomplished easily by means of the stethoscope,

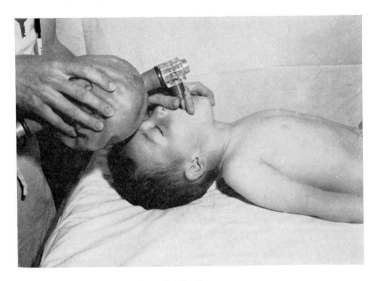

Fig. 28-7. Ventilation with bag and endotracheal tube.

which is being used to monitor respiratory exchange. In apneic patients of any age a slowing heart rate is a definite indication for immediate endotracheal intubation and direct oxygenation if this has not already been accomplished.

DIAGNOSTIC AND THERAPEUTIC CONSIDERATIONS

During all phases of resuscitation one must continually evaluate and re-evaluate the situation. At the beginning, as the first simple steps are being applied, one summons any available help and information in order to clarify the cause of the incident. If resuscitation is not immediately effective, one should look for an explanation and shape subsequent efforts as indicated by the situation.

The principal underlying causes of respiratory arrest may differ significantly. It is of utmost importance to determine at once whether the child was in terminal state of incurable disease, had a known lesion of the central nervous system, a metabolic disorder, or some cardiovascular or pulmonary pathology.

One's attention usually is fixed upon cardiorespiratory problems as the most probable cause. Here one must bear in mind that excessive ventilatory pressure can be dangerous if the patient has diaphragmatic hernia, pneumothorax, or cystic lung (Fig. 28-8). Absent breath sounds should suggest immediate roentgen-ray examination to confirm such a diagnosis.

Cardiac failure and respiratory failure may occur simultaneously, and prompt cardiac resuscitation will be essential for recovery. Methods of cardiac resuscitation have been described in the previous chapter.

The spot diagnosis of underlying cardiac lesions is often difficult during cardiorespiratory emergencies, but an electrocardiograph should be one of the first tools to be used in such situations for aid in recognizing changing cardiac responses as well as organic lesions.

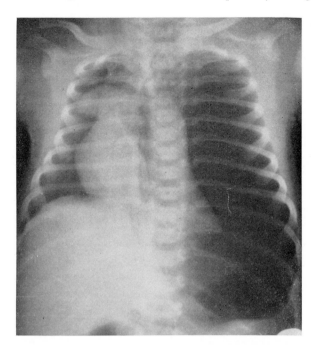

Fig. 28-8. Pneumothorax is always a potential complication of ventilatory assistance.

In addition to determining and treating the principal underlying cause, one must consider other contributing factors, many of which may actually be aggravated during resuscitation. Chief among these are acidosis, loss of body heat, hypovolemia, and hypoglycemia.

Acidosis. If hypoxia preceded the respiratory emergency, or if respiration fails to return from any cause within 5 minutes, heparinized arterial blood should be analyzed for pH, pO_2, and pCO_2. Respiratory acidosis may be treated most promptly by use of sodium bicarbonate (4 mEq./kg. should raise pH by 0.1). Tris (hydroxymethyl) aminomethane (150 mg./kg.) may be used, but it carries the danger of causing respiratory depression and hypoglycemia.

Loss of body heat. One of the most frequent secondary factors complicating resuscitation is loss of body heat. Excessive exposure of the patient during resuscitative efforts is commonplace, and body temperature often drops to 90° to 92° F., thereby greatly reducing the chances of recovery. Should such a fall in temperature occur, warming must be accomplished quickly but safely. Tissue that is poorly circulated burns more easily than normal tissue, and the temperature of warming materials should not be higher than 100° F.

Hypovolemia. Hypovolemia often goes unnoticed in weak infants who have obvious respiratory distress. Since this is easily corrected, its early recognition is most valuable.

Hypoglycemia. Hypoglycemia often is present at birth in premature infants, and it complicates many pathologic states such as diabetes and erythroblastosis.[3] In all age groups it develops rapidly in the presence of hypoxia, acidosis, and hypothermia. Here, again, treatment is simple and may be of critical importance. Intravenous administration of 50% glucose should be effective rapidly and may be supplemented by an infusion as indicated. Reasonable dosage varies between 3 ml. for a neonate and 50 ml. for an adult.

ADDITIONAL MEASURES IN RESPIRATORY RESUSCITATION

The causes, prevention, and treatment of respiratory distress in patients of all ages, especially that of asphyxia neonatorum, have been profusely reported, and articles by Apgar and associates,[4,5] Cook and associates,[6] Flagg,[7] and Little and associates,[8,9] should be consulted for details and further references. In these studies numerous additional methods of resuscitation are recommended or evaluated, but few add significantly to the simple emergency measures outlined previously.

Ventilating devices. One-phase positive pressure ventilators such as the Kreiselman, Emerson, and Bennett machines are endorsed as reliable when used with maximum pressures not exceeding 22 to 25 cm. H_2O and when cycling at normal respiratory rates. For treatment of mild hypoventilation such devices are preferable to manual artificial resuscitation and emergency mouth-to-mouth techniques; consequently, either a mechanical resuscitator or appropriate anesthetic apparatus should be maintained in all delivery and operating rooms.

Although there has been general acceptance of 25 cm. H_2O as the safe limit of positive pressure, Day and associates[10] recommended short bursts (0.1 second) of considerably higher pressure (40 cm. H_2O). The merits of this system have not been proved. Two-phase negative-and-positive pressure ventilators have not been found to be of added value.

Tank respirators. The Drinker tank respirator is effective for adults and small children but is unsatisfactory for newborn infants. The Bloxsom air lock has been found relatively ineffective.[11]

Electrophrenic respiration. Technical difficulty and unconvincing results have led to general abandonment of phrenic nerve stimulation in respiratory depression.

Artificial resuscitation. Body bending and other maneuvers have been condemned in infant resuscitation, but various techniques may be helpful in children and adults. During the past 15 years preference passed from the Schafer prone pressure technique to the Holger-Nielsen arm-lift method, and more recently evidence has shown that the mouth-to-mouth technique may be most effective when properly performed.[12,13]

Respiratory stimulants. The use of carbon dioxide and such analeptic drugs as nikethamide (Coramine), alpha lobeline, and pictrotoxin has long been considered obsolete and unphysiologic by most anesthesiologists. During prolonged ventilation with oxygen, however, it is possible that the addition of carbon dioxide might have a beneficial effect upon cerebral circulation. Furthermore, those persistent individuals who have continued to use nikethamide now are encouraged by the report of Dulfano and Segal,[14] who found this drug truly effective.

Recently doxapram hydrochloride has been reported to increase ventilation in the depressed postoperative state.[15,16] Its value in resuscitative procedures is questionable.

Narcotic antagonist. When narcotics contribute to respiratory depression, antagonists such as nalorphine or levallorphan should be employed (p. 437).

The Eve method. Although rocking or tilting of adult patients supplies sufficient exchange to be used for effective treatment of intercostal paralysis, infants are not benefited significantly, and reliance cannot be placed upon infant bassinets fitted with rocking mechanisms.

Gastric suction following cesarean section. Critical analysis of the value of gastric suction for infants delivered by cesarean section has failed to confirm the importance of this procedure.[4]

PROBLEMS OF PROLONGED RESPIRATORY FAILURE

If spontaneous respiration does not return, it is natural to consider going on to the use of a mechanical ventilating device. Before taking this step, three major problems arise; these are diagnostic, ethical, and practical. Diagnosis may be evident from the onset of the situation. If not, it is certainly advisable to call in all available help before embarking upon a long-term course that may prove hopeless. The diagnosis of death itself is difficult when heart and respiration are being assisted.

This brings up the ethical problem: Is an attempt to prolong this life justified? In the presence of irreparable brain damage through trauma, hypoxia, fever, or pressure, one certainly is not justified in the indefinite support of life by use of artificial ventilating devices.

If one believes that ventilatory assistance *is* indicated, one then faces the practical problems of the choice of ventilator and the decision between use of endotracheal tube or tracheostomy. These are discussed in Chapter 29.

Hypothermia. The concept that cooling would decrease oxygen demand and thereby be of value in resuscitation has long been an inviting one. It has been shown, however, that even in the neonate, the unanesthetized human responds to cooling by increased oxygen utilization, whether by muscular activity[17] or catechol release.[18] Miller and Miller[19] have clung to the idea that deeply hypoxic infants (white asphyxia) who cannot produce the normal response to cold might profit by hypothermic therapy. Although there are few adherent to their theory, they report very interesting results in survival studies of asphyxiated puppies. These follow in summary:

Subjects *Asphyxiated, warm puppies*	Percent increase in survival *Control*
1. Treated with THAM	117.1%
2. Treated with THAM and glucose	168.4%
3. Treated with cooling to 15%	654.5%
4. Treated with THAM, glucose, and cooling	1,104.2%

Hyperbaric oxygenation. Along similar lines, there is theoretic support for the use of hyperbaric oxygen therapy in resuscitation.[20] Here, again, clinical trials have proved disappointing. The hypoxic patient whose tissue oxygen is considerably below 50 mm. Hg will profit as much by exposure to 600 mm. Hg

(100% oxygen at normal pressure) as at 2,000 mm. Hg (100% oxygen at 3 atmospheres). (See next chapter.)

USE OF TRACHEOSTOMY OR PROLONGED ENDOTRACHEAL INTUBATION

In severe upper airway obstruction, tracheostomy formerly was the procedure employed when all others failed. At present one has the choice of using tracheostomy or endotracheal intubation for many of these problems. As yet, true evaluation of relative merits cannot be made. For this moment, the problem to be discussed is not which method to use but when, in the course of increasing airway difficulties, it becomes necessary to perform either maneuver.

Indications for tracheostomy or intubation. In many discussions of the indications for tracheostomy, the underlying diseases and pathologic conditions have been listed,[21,22] e.g., neuromuscular disorders, airway obstruction, excessive secretions, etc. True indications consist of the signs that determine when one should take the definite step of establishing an improved airway. Increasing stridor, retraction, hoarseness, and labored respiration are suggestive but not definitive. More definite signs are those that show failure of compensation and the appearance of true hypoxia or CO_2 excess. These include increasing restlessness, significant pulse elevation, dulled responses, refusal to eat or drink, and cyanosis in 40% oxygen. Blood gas alterations are even more definitive. If pH falls below 7.25, pO_2 below 50 mm. Hg, or if pCO_2 exceeds 65 mm. Hg,[23] these are real indications for tracheostomy or intubation.

Choice between tracheostomy or prolonged intubation. The current interest in the relative value of tracheostomy versus prolonged intubation is tremendous, and deservedly so. The wrong choice can be crippling or fatal. Thus far we can make general statements only.

Tracheostomy entails a true operation with local or usually general anesthesia. Decision is likely to be delayed because of the hazards involved in a sick child. The operation is not easy and may involve bleeding, airway obstruction, and mediastinal emphysema. Maintenance of tracheostomy often is complicated by mechanical problems with the tube, accidental extubation, bleeding, and especially infection. Extubation, especially in infants, entails problems in reaccommodation to normal breathing, and postoperative scarring may occur. These disadvantages led to the enthusiastic adoption of nasotracheal intubation as a substitute.[24-26] After some five years of trial, the advantages and disadvantages of intubation are coming into clearer view. It is easily and quickly performed and usually entails less hesitation to make the decision. The maneuver is simpler and safer than tracheostomy. However, complications may be of real concern.[27-29] Continued intubation requires more sedation of the patient, and consequently greater depression, obstruction of the lumen is of greater danger, especially in small infants, and both immediate and late postextubation lesions have been very distressing. Subglottic membranes frequently have been found, as well as vocal cord damage, while severe tracheal stenosis requiring permanent tracheostomy has occurred in several patients following relatively minor diseases.[30-32] These have been real tragedies.

Both techniques have their ardent champions. The nonbiased view seems to be that establishment of an airway for up to 3 or 4 days is usually an indication for nasotracheal intubation. The presence of an inflammatory process such as croup probably will increase the chance of an irritative reaction, as will any patient who moves excessively. Infants tolerate inlying tubes better than older patients, while they are poorer subjects for tracheostomy. Individual experience also is a factor. A meticulous team with strict aseptic technique will have fewer complications. Our experience to date includes an infant and a 14-year-old boy, both of whom tolerated nasal intubation for 6 weeks without airway complications.

When faced with the problem of tracheostomy or intubation, it seems reasonable to start with intubation, which usually must be performed prior to operative tracheostomy. If the endotracheal tube is easily tolerated, it may be left in for a more extended time. If the patient appears to fight it and if suctioning is difficult, 3 or 4 days' trial may be sufficient, and the advantage of tracheostomy will become obvious.

REFERENCES

1. Proctor, D. F., and Safar, P.: In Safar, P., editor: Management of airway obstruction in respiratory therapy, Philadelphia, 1965, F. A. Davis Co.
2. Safar, P.: Ventilatory efficiency of mouth-to-mouth artificial respiration, J.A.M.A. **167:**335-341, 1958.
3. Hazeltine, F. G.: Hypoglycemia and erythroblastosis, Pediatrics **39:**696-700, 1967.
4. Apgar, V.: Infant resuscitation, Postgrad. Med. **19:**447-450, 1956.
5. Apgar, V., Girdany, B. R., McIntosh, R., and Taylor, H. C., Jr.: Neonatal anoxia. I. Study of relation of oxygenation at birth to intellectual development, Pediatrics **15:**653-661, 1955.
6. Cook, C. D., Lucey, J. F., Drorbaugh, J. E., Segal, S., Sutherland, J. M., and Smith, C. A.: Apnea and respiratory distress in the newborn infant, New Eng. J. Med. **254:**562-568, 651-657, 1956.
7. Flagg, P. J.: Asphyxia neonatorum. The pivot upon which turns the movement to prevent asphyxial death, Surg. Gynec. Obstet. **67:**153-162, 1938.
8. Little, D. M., Hampton, L. J., and White, M. L.: Asphyxia neonatorum: the syndrome, its prevention, and its treatment, Anesthesiology **13:**518-539, 1952.
9. Little, D. M., and Tovell, R. M.: Collective review: the physiological basis for resuscitation of the newborn, Internat. Abstr. Surg. **86:**417-428, 1948.
10. Day, R., Goodfellow, A. M., Apgar, V., and Beck, G. J.: Pressure-time relations in safe correction of atelectasis in animal lungs, Pediatrics **10:**593-602, 1952.
11. Apgar, V., and Kreiselman, J.: Studies on resuscitation: experimental evaluation of Bloxsom air lock, Amer. J. Obstet. Gynec. **65:**45-52, 1953.
12. Elam, J. O., Brown, E. S., and Elder, J. D., Jr.: Artificial respiration by mouth-to-mask method: study of respiratory gas exchange of paralyzed patients ventilated by operator's expired air, New Eng. J. Med. **250:**749-754, 1954.
13. Gordon, A. S., Frye, C. W., Gittelson, L., Sadove, M. S., and Beattie, E. J.: Mouth-to-mouth versus manual artificial respiration for children and adults, J.A.M.A. **167:**320-334, 1958.
14. Dulfano, M. J., and Segal, M. S.: Nikethamide as a respiratory analeptic, J.A.M.A. **185:**69-74, 1963.
15. Noe, F. E.: Respiratory stimulation with doxapram hydrochloride during the anesthesia recovery period, Anesth. Analg. **45:**479-483, 1966.
16. Stephen, C. R., and Talton, I.: Investigation of doxapram as a postanesthetic respiratory stimulant, Anesth. Analg. **43:**628-640, 1964.
17. Adamsons, K., and Towell, M. E.: Thermal hemeostasis in the fetus and newborn, Anesthesiology **26:**531-548, 1965.

18. Stern, I., Lees, M. H., and Leduc, J.: Temperature, oxygen and catecholamine excretion in newborn infants, Pediatrics **36**:367-374, 1965.
19. Miller, J. A., and Miller, F. S.: Interactions between hypothermia and hypoxia-hypercapnia in neonates, Fed. Proc. **25**:1338-1341, 1966.
20. MacDowall, D. G.: Hyperbaric oxygen in relation to circulatory and respiratory emergencies, Brit. J. Anaesth. **36**:563-571, 1964.
21. Head, J. M.: Tracheostomy in the management of respiratory problems, New Eng. J. Med. **264**:587-591, 1961.
22. Engineer, E. H.: Tracheostomy in children-indications, anesthetic management and complications. In Smith, R. M., editor: Pediatric anesthesia, Boston, 1962, Little, Brown & Co.
23. Downes, J. J., Striker, T. W., and Stool, S.: Complications of nasotracheal intubation in children with croup, New Eng. J. Med. **274**:226-227, 1966.
24. Branstater, B.: Prolonged intubation, an alternative to tracheostomy in children. Proceedings First European Congress of Anaesthesiology, Vienna, Paper 106, 1962.
25. MacDonald, I. H., and Stocks, J. G.: Prolonged nasotracheal intubation: a review of its development in a paediatric hospital, Brit. J. Anaesth. **37**:161-172, 1965.
26. Reid, D. H. S., and Tunstall, M. E.: Treatment of respiratory distress syndrome of newborn with nasotracheal intubation and intermittent positive pressure respiration, Lancet **1**:1196-1197, 1965.
27. Allen, T. H., and Steven, I. M.: Prolonged endotracheal intubation in infants and children, Brit. J. Anaesth. **37**:566-573, 1965.
28. Harrison, G. A., and Tonkin, J. P.: Laryngeal complications of prolonged endotracheal intubation, Med. J. Australia **2**:709-710, 1965; abstract in Survey Anesth. **10**:566-567, 1966.
29. Fearon, B., MacDonald, R. E., Smith, C., and Mitchell, D.: Airway problems in children following prolonged endotracheal intubation, Ann. Otol. **75**:975-987, 1966.
30. Rees, G. J., and Owen-Thomas, J. B.: A technique of pulmonary ventilation with a nasotracheal tube, Brit. J. Anaesth. **38**:901-906, 1966.
31. MacDonald, I. H., and Steven, I. M.: Prolonged endotracheal intubation in infants and children, Brit. J. Anaesth. **37**:161-172, 1965; abstract in Survey Anesth. **10**:54-55, 1966.
32. Markham, W. G., Blackwood, M. J. A., and Conn, A. W.: Prolonged nasotracheal intubation in infants and children, Canad. Anaesth. Soc. J. **14**:11-22, 1967.

Chapter 29

Oxygen and respiratory therapy

The administration of oxygen and respiratory therapy has become an increasingly complicated field of medicine that now encompasses aspects of internal medicine, anesthesiology, physiotherapy, and surgery. The responsibility for the organization and activation of this work has largely fallen upon the anesthesiologist. In larger hospitals it has been expedient to have a corps of nurses and technicians to maintain, store, and assemble apparatus and to attend to details of therapy. Such therapy, however, usually continues to be supervised by the anesthesiologists.

Intensive care units in which oxygen administration and respiratory therapy play a basic role also may be largely dependent upon the anesthesiologist for direction.

Pediatric patients probably have more acute and more varied respiratory problems than do adults. Apparatus and techniques must be adapted to the special demands of size, behavior, and pathology.

THE ADMINISTRATION OF OXYGEN

The specific indications for oxygen therapy are poorly defined. Oxygen is undoubtedly the most misused of all our medicinal agents and in a great many cases is ordered unnecessarily, administered inefficiently, or used too long. When needed, it is of utmost importance that it be administered with maximal effect.

Actually it is not the disease but the child's clinical condition that determines his need for oxygen therapy.[1] Regardless of the diagnosis, the use of oxygen will be indicated whenever the need becomes evident or suspected. Signs of increasing oxygen want that may be seen in infants and children are tachycardia, restlessness, anorexia, rapid respiration, flaring nostrils, and elevation of blood pressure, to be followed by falling blood pressure, cyanosis, coma, bradycardia, gasping, irregular respiration, and death.

In the absence of these signs of acute hypoxia, the presence of other clinical conditions should be taken as indications for prophylactic use of oxygen. These include various forms of respiratory obstruction and depression, acute infectious disease, and hyperpyrexia, as well as cardiac failure and circulatory depression.

METHODS OF OXYGEN THERAPY IN PEDIATRICS

Mask, tent, or nasal catheter may be used for adult oxygen therapy,[2] but with children the apparatus is determined largely by the age and size of the patient.

Newborn babies and small infants are most suitably treated in enclosed plastic cubicles such as the Isolette or the Armstrong baby incubator, which may be warmed, humidified, or oxygenated, as desired (Fig. 29-1). It should be noted that infants who have received ether should not be placed in a heated incubator

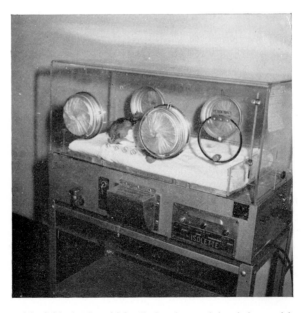

Fig. 29-1. Incubator with rigid plastic cubicle (Isolette), supplying infants with oxygen, humidity, and warmth.

until 2 hours after operation, since ether, if heated by a warming element, may decompose to give off formaldehyde.[3] Oxygen and vapor may be administered to larger infants and small children by means of a plastic canopy tent (Croupette), which is equipped with a humidifying device (Fig. 29-2). If the child is small, he can be completely enclosed by the canopy; when larger children are treated, only the head and shoulders are covered.

For children of school age a small motorless tent (Plymouth tent) has been found to be very satisfactory—it allows patients to sit up yet still have a relatively small canopy in which adequate oxygen concentrations can be maintained (Fig. 29-3). Oxygen is circulated in this tent by a Venturi jet. This tent is especially useful following thoracic operations and in treating children with pneumonia, cardiac failure, or peritonitis.

Infants and small children will rarely tolerate the use of an oxygen mask when awake, and it is extremely difficult to keep masks in position when they are asleep. Children who are very ill or who are recovering from anesthesia will often tolerate the short plastic nasal tubes mounted on a light harness that may be strapped to the face, but enclosed cubicles or tents seem preferable for oxygen therapy for most young patients.

Starting treatment. The physician who orders oxygen therapy should specify the concentration that is to be maintained in the tent or cubicle. When an infant is placed is a small plastic cubicle, the oxygen may be started at 10 L. per minute for 3 or 4 minutes. The oxygen concentration is then tested, and the flow rate is adjusted accordingly. Usually a flow rate of 3 or 4 L. per minute is satisfactory for maintenance.

If oxygen therapy is needed, it should be administered rationally, and consequently tent concentration should be measured at least twice daily and more

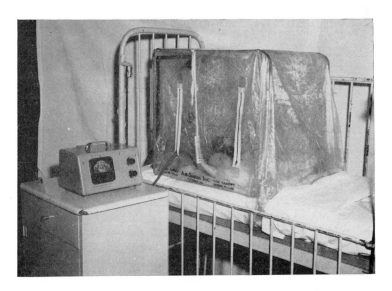

Fig. 29-2. Plastic canopy tent (Croupette) for administration of oxygen and vapor.

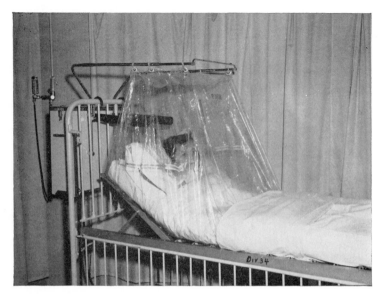

Fig. 29-3. Motorless oxygen tent for larger children.

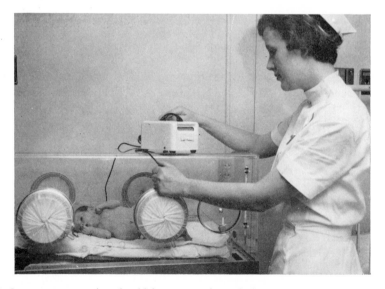

Fig. 29-4. Oxygen concentration should be measured regularly.

often if patients are in critical condition (Fig. 29-4). To be of benefit the concentration should be above 40%. Before exposing small newborn babies to high concentrations of oxygen, however, one should consider the danger of retrolental fibroplasia (p. 484). For most conditions in which there is no obstructive pulmonary disease, an oxygen concentration of 40% to 60% is desirable.

When children are to be placed in larger tents, the oxygen should be turned to 20 L. per minute for several minutes in order to build up a suitable concentration before the child is placed under the canopy. Then the flow may be regulated at 8 to 10 L. or more per minute as indicated.

Although there are several methods of determining oxygen concentration, it is most easily measured by use of the Pauling[4] oxygen analyzer. The basic principle upon which this instrument acts is the paramagnetic property of oxygen. Since this analyzer is powered by a battery, it may be used under all conditions.

Removal of patients from oxygen tent. Oxygen therapy should not be terminated until signs of respiratory distress are relieved and there is significant improvement in the underlying disease. Then the patient is taken out of the tent for a short trial period and is observed for appearance of pulse elevation, respiratory distress, or cyanosis. It is usually best to put the child back in the tent and to extend the trial periods gradually. It is also advisable to keep him in the tent at night during the weaning period.

COMPLICATIONS OF OXYGEN THERAPY

When an enclosed tent or cubicle is being used, inadequate oxygen supply and maintenance may result in *asphyxia, carbon dioxide intoxication,* or *overheating.* With any form of oxygen therapy there is increased danger of *fire and explosion,* and appropriate precautions are indicated. If nasopharyngeal catheters are used, oxygen may pass down the esophagus, causing *distention or rupture of the stomach.* For this reason nasopharyngeal catheters have largely been abandoned in oxygen therapy.

As emphasized by Saklad,[1] prolonged administration of high concentrations of oxygen by direct nasal or endotracheal insufflation will cause *drying and irritation of respiratory membranes* unless humidification is provided. In addition to these hazards that are always present, several specific complications may occur.

Oxygen toxicity. Adverse effects of high concentrations of oxygen have been noted since the time of Bert and Lavoisier.[5] An inflammatory reaction of the lungs and respiratory tract was reported by Smith, and this lesion is still known as the Lorraine Smith effect.[5] Although Behnke and associates[7] believed it was necessary to be exposed to very high concentration of oxygen (98% to 99%) to develop oxygen toxicity, Comroe and associates[8] found that normal males would develop substernal distress after breathing 50% to 75% oxygen for several hours. It has been shown that very short interruptions in exposure to high oxygen concentration will prevent the development of symptoms.

The development of toxic effects of hyperoxia depends upon the partial pressure of oxygen to which the subject is exposed and the duration of the exposure. If the partial pressure of oxygen is maintained at less than 150 mm. Hg, it is believed that oxygen toxicity will not occur.

When patients have normal lungs, a 60% concentration of oxygen is thought to be the maximum that can be used with safety. It should be emphasized, however, that in many conditions pulmonary pathology prevents normal oxygen uptake, and patients will require 60% to 100% oxygen for survival.

With prolonged inspiration of 100% oxygen at normal atmospheric pressure, symptoms most commonly noted have been substernal distress, dyspnea, and nausea. These are due primarily to pulmonary irritation.[6-8] Pathologic examination shows atelectasis, pneumonitis, and leukyocytic infiltration, and there is definite decrease in pulmonary compliance. The danger is slight when patients are merely receiving therapy in the form of mask, tent, or nasal catheter, but it becomes of real significance during ventilator therapy.

The use of hyperbaric oxygen as a form of therapy has demonstrated that with exposure to much higher partial pressures of oxygen symptoms of central nervous system will predominate. Convulsions occur with 2-hour exposure at 3 atmospheres (pO_2 approximately 2,000 mm. Hg).[8,9]

Retrolental fibroplasia. For some time it has been known that if premature infants are placed in high concentrations of oxygen (over 60%) and allowed to remain in it for over 24 hours, a resultant fibrous overgrowth of the posterior surface of the optic lens may occur, causing blindness.[10] Following the recognition of this hazard, the incidence of retrolental fibroplasia was greatly reduced.[11] Recently further evidence has suggested that some infants show increased sensitivity, and even 40% oxygen is not always safe.[12]

Here again it should be clearly understood that when infants have obstructive pulmonary pathology such as respiratory distress syndrome or pneumonia one should not hesitate to give any concentration that is required to provide adequate oxygenation of the blood. If oxygen concentration is limited to 60% in such cases, many will die of hypoxia.

Carbon dioxide narcosis. The syndrome known as carbon dioxide narcosis is most frequently encountered in emphysematous adults.[13,14] However, it may also occur in children. When a child has severe asthma and ventilation is seriously impaired, the alveolar concentration of carbon dioxide gradually is elevated to abnormally high levels. The respiratory center becomes insensitive to the high concentration of carbon dioxide and responds only to hypoxia. If such a child is put into an oxygen tent, the oxygen requirement is exceeded, and the child's stimulus to breathe will be removed. As a result, ventilation will be sharply decreased, and carbon dioxide will be allowed to reach stupefying levels. A 6-year-old girl demonstrated this reaction very dramatically. She came to the hospital in severe status asthmaticus. She was dusky and breathing with great difficulty, but she was quite rational. Upon being placed in an oxygen tent her color promptly improved; she ceased to struggle for breath but became wildly delirious. On removal from the oxygen tent she regained her rationality and also her dyspnea and cyanosis. The correct treatment, of course, would have been to ventilate the child with room air.

HUMIDIFICATION AND AEROSOL THERAPY

Although many aspects of oxygen therapy have become relatively well standardized, that of humidification and aerosol therapy is poorly understood by many clinicians. The review by Cushing and Miller[15] offers an excellent coverage of this subject, and details of measurement of humidity are described by Dery and associates.[16]

Indications. It is well known that breathing increased concentrations of oxygen will cause drying of the respiratory tract, thickening of secretions, impairment of ciliary activity, and irritation of tracheobronchial mucosa. It is quite possible that it is this drying rather than the high concentration of oxygen that causes substernal distress, previously ascribed to oxygen toxicity. For prevention of these conditions, humidification is indicated with the use of most forms of oxygen therapy and is mandatory when oxygen is applied directly, as in nasal administration or by means of endotracheal tube or tracheostomy.

Humidification also is employed therapeutically for both acute and chronic types of respiratory disease, especially those involving inflammation and thickened secretions. The study of the flow of fluid material, dignified by the term rheology, has been vigorously applied to problems of liquefying tracheobronchial secretions.

There is reasonable doubt in the minds of many clinicians whether supersaturated vapor in the form of aerosol or fog is preferable to warm saturated air. This doubt is fortified if one has taken a deep inspiration of a concentrated aerosol that resulted in a severe coughing spasm.

There is also disagreement concerning the advantage of warming the vapor that the patient inhales. In the days of croup tents, when febrile children were enclosed in a hot, saturated atmosphere, the child's temperature often would become even more elevated. It is now generally agreed that warming the vapor is an essential part of humidification; however, if a child has fever, it is important to avoid any technique that warms his environment. Another fundamental question yet to be settled is whether saline or distilled water should be the basic humidifying fluid. Using puppies as subjects, Modell[17] has shown that inhalation of saline vapor will cause pulmonary abscess, while water vapor does not; however, both fluids are commonly employed.

Many of the terms used in this field have been somewhat confusing. It should be pointed out that a *humidifier* increases the moisture content in the air and can produce saturated air, but it will not cause a fog or droplets. A *nebulizer,* however, produces droplets, thereby making a fog or mist, also called an aerosol. The droplet size is important, because to penetrate beyond the larger bronchi the particle size should be less than 5 μ in diameter.

There are several types of nebulizers that are useful in ventilatory therapy. The original Mistogen[18] apparatus (Fig. 29-5) is a portable unit that generates an unwarmed mist with a particle size of 1 to 5 μ diameter. Other nebulizers[19] are now manufactured that deliver heated mist of similar particle size and may be adapted to anesthesia apparatus, tracheostomy tubes, or oxygen tents.

The recently developed ultrasonic nebulizers[20,21] create a dense fog of small particle size. These nebulizers are especially useful in preventing accumulation of secretions in endotracheal tubes during prolonged therapy.

Aerosol medication. The administration of aerosolized drugs for either local or general effect has been given considerable trial. Antibiotics were used for children with cystic fibrosis,[22] bronchodilators for asthmatics,[23] and various mucolytic and detergent drugs for symptomatic treatment of airway obstruction.

Antibiotic therapy has proved more effective by other routes. Early en-

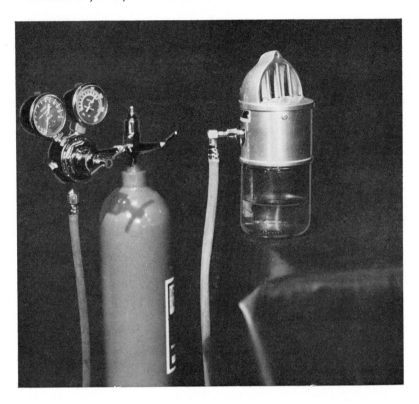

Fig. 29-5. Portable nebulizer for use in tents or cubicles.

thusiasm for detergents and wetting agents has not been substantiated; in fact some of these materials actually reduce pulmonary compliance, whereas enzymatic products such as chymotrypsin have been found to cause metaplasia of mucous membranes or actual digestion of local tissues.

There is some evidence that a mixture of ascorbic acid, sodium percarbonate, and copper sulfate*[24] is safe and effective as a proteolytic agent. N-acetyl cysteine†[25] also acts as a mucolytic agent and has been used both as an aerosol and a tracheal wash in patients with cystic fibrosis. The latter drug is moderately effective but also is somewhat irritant.

Bronchodilating agents probably have been more successful than other aerosols. Among these isoproterenol has been particularly effective in controlling asthmatic bronchospasm with minimal side effects.

MEDICAL AND SURGICAL APPLICATION OF HYPERBARIC OXYGEN

A resurgence of enthusiasm for the clinical application of hyperbaric oxygen was initiated by Boerema and associates[26] in Holland and by Illingworth and as-

---

*Available as Ascoxal, Astra Pharmaceutical Products, Inc., Worcester, Mass.
†Mead-Johnson Laboratories, Evansville, Ind.

sociates[27] in Scotland. Following their reported success in connection with gas gangrene, carbon monoxide poisoning, and vascular disease, it appeared that there were many phases of medicine in which increased oxygen could be tremendously beneficial.

In pediatric medicine the use of hyperbaric oxygen was attempted in treatment of respiratory distress syndrome. Hutchison and associates[28] have placed apneic cyanotic infants in a small chamber, without any method of artificial ventilation or airway control, and observed improvement in color and initiation of respiration. Dawes[29] has shown that an apneic subject is more successfully resuscitated by endotracheal ventilation with oxygen at normal pressure than by unattended therapy at increased pressure. Cochran[30] also has shown that infants with respiratory distress syndrome do not show improved survival by unassisted exposure in hyperbaric oxygen. Thus far no one has made a fair evaluation of the treatment of respiratory distress syndrome with hyperbaric oxygenation when used in combination with airway control and standard resuscitative therapy. At present the future application of oxygen at increased pressure does not appear to be indicated, inasmuch as exposure of the neonatal lung to high partial pressures of oxygen of itself causes histologic changes much like those seen in respiratory distress syndrome.

Individual attempts have been made to treat other pulmonary lesions with hyperbaric oxygenation. These include pneumonia and various forms of pneumonitis. Although one successful application in this general field has been reported, there have been many failures, and it does not appear to be promising.

In the treatment of anaerobic infections, hyperbaric oxygen has shown its greatest value in controlling gas gangrene,[31] while it has been of questionable value in the therapy of septic shock[32] and quite useless for treatment of tetanus. In gas gangrene the duration of action of the exotoxin is only about one hour. Although the organisms are not killed, toxin formation is arrested, and the effect on the patient is one of almost immediate improvement. Usually the patient is treated 90 minutes at 3 atmospheres, at which time initial debridement is performed. Subsequently one or two more treatments of 30 to 45 minutes are advised during the first 24 hours, after which further therapy may consist of 2 to 3 more exposures, but often these will not be necessary. The results have been overwhelmingly convincing that lives are saved and that amputation and other sacrifice of tissue are greatly reduced.

In the case of tetanus, the exotoxin rapidly becomes fixed in the nervous tissue, and increased partial pressure of oxygen does not appear to affect it.

Congenital heart lesions. In our experience by far the greatest number of children treated under hyperbaric oxygen have been infants and small children who required operation for congenital heart defects. These lesions involve either severe cyanosis or acyanotic disease with acute failure.

Operation usually involves construction of some form of shunt during which blood flow to one lung usually must be interrupted, but may involve complete occlusion of cardiac inflow. The latter operation could be performed using extracorporeal circulation, but the problems involved in small infants are increased greatly. By raising the partial pressure of oxygen, it is possible to increase the oxygen saturation of these infants significantly[33] and avoid use of extracorporeal circulation. Results show that the risk to the child is decreased considerably when compared to those children operated upon at normal barometric pressure. Thus far over 250 infants and small children have undergone surgical correction of congenital heart lesions in our hospital.[34,35] Details of their management are described in Chapter 18.

PROLONGED VENTILATORY ASSISTANCE WITH INTERMITTENT POSITIVE PRESSURE APPARATUS

The most important problem associated with pediatric anesthesia today unquestionably is that of maintaining oxygenation in patients during a period in which the lungs are rendered inadequate by operation or disease. The solution to this problem is also the solution to the greatest cause of infant mortality in this country, the respiratory distress syndrome.

Rapidly growing enthusiasm in this field is producing real improvement, but there is much to be learned. One underlying fact has been generally recognized. The answer does not lie in the development of a single piece of apparatus, but in the establishment of a team of dedicated individuals in each hospital who will accept complete responsibility for patients in respiratory failure. Several such teams have already grown up within the country, and their results are convincing.

Indications. Prolonged ventilatory assistance is used in numerous situations involving actual or threatened respiratory failure. At present our most frequent use of mechanical ventilators is in postoperative open-heart surgery.

When patients have required pump-oxygenator support for over 90 minutes, or have severely damaged hearts, postoperative ventilatory support is usually instituted. [35,36]

Postoperative ventilatory support is occasionally required following destructive neurosurgery, although this is considerably less common.

Nonsurgical conditions involving prolonged assistance include respiratory distress syndrome, Guillain-Barré disease, status asthmaticus, pneumonia, tetanus, and other pulmonary or neuromuscular disorders and traumatic conditions.

The actual indications for the institution of ventilatory assistance are not easily defined but in many respects are similar to those that have been used for tracheostomy. Specifically they are the signs of respiratory failure and include rapid respiration, subcostal retraction, tachycardia, increased secretions, decreased tidal volume, decreased mental acuity and response to pain, and cyanosis in 40% oxygen. In discussing therapy for status asthmaticus, Downes and Wood[37] list the preceding signs and state that the presence of any three constitute definite indication for ventilatory assistance. Blood gas determinations offer more definite guidance. Most agree that $pO_2 < 40$, $pCO_2 > 65$ and pH under 7.25 indicate need for active respiratory assistance.

Numerous ventilating devices have been developed, many of which are adaptable to children. Apparatus for infants has been more difficult to perfect due to infants' rapid respiration, greater resistance to control, small tidal volume, and their sudden development of pressure.[38,39]

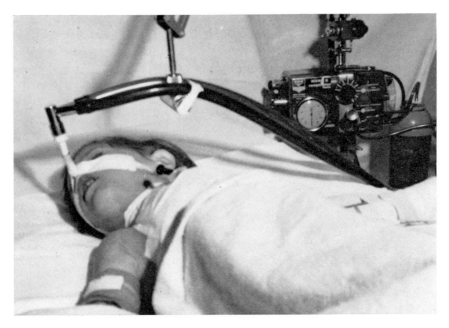

Fig. 29-6. Two-year-old child receiving ventilatory support using Bird Mark 8 via nasoendo-tracheal tube.

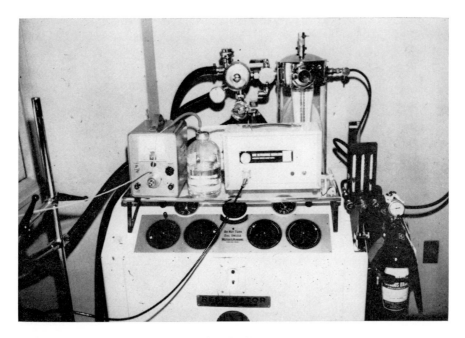

Fig. 29-7. Engström ventilator with ultrasonic nebulizer.

Ventilators may be classified as pressure-limited (Bird, Bennett) or volume-limited (Engström, Emerson), but Norlander and Engström[40] stress the importance of power curves. Pressure-limited devices can be used to assist respiration, while volume-controlled devices must control respiration (Figs. 29-6 and 29-7).

Starting ventilatory assistance. The actual choice of mechanical ventilator will be affected by practical as well as theoretical factors. The location where treatment is to be carried out is important. A central intensive therapy unit is preferable, but newborn infants should be kept in a separate area. Unless separated areas are permanently equipped with ventilators, the portable units will be more practical for short-term use. Who is to supervise the unit is also important, for simplicity will be essential if untrained personnel are to be in control.

The size and age of the patient are to be considered. In general, pressure-limited devices have been used more frequently in smaller infants, due probably to difficulty in controlling infant respiration.[38]

A real consideration is the presence or absence of lung pathology. When lungs have normal compliance, pressure-limited ventilators are reliable, but with changing resistance they do not deliver predictable volumes of oxygen or air.

The physical condition of the child plays an important part in planning respiratory care. With severe pulmonary disease the work of breathing will be increased greatly. The energy required to initiate inspiration (or trip an assisting ventilator) may constitute half of the total work of breathing; therefore, in such patients it is far better to employ a ventilator with total control of respiration. Infants with respiratory distress syndrome, children with asthma, and infants or children with pulmonary hypertension are examples of those with decreased pulmonary compliance who may need increased and variable pressure to deliver adequate volumes of gas.

The expected duration of mechanical assistance is often a factor in choosing a ventilator. If assistance is planned only for a few hours while a patient is regaining full ventilatory power, it may seem preferable to allow the patient to continue spontaneous breathing; consequently, a pressure-limited apparatus would be used, and respiration would be assisted rather than controlled. If a patient is expected to need assistance for several days, complete control on a volume-limited machine would be more practical.

In last analysis, the best way to choose a respirator is to make a reasonable guess and try it; then if it cannot be made to suit the patient, try another type. For some reason each situation is different, and a method that succeeded once may fail completely on the second attempt.

A child of 3 or more years of age may be treated much like an adult in respect to ventilatory care. As an example, consider a child who has just undergone open correction of tetralogy of Fallot under curare–nitrous oxide anesthesia. It is decided to support respiration for 12 to 24 hours or until he appears well stabilized. A volume-controlled respirator is chosen, and here the Emerson would be our present choice because of greater simplicity and equal effectiveness. An uncuffed nasoendotracheal tube is inserted. The child remains curarized at the end of the operation. The ventilator is turned on and set at a rate of 24 per minute and a tidal volume of 250. This is intentionally in excess of his predicted tidal volume, to allow for dead space and air compression in the ventilator.[41] Oxygen is added to give a 40% mixture. The chest is observed to expand evenly, and breath sounds are satisfactory by auscultation. After 15 minutes blood gases are drawn, and the ventilator action is altered as indicated. Most frequently it is found that the patient is being hyperventilated. Although mild hyperventilation is desirable, pO_2 above 150 is believed to invite oxygen toxicity, while pCO_2 below 25 may lead to cerebral vasoconstriction. The desired blood gas levels are pO_2 100 to 150 mm. Hg, pCO_2 25 to 35 mm. Hg, and pH 7.35 to 7.55.

Special attention must be given to the endotracheal tube. Suctioning of tube and trachea is carried out under strict sterile technique when secretions are present. The ventilatory gases must be humidified to prevent occlusion of the tube by dried secretions. This is accomplished best by use of an ultrasonic humidifier, using distilled water. Should ventilatory assistance be required for a prolonged period, one must decide between changing the tube or performing tracheostomy. The conservative approach is to tracheostomize patients after 3 days of intubation, but much evidence is available to show this to be un-necessary.[42,43]

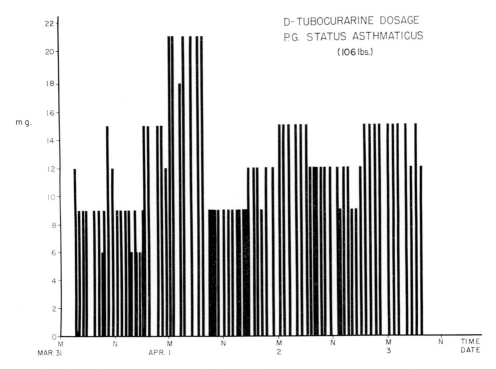

Fig. 29-8. Chart of *d*-tubocurarine required by 106-lb. boy during 3½ days of ventilatory therapy for status asthmaticus.

The chief problem may be to keep the child from resisting the ventilator. Older patients can usually be controlled by simple hyperventilation. Further control may be obtained by the use of repeated small doses of *d*-tubocurarine, by the addition of nitrous oxide in 50% mixture, or by the use of morphine[44] (Fig. 29-8).

It is especially desirable to avoid tracheostomy in infants. Fortunately, nasotracheal intubation may be continued for more prolonged periods because babies tolerate the tube more easily than older patients. The chief difficulty will be in preventing occlusion of the tube. Again, humidification with ultrasonic nebulization will give reassurance that the tube will remain patent. Unless this nebulizer is run at one-half volume, however, the infant may become over-

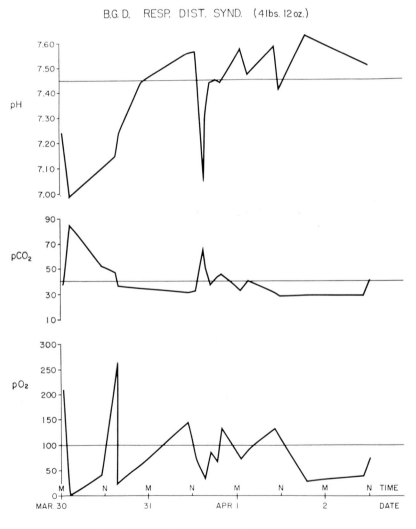

Fig. 29-9. Blood gases in 4-lb. infant with respiratory distress syndrome during ventilatory support with Emerson ventilator. Sudden drop in pH at midpoint caused by accidental extubation.

hydrated. This must be checked by daily weighing. When infants are artificially ventilated, an intelligent attendant must remain at the bedside at all times, since the apparatus may require repeated adjustment in response to the infant's changing condition.

In addition to airway obstruction, atelectasis, pneumonia, and pneumothorax are the great dangers of children during artificial ventilation. If tracheostomized, local infection is added to this list. Change of position, chest physiotherapy, frequent roentgen-ray examination, and sterile technique will help reduce complications. Warmth is essential, as well as nutritional and fluid maintenance.

Both morphine and relaxants will cause blood pressure depression in poor-risk patients and must be used in approximately one-fourth the usual dosage.

The proper time to terminate artificial ventilation is not easily fixed. Several factors are mandatory. The patient should be warm, in fluid and nutritional balance, and with adequate cardiovascular stability. He should be alert and able to respond to commands, and his vital capacity should be at least three times his tidal volume.[45] It is often helpful to "wean" the patient from the volume-limited respirator to a pressure-limited device that allows him to breathe spontaneously. It may be preferable to try the child off the respirator for periods of 10 to 20 minutes at a time and gradually prolong these periods. It is also advisable to avoid this transition either late in the day or on weekends, when the hospital is more likely to be inadequately staffed.

MECHANICAL VENTILATION FOR INFANTS

The problem of artificial respiration for infants is more difficult to solve. Controlled respiration with volume-limited devices can be carried out. The Engström ventilator has been employed extensively in Scandinavia for infants of all ages, using a special nomogram to determine flow rates.[40,46] Infants' respiration is less easily controlled, and one usually must make the choice between using assisted respiration with the pressure-limited Bird Q circle or double Venturi, or else using a volume-controlled device and a muscle relaxant (Fig. 29-9). We are becoming more convinced that the latter method is more reliable, especially when infants have pulmonary pathology. Considerable effort has been spent in developing ventilators especially suited to infants.[47-49] Silverman converted the Air-Shields Isolette* into a ventilator resembling the early tank respirator with a diaphragm at the neck. The purpose of this apparatus is to avoid endotracheal intubation. It has been moderately successful, but irritation of the skin by the neck collar has been difficult to overcome. The machine has a delicate sensing device and may be used as an assistor.

The more complex Bourns† ventilator has been developed recently. The infant is held in a fixed cradle, that turns automatically to alter his position. It requires endotracheal intubation, but it, too, has a fine sensing device that enables the child to cycle the ventilator with a negligible amount of expended work.

The Harvard animal pump, a small piston, volume-controlled ventilator, has also been effectively adapted for use in small infants.

*Air-Shields Co., Hatboro, Pa.
†Bourns, Inc., Ames, Iowa.

Again it must be stressed that in order to attain success with any ventilator, one must expect to devote full time to this one project.

REFERENCES

1. Saklad, M.: Inhalation therapy and resuscitation, Springfield, Ill., 1953, Charles C Thomas, Publisher.
2. Winchell, S. W.: Inhalation of oxygen. In Safar, P., editor: Respiratory therapy, Philadelphia, 1965, F. A. Davis Co.
3. Mendenhall, M. K., Jenicek, J. A., and Bryant, J. N.: Thermal decomposition of ether in the infant incubator, J.A.M.A. 173:651-653, 1960.
4. Pauling, L., Wood, R. E., and Sturdivant, J. H.: An instrument for determining the partial pressure of oxygen in a gas, Science 103:338, 1946.
5. Garrison, F. H.: An introduction to the history of medicine, Philadelphia, 1921, W. B. Saunders Co.
6. Comroe, J. H., Jr., and Dripps, R. D.: The physiological basis for oxygen therapy, Springfield, Ill., 1950, Charles C Thomas, Publisher.
7. Behnke, A. R., Shaw, L. A., Shilling, C. W., Thompson, R. D., and Messer, A. C.: Studies on the effects of high oxygen pressure, Amer. J. Physiol. 107:13-28, 1934.
8. Comroe, J. H., Jr., Dripps, R. D., Dumke, P. R., and Deming, M.: Oxygen toxicity, J.A.M.A. 128:710-717, 1945.
9. Lambertsen, C. J., Stroud, M. W., Gould, R. A., Kough, R. H., Ewing, J. H., and Schmidt, C. F.: Oxygen toxicity; respiratory responses of normal man to inhalation of 6 to 100 per cent oxygen under 3.5 atmospheres pressure, J. Appl. Physiol. 5:487-494, 1953.
10. Terry, T. L.: Extreme prematurity and fibroplastic overgrowth of persistent vascular sheath behind each crystalline lens: preliminary report, Amer. J. Ophth. 25:203-204, 1942.
11. Parmelee, A. H., Jr., Pilger, I. S., and Austin, W. O.: Retrolental fibroplasia: a reduction in incidence following a decrease in use of oxygen therapy for premature infants, California Med. 84:424-426, 1956.
12. Zacharias, L.: Unpublished data.
13. Calloway, J. J., and McKusick, V. A.: Carbon-dioxide intoxication in emphysema; emergency treatment by artificial pneumoperitoneum, New Eng. J. Med. 245:9-13, 1951.
14. Lovejoy, F. W., Jr., Yu, P., Nye, R., Jr., Joos, H. A., and Simpson, J. H.: Pulmonary hypertension: physiological studies in 3 cases of carbon-dioxide narcosis treated by artificial respiration, Amer. J. Med. 16:4-11, 1954.
15. Cushing, I. E., and Miller, W. F.: Nebulization therapy. In Safar, P., editor: Respiratory therapy, Philadelphia, 1965, F. A. Davis Co.
16. Dery, R., Pelletier, J., Jacques, A., Clavet, M., and Houde, J. J.: Humidity in anesthesiology, I. A modified dew-point hygrometer, Canad. Anaesth. Soc. J. 14:104-112, 1962.
17. Modell, J. H., Giammona, S. T., and Davis, J. H.: Effect of chronic exposure to untrasonic aerosols on the lung, Anesthesiology 28:680, 1967.
18. Denton, R., and Smith, R. M.: Portable humidifying unit. II. Large capacity metal nebulizer, Amer. J. Dis. Child. 82:433-438, 1951.
19. Wynands, J. E.: A simple method of humidifying gases, Canad. Anaesth. Soc. J. 13:403-405, 1966.
20. Herzog, P., Norlander, O. P., and Engström, C. G.: Ultrasonic generation of aerosol for the humidification of inspired gas during volume-controlled ventilation, Acta Anaesth. Scand. 8:79-84, 1964.
21. Stevens, H. R., and Albrecht, N. B.: Assessment of ultrasonic nebulization, Anesthesiology 27:648-653, 1966.
22. Smith, R. M.: Inhalational therapy in pediatrics, Anesthesiology 23:548-558, 1962.
23. Abramson, H. A.: Improved inhalation therapy of asthma, Arch. Phys. Ther. 21:612-615, 1940.
24. Palmer, K. N. V.: New mucolytic agent by aerosol for inhalation in chronic bronchitis, Lancet 2:802, 1961.

25. Webb, W. R.: Clinical evaluation of a new mucolytic agent, acetyl-cysteine, J. Thorac. Cardiov. Surg. 44:330-343, 1962.

26. Boerema, I., Brummelkamp, W. H., and Meijne Amsterdam, N. G., editors: Clinical application of hyperbaric oxygen, New York, 1964, Elsevier Publishing Co.

27. Illingworth, C. F., Smith, G., Lawson, D. D., Ledingham, A. McA., Sharp, G. R., Griffiths, J. C., and Henderson, C. I.: Surgical and physiological observations in a experimental pressure chamber, Brit. J. Surg. 49:222-227, 1961.

28. Hutchison, J. H., Kerr, M. M., McPhail, F. M., and Douglas, T. A.: Studies in the treatment of the pulmonary syndrome of the newborn, Lancet 2:465, 1962.

29. Cross, K. W., and Dawes, G. S.: Apnoea in hyperbaric oxygen, Lancet 1:47-48, 1967.

30. Cochran, W. E., Levison, H., Muirhead, D. M., Boston, R. W., Wang, C. C. S., and Smith, C. A.: A clinical trial of high oxygen pressure for the respiratory distress syndrome, New Eng. J. Med. 272:347-351, 1965.

31. Bernhard, W. F.: Current concepts. Hyperbaric oxygenation, New Eng. J. Med. 271:562-564, 1964.

32. Ollodart, R., and Blair, E.: High pressure oxygen as an adjunct in experimental bacteremic shock, J.A.M.A. 191:736-739, 1965.

33. Bernhard, W. F., Tank, E., Fritelli, G., and Gross, R. E.: The feasibility of hypothermic perfusion under hyperbaric conditions in the surgical management of infants with cyanotic congenital heart disease, J. Thorac. Cardiov. Surg. 46:651-664, 1963.

34. Smith, R. M., Crocker, D., and Adams, J. G., Jr.: Anesthetic management of patients during surgery under hyperbaric oxygenation, Anesth. Analg. 43:766-776, 1964.

35. Dammann, J. F., Jr., Thung, N., Christlieb, I. J., Littlefield, J. B., and Muller, W. H., Jr.: The management of the severely ill patient after open heart surgery, J. Thorac. Cardiov. Surg. 45:80-90, 1963.

36. Brown, K., Johnston, A. E., and Conn, A. W.: Respiratory insufficiency and its treatment following paediatric cardiovascular surgery, Canad. Anaesth. Soc. J. 13:342-361, 1966.

37. Downes, J. J., and Wood, D. W.: Mechanical ventilation in the management of status asthmaticus in children. In Eckenhoff, J. E., editor: Science and practice in anesthesia, Philadelphia, 1965, J. B. Lippincott Co.

38. Ahlgren, E. W., and Stephen, C. R.: Mechanical ventilation of the infant, Anesthesiology 27:692-694, 1966.

39. Ahlgren, E. W., and Stephen, C. R.: Experience in the management of hyaline membrane disease with a new mechanical ventilator, Anesthesiology 28:237-238, 1967.

40. Norlander, O. P., and Engström, C. G.: Volume-controlled respirators, Ann. N. Y. Acad. Sci. 121:766-780, 1965.

41. Robbins, L., Crocker, D., and Smith, R. M.: Tidal volume losses of volume-limited ventilators, Anesth. Analg. 46:428-431, 1967.

42. MacDonald, I. H., and Stocks, J. G.: Prolonged nasotracheal intubation: a review of its development in a paediatric hospital, Brit. J. Anaesth. 37:161-173, 1965.

43. Rees, G. J., and Owen-Thomas, J. B.: A technique of pulmonary ventilation with a nasotracheal tube, Brit. J. Anaesth. 38:901-906, 1966.

44. Safar, P., and Kunkel, H. G.: Prolonged artificial ventilation. In Safar, P., editor: Respiratory therapy, Philadelphia, 1965, F. A. Davis Co.

45. Bendixen, H. H., Egbert, L. D., Hedley-Whyte, J., Laver, M. B., and Pontoppidan, H.: Respiratory care, St. Louis, 1965, The C. V. Mosby Co.

46. Grenvik, A.: Respiratory, circulatory and metabolic effects of respiratory treatment. A clinical study in postoperative thoracic surgical patients, Acta Anaesth. Scand., supp. 19, 1966.

47. Okmian, L. G.: Artificial ventilation by respirator for newborn infants during anaesthesia, Acta Anaesth. Scand. 7:31-57, 1963.

48. Thomas, D. V., and Fletcher, G.: Prolonged respirator use in newborn pulmonary insufficiency, J.A.M.A. 193:183-189, 1965.

49. McCaughey, T. J., Kuwabara, S., and Fund, H.: Respiratory distress syndrome of the newborn: a critique of current management of the ventilation-oxygenation problem, Canad. Anaesth. Soc. J. 13:476-494, 1966.

Chapter 30

Mortality in pediatric surgery and anesthesia

It has been suggested repeatedly that pediatric anesthesia carries a disproportionately high mortality. Statistical reports from the University of Wisconsin[1] and the study of Beecher and Todd[2] show anesthetic deaths to be higher in the first decade than in any other until the seventh decade is reached. Similarly, studies on cardiac arrest reported by Stephenson, Reid, and Hinton[3] and by Rackow, Salanitre, and Green[4] point to an alarmingly high incidence of this complication during pediatric anesthesia.

Clinical reports[5-7] strengthen the impression that anesthetic deaths are surprisingly common among children and that many of them have been preventable. Certain errors have been noticed to recur repeatedly.[8] Among these, the most common are failure to provide adequate equipment, improper preparation of children with perforated appendix, unrecognized shock, and death caused by aspiration of vomitus.

The value of statistical analysis is limited, and figures definitely may be misleading, but it appears that an attempt should be made to study all available material in order to clarify the existing situation.

It seems desirable first to present only factual data to show the number of children who died during or following surgery, with their age, type of surgery, and time of death. Such knowledge is fundamental in studying operative mortality and may be presented without involving the interpretation of statistical data. With some idea of the basic conditions in mind, it may then be possible to venture out onto less certain ground in order to determine whether some of these deaths were preventable and, if so, to find methods of preventing them.

Most information concerning mortality in pediatric surgery and anesthesia has come from reports of relatively small numbers of cases. To provide a larger series, figures are presented on the operative and postoperative mortality at the Children's Hospital Medical Center of Boston in 12 years of anesthesia involving a total of 69,977 patients. Consideration is devoted chiefly to the 54,737 children in this series who were under 10 years of age.

OVER-ALL MORTALITY DURING THE FIRST TWO DECADES

During 12 years studied, 1954 through 1960 and 1962 through 1966, a total of 54,737 operations were performed on infants and children under 10 years of age. A total of 849 patients were known to have died *within a year following operation.* The yearly mortality varied between 1.1% and 1.9%, and the average mortality was 1.5% (Table 30-1).

Table 30-1. *Operative and postoperative mortality in children under 10 years of age at the Children's Hospital Medical Center, Boston*

	1954	1955	1956	1957	1958	1959	
Number of operations	3,516	3,424	4,013	4,013	4,301	4,419	
Deaths	67	58	54	70	83	85	
Percent mortality	1.9	1.3	1.3	1.6	1.8	1.9	

	1960	1962	1963	1964	1965	1966	*Total*
Number of operations	4,512	4,340	4,874	5,098	5,627	6,159	54,737
Deaths	78	69	71	74	71	69	849
Percent mortality	1.7	1.6	1.5	1.5	1.2	1.1	1.5

Table 30-2. *Operative and postoperative mortality in patients 10 to 20 years of age at the Children's Hospital Medical Center, Boston*

	1954	1955	1956	1957	1958	1959	
Number of operations	684	655	867	1,455	1,462	1,036	
Deaths	6	3	3	6	13	23	
Percent mortality	0.9	0.5	0.3	0.4	0.9	2.1	

	1960	1962	1963	1964	1965	1966	*Total/Average*
Number of operations	1,024	1,335	1,491	1,724	1,760	1,746	15,240
Deaths	25	21	9	10	14	15	148
Percent mortality	1.1	1.6	0.5	0.6	1.0	1.0	0.9

Because a small but appreciable amount of surgery is performed upon older children at the Children's Hospital, figures for mortality in these patients are added (Table 30-2).

Data from Tables 30-1 and 30-2 show that during the years studied the mortality in children under 10 years of age, 1.5%, was not excessive and remained fairly stable. The mortality in patients in the second decade was less than that for children under 10 years of age in the years 1954 through 1958. The sharp rise in mortality shown following 1958 was due primarily to the establishment of open-heart surgery, which introduced a much larger number of poor-risk patients into the older age group. Fortunately, the trend was quickly changed and fell back to previous low rates.

RELATION OF MORTALITY TO AGE DURING THE FIRST DECADE

The figures are more remarkable when the individual years of the first decade are examined (Table 30-3).

It at once appears that the first year of life is the most critical. In this series deaths in infants under 1 year of age totaled 495, well over half the number for the entire first 10-year period and at least eight times as many as during any other year of this decade. It is interesting to notice, however, that twice or three times as many operations were performed on infants under 1 year of age than upon children during any other year in the first decade. The mortality percentage, although not expressive of an eight-to-one relationship in absolute numbers, still shows at least a two-to-one ratio to the mortality of subsequent years.

A closer look at the statistics of the first year of life shows that although the

Table 30-3. *Operative and postoperative mortality in children under 10 years of age at the Children's Hospital Medical Center, Boston, as related to age in years*

	Age in years										
	0-1	1-2	2-3	3-4	4-5	5-6	6-7	7-8	8-9	9-10	Total
Operations	11,817	6,080	5,284	5,491	5,654	5,546	4,418	3,897	3,475	3,075	54,737
Deaths	495	61	51	40	39	37	32	36	28	30	849
Percent mortality	4.0	1.0	1.0	0.7	0.7	0.7	0.7	0.9	0.8	1.0	1.7

Table 30-4. *Operative and postoperative mortality during the first year of life at the Children's Hospital Medical Center, Boston, 1954 through 1960 and 1962 through 1966*

	Age				
	0-7 days	7 days-1 mo.	1-6 mo.	6-12 mo.	Total
Deaths	218	95	128	54	495

mortality throughout the whole year is considerably higher than in succeeding years, that in the *first week of life* is far in excess of any other period (Table 30-4).

The deaths that occur in the first week of life amount to approximately one half of the deaths of the first year and to more than one fourth of the total for the first 10 years of life.

MORTALITY RELATED TO TYPE OF SURGERY

The relationship of mortality to the type of surgery deserves consideration. In gross figures, 85% of all deaths were divided between thoracic, abdominal, and neurosurgery (Table 30-5). Thoracic surgery was associated with both the greatest number of deaths and the highest percentage rate.

Table 30-5. *Mortality related to type of surgery in patients under 10 years of age at the Children's Hospital Medical Center, Boston*

Type of surgery	Operations	Deaths	Percent
Thoracic surgery	4,068	356	8.7
Plastic surgery	4,491	3	0.07
Abdominal surgery	13,030	232	1.8
Other general surgery	6,516	102	1.5
Neurosurgery	3,338	141	4.0
Orthopedic surgery	6,147	4	0.07
Ear, nose, and throat surgery	7,223	11*	0.15
Dental surgery	1,488	0	0
Miscellaneous minor	8,436	0	0
Total	54,737	849	

*None of these deaths was associated with tonsillectomy.

Table 30-6. *Lesions in infants who died in the first week of life at the Children's Hospital Medical Center, Boston, 1954 through 1960 and 1962 through 1966*

Surgical lesion	Fatal cases	Premature infants	Infants having other congenital anomalies
Cardiovascular	11	2	2
Tracheoesophageal fistula with esophageal atresia	54	26	28
Diaphragmatic hernia	14	0	7
Omphalocele	31	7	15
Meconeum ileus	18	4	0
Other types of intestinal obstruction	46	29	17
Imperforate anus	11	3	6
Teratoma	2	1	0
Miscellaneous	11	1	7
Total	218	73	82

TYPES OF LESIONS IN INFANTS
WHO DIED DURING THE FIRST WEEK OF LIFE

Since the highest mortality occurred in infants operated upon during their first week of life, it is interesting to see what pathologic lesions occurred in this group. This information is listed in Table 30-6. In addition, figures are added showing the incidence of coexisting prematurity and of coexisting multiple congenital anomalies. Both of these factors were common in this group and were important in raising the toll of death.

PREOPERATIVE CONDITION OF PATIENTS

The preoperative physical condition of all patients in this study (Table 30-7) was rated according to the standards suggested by Saklad in 1941,[9] and revised by the 1962 House of Delegates of the American Society of Anesthesiologists as follows:

A.S.A. classification of physical status

1. A normal healthy patient.
2. A patient with mild systemic disease.
3. A patient with a severe systemic disease that limits activity, but is not incapacitating.
4. A patient with an incapacitating systemic disease that is a constant threat to life.
5. A moribund patient not expected to survive 24 hours with or without operation.

To denote an emergency operation in any class, the number will be followed by the letter E.

It is interesting to see that in the 849 patients who died, none were in Class

Table 30-7. *Preoperative condition of children under 10 years of age who died during or after operation at the Children's Hospital Medical Center, Boston, 1954 through 1960 and 1962 through 1966*

Age	1	1E	2	2E	3	3E	4	4E	5	5E	Total
0-7 days				2	10	20	62	76	15	33	218
1 wk.-1 mo.			1	1	4	2	37	37	8	5	95
1-6 mo.			1		7	4	75	27	7	7	128
6 mo.-1 yr.					1	2	38	10	3		54
1-2 yr.			1		7	4	35	9	2	3	61
2-3 yr.					5	7	20	14	3	2	51
3-4 yr.					3	2	22	7	3	3	40
4-5 yr.					4	2	18	10	5		39
5-6 yr.			1		6	2	22	3	2	1	37
6-7 yr.			1			1	23	6		1	32
7-8 yr.					1		28	5	1	1	36
8-9 yr.					2	1	23	2			28
9-10 yr.					1	1	18	5	3	2	30
Total			4	4	51	48	421	211	53	58	849

1 or Class 1E, while the vast majority were definitely poor-risk patients. The greatest number of deaths in all patients fell into Class 4 or Class 4E. In general these represented children with severe cardiac disease, while the neurosurgical patients more frequently were in Class 3. During early infancy it is seen that there is a relative increase in Class 5, and in the emergency groups of both Class 4 and Class 5.

In order to show the incidence of different classes of physical status in the general population of the patients coming to operation, a tabulation was made of all patients coming to operation in 1956 (Table 30-8). The large number of patients in Classes 1 and 2 and the virtual absence of mortality in these classes show that the operative and anesthetic mortality in normal good-risk infants and children should be no more than one in 3 or 4 thousand. Over 12 years our series showed only 8 deaths in these two groups, which totaled approximately 42,000 patients. Anesthesia was not involved in any of these 8 deaths.

TIME OF DEATH

Eighty-four of the patients under 10 years of age died during operation (Table 30-9). Seven hundred sixty-five deaths occurred at times varying from the immediate postoperative period to 12 months after operation.

At the present time concern has shifted from the intraoperative period to the 48 hours immediately following operation. During operation respiration and circulation can be controlled or supported through all but the grossest insults, while the early postoperative period finds the patient struggling weakly to reestablish his own stability. The fact that 386 patients died in this period confirms the importance of this situation.

Although it would be pleasant to assume that anesthesia could not play a part

Table 30-8. *Preoperative condition of all children operated upon during 1956 at the Children's Hospital Medical Center, Boston*

Age	Condition										
	1	*1E*	*2*	*2E*	*3*	*3E*	*4*	*4E*	*5*	*5E*	*Total*
0-7 days	4	1	8	0	12	14	2	35	2	2	80
7 days-1 mo.	40	5	20	7	18	10	4	4		3	111
1 mo.-6 mo.	318	7	137	5	49	8	11	6		1	542
6 mo.-1 yr.	144	5	66	4	24	7	5	5	1		261
1-2 yr.	259	15	106	8	38	6	6	4	2		444
2-3 yr.	206	13	102	7	42	3	4	2			379
3-4 yr.	206	15	124	8	34	4	7	3			401
4-5 yr.	223	9	103	6	26	2	4	1			374
5-6 yr.	228	16	117	12	24	8	6	3			414
6-7 yr.	145	14	100	5	20	2	5	1			292
7-8 yr.	131	12	66	6	17	2	4				238
8-9 yr.	151	18	52	8	18	6	2	2	1		258
9-10 yr.	118	17	63	6	12	1	1	1		1	219
Total	2173	147	1064	82	334	73	61	67	6	6	4013

Table 30-9. *Time of death of 849 children who died during or after operation at the Children's Hospital Medical Center, Boston*

Time	Number
During operation	84
Operative day	197
First postoperative day	118
Second postoperative day	73
Third postoperative day	52
Fourth postoperative day	29
Fifth postoperative day	24
Sixth postoperative day	12
Seventh postoperative day	17
Eighth postoperative day	8
Ninth postoperative day	10
Tenth postoperative day	15
11 days to 1 month postoperative	103
1 to 2 months postoperative	43
2 to 3 months postoperative	24
3 to 12 months postoperative	34

in any death that occurred after the early postoperative period, this certainly is not possible. Most anesthetic deaths probably do occur during or shortly after operation, but a patient who is exposed to moderate hypoxia during anesthesia may live on in a decerebrate state and die weeks or even months later. Consequently, since anesthesia can never be excluded as a factor in postoperative deaths purely on the basis of elapsed time, all deaths occurring within 1 year after operation are recorded. In this series anesthesia did not appear to play a part in any death that occurred more than 9 days following operation.

PATIENTS WHO DIED DURING OPERATION

The anesthesia must always be scrutinized when patients die during operation. Of 84 patients in this series who died during surgery, over half were undergoing thoracic or thoracoabdominal procedures. Age again played a part, since 47 of 84 children were less than 1 year old.

Hemorrhage was obviously the greatest cause of death in the operating room and was associated with 40 of the fatalities. Simple exsanguination occurred rarely, however, since all the patients who died from hemorrhage were receiving blood at the time. In most instances hemorrhage appeared to be the initial factor, to be followed by a complex series of events leading to disaster.

There were 2 children being operated upon for patent ductus arteriosus and 1 undergoing removal of a thoracoabdominal tumor whose deaths appeared to be the result of rapid blood loss alone. The deaths of 3 children during neurosurgery were caused by hemorrhage plus major intracranial pathology due to trauma or tumor. The remaining 18 deaths in which hemorrhage occurred involved further problems. In several instances blood loss was corrected rapidly, but the presence of severe cardiac anomalies and myocardial weakness appeared to prevent recovery of normal heart action. Several patients died after massive blood replacement. In the case of another child blood loss was replaced and calcium chloride was given to prevent citrate toxicity. Death occurred immediately after the administration of calcium. Because this child had been receiving digitalis, it was believed that the death might have been due to potentiation of the digitalis effect by rapid administration of calcium.

Anesthesia was believed to have played a leading part in the deaths of 5 patients who died during operation: a newborn infant and 4 older children, 1, 5, 5, and 6 years of age. Details concerning these patients are given later. This widely spaced incidence does not suggest that death from anesthesia showed any particular relationship to the age of the patient.

CAUSES OF DEATH

Having examined the mortality statistics from several viewpoints, one can evaluate the causes of death more fairly. The causes may be grouped under four headings: (1) hebdomadal or perinatal factors, (2) disease, (3) surgery, and (4) anesthesia.

Perinatal factors. Death in the first week of life has always been disproportionately high, in patients on whom operations have not been performed as well as in those operated upon. This perinatal period has attracted considerable attention recently since mortality during this period has failed to show appreciable reduction. Bundesen,[10] in discussing nonsurgical mortality, states that 95% of deaths during the first year of life occur in the first week after birth. The outstanding causes are prematurity, congenital anomalies, respiratory inadequacy, and birth trauma. The figures in our series of patients operated upon paint a similar picture, inasmuch as the predominant portion of operative deaths occur in the first week and are heavily affected by prematurity, multiple congenital anomalies, intracranial hemorrhage, and infection.

Disease. Disease in the patient actually includes the factor of perinatal weakness but, in addition, extends throughout the whole decade. As shown by the data in Table 30-7, the child's primary disease was the major factor in many of the deaths and a heavily contributing factor in nearly all of the deaths since very few of the children who died were in fair or good preoperative condition. This was especially true in the neurosurgical deaths, a large number of which were caused by malignant tumors.

Surgery. When one tries to designate the deaths due to errors in technique or judgment in either surgery or anesthesia, one at once gets into difficulty. Very few deaths can be attributed to any single factor. Suffice it to say that the surgeons are faced with innumerable problems, many of insurmountable proportions. In infants and small children significant blood loss occurs rapidly, and transfusion not only entails the problem of exact replacement but also associated complications of transfusion reaction not clearly defined. In the series of cases presented hemorrhage was obviously the major surgical problem during the operative period and was the greatest factor in mortality in patients operated upon for congenital heart disease and tumor.

In the postoperative period such factors as wound infection and thrombosis, which are prominent complications following operations in adults, play little part in pediatric mortality. One of the greatest surgical problems is the management of infants after operation for intestinal obstruction because ileus and bowel stasis often persist after the anatomic obstruction is relieved. Repeated operations and prolonged maintenance of premature infants on parenteral therapy present problems that are appreciated only by members of the surgical house staff.

Anesthesia. It is also difficult to state which patients died because of anesthesia, but in the 69,977 children under 10 years of age to whom anesthetics were administered, 10 deaths occurred in which anesthesia was considered to have played the principal or a major contributing part, although the evidence is not clear-cut in all cases. These cases have been referred to already, but they deserve full description, which follows:

1. *J. B.—Condition 3 (1956).* This 6-week-old infant was found to have a slightly enlarged head. He was diagnosed as hydrocephalic and was operated upon for removal of a kidney and the performance of lumboureteral shunt. Anesthesia was performed with trifluoroethylvinyl ether (Fluoromar), starting with the open-drop technique and then, after intubation, using endotracheal insufflation via a Y nonrebreathing tube. The level was uneven, and the patient entered a light plane of anesthesia several times but never appeared to be in critical conditon. He awoke and cried within an hour after operation and appeared normal until 4 hours after operation. At this time he vomited and aspirated and then developed hypotension. His airway was cleared, he was given blood, and he appeared much improved. However, shortly afterward (about 8 hours following operation) he suddenly developed pulmonary edema and died.

    Many operations of this type had previously been performed successfully under ether. Because of the unsatisfactory behavior of the patient during anesthesia with Fluoromar, the agent and the technique were indicated as the probable cause of the fatal pulmonary complications, and death was termed a preventable one. Actually, the postoperative vomiting and aspiration would appear the most probable cause.

2. *C. M.—Condition 4 (1955).* This boy 2 years, 9 months of age was suspected of having leukemia and was to undergo iliac marrow biopsy. Anesthesia was induced with nitrous oxide, divinyl ether, and ether. During induction the boy developed crowing respiration and then vomited and aspirated thick, fluid material. His color remained good; an endotracheal tube was passed without difficulty, but it was necessary to apply extensive suction during and after the operation. The night following operation his temperature was 103° F., his lips were swollen, and respiration was noisy and became increasingly obstructed. Tracheostomy relieved him, but his general condition became progressively worse. The larynx and trachea became involved in a necrotizing infection. Gross hematuria and tarry stools also developed. Death occurred 6 days after the initial iliac biopsy, apparently because of overwhelming infection. Anesthetic management in allowing the child to vomit was the major factor originating these events. This was considered a preventable complication, but there was some ques-

tion as to whether the blood dyscrasia might have explained the lack of resistance to the infection. This patient was the only one in our series who died following a minor operation.

3. *M. E. F.—Condition 4E (1957).* This 1-day-old baby was admitted for excision of a huge sacrococcygeal teratoma. Anesthesia was induced with divinyl ether and ether, and the infant was intubated and maintained on a Y nonrebreathing apparatus with ether insufflation. There was continued difficulty in positioning the infant so that he could be ventilated adequately and at the same time allow the surgeon a satisfactory field. After 90 minutes the infant died as a result of both shock and hypoventilation. The problems involved here were extremely difficult, but death might have been prevented if a suitable position for the infant could have been found and if the blood volume could have been maintained.

4. *D. G.—Condition 4 (1958).* Anesthesia appeared to be a major factor in precipitating the death of this boy, 1 year, 11 months of age, although he was definitely a severe risk before operation. In addition to coarctation of the aorta he had mitral stenosis, pulmonary hypertension, tricuspid atresia, endocardial sclerosis, and asthma. Induction under cyclopropane and ether was prolonged, and vomiting occurred. Irregular, tugging respiration developed and could not be overcome. The operation progressed and the aorta was clamped preparatory to excision of the coarctation. At this point the child's heart stopped and could not be resuscitated.

One will never know whether this child could have tolerated clamping of his aorta under any conditions, but the prolonged difficulty with ventilation prior to aortic occlusion was definitely abnormal. The associated hypoxia and carbon dioxide excess may well have sensitized the patient so that the sudden elevation of arterial pressure occasioned by the aortic occlusion could have caused abrupt cardiac asystole.

5. *B. G. R.—Condition 4E (1956).* This newborn infant had a large diaphragmatic hernia that was reduced under endotracheal cyclopropane anesthesia administered by the to-and-fro system. Repeated but unsuccessful attempts were made by the anesthetist to inflate the unexpanded lung. The operation was completed, and the infant appeared to be in good condition. The following night, however, he developed bilateral pneumothorax and died. It seemed probable that during attempts to expand the lung both lungs had been damaged. This was considered a preventable anesthetic death.

6. *D. J.—Condition 5E (1957).* This 6-year-old boy had acute glomerulonephritis and uremia (NPN 273) and was to be dialyzed by means of the artificial kidney. Before being subjected to this complicated procedure the patient was to undergo cystoscopy to rule out an obstructive lesion of the lower genitourinary tract. Since he was semicomatose, it was thought that light nitrous oxide analgesia would be indicated in the presence of roentgen-ray treatment.

After 15 minutes of anesthesia an arrhythmia was noted, followed by cessation of cardiac beat. The chest was opened and the heart was found to be in fibrillation. After 2 hours of massage and attempts to resuscitate and defibrillate the heart, a normal beat was obtained at 100 per minute, with blood pressure 85/50. This was of short duration, however, for cardiac action weakened and ceased an hour later.

Due to the advanced renal disease this patient did not have long to live, and the death was not considered a preventable one. Anesthesia appeared to precipitate the death, however, and consequently must be classed as a major contributing factor.

7. *S. A. D.—Condition 3 (1958)*. This girl 2 years, 5 months of age was admitted with patent ductus arteriosus. There were prolonged induction and technical difficulty with intubation followed by inadequate ventilation due to a leak in apparatus. There was postoperative convulsion, the temperature rose to 104° F., and death followed 48 hours later.

8. *S. R.—Condition 4 (1960)*. This 5-year-old boy had transposition of the great vessels and a markedly enlarged heart. Cyclopropane induction and intubation were uneventful. Intramuscular and intravenous succinylcholine was added. A total of 20 mg. was administered when cardiac standstill occurred. The chest was opened and the heart massaged at once, but no response could be obtained.

Increased sensitivity to anesthetics and failure to regain functional activity have been noted in several patients with severe cardiac lesions. Cyclopropane has shown rapid and marked depressant effect in such cases.

9. *L.P.H.—Condition 4 (1959)*. This 3-month-old child had a right lung abscess. Induction with cyclopropane was complicated by copious secretions and repeated raising of thick pus. Pneumonectomy was performed, but the airway was impeded throughout and the color was dusky at intervals. Pulse and blood pressure were poor postoperatively; cardiac standstill occurred 1 hour after operation. The patient did not respond to open cardiac massage or defibrillator.

10. *B. B. C.—Condition 4 (1959)*. This 1-month-old infant had coarctation of the aorta and hypoplastic aortic arch. To-and-fro cyclopropane anesthesia was tolerated satisfactorily until the chest and pericardium were opened. Complete auriculoventricular block occurred and could not be controlled with pacemaker or cardiotonic agents. The mechanism of this event was not obvious, but it is probable that the depth of anesthesia was a major factor.

11. *B. K.—Condition 4 (1964)*. This cachectic-appearing 5-year-old child was born with severe omphalocele that had been repaired only by skin closure. At operation a large mass, including liver and other viscera, protruded anterior to the unyielding rectus muscles. The repair was attempted under endotracheal cyclopropane. During completion of the operation relatively deep anesthesia was required to facilitate closure. Sudden irreversible cardiovascular collapse occurred, probably due to depth of anesthesia plus obstructed vena caval flow and general bodily debility.

SUMMARY

The present survey brings out several points:

1. The high mortality associated with pediatric anesthesia and surgery is due chiefly to complicating factors at early infancy.

2. In this series infants and children with incapacitating cardiac lesions contributed a large factor.

3. The greatest problem affecting all age groups was hemorrhage; however, the mechanism of death associated with blood loss often remained obscure.

4. The *normal* child does not present an increased anesthetic or operative risk.

5. In a series of 69,977 cases, 11 deaths were thought either to have been due to anesthesia entirely or to have been precipitated by anesthesia.

6. Although anesthesia undoubtedly played a contributing role in many other deaths, it was not obvious.

7. No anesthetic or technique could be singled out as being more dangerous than others by these figures. The evidence in the death under fluroxene was certainly unconvincing. (The death described under halothane in Chapter 27 occurred too recently to be included in the statistical survey.)

8. Mortality may be reduced by elimination of preventable errors in equipment, patient preparation, and anesthetic technique.

REFERENCES

1. Annual Statistical Reports, Department of Anesthesia, Wisconsin General Hospital, 1954-1962.
2. Beecher, H. K., and Todd, D. P.: A study of the deaths associated with anesthesia and surgery, Ann. Surg. **140:**2-34, 1954.
3. Stephenson, H. E., Jr., Reid, L. C., and Hinton, J. W.: Some common denominators in 1200 cases of cardiac arrest, Ann. Surg. **137:**731-744, 1953.
4. Rackow, H., Salanitre, E., and Green, L. T.: Frequency of cardiac arrest associated with anesthesia in infants and children, Pediatrics **28:**697-704, 1961.
5. West, J. P.: Cardiac arrest during anesthesia and surgery, an analysis of 30 cases, Ann. Surg. **140:**623-629, 1954.
6. Bergner, R. P.: Cardiac arrest; some etiologic considerations, with reports of seventeen cases, Anesthesiology **16:**177-189, 1955.
7. Dornette, W. H. L., and Orth, O. S.: Death in the operating room, Anesth. Analg. **35:**545-569, 1956.
8. Smith, R. M.: Some reasons for the high mortality in pediatric anesthesia, New York J. Med. **56:**2212-2216, 1956.
9. Saklad, M.: Grading of patients for surgical procedures, Anesthesiology **2:**281-284, 1941.
10. Bundesen, H. N.: Effective reduction of needless hebdomadal deaths in hospitals, J.A.M.A. **157:**1384-1399, 1955.

Chapter 31

Legal aspects of pediatric anesthesia

Preoperative period
 Permission for anesthesia
 Written orders
 Identification of patients
 Responsibility for bodily harm
 Equipment
 Precautions and preventive devices
Operative period
 Physical injury
 Explosions
 Complications of infusion of fluid and blood
 Anesthetic death
Postoperative period

Anesthetists must be increasingly aware of the possibility of legal suit in case of accidents or various types of complications. For this reason it seems advisable to call attention to a number of details that may have special bearing on this aspect. These may pertain to the preoperative, operative, or postoperative phases of management and may be of importance primarily when dealing with children or may be of concern in patients of all ages.

Most details merely consist of points that are essential in complete care of the patient. In some instances, however, it appears that unusual or extreme precautions must be taken simply for the sake of legal protection.

PREOPERATIVE PERIOD

Any anesthetist should realize the danger of taking shortcuts. Inadequate knowledge of the patient's history and physical condition borders on professional negligence.

One certainly must be aware of past illnesses, operations, and metabolic disorders. In addition, there may be sensitivity to therapeutic agents or recent use of steroids or depressants that can complicate anesthesia and recovery. For the

508

best interests of all concerned, history, physical, and laboratory reports should all be entered in the patient's chart prior to anesthesia. In certain circumstances omissions are excusable. Obviously it would not appear reasonable to delay splenectomy for ruptured spleen simply because of inability to procure a urine sample. A point that does cause disagreement is whether well children require blood and urine examination prior to tonsillectomy. Since the hematocrit is easily and quickly determined, there seems little excuse for omitting it. On the other hand, if a child who has been carefully attended medically and has had no signs of renal disease is unable to pass a specimen, it seems reasonable to proceed without it. Tests for bleeding and clotting time are unreliable and are certainly not indicated as a standard preoperative procedure.

Permission for anesthesia. When children are to be operated upon, it is necessary to have the written permission of the parents.[1] In case of serious emergency the hospital administrator may assume this responsibility if the parents cannot be located.

Jehovah's Witnesses. Children whose parents belong to the Jehovah's Witnesses sect may allow permission to operate but deny permission to use blood or blood fractions. If the physician cannot persuade the parents to allow transfusion he can refuse to treat the patient, or he can proceed and use blood substitutes. The latter course usually is possible. It does not appear advisable to act against the faith or specific instruction of any mature individual. In the case of an emergency, when the parent has not stated any specific terms, it is often considered reasonable to act on the judgment of a predetermined council of three chiefs of service.

Use of new and nonapproved drugs. Permission also must explicitly be granted for use of any new drugs or anesthetic agents.

Written orders. Orders for medication, especially for sedative or narcotic agents, should be written and signed by the physician, and the exact amount should be clearly specified. To minimize the danger of errors in measuring fractional doses for children, it is best to use diluted agents that can be measured more accurately.

Identification of patients. It is extremely easy to mistake one infant or sleeping child for another, and the results in the operating room might be most unfortunate for all concerned. Beds should be well marked, and all patients should wear identifying bracelets or name tags at all times.

Responsibility for bodily harm. Once the anesthetist takes charge of a child he must be sure that the child is never left unguarded. Dangers exist whether the child is awake or asleep. He may turn quickly and roll off a litter, vomit and aspirate, or try to stand and fall against the side of his crib. During pediatric operations the anesthetist should plan to stay at the head of the table and not assume responsibility for infusions, the positioning of lights, and other operating room functions.

Equipment. An anesthetist certainly invites disaster if he undertakes anesthesia without adequate equipment. This applies primarily to apparatus for resuscitation and the treatment of complications, including suction apparatus, airways, endotracheal tubes, and laryngoscopes.

If accidents occur that are traced to the use of faulty or unsafe equipment, the anesthetist may expect to be held accountable. This has been brought out in several cases in which the preparation of materials for spinal anesthesia has been questioned.

Precautions and preventive devices. The interchanging of nitrous oxide and oxygen tanks or connections has caused several deaths. The pin-index system has been devised to prevent such errors, and its adoption is advised for protection of both patient and anesthetist.

The fail-safe mechanisms, whereby nitrous oxide will be automatically shut off by failure of oxygen supply, is highly recommended in view of the wide usage of nitrous oxide–oxygen mixtures.

OPERATIVE PERIOD

Physical injury. A number of complications may occur while patients are under anesthesia unless meticulous care is taken to avoid them. Ether burns of the eyes or face, pressure necrosis of the face or other areas, and nerve damage due to pressure or faulty positioning on the operating table are but a few of the disturbing accidents that may happen.

The use of hot-water bottles, water mattresses, ice, and other temperature-regulating devices may result in tissue injury against which infants and anesthetized patients have little defense.

Damage to the teeth and mouth occasionally occurs in connection with endotracheal intubation or the use of oropharyngeal airways. When teeth are weakened by large cavities or are loosened prior to anesthesia and then become broken or dislodged during accepted procedures of intubation, the anesthetist certainly should not be held responsible. Graves[2] states that all patients must assume the risk of dental trauma as being one of the necessary hazards of the operation. This appears to be reasonable. If however, a tooth is dislodged, the anesthetist must locate it. If it has been swallowed, it may be allowed to pass through the intestinal tract, but if it has been aspirated, steps should be taken for its immediate recovery.

Explosions. Standard precautions for use of explosive anesthetic agents have been well defined and need not be repeated here. The time seems to be approaching when no flammable agents will be used, especially in the presence of any explosive hazard. At present, however, occasional use of ether for bronchoscopy and a few similar situations still may be justifiable in pediatric anesthesia.

Complications of infusion of fluid and blood. Incorrect cross matching of blood has been the reason for several suits. Other complications consist of strapping a limb too tightly to a padded board, admission of air embolism via pumping apparatus,[3] or drowning patients by inadvertent administration of excessive amounts of fluid or blood. All of these complications occur more easily in children and infants. Since children are usually successful in dislodging intravenous needles inserted in the antecubital space, this area should be avoided if possible as a site of percutaneous infusion.

Infusions of potentially irritant fluids must be observed most carefully, for a dislodged needle may be followed by severe tissue destruction (Fig. 31-1).

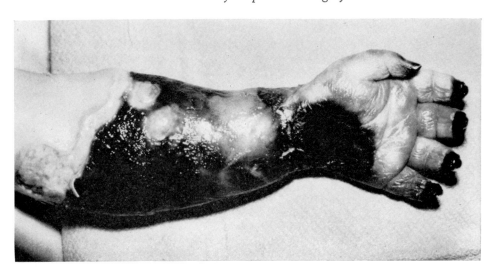

Fig. 31-1. Necrosis of forearm following iatrogenic arterial injury in a 6-month-old infant.

Anesthetic death. This term has been used extensively to include all patients who die in the operating room, regardless of the cause. With the present readiness of laymen to seize upon our less successful results, it should be used only when it means that death was caused by error in judgment or technique of the anesthetist. The decision as to whether a death was due to the anesthetic, surgery, the disease, or a combination of factors can be decided only by a group of physicians who have had experience in considering such matters, some of whom were familiar with the individual case.

POSTOPERATIVE PERIOD

Serious complications may occur during recovery unless strict precautions are observed. If left unattended, a child may suddenly regurgitate and aspirate stomach contents or his tongue may fall back and completely obstruct his airway. Should morbidity or mortality result from such obviously preventable situations, the anesthetist might well be one of those held responsible. The best way to avoid such risks is to have a well-equipped and supervised Recovery Room in which to care for all patients at least until they are out of danger of shock, are breathing normally, and have regained their protective reflexes.

Although children have fewer postoperative anesthetic complications than do adults, these may develop rapidly and entail considerable danger. Postoperative tracheitis is perhaps the best example of such a complication and is one for which the anesthetist might be held responsible if neglect or improper technique is involved. Since this is rarely the case, postoperative tracheitis following legitimate use of endotracheal anesthesia would hardly be just cause for suit. Barton,[4] in discussing the medicolegal aspects of intubation granuloma, also believes that postoperative irritation of the larynx does not of necessity reflect unfavorably upon the anesthetist.

The best way to prevent litigation of all types is to know the patient well and to watch him closely. During the postoperative phase this is especially important. The anesthetist can do much to prevent complications, and, should they occur, he can help to control them and to explain their origin to the patient or his parents. Such treatment dissolves the ill-will that underlies many lawsuits and, in addition, represents good medical practice.

REFERENCES

1. Wasmuth, C. E., and Oleck, H. L.: The privilege of consent, Anesth. Analg. **36:**51-54, 1957.
2. Graves, H. B.: The medicolegal responsibilities of the anaesthetist, Canad. Anaesth. Soc. J. **4:**428-434, 1957.
3. Camps, F. E.: Medicolegal investigations of some deaths occurring during anesthesia, New Eng. J. Med. **253:**643-646, 1955.
4. Barton, R. T.: Medicolegal aspects of intubation granuloma, J.A.M.A. **166:**1821-1823, 1958.

Additional references

Overton, P. R.: Rule of "respondeat superior," J.A.M.A. **163:**847-852, 1957.
Stetler, C. J., and Moritz, A. R.: Doctor and patient and the law, ed. 4, St. Louis, 1962, The C. V. Mosby Co.
Tarrow, A. B.: Medicolegal aspects of anesthesiology, Anesth. Analg. **36:**64-71, 1957.

Index